OXFORD MEDICAL PUBLICATIONS

Oxford Handbook of
Emergency Medicine

Published and forthcoming Oxford Handbooks

Oxford Handbook for the Foundation Programme 3e
Oxford Handbook of Acute Medicine 3e
Oxford Handbook of Anaesthesia 3e
Oxford Handbook of Applied Dental Sciences
Oxford Handbook of Cardiology 2e
Oxford Handbook of Clinical and Laboratory Investigation 3e
Oxford Handbook of Clinical Dentistry 5e
Oxford Handbook of Clinical Diagnosis 2e
Oxford Handbook of Clinical Examination and Practical Skills
Oxford Handbook of Clinical Haematology 3e
Oxford Handbook of Clinical Immunology and Allergy 2e
Oxford Handbook of Clinical Medicine - Mini Edition 8e
Oxford Handbook of Clinical Medicine 8e
Oxford Handbook of Clinical Pharmacy
Oxford Handbook of Clinical Rehabilitation 2e
Oxford Handbook of Clinical Specialties 8e
Oxford Handbook of Clinical Surgery 3e
Oxford Handbook of Complementary Medicine
Oxford Handbook of Critical Care 3e
Oxford Handbook of Dental Patient Care 2e
Oxford Handbook of Dialysis 3e
Oxford Handbook of Emergency Medicine 4e
Oxford Handbook of Endocrinology and Diabetes 2e
Oxford Handbook of ENT and Head and Neck Surgery
Oxford Handbook of Expedition and Wilderness Medicine
Oxford Handbook of Forensic Medicine
Oxford Handbook of Gastroenterology & Hepatology 2e
Oxford Handbook of General Practice 3e
Oxford Handbook of Genetics
Oxford Handbook of Genitourinary Medicine, HIV and AIDS 2e
Oxford Handbook of Geriatric Medicine
Oxford Handbook of Infectious Diseases and Microbiology
Oxford Handbook of Key Clinical Evidence
Oxford Handbook of Medical Dermatology
Oxford Handbook of Medical Sciences
Oxford Handbook of Medical Statistics
Oxford Handbook of Nephrology and Hypertension
Oxford Handbook of Neurology
Oxford Handbook of Nutrition and Dietetics
Oxford Handbook of Obstetrics and Gynaecology 2e
Oxford Handbook of Occupational Health
Oxford Handbook of Oncology 3e
Oxford Handbook of Ophthalmology 2e
Oxford Handbook of Paediatrics
Oxford Handbook of Pain Management
Oxford Handbook of Palliative Care 2e
Oxford Handbook of Practical Drug Therapy 2e
Oxford Handbook of Pre-Hospital Care
Oxford Handbook of Psychiatry 2e
Oxford Handbook of Public Health Practice 2e
Oxford Handbook of Reproductive Medicine & Family Planning
Oxford Handbook of Respiratory Medicine 2e
Oxford Handbook of Rheumatology 3e
Oxford Handbook of Sport and Exercise Medicine
Oxford Handbook of Tropical Medicine 3e
Oxford Handbook of Urology 2e

Oxford Handbook of
Emergency Medicine

Fourth edition

Jonathan P. Wyatt

Consultant in Emergency Medicine and
Forensic Physician
Royal Cornwall Hospital, Truro, UK

Robin N. Illingworth

Consultant in Emergency Medicine
St James's University Hospital, Leeds, UK

Colin A. Graham

Professor of Emergency Medicine
Chinese University of Hong Kong,
Hong Kong SAR, China

Kerstin Hogg

Clinical Research Fellow,
The Ottawa Hospital, Ottawa, Canada

with senior international advisors:

Michael J. Clancy

Consultant in Emergency Medicine
Southampton General Hospital,
Southampton, UK

Colin E. Robertson

Professor of Emergency Medicine
Royal Infirmary, Edinburgh, UK

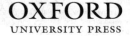

OXFORD
UNIVERSITY PRESS

OXFORD
UNIVERSITY PRESS

Great Clarendon Street, Oxford OX2 6DP

Oxford University Press is a department of the University of Oxford.
It furthers the University's objective of excellence in research, scholarship,
and education by publishing worldwide in

Oxford New York

Auckland Cape Town Dar es Salaam Hong Kong Karachi
Kuala Lumpur Madrid Melbourne Mexico City Nairobi
New Delhi Shanghai Taipei Toronto

With offices in

Argentina Austria Brazil Chile Czech Republic France Greece
Guatemala Hungary Italy Japan Poland Portugal Singapore
South Korea Switzerland Thailand Turkey Ukraine Vietnam

Oxford is a registered trade mark of Oxford University Press
in the UK and in certain other countries

Published in the United States
by Oxford University Press Inc., New York

© Oxford University Press, 2012

The moral rights of the authors have been asserted
Database right Oxford University Press (maker)

First edition published 1999
Second edition published 2005
Third edition published 2006
Fourth edition published 2012

British Library Cataloguing in Publication Data
Data available

Library of Congress Cataloging-in-Publication-Data
Data available

Typeset by Cenveo, Bangalore, India
Printed in China
on acid-free paper by
C & C Offset Printing Co., Ltd.

ISBN 978–0–19–958956–2

10 9 8 7 6 5 4 3 2

Oxford University Press makes no representation, express or implied, that the
drug dosages in this book are correct. Readers must therefore always check the
product information and clinical procedures with the most up-to-date published
product information and data sheets provided by the manufacturers and the most
recent codes of conduct and safety regulations. The authors and publishers do not
accept responsibility or legal liability for any errors in the text or for the misuse or
misapplication of material in this work. Except where otherwise stated, drug dosages
and recommendations are for the non-pregnant adult who is not breastfeeding.

Dedicated to Dr Robin Mitchell (1964–2010)
Emergency Physician in Christchurch, Edinburgh and Auckland.
Outstanding clinician and teacher, tremendous colleague and friend.

Contents

Abbreviations and symbols

°	degrees
≈	approximately
+ve	positive
−ve	negative
±	plus or minus
↑	increase(d)
↓	decrease(d)
ABC	airway, breathing, circulation
ABG	arterial blood gas
AC	acromio-clavicular
ACE	angiotensin-converting enzyme
ACTH	adrenocorticotropic hormone
ACS	acute coronary syndrome
AF	atrial fibrillation
AIDS	acquired immune deficiency syndrome
AIO	Ambulance incident officer
AIS	abbreviated injury scale
ALS	advanced life support
ALT	alanine aminotransferase
ALTE	apparently life-threatening event
AP	antero-posterior
APLS	Advanced Paediatric Life Support
APTT	activated partial thromboplastin time
ARDS	adult respiratory distress syndrome
ARF	acute renal failure
AST	aspartate transaminase
ATLS	advanced trauma life support
AV	atrio-ventricular
bd	twice daily
BKPOP	below knee Plaster of Paris
BKWPOP	below knee walking Plaster of Paris
BLS	basic life support
BMG	bedside strip measurement of venous/capillary blood glucose
BNF	*British National Formulary*
BNFC	*British National Formulary for Children*

BP	blood pressure
BTS	British Thoracic Society
BZP	benzylpiperazine
CBRN	chemical, biological, radiological, nuclear
CCU	critical care unit
CK	creatine kinase
cm	centimetre(s)
CMV	cytomegalovirus
CN	chloroacetophenone
CNS	central nervous system
CO	carbon monoxide
CO_2	carbon dioxide
COHb	carboxyhaemoglobin
COPD	chronic obstructive pulmonary disease
CPAP	continuous positive airways pressure
CPR	cardiopulmonary resuscitation
CRF	chronic renal failure
CRP	C-reactive protein
CSF	cerebrospinal fluid
CT	computed tomography
CTPA	computed tomography pulmonary angiography
CVP	central venous pressure
CVS	cardiovascular system
CXR	chest X-ray
DIC	disseminated intravascular coagulation
DIPJ	distal interphalangeal joint
DKA	diabetic ketoacidosis
dL	decilitre
DPL	diagnostic peritoneal lavage
DPT	diphtheria, pertussis, and tetanus
DSH	deliberate self-harm
DVT	deep venous thrombosis
EBV	Epstein–Barr virus
ECG	electrocardiogram
ECT	electroconvulsive therapy
ED	emergency department
EEG	electroencephalogram
EMLA	eutectic mixture of local anaesthetics
ENT	ear, nose and throat
EPAP	expiratory positive airway pressure

ESR	erythrocyte sedimentation rate
ET	endotracheal
$ETCO_2$	end-tidal carbon dioxide
FAST	focused assessment with sonography for trauma
FB	foreign body
FBC	full blood count
FFP	fresh frozen plasma
FG	French Gauge
FiO_2	inspired oxygen concentration
FOB	faecal occult blood
G6-PD	glucose 6-phosphate dehydrogenase
g	gram(s)
G	gauge
GA	general anaesthetic
GCS	Glasgow Coma Score
GFR	glomerular filtration rate
GI	gastrointestinal
GHB	gammahydroxybutyrate
GMC	General Medical Council
GP	general practitioner
GTN	glyceryl trinitrate
GU	genitourinary
5HT	5-hydroxytryptamine
HATI	human anti-tetanus immunoglobulin
Hb	haemoglobin
HCG	human chorionic gonadotrophin
HCM	hypertrophic cardiomyopathy
Hct	haematocrit
HDU	high dependency unit
HHS	hyperosmolar hyperglycaemic state
HIV	human immunodeficiency virus
HONK	hyperosmolar non-ketotic hyperglycaemia
hr	hour/s
HTLV	human T-cell lymphotropic virus
ICP	intracranial pressure
ICU	intensive care unit
IDDM	insulin dependent diabetes mellitus
IHD	ischaemic heart disease
IM	intramuscular
INR	international normalized ratio (of prothrombin time)

IO	intra-osseous
IPAP	inspiratory positive airway pressure
IPg	interphalangeal
IPPV	intermittent positive pressure ventilation
ISS	injury severity score
ITP	idiopathic thrombocytopenic purpura
IUCD	intrauterine contraceptive device
IV	intravenous
IVI	intravenous infusion
IVRA	intravenous regional anaesthesia
IVU	intravenous urography
JVP	jugular venous pressure
KE	kinetic energy
kPa	kiloPascal(s) pressure
KUB	X-ray covering the area of kidneys, ureters and bladder
L	litre(s)
LA	local anaesthetic
LAD	left axis deviation
LBBB	left bundle branch block
LDH	lactate dehydrogenase
LET	lidocaine epinephrine tetracaine
LFTs	liver function tests
LMA	laryngeal mask airway
LMP	last menstrual period
LMWH	low molecular weight heparin
LP	lumbar puncture
LSD	lysergic acid diethylamide
LV	left ventricular
LVF	left ventricular failure
LVH	left venticular hypertrophy
m	metre(s)
MAOI	monoamine oxidase inhibitor
MAST	military anti-shock trousers
max	maximum
MC	metacarpal
MCA	Mental Capacity Act
MCPJ	metacarpophalangeal joint
MDU	Medical Defence Union
MI	myocardial infarction
min	minute/s

MIO	medical incident officer
mL	millilitre(s)
mmHg	millimetres of mercury pressure
mmol	millimoles
MMR	mumps, measles, and rubella
MRI	magnetic resonance imaging
MRSA	meticillin resistant *Staphylococcus aureus*
MS	multiple sclerosis
MSU	mid-stream specimen of urine
MT	metatarsal
MTPJ	metatarsophalangeal joint
MUA	manipulation under anaesthetic
NAC	*N*-acetyl cysteine
NAI	non-accidental injury
ND	notifiable disease
NG	nasogastric
NHS	National Health Service
NIV	non-invasive ventilation
NO	nitrous oxide
NSAID	non-steroidal anti-inflammatory drug
NSTEMI	non-ST segment elevation myocardial infarction
NWBPOP	non-weight-bearing Plaster of Paris
O_2	oxygen
OA	osteoarthritis
OCP	oral contraceptive pill
od	once daily
OPG	orthopantomogram
ORIF	open reduction and internal fixation
ORT	oral replacement therapy
PA	postero-anterior
PACS	picture archiving and communication system
PAN	polyarteritis nodosa
PCI	percutaneous coronary intervention
pCO_2	arterial partial pressure of carbon dioxide
PCR	polymerase chain reaction
PE	pulmonary embolus
PEA	pulseless electrical activity
PEEP	positive end-expiratory pressure
PEFR	peak expiratory flow rate
PGL	persistent generalized lymphadenopathy

PICU	paediatric intensive care unit
PID	pelvic inflammatory disease
PIPJ	proximal interphalangeal joint
PO	per os (orally/by mouth)
pO_2	arterial partial pressure of oxygen
POP	plaster of Paris
PPE	personal protective equipment
PPI	proton pump inhibitor
PR	per rectum
PRF	patient report form
PRN	pro re nata (as required)
PSP	primary spontaneous pneumothorax
PV	per vaginam
qds	four times a day
RA	rheumatoid arthritis
RAD	right axis deviation
RBBB	right bundle branch block
RBC	red blood cells
Rh	Rhesus
ROSC	restoration of spontaneous circulation
RR	respiratory rate
RSI	rapid sequence induction/intubation
RSV	respiratory syncytial virus
rtPA	recombinant tissue plasminogen activator
RTS	revised trauma score
RV	right ventricular
SA	sino-atrial
SARS	severe acute respiratory syndrome
SC	subcutaneous
SCIWORA	spinal cord injury without radiographic abnormality
sec	second(s)
SIDS	sudden infant death syndrome
SIGN	Scottish Intercollegiate Guidelines Network
SIRS	systemic inflammatory response syndrome
SL	sublingual
SLE	systemic lupus erythematosus
SpO_2	arterial oxygen saturation
SSP	secondary spontaneous pneumothorax
SSRI	selective serotonin re-uptake inhibitor
STD	sexually transmitted disease

STEMI	ST segment elevation myocardial infarction
SVT	supraventricular tachycardia
$T°$	temperature
T_3	tri-iodothyronine
T_4	thyroxine
TAC	tetracaine, adrenaline and cocaine
TB	tuberculosis
tds	three times a day
TFTs	thyroid function tests
TIA	transient ischaemic attack
TIMI	thrombolysis in myocardial infarction
tPA	tissue plasminogen actvator
TSH	thyroid stimulating hormone
u/U	unit(s)
U&E	urea and electrolytes
URTI	upper respiratory tract infection
USS	ultrasound scan
UTI	urinary tract infection
V	volts
VA	visual acuity
VF	ventricular fibrillation
VHF	viral hemorrhagic fever
V/Q	ventilation/perfusion (scan)
VT	ventricular tachycardia
WB	weight-bear(ing)
WBC	white blood cells
WCC	white cell count
WHO	World Health Organization
WPW	Wolff Parkinson White (syndrome)

Normal values

Note that 'normal' values in adults may vary slightly between labs.

Normal values in pregnancy are shown in 📖 The pregnant patient, p.576.

Arterial blood gas analysis

H^+	35–45 nanomol/L
pH	7.35–7.45
pO_2 (on air)	>10.6 kPa, 75–100 mmHg
pCO_2	4.5–6.0 kPa, 35–45 mmHg
bicarbonate	24–28 mmol/L
base excess	±2 mmol/L

Biochemistry

alanine aminotransferase (ALT)	5–35 iu/L
albumin	35–50 g/L
alkaline phosphatase	30–300 iu/L
amylase	0–180 Somogyi U/dL
aspartate transaminase (AST)	5–35 iu/L
bicarbonate	24–30 mmol/L
bilirubin	3–17 micromol/L
calcium (total)	2.12–2.65 mmol/L
calcium (ionized)	1–1.25 mmol/L
chloride	95–105 mmol/L
creatine kinase (CK)	25–195 iu/L
creatinine	70–150 micromol/L
C-reactive protein (CRP)	<10 mg/L
glucose (fasting)	3.5–5.5 mmol/L
γ glutamyl transpeptidase (♂)	11–51 IU/L
(♀)	7–33 IU/L
magnesium	0.75–1.05 mmol/L
osmolality	278–305 mosmol/kg
potassium	3.5–5.0 mmol/L
sodium	135–145 mmol/L
urea	2.5–6.7 mmol/L
urate (♀)	150–390 micromol/L
(♂)	210–480 micromol/L

Haematology

RBC (women)	$3.9–5.6 \times 10^{12}$/L
(men)	$4.5–6.5 \times 10^{12}$/L
Hb (women)	11.5–16.0g/dL
(men)	13.5–18.0g/dL
Hct (women)	0.37–0.47
(men)	0.40–0.54
MCV	76–96 femtoL
WCC	$4.0–11.0 \times 10^9$/L
neutrophils	$2.0–7.5 \times 10^9$/L (40–75% of WCC)
lymphocytes	$1.5–4.0 \times 10^9$/L (20–40% of WCC)
monocytes	$0.2–0.8 \times 10^9$/L (2–10% of WCC)
eosinophils	$0.04–0.40 \times 10^9$/L (1–6% of WCC)
basophils	$<0.1 \times 10^9$/L (<1% of WCC)
platelets	$150–400 \times 10^9$/L
prothrombin time (factors I, II, VII, X)	12–15sec
APTT (factors VII, IX, XI, XII)	23–42sec

International Normalized Ratio (INR) therapeutic targets

2.0–3.0	(for treating DVT, pulmonary embolism)
2.5–3.5	(embolism prophylaxis for AF)
3.0–4.5	(recurrent thrombo-embolic disease, arterial grafts & prosthetic valves)
ESR (women)	$< {}^{(\text{age in years}+10)}/_2$ mm/hr
(men)	$< {}^{(\text{age in years})}/_2$ mm/hr

Metric conversion

Length

1m = 3 feet 3.4 inches	1 foot = 0.3048m
1cm = 0.394 inch	1 inch = 25.4mm

Weight

1kg = 2.20 pounds	1 stone = 6.35kg
1g = 15.4 grains	1 pound = 0.454kg
	1 ounce = 28.4g

Volume

1 L = 1.76 UK pints = 2.11 US liquid pints
1 UK pint = 20 fluid ounces = 0.568 L
1 US liquid pint = 16 fluid ounces = 0.473 L
1 teaspoon ≈ 5mL
1 tablespoon ≈ 15mL

Temperature

$T°$ in °C = ($T°$ in Fahrenheit − 32) $\times \frac{5}{9}$

Pressure

1kPa = 7.5mmHg

Acknowledgements

A number of people provided comments, help and moral support. Special thanks are due to Dr Phil Munro. We also wish to thank:

Miss Sehlah Abassi, Mr David Alao, Dr Matt Baker, Dr Joan Barber, Dr Ruth Beach, Mr Dewald Behrens, Dr Ash Bhatia, Dr Angela Bonnar, Dr Rachel Broadley, Dr Chris Brown, Mrs Debra Clayton, Mr Jon Davies, Dr Kate Evans, Dr James Falconer, Miss Paula Fitzpatrick, Mrs Jennifer Flemen, Dr Adrian Flynn, Dr Debbie Galbraith, Mr Blair Graham, Dr Catherine Guly, Mr Chris Hadfield, Dr Steve Halford, Mr Andrew Harrower, Miss Emily Hotton, Mr Jim Huntley, Mrs Eileen Hutchison, Mr Nicholas Hyatt, Dr Karen Illingworth, Mr Ian Kelly, Mr Jacques Kerr, Dr Alastair Kidd, Dr Paul Leonard, Mr Malcolm Lewis, Mr AF Mabrook, Dr Simon Mardel, Dr Nick Mathiew, Ms Carolyn Meikle, Dr Louisa Mitchell, Dr Claudia Murton, Dr Louisa Pieterse, Dr Stephanie Prince, Dr Laura Robertson, Miss Katharine Robinson, Dr Andrew Sampson, Mr Tom Scott, Dr Simon Scott-Hayward, Ms Karen Sim, Mr Toby Slade, Dr Timothy Squires, Mr Ashleigh Stone, Dr Luke Summers, Dr Rob Taylor, Dr Ross Vanstone, Ms Fiona Wardlaw, Dr Mike Wells, Mr Ken Woodburn, Mrs Polly Wyatt.

General approach

The emergency department

The role of the emergency department

The emergency department (ED) occupies a key position in terms of the interface between primary and secondary care. It has a high public profile. Many patients attend without referral, but some are referred by NHS Direct, minor injury units, general practitioners (GPs), and other medical practitioners. The ED manages patients with a huge variety of medical problems. Many of the patients who attend have painful and/or distressing disorders of recent origin.

Priorities are:
• To make life-saving interventions.
• To provide analgesia.
• To identify relevant issues, investigations, and commence treatment.
• To decide upon need for admission or discharge.

ED staff work as a team. Traditional roles are often blurred, with the important issue being what clinical skills a member of staff is capable of.

ED staff include:
• Nurses (including nurse practitioners, nurse consultants, health care assistants).
• Doctors (permanent and fixed-term).
• Reception and administrative staff (receptionists, secretaries, managers).
• Radiographers, including reporting radiographers.
• Other specialist staff (eg psychiatric liaison nurses, plaster technicians, physiotherapists, paramedic practitioners, physician assistants, occupational therapists, clinic/ED ward staff).
• Supporting staff (security, porters, cleaners, police).

Physical resources

A principal focus of the ED is to provide immediate resuscitation for patients who present with emergency conditions. In terms of sheer numbers, more patients attend with minor conditions and injuries, often presenting quite a challenge for them to be seen and treated in a timely fashion. Different departments have systems to suit their own particular needs, but most have a resuscitation room, an area for patients on trolleys, and an area for ambulant patients with less serious problems or injuries. Paediatric patients are seen in a separate area from adults. In addition, every ED requires facilities for applying casts, exploring and suturing wounds, obtaining X-rays, and examining patients with eye problems.

Discharge from the ED

To work efficiently, the overall hospital system needs to enable easy flow of patients out of the ED. Options available for continuing care of patients who leave the ED, include:
• Discharge home with no follow-up.
• Discharge home with GP and/or other community support/follow-up.
• Discharge with hospital clinic follow-up arranged.
• Admission to hospital for further investigation and treatment.
• Transfer to another hospital with more specialist facilities.

Emergency department staff beyond the emergency department

In addition to their roles in providing direct clinical care in their departments, many ED staff provide related clinical care in other settings and ways:

- *Short stay wards* (sometimes called clinical decision units) where emergency care can be continued by ED staff. The intention is for admissions to these units to be short: most of the patients admitted to such wards are observed for relatively short periods (<24hr) and undergo assessments at an early stage to decide about the need for discharge or longer-term admission.
- *Outpatient clinics* enable patients with a variety of clinical problems (eg burns, soft tissue injuries, and infections) to be followed up by ED staff.
- *Planned theatre lists* run by ED specialists are used by some hospitals to manage some simple fractures (eg angulated distal radial fractures).
- *Telemedicine advice* to satellite and minor injury units.

Emergency medicine in other settings

As the delivery of emergency care continues to develop, patients with emergency problems are now receiving assessment and treatment in a variety of settings. These include minor injury units, acute medical assessment units and walk-in centres. Traditional distinctions between emergency medicine, acute medicine, and primary care have become blurred.

Note keeping

General aspects

It is impossible to over-emphasize the importance of note keeping. Doctors and nurse practitioners each treat hundreds of patients every month. With the passage of time, it is impossible to remember all aspects relating to these cases, yet it may be necessary to give evidence in court about them years after the event. The only reference will be the notes made much earlier. Medicolegally, the ED record is the prime source of evidence in negligence cases. If the notes are deficient, it may not be feasible to defend a claim even if negligence has not occurred. A court may consider that the standard of the notes reflects the general standard of care. Sloppy, illegible, or incomplete notes reflect badly on the individual. In contrast, if notes are neat, legible, appropriate, and detailed, those reviewing the case will naturally expect the general standards of care, in terms of history taking, examination, and level of knowledge, to be competent.

The *Data Protection and Access to Medical Records Acts* give patients right of access to their medical notes. Remember, whenever writing notes, that the patient may in the future read exactly what has been written. Follow the basic general rules listed below.

Layout

Follow a standard outline:

Presenting complaint Indicate from whom the history has been obtained (eg the patient, a relative, or ambulance personnel). Avoid attributing events to certain individuals (eg patient was struck by 'Joe Bloggs').

Previous relevant history Note recent ED attendances. Include family and social history. An elderly woman with a Colles' fracture of her dominant hand may be able to manage at home with routine follow-up provided she is normally in good health, and has good family or other support, but if she lives alone in precarious social conditions without such support, then admission on 'social grounds' may be required.

Current medications Remember to ask about non-prescribed drugs (including recreational, herbal, and homeopathic). Women may not volunteer the oral contraceptive pill (OCP) as 'medication' unless specifically asked. Enquire about allergies to medications and document the nature of this reaction.

Examination findings As well as +ve features, document relevant −ve findings (eg the absence of neck stiffness in a patient with headache and pyrexia). Always document the side of the patient which has been injured. For upper limb injuries, note whether the patient is left or right handed. Use 'left' and 'right', not 'L' and 'R'. Document if a patient is abusive or aggressive, but avoid non-medical, judgemental terms (eg 'drunk').

Investigation findings Record clearly.

Working diagnosis For patients being admitted, this may be a differential diagnostic list. Sometimes a problem list can help.

Treatment given Document drugs, including dose, time, and route of administration (see current *British National Formulary* (*BNF*) for guidance). Include medications given in the ED, as well as therapy to be continued (eg course of antibiotics). Note the number and type of sutures or staples used for wound closure (eg '5 × 6/0 nylon sutures').

Advice and follow-up arrangements Document if the patient and/or relative is given preprinted instructions (eg 'POP care'). Indicate when/ if the patient needs to be reviewed (eg 'see GP in 5 days for suture removal') or other arrangement (eg 'Fracture clinic in one week').

Record advice about when/why the patient should return for review, especially if there is a risk of a rare but serious complication (eg for low back pain 'see GP if not better in 1 week. Return to the ED at once if bladder/bowel problem or numb groin/bottom' that might be features of cauda equina syndrome).

Basic rules

- Write legibly in ballpoint pen, ideally black, which photocopies well.
- Always date and time the notes.
- Sign the notes, and print your name and status below.
- Make your notes concise and to the point.
- Use simple line drawings or preprinted sheets for wound/injury descriptions.
- Avoid idiosyncratic abbreviations.
- *Never* make rude or judgemental comments.
- *Always* document the name, grade, and specialty of any doctor from whom you have received advice.
- When referring or handing a patient over, *always* document the time of referral/handover, together with the name, grade, and specialty of the receiving doctor.
- Inform the GP by letter (📖 Liaising with GPs, p.10), even if the patient is admitted. Most EDs have computerized systems that generate such letters. In complex cases, send also a copy of ED notes, with results of investigations.

Pro formas

Increasing emphasis on evidence-based guidelines and protocols has been associated with the introduction of protocols for many patient presentations and conditions. Bear in mind the fact that, for some patients, satisfactory completion of a pro forma may not adequately capture all of the information required.

Electronic records

In an electronic age, there has been an understandable move towards trying to introduce electronic patient records. The potential advantages are obvious, particularly in relation to rapidly ascertaining past medical history. When completing electronic records, practitioners need to follow the same principles as those outlined above for written records.

Access to old records can make a huge contribution to decision making. One potential advantage of electronic records is that they can be accessed rapidly (compared with older systems requiring a porter to search through the medical records store and retrieve paper-based notes).

Radiological requests

'I am glad to say that in this country there is no need to carry out unnecessary tests as a form of insurance. It is not in this country desirable, or indeed necessary, that over protective and over examination work should be done, merely and purely and simply as I say to protect oneself against possible litigation'—Judge Fallon, quoted by Oscar Craig, Chairman Cases Committee, Medical Protection Society.

Requesting investigations

The Royal College of Radiologists' booklet '*Making the Best Use of a Department of Clinical Radiology: Guidelines for Doctors*' (6th edn, London, RCR, 2007) contains very useful information and is strongly recommended.

General aspects

- An X-ray is no substitute for careful, thorough clinical examination. It is usually unnecessary to request X-rays to confirm the clinical diagnosis of uncomplicated fractures of the nose, coccyx, a single rib, or toes (other than the big toe).
- If in doubt about the need for X-rays or the specific test required, consider relevant guidelines (eg Ottawa rules for ankle injuries, 📖 p.484) and/or discuss with senior ED staff or radiologist.
- When requesting X-rays, describe the indication/mechanism of injury, clinical findings, including the side involved (right or left—spelt out in full, not abbreviated) and the suspected clinical diagnosis. This is important for the radiologist reporting the films without the advantage of being able to examine the patient.
- Do not worry about specifying exactly which X-ray views are required. The radiographer will know the standard views that are needed, based on the information provided (eg AP + simplified apical oblique views for a patient with suspected anterior shoulder dislocation). In unusual cases, discuss with senior ED staff, radiographer, or radiologist.
- Always consider the possibility of pregnancy in women of child-bearing age before requesting an X-ray of the abdomen, pelvis, lumbar spine, hips, or thighs. If the clinical indication for X-ray is overriding, tell the radiographer, who will attempt to shield the foetus/gonads. If the risks/benefits of X-rays in pregnant or possibly pregnant women are not obvious, consult senior ED or radiology staff.

X-ray reporting system

Many hospitals have systems so that all ED X-rays are reported by a specialist within 24hr. Reports of any missed abnormalities are returned with the X-rays to the ED for the attention of senior staff, so that appropriate action can be taken.

System for identifying abnormalities

In addition to the formal reporting system described above, a system is commonly used whereby the radiographer taking the films applies a sticky 'red dot' to hard copy X-ray films and/or request card or to the equivalent electronic image if they identify an abnormality. This alerts other clinical staff to the possibility of abnormal findings.

Triage

The nature of ED work means that a sorting system is required to ensure that patients with the most immediately life-threatening conditions are seen first. A triage process aims to categorize patients based on their medical need and the available departmental resources. One most commonly used process in the UK is the National Triage Scale (Table 1.1).

Table 1.1		
National Triage Scale	**Colour**	**Time to be seen by doctor**
1 Immediate	Red	Immediately
2 Very urgent	Orange	Within 5–10 min
3 Urgent	Yellow	Within 1 hr
4 Standard	Green	Within 2 hr
5 Non-urgent	Blue	Within 4 hr

As soon as a patient arrives in the ED he/she should be assessed by a dedicated triage nurse (a senior, experienced individual with considerable common sense). This nurse should provide any immediate interventions needed (eg elevating injured limbs, applying ice packs or splints, and giving analgesia) and initiate investigations to speed the patient's journey through the department (eg ordering appropriate X-rays). Patients should not have to wait to be triaged. It is a brief assessment which should take no more than a few minutes.

Three points require emphasis:
- Triage is a dynamic process. The urgency (and hence triage category) with which a patient requires to be seen may change with time. For example a middle-aged man who hobbles in with an inversion ankle injury is likely to be placed in triage category 4 (green). If in the waiting room he becomes pale, sweaty, and complains of chest discomfort, he would require prompt re-triage into category 2 (orange).
- Placement in a triage category does not imply a diagnosis, or even the lethality of a condition (eg an elderly patient with colicky abdominal discomfort, vomiting, and absolute constipation would normally be placed in category 3 (yellow) and a possible diagnosis would be bowel obstruction). The cause may be a neoplasm which has already metastasized and is hence likely to be ultimately fatal.
- Triage has its own problems. In particular, patients in non-urgent categories may wait inordinately long periods of time, whilst patients who have presented later, but with conditions perceived to be more urgent, are seen before them. Patients need to be aware of this and to be informed of likely waiting times. Uncomplaining elderly patients can often be poorly served by the process.

Discharge, referral, and handover

Most patients seen in the ED are examined, investigated, treated, and discharged home, either with no follow-up, or advice to see their GP (for suture removal, wound checks, etc.). Give these patients (and/or attending relative/friend) clear instructions on when to attend the GP's surgery and an indication of the likely course of events, as well as any features that they should look out for to prompt them to seek medical help prior to this. *Formal written instructions* are particularly useful for patients with minor head injury (📖 p.367) and those with limbs in POP or other forms of cast immobilization (📖 Casts and their problems, p.424).

The referral of patients to an inpatient team can cause considerable anxiety, misunderstanding, and potential conflict between ED staff and other disciplines. Before making the referral the following should be considered.

Is it appropriate to refer this patient to the inpatient team?

Usually, this will be obvious. For example, a middle-aged man with a history of crushing chest pain and an ECG showing an acute MI clearly requires urgent management in the ED, and rapid admission for further investigation and treatment. Similarly, an elderly lady who has fallen, is unable to weight-bear and has a fractured neck of femur will require analgesia, inpatient care and surgery.

However, difficult situations occur where the clinical situation is less clear; for example, if a man experienced 4–5min of atypical chest pain, has a normal ECG and chest X-ray (CXR), and is anxious to go home. Or a lady has no apparent fracture on X-ray, but cannot weight-bear.

Is there appropriate information to make this decision?

This requires a balance between availability, time, and appropriateness. In general, simple investigations which rapidly give the diagnosis, or clues to it, are all that are needed. These include electrocardiogram (ECGs), arterial blood gas (ABG), and plain X-rays. It is relatively unusual to have to wait for the results of investigations such as full blood count (FBC), urea & electrolytes (U&E), and liver function tests (LFTs) before referring a patient, since these rarely alter the immediate management. Simple trolley-side investigations are often of great value, for example, stix estimations of blood glucose (BMG) and urinalysis. If complicated investigations are needed, then referral for inpatient or outpatient specialist care is often required.

Has the patient had appropriate treatment pending the admission?

Do not forget, or delay, analgesia. Treat every patient in pain appropriately as soon as possible. A patient does not have to 'earn' analgesia. Never delay analgesia to allow further examination or investigation. Concern regarding masking of signs or symptoms (for example, in a patient with an acute abdomen) is inhumane and incorrect.

How to refer patients

Referral is often by telephone, and this can create problems:
- Introduce yourself and ask for the name and grade of the specialist.
- Give a clear, concise summary of the history, investigations, and treatment that you have already undertaken.
- Early in the discussion say clearly whether you are making a referral for admission or a request for a specialist opinion. With ever increasing pressure on hospital beds, inpatient teams can be reluctant to come and see patients, and may appear to be happier to give advice over the phone to avoid admission. If, in your view, the patient needs to be admitted, then clearly indicate this. If, for whatever reason, this is declined, do not get cross, rude, or aggressive, but contact senior ED medical staff to speak to the specialist team.
- When the specialist team comes to see the patient, or the patient is admitted directly to a ward, the ED notes need to be complete and legible. Make sure that there is a list of the investigations already performed, together with the available results and crucially, a list of investigations whose results remain outstanding. The latter is essential to ensure continuity of care and to prevent an important result 'falling through the net'. Similarly, summarize treatment already given and the response. In an emergency, do not delay referral or treatment merely to complete the notes, but complete them at the earliest opportunity.
- Encourage inpatient specialists who attend patients to write their findings and management plan in the notes, adding a signature and the time/date.

Handing over patients

Dangers of handing over

Handing over a patient to a colleague, because your shift has ended and you are going home, is fraught with danger. It is easy for patients to be neglected, or receive sub-optimal or delayed treatment. It is safest to complete to the point of discharge or referral to an inpatient team every patient that you are seeing at the end of a shift. Occasionally this may not be possible (eg if there is a delay in obtaining an X-ray or other investigation). In these situations, hand over the patient carefully to the doctor who is taking over and inform the nursing staff of this.

How to hand over

Include in the handover relevant aspects of history and examination performed, the investigation results, and the treatment undertaken. Sign and aim to complete records on the patient as soon as possible. Note the time of hand over, and the name of the doctor or nurse handed over to. When accepting a 'handed-over patient' at the start of a shift, spend time establishing exactly what has happened so far. Finally, it is courteous (and will prevent problems) to tell the patient that their further care will be performed by another doctor or nurse.

Liaising with GPs

Despite changes in the way that care (particularly out of hours) is delivered, GPs still have a pivotal role in co-ordinating medical care. Often the GP will know more than anyone about the past history, social and family situation, and recent events of their patient's management. Therefore, contact the GP when these aspects are relevant to the patient's ED attendance, or where considerations of admission or discharge are concerned.

Every attendance is followed routinely by a letter to the GP detailing the reason(s) for presentation, clinical findings and relevant investigations, treatment given, and follow-up arrangements.

If a patient dies, contact the GP without delay—to provide a medical contact and assistance to the bereaved family, to prevent embarrassing experiences (eg letters requesting clinic attendances), and out of courtesy, because the GP is the patient's primary medical attendant. Finally, the GP may be asked to issue a death certificate by the Coroner (in Scotland, the Procurator Fiscal) following further enquiries.

Always contact the GP prior to the discharge of a patient where early follow-up (ie within the next 24–72hr) is required. This may occur with elderly patients where there is uncertainty about the home situation and their ability to manage. A typical example is an elderly lady with a Colles' fracture of her dominant wrist who lives alone. The ED management of this patient is relatively simple (📖 p.444). However, merely manipulating a Colles' fracture into a good position, supporting it in an adequate cast, and providing analgesia, is only one facet of care. The GP may know that the lady has supportive relatives or neighbours who will help with shopping and cooking, and will help her to bath and dress. The GP and the primary care team may be able to supplement existing support and check that the patient is coping. Equally, the GP may indicate that with additional home support (eg home helps, meals, district nurses), the patient could manage. Alternatively, the GP may indicate that the Colles' fracture merely represents the final event in an increasingly fragile home situation and that the patient will require hospital admission, at least in the short-term.

For the same reasons, a GP who refers a patient to the ED and indicates that the patient requires admission does so in the full knowledge of that patient's circumstances. Always contact the GP if it is contemplated that the patient is to be discharged—preferably after senior medical consultation.

Finally, remember that GPs are also under considerable pressure. Some situations may appear to reflect the fact that a patient has been referred inappropriately or the patient may report that they have tried to contact their GP unsuccessfully. Rather than irately ringing the practice and antagonizing them, inform the ED consultant who can raise this constructively and appropriately in a suitable environment.

Telephone advice

Many departments receive calls from patients, parents, and other carers for advice. Approach these calls in exactly the same way as a face-to-face consultation. Formally document details of the call, including:

- Date and time of the call.
- The caller's telephone number.
- The caller's relationship to the patient.
- The patient's name, age, and sex.
- The nature of the problem.
- The advice given.

As with all notes, date, time, and sign these notes.

NHS Direct

In England and Wales *NHS Direct* provides a 24-hr, 7-day a week telephone service providing information and advice on health matters. It is staffed by nurses who respond according to protocols.

The telephone number for *NHS Direct* is *0845 4647*.

The equivalent service in Scotland is *NHS24* tel. *08454 242424*.

These services have internet websites at www.nhsdirect.nhs.uk and www.nhs24.com

Telephone advice calls from other health professionals

Occasionally, other health professionals request advice regarding the management of patients in their care. Such advice should be given by experienced ED staff.

Telemedicine

Increasingly, emergency health care is provided by integrated networks, which include EDs, minor injuries units, radiology departments, and GP surgeries connected by telemedicine links. This has advantages in remote or rural settings, enabling a wide range of injuries and other emergencies to be diagnosed and treated locally. The combination of video and teleradiology may allow a decision to be made and explained directly to the patient. A typical example is whether a patient with an isolated Colles' fracture needs to have a manipulation of the fracture. Expertise is required to undertake telemedicine consultations safely. This specialist advice should be given by senior ED staff, and careful documentation is crucial.

Liaising with the ambulance crew

Paramedics and ED staff have a close professional relationship. Paramedics and ambulance staff are professionals who work in conditions that are often difficult and sometimes dangerous. It is worth taking an off-duty day to accompany a crew during their shift to see the problems they face.

A benefit of paramedic training has been to bring ambulance staff into the ED to work with medical and nursing staff, and to foster the communication and rapport essential for good patient management.

In the UK, a patient brought to an ED by ambulance will routinely have a patient report form (PRF) (see Fig. 1.1). This is completed by the crew at the scene and in transit, and given to reception or nursing staff on arrival. The information on these forms can be invaluable. In particular, the time intervals between the receipt of the 999 call, and arrival at the scene and at hospital, provide a time framework within which changes in the patient's clinical condition can be placed and interpreted.

The initial at-scene assessment will include details of the use of seat belts, airbags, crash helmets, etc., and is particularly valuable when amplified by specifically asking the crew about their interpretation of the event, likely speeds involved, types of vehicle, etc.

The clinical features of the Glasgow Coma Score (GCS), pulse rate, blood pressure (BP), and respiratory rate form baseline values from which trends and response to treatment can be judged. Useful aspects in the history/ comments section include previous complaints, current medications, etc., which the crew may have obtained from the patient, relatives, or friends. The PRF will also contain important information about oxygen, drugs, IV fluids administered, and the response to these interventions. Before the crew leave the department, confirm that they have provided all relevant information.

Do not be judgemental about the crew's performance. Remember the constraints under which they operate. Without the benefits of a warm environment, good lighting, and sophisticated equipment, it can be exceedingly difficult to make accurate assessments of illness or injury severity, or to perform otherwise simple tasks (eg airway management and intravenous (IV) cannulation).

Do not dismiss the overall assessment of a patient made by an experienced crew. While the ultimate diagnosis may not be clear (a situation which pertains equally in the ED), their evaluation of the potential for life-threatening events is often extremely perceptive. Equally, take heed of their description of crash scenes. They will have seen far more than most ED staff, so accept their greater experience.

Most ambulance staff are keen to obtain feedback, both about specific cases and general aspects of medical care. Like everyone, they are interested in their patients. A few words as to what happened to Mrs Smith who was brought in last week and her subsequent clinical course is a friendly and easy way of providing informal feedback, and helps to cement the professional relationship between the ambulance service and the ED.

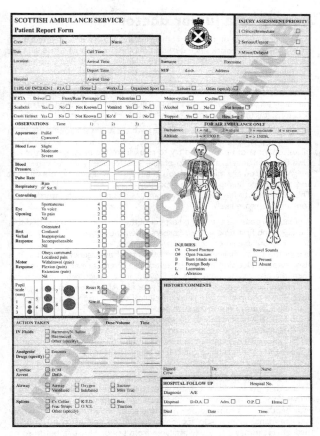

Fig. 1.1 An example of a patient reporting form. Reproduced with kind permission from the Scottish Ambulance Service.

Coping as a junior doctor

Although many junior doctors coming to the ED have completed more than 12 months of work since qualification, the prospect of working at the 'sharp end' can be accompanied by trepidation. As with many potentially worrying situations in life, reality is not as terrifying as its anticipation. The number of hours worked may not appear long in comparison with other posts, but do not assume that this makes an ED job 'easy'. Being on duty inevitably involves much time standing, walking, working, thinking, and making decisions. It is unusual to come off-shift without feeling physically tired.

Active young doctors can usually cope with these physical demands, but a demanding professional life and demanding social life are rarely compatible. Make the most of time off and try to relax from the pressures of the job. One function of relaxation is to enable you to face work refreshed and invigorated. You are mistaken if you believe that you can stay out all night and then work unimpaired the next day. Tired doctors make mistakes. They also tend to have less patience and, as a consequence, interpersonal conflicts are more likely.

A greater problem is the mental aspect of the job. Doctors often find that the ED is the first time in their careers when they have to make unequivocal decisions based on their own assessment and investigations. This is one of the great challenges and excitements of emergency medicine. It is also a worry. Decision-making is central to ED practice and, with experience, the process becomes easier. Developing a structured approach can pre-empt many problems and simplify your life. After taking an appropriate history and completing the relevant clinical examination of a patient, ask yourself a series of questions such as:

• Do I know what is likely to be wrong with this patient?
• What investigations are required to confirm the diagnosis?
• Do I know what treatment is needed and have I got the skills needed?
• Does this patient require referral to an inpatient team (📖 p.8)?
• If not, do they need to be reviewed in the ED or another specialist clinic?

The wide spectrum of problems with which ED patients can present means that no individual can be expert in every possible condition. It is therefore as important to recognize and accept when you are out of your depth as it is to make decisions and treat patients whom you know you can manage. Seek help appropriately and do not just try to muddle through. Help may be readily available from senior ED staff, but in some departments direct contact with a specialist team is required. One of the most difficult situations is where a specialist either refuses to come to see the patient or gives telephone advice that is clearly inappropriate. You must always act as the patient's advocate. If you refer a patient with a fractured neck of femur, and the telephone message from the inpatient team is 'bring him back to the Fracture Clinic in one week', it is clearly wrong to carry this out. First, check that the doctor has understood the details of the patient's condition and your concerns. More conflict and aggravation is caused by communication errors (usually involving second-hand telephone messages) than by anything else. If the situation remains unresolved, consult senior ED staff. Whatever happens, never lose your cool in public and always put your patient's interests first.

Learning in the ED

Try to learn something new every day. Keep a note of patients with interesting or unusual problems, and later check what happened to them. Ask senior staff for advice. Use the ED reference books. Try to note all new conditions seen during a shift and read about them later.

Staff interaction

The nature of the job, the patients, and the diversity of staff involved means that a considerable degree of camaraderie exists. For an outsider, this can initially be daunting. Junior medical staff are likely to work for 4–12 months in the department. Other staff may have spent a lifetime there with long-established friendships (or sometimes animosities). Respect their position and experience, learn from them.

The nub of this is an understanding that the role of one individual and that of other individuals in the department are inextricably linked. Any junior (or senior) doctor who feels that they are the most important individual in their working environment will have an extremely uncomfortable professional existence. In the ED, every member of staff has a role. Your professionalism should dictate that you respect this. Only in this way will you gain reciprocal respect from other staff members.

Never consider any job 'beneath you' or someone else's responsibility. Patients come before pride. So, if portering staff are rushed off their feet and you are unoccupied, wheel a patient to X-ray yourself—it will improve your standing with your colleagues and help the patient.

Shifts

Rule 1 Never be late for your shift.

Rule 2 If, for whatever reason, you are unable to work a shift, let the senior staff in the ED know as soon as possible.

Ensure that you take a break. Two or three short breaks in an 8-hr shift are better than one long one. Remember to eat and maintain your fluid intake. Shift working may mean that you will work sometimes with familiar faces and perhaps occasionally with individuals with whom you find social contact uncomfortable. Put these considerations aside while you are at work, for the sake of the patients and your peace of mind.

If you can't cope

Finally, if you feel that you are unable to manage or that the pressure of the job is too great—*tell someone*. Don't bottle it up, try to ignore it, or assume that it reflects inadequacy. It doesn't. Everyone, at some time, has feelings of inability to cope. Trying to disguise or deny the situation is unfair to yourself, your colleagues, and your patients. You need to tell someone and discuss things. Do it now. Talk to your consultant. If you cannot face him or her, talk to your GP or another senior member of staff—but talk to someone who can help you.

The *BMA Counselling Service for Doctors* (tel: 08459 200169) provides a confidential counselling service 24 hr a day, 365 days of the year to discuss personal, emotional, and work-related problems. The Doctors' Support Network (www.dsn.org.uk) and Doctors' Support Line (tel: 0844 395 3010) are also useful resources.

Inappropriate attenders

This is an emotive and ill-defined term. Depending upon the department, such patients could comprise 4–20% of attendances.

The perception as to whether it is appropriate to go to an ED or attend a GP will vary between the patient, GP, and ED staff. Appropriateness is not simply related to the symptoms, diagnosis, or the time interval involved. It may not necessarily be related to the need for investigation. For example, not all patients who require an X-ray necessarily have to attend an ED. Further blurring of 'appropriate' and 'inappropriate' groups relates to the geographical location of the ED. In rural areas, GPs frequently perform procedures such as suturing. In urban areas, these arrangements are less common. For ill-defined reasons, patients often perceive that they should only contact their GP during 'office' hours, and outside these times may attend an ED with primary care complaints.

It is clearly inappropriate to come to an ED simply because of a real or perceived difficulty in accessing primary care. Nevertheless, the term 'inappropriate attendance' is a pejorative one—it is better to use the phrase 'primary care patients'. It must be recognized that primary care problems are best dealt with by GPs. Many departments try to prevent this primary care workload presenting to the ED. Some departments tackle the problem by having GPs working alongside ED staff.

Managing inappropriate attenders

Only through a continual process of patient education will these problems be resolved. Initiatives include nurse practitioner minor injury units and hospital-based primary care services. Evaluations are underway but, to function effectively, such services require adequate funding and staffing.

It can sometimes be difficult to deal with primary care problems in the ED. After an appropriate history and examination, it may be necessary to explain to patients that they will have to attend their own GP. This may need direct contact between the ED and the practice to facilitate this.

Inappropriate referrals

Sometimes, it may appear that another health professional (eg GP, emergency nurse practitioner, nurse at NHS Direct) has referred a patient to the ED inappropriately. Avoid making such judgements. Treat patients on their merits, but mention the issue to your consultant. Remember that the information available to the referring clinician at the time of the prehospital consultation is likely to have been different to that available at the time of ED attendance.

The patient with a label

Some patients will have been referred by another medical practitioner, usually a GP. The accompanying letter may include a presumptive diagnosis. The details in the letter are often extremely helpful, but do not assume the diagnosis is necessarily correct. Take particular care with patients who re-attend following an earlier attendance. The situation may have changed since the previous doctor saw the patient. Clinical signs may have developed or regressed. The patient may have not given the referring doctor and ED staff the same history. Do not pre-judge the problem: start with an open mind. Apply common sense, however. Keep any previous history in mind. For example, assume that a patient with a known abdominal aortic aneurysm who collapses with sudden, severe, abdominal pain, signs of hypovolaemic shock, and a tender pulsatile mass in the abdomen, to have a ruptured abdominal aortic aneurysm, rather than intestinal obstruction. The patient's *previous ED and hospital case notes* are invaluable and will often give useful information and allow, for example, ECG comparisons, aiding the diagnostic process. A call to the GP can also provide useful background, which they may not have had time to include in their referral letter or may have excluded for confidentiality or other reasons.

Self-labelled patients

Take care with patients who label themselves. Those with chronic or unusual diseases often know significantly more about their conditions than ED staff! In such situations, take special notice of comments and advice from the patient and/or their relatives. Do not resent this or see it as a professional affront—rapport with the patient will increase markedly and management will usually be easier.

Regular attenders

Every ED has a group of 'regular' patients who, with time, become physically and sometimes emotionally attached to the department. Some have underlying psychiatric illnesses, often with 'inadequate' personalities. Some are homeless. Regular attenders frequently use the ED as a source of primary care. As outlined above, make attempts to direct them to appropriate facilities, because the ED is unsuited to the management of chronic illness, and is unable to provide the continuing medical and nursing support that these patients require.

Repeated presentations with apparently trivial complaints or with the same complaint often tax the patience of ED staff. This is heightened if the presentations are provoked or aggravated by alcohol intake. Remember, however, that these patients can and do suffer from the same acute events as everyone else. Keep an open mind, diagnostically and in attitude to the patient. Just because he/she has returned for the third time in as many days complaining of chest pain, does not mean that on this occasion he does not have an acute MI! Maintain adequate documentation for each attendance. Occasionally, especially with intractable re-attenders, a joint meeting between the social work team, GP, ED consultant and psychiatric services is required to provide a definitive framework for both the patient and the medical services. For some patients, it will be possible to follow a plan of action for ED presentations with a particular complaint.

The patient you dislike

General approach

Accept the patient as he or she is, regardless of behaviour, class, religion, social lifestyle, or colour. Given human nature, there will inevitably be some patients whom you immediately dislike or find difficult. The feeling is often mutual. Many factors that cause patients to present to the ED may aggravate the situation. These include their current medical condition, their past experiences in hospitals, their social situation, and any concurrent use of alcohol and/or other drugs. Your approach and state of mind during the consultation play a major role. This will be influenced by whether the department is busy, how much sleep you have had recently, and when you last had a break for coffee or food.

Given the nature of ED workload and turnover, conflict slows down the process and makes it more likely that you will make clinical errors. Many potential conflicts can be avoided by an open, pleasant approach. Introduce yourself politely to the patient. Use body language to reduce a potentially aggressive response.

The patient's perspective

Put yourself in the patient's position. Any patient marched up to by a doctor who has their hands on hips, a glaring expression, and the demand 'Well, what's wrong with you now?' will retort aggressively.

Defusing a volatile situation

Most complaints and aggression occur when the department is busy and waiting times are long. Patients understand the pressures medical and nursing staff have to work under, and a simple, 'I am sorry you have had to wait so long, but we have had a number of emergencies elsewhere in the department', does much to diffuse potential conflict and will often mean that the patient starts to sympathize with you as a young, overworked practitioner!

There is never any excuse for rude, abusive, or aggressive behaviour to a patient. If you are rude, complaints will invariably follow and more importantly, the patient will not have received the appropriate treatment for their condition. It may be necessary to hand care of a patient to a colleague if an unresolvable conflict has arisen.

Management of the violent patient is considered in detail on p.610.

Special patient groups

Attending the ED is difficult enough, but can be even more so for certain 'special' patient groups. It is important that ED staff are sensitive to the needs of these groups and that there are systems in place to help them in what may be regarded as an intimidating atmosphere. The following list is far from exhaustive, but includes some important groups who require particular consideration:

- *Children*: they are such an 'obvious' and large 'minority' group that they receive special attention to suit their particular needs (see 📖 Paediatric emergencies, p.630).
- *Pregnant women*: see 📖 Obstetrics and gynaecology, p.563.
- *Those with mental health problems*: see 📖 Psychiatry, p.601.
- *The elderly*: who often have multiple medical problems and live in socially precarious circumstances.
- Patients with Alzheimer's disease and other states associated with chronic confusion.
- *Those with learning difficulties*: 📖 p.21.
- Patients with hearing problems.
- The visually impaired.
- *Those who do not speak or understand English*: arrangements should be in place to enable the use of interpreters.
- *Patients with certain cultural or religious beliefs (particularly amongst 'minority groups')*: these can impact significantly upon a variety of situations (eg after unsuccessful resuscitation for cardiac arrest— 📖 Breaking bad news, p.24).
- Those who are homeless or are away from home, friends, and family (eg holiday makers).
- Those who have drug/alcohol dependency.

Isn't everyone special?

Taken at face value, the concept that certain groups of patients are 'special' and so require special attention does not meet with universal approval. There is a good argument that every patient deserves the best possible care. Whilst this is true, it is also obvious that certain patients do have additional needs that need to be considered. Many of these additional needs relate to effective communication. There are some tremendous resources available that can help practitioners to overcome communication difficulties (eg www.communicationpeople.co.uk).

Discharging the elderly patient

There are no set predisposing factors that determine patients most at risk following discharge. Those that affect the chance of difficulties at home include the current medical problem, underlying functional and social factors.

Risk indicators

Multiple pathologies and atypical symptoms render this group more vulnerable to the physical, functional, and social effects of acute illness. Past medical history and pre-admission status are especially important determinants for patients with dementia or psychiatric illness. There may be evidence of recently changed circumstances, a recent bereavement, a change in medical or physical condition, increasing confusion, or unusual behaviour. The patient may not be able to afford adequate food or heating. Community services may not be aware that support is needed or help may have been offered, but refused.

Other important indicators are:
• Those living alone.
• Absence of close family support or community services.
• Unsuitable home circumstances (eg external or internal stairs).
• Difficulty with mobility.

Determining those unable to cope

Look for evidence of self-neglect that suggests that the elderly person is having difficulty coping at home (eg poor personal hygiene, unclean or unsuitable clothing). Evidence of recent weight loss may suggest difficulties with food preparation or eating, unavailability of food, or may be due to serious pathology, such as a malignancy or tuberculosis. Signs of old bruising or other minor injuries may be consistent with frequent falls. Shortness of breath and any condition producing impaired mobility are important factors.

Falls are a common problem of old age and require careful analysis, perhaps at a special 'Falls' clinic. Correctable factors include damaged walking aids, loose rugs, poor lighting, or unsuitable footwear or glasses. Common medical causes include cerebrovascular disease, arthritis, and side-effects of drugs.

Many elderly people claim that they can cope at home when they are unable to do so. If in doubt, ask relatives, the GP, and community support agencies. They may give helpful insight into the patient's mental state, which can be investigated/assessed further, whether it be a cognitive or reactive condition.

The decision to discharge

Hospital admission for an elderly person is a frightening experience and can lead to confusion and disorientation. If circumstances allow, discharge home is often a more appropriate outcome. If there are concerns regarding their functional ability and mobility, ask for an *occupational therapy* and/or *physiotherapy* assessment with, if appropriate, a home assessment. The elderly person is best seen in their home environment with familiar surroundings, especially if there is evidence of cognitive deficit. The provision of equipment and recommendations for adaptations can be made at this point if required. A wide range of community services including district nurse, health visitor, home help, crisis care, social work, hospital discharge, and rapid response therapy teams can be contacted to provide immediate follow-up and support and play a crucial role in preventing later breakdowns in home circumstances and unnecessary admissions for social reasons.

The patient with learning difficulties

Patients with learning difficulties use the healthcare system more than the general population. Unfortunately, many healthcare professionals have little experience with these patients. However, understanding common illness patterns and using different techniques in communication can result in a successful consultation. Patients with learning difficulties often have complex health needs. There are many barriers to assessing health care, which may lead to later presentations of illness. Patients may have a high tolerance of pain—take this into consideration when examining them.

Associated health problems

Patients with learning difficulties have a higher incidence of certain problems:

- Visual and hearing impairment.
- Poor dental health.
- Swallowing problems.
- Gastro-oesophageal reflux disease.
- Constipation.
- Urinary tract and other infections.
- Epilepsy.
- Mental health problems (↑ incidence of depression, anxiety disorders, schizophrenia, delirium, and dementia), with specific syndromes having their own particular associations (eg Down's is associated with depression and dementia; Prader–Willi with affective psychosis).
- Behavioural problems (eg Prader–Willi, Angelman syndrome).

Leading causes of death

These include pneumonia (relating to reflux, aspiration, swallowing, and feeding problems) and congenital heart disease.

The patient's perspective

Past experiences of hospital are likely to have a big impact on the patient's reaction to his/her current situation. Most patients have problems with expression, comprehension, and social communication. They find it difficult to describe symptoms—behavioural change may the best indication that something is wrong.

Tips for communication

- Explain the consultation process before starting.
- Speak first to the patient, then to the carer.
- Use open questions, then re-phrase to check again.
- Aim to use language that the patient understands, modifying this according to comprehension.
- Patients may have difficulties with time, so try to relate symptoms to real life temporal events (eg 'did the pain start before lunch?')
- They may not make a connection between something that they have done and feeling ill (eg several questions may be required in order to establish that they have ingested something).
- Take particular note of what the carer has to say—information from someone who knows the patient well is invaluable.

Patient transfer

The need to transfer

When patients have problems that exceed the capabilities of a hospital and/or its personnel, transfer to another hospital may be needed.

Timing the transfer

Do not commence any transfer until life-threatening problems have been identified and managed, and a secondary survey has been completed. Once the decision to transfer has been made, do not waste time performing non-essential diagnostic procedures that do not change the immediate plan of care. First, secure the airway (with tracheal intubation if necessary). Ensure that patients with pneumothoraces and chest injuries likely to be associated with pneumothoraces have intercostal drains inserted prior to transfer. This is particularly important before sending a patient by helicopter or fixed wing transfer. Consider the need to insert a urinary catheter and a gastric tube.

Arranging the transfer

Speak directly to the doctor at the receiving hospital. Provide the following details by telephone or telemedicine link:
- Details of the patient (full name, age, and date of birth).
- A brief history of the onset of symptoms/injury.
- The pre-hospital findings and treatment.
- The initial findings, diagnosis, and treatment in the ED and the response to treatment.

Write down the name of the doctor responsible for the initial reception of the patient after transfer. Establish precisely where within the receiving hospital the patient is to be taken. Where possible, prepare the receiving unit by sending details ahead by fax/email. Pre-printed forms can help in structuring the relevant details and avoiding omissions.

Preparing for transfer

Transfer team

If the patient to be transferred may require advanced airway care, ensure they are accompanied by a doctor who can provide this. The accompanying nurse should be trained in resuscitation with a good knowledge of the equipment used during transfer.

Equipment

'Transfer cases' containing a standardized list of equipment must be immediately available and regularly checked. Take all the emergency equipment and drugs that might prove necessary to maintain the 'Airway', 'Breathing' and 'Circulation' (ABC) during transfer. In particular, take at least twice the amount of O_2 estimated to be necessary (a standard 'F' cylinder contains 1360 L of O_2 and will therefore last <3hr running at 10L/min). Before leaving, ensure that the patient and stretcher are well-secured within the ambulance. Send all cross-matched blood (in a suitably insulated container) with the patient.

Monitoring during transfer

Minimum monitoring during transfer includes ECG monitoring, pulse oximetry, and non-invasive BP measurement. If the patient is intubated and ventilated, end-tidal carbon dioxide (CO_2) monitoring is mandatory. An intra-arterial line is recommended, to monitor BP during the journey. Make allowances for limited battery life on long transfers: spare batteries may be needed. Plug monitors and other equipment into the mains supply whenever possible.

Accompanying documentation

Include the following:
- *Patient details*: name, date of birth, address, next of kin, telephone numbers, hospital number, GP.
- History, examination findings, and results of investigations (including X-ray films).
- Type and volume of all fluids infused (including pre-hospital).
- Management including drugs given (type, route, and time of administration), practical procedures performed.
- Response to treatment, including serial measurements of vital signs.
- Name of referring and receiving doctors, their hospitals, and telephone numbers.

Some departments use standard forms to ensure that important information is complete.

The relatives

Keep the patient's relatives informed throughout. Explain where and why the patient is going. Document what they have been told. Arrange transport for relatives to the receiving hospital.

Before leaving

Prior to transfer, re-examine the patient. Check that the airway is protected, ventilation is satisfactory, chest drains are working, IV cannulae patent and well secured, and that the spine is appropriately immobilized, but pressure areas protected. Ensure that the patient is well-covered to prevent heat loss. Inform the receiving hospital when the patient has left and give an estimated time of arrival.

After leaving

Communicate to the receiving hospital the results of any investigations that become available after the patient has left. Contact the receiving doctor afterwards to confirm that the transfer was completed satisfactorily and to obtain feedback.

Intra-hospital transfers

In many respects, the only difference between intra- and inter-hospital transfers is the distance. The principles involved in organizing a transfer are the same, whether the patient is to be conveyed to the computed tomography (CT) scanner down the corridor, or to the regional neurosurgical unit miles away.

Breaking bad news

A proportion of patients presenting to the ED have life-threatening conditions and some will die in the department. Often, the event will be sudden and unexpected by family and friends. It may already involve other family members (eg in the context of a road traffic collision). In contrast to hospital inpatients or those in general practice, an opportunity to forewarn relatives as to what has happened or the eventual outcome is unlikely. The relatives may already be distressed after witnessing the incident or collapse, and may have been directly involved in providing first aid.

It is inappropriate for junior hospital staff without suitable experience to speak with distressed or bereaved relatives. The task must be undertaken by someone with sufficient seniority and authority, who also has the skills of communication and empathy. The most important component is time.

Reception

Relatives usually arrive separately and after the patient. Anticipate this by designating a member of staff to meet them and show them to a relatives' room, which should afford privacy, comfortable seating, an outside telephone line, tea, coffee, and toilet facilities. Paper tissues, some magazines, and toys for small children are useful.

While the relatives are waiting, a designated nurse should stay with them to act as a link with the department and the team caring for the patient. This nurse can pre-warn relatives of the life-threatening nature of the patient's condition and assist in building (an albeit short) relationship between staff and relatives. The link nurse should also check that important details have been recorded correctly, eg the patient's name, address, date of birth, religion (in case last rites are required), next of kin (name, relationship to patient, address and phone no.), and the patient's GP. This information should be collected as soon as possible, since later the relatives may be too upset to remember all these details or it may be difficult to ask for them.

Breaking the news

Irrespective of who performs this task, remember a number of points. If you are the person who informs the relatives, ensure the link nurse is with you. After leaving the resuscitation room or clinical area, allow a minute or two of preparation to make yourself presentable, checking clothing for bloodstains, etc. Confirm that you know the patient's name. Enter the room, introduce yourself, and sit or kneel by the relatives so that you are at their physical level. Ensure that you speak with the correct relatives and identify who is who. Speak slowly, keep your sentences short and non-technical. Do not hedge around the subject. In their emotional turmoil, relatives very often misconstrue information. Therefore, you may need to re-emphasize the important aspects.

For many critically ill patients, their ultimate prognosis cannot be determined in the ED. In these situations, do not raise unrealistic expectations or false hopes, but be honest and direct with the relatives and the patients.

If the patient has died, then use the words 'death' or 'dead'. Do not use euphemisms such as 'passed away', or 'gone to a better place'.

After giving the news, allow relatives a few minutes to collect their thoughts and ask questions. In some cases, these may be unanswerable. It is better to say 'we don't yet know', rather than confuse or give platitudinous answers.

Common responses to bad news or bereavement include emotional distress, denial, guilt, and aggression. The feelings of guilt and anger can be particularly difficult to come to terms with, and relatives may torture themselves with the idea that if only their actions had been different, the situation would never have arisen, or the clinical outcome would have been different.

Relatives seeing patients

Many relatives wish to see or touch their loved ones, however briefly. Television and cinema have prepared much of the population for the sights and sounds in the ED. In some departments, relatives are encouraged to be present in the resuscitation room. In selected situations the stratagem has benefits. If the relatives are present during resuscitation, it is essential that the link nurse is present with the relatives to provide support, explain what is happening, and accompany them if they wish to leave.

More frequently, the relatives can see the patient in the resuscitation room briefly or while they are leaving the ED (eg to go to CT scan room or theatre). Even a few seconds, a few words, and a cuddle can be immensely rewarding for both relative and patient. The link nurse can give guidance beforehand as to the presence of injuries (especially those involving the face), monitors, drips, and equipment, to diminish any threatening impact that these may have.

When death occurs

Even before death has occurred, involvement of religious leaders is valuable. As early as possible, inform the hospital chaplain, who can provide invaluable help to relatives and staff.

When a patient has died, offer the relatives the opportunity to see the body. This contact, which should be in a private quiet room, can greatly assist in the grieving process. With careful preparation, most patients who have died from multiple injuries can be seen by relatives in this fashion.

Remember that followers of some faiths, such as Muslims and Hindus, have important procedures and rituals to be followed after death, although these may not always be feasible after a sudden death, especially from trauma. In such situations, discuss the matter with the Coroner's or Procurator Fiscal's officer, and obtain help from an appropriate religious leader to look after the bereaved relatives.

What to do after a death

Who to contact

Any suspicious death must be immediately reported to the Police who will liaise directly with the Coroner or Procurator Fiscal (in Scotland).

Following all deaths in the ED, a number of important contacts must be made as soon as possible:
- *Informing the next of kin*: if the relatives are not already present in ED, it may be necessary to ask the Police for assistance.
- Notifying the Coroner (Procurator Fiscal in Scotland).
- Informing the patient's GP.
- Cancelling hospital outpatient appointments.
- Informing social work and health visitor teams as appropriate.

Ensure deceased's relatives are given information about the process for death certification and registration, and how to organize funeral arrangements. Most EDs have useful leaflets that cover these matters and can answer many questions. Some departments have formal arrangements for counselling after bereavement. Often the GP is the best individual to co-ordinate bereavement care, but in any event, give the relatives a telephone number for the ED so they can speak to a senior nurse or doctor if they need further information or help.

Information for the Coroner or Procurator Fiscal

Report sudden deaths as soon as possible to the Coroner (in Scotland the Procurator Fiscal). It is helpful to give the following information if it is available:
- Patient's name, address, date of birth.
- Next of kin (name, relationship, address, phone no.).
- Patient's GP.
- Date and time of patient's arrival in the ED.
- Date and time of patient's death.
- Name and job title of doctor who pronounced death.
- Details of the incident, injuries, or illness.
- Relevant past medical history.
- When the patient last saw a doctor (the Coroner may be happy for a GP or hospital doctor to write a death certificate if they saw the patient recently for the condition that caused death, eg a patient with known terminal cancer).
- *The patient's religion*: some faiths may wish to arrange burial before the next sunset, but this may not be feasible after a sudden death.
- Anything else that is important, eg difficulties in communication with the next of kin due to language or deafness.

Looking after the staff

The death of a patient or the management of patients with critical illness inevitably affects the ED staff. This is particularly so when some aspect of the event reminds staff of their own situation or relatives. These episodes often occur at the busiest times and when everyone in the ED is working under pressure.

One of the most difficult situations is to have to inform parents of the death of their child and help them in the initial grieving process, and then return to the busy department where many people are waiting with increasingly strident demands. It would be easy to respond that such individuals, with injuries or illnesses that are minor or present for days or weeks, are time-wasting. However, this approach will lead to conflict and is unfair to all concerned. Instead, take 5–10min for a break in the staff room before returning to the fray. Remember that in these circumstances you too are a patient. Even senior and experienced staff may be distressed after difficult resuscitation situations and may require support.

Organ donation

There is considerable potential to assist with the process of organ/tissue donation in the ED. However, the possibility of organ donation is sadly often overlooked in the ED. Many patients who die after unexpected cardiac arrest are potential donors of corneal tissue and heart valves. Kidneys may also be retrieved from some patients who have died in the ED, if a protocol for this has been arranged with the transplant team and the local Coroner or Procurator Fiscal. Many other patients who are moribund, intubated and ventilated (eg following massive subarachnoid haemorrhage) may be identified as potential donors of other tissues also. Consider the possibility of organ donation in patients who die in the ED or who are moribund with no hope of survival. Most hospitals have specialist organ donation nurses (previously known as 'donor transplant coordinators') who will educate, advise and assist with the process of organ donation. Useful information about organ/tissue transplantation is available on the website of the British Transplantation Society (www.bts. org.uk).

Medicolegal aspects: avoiding trouble

Medicolegal problems are relatively common in the ED. Many of these problems may be avoided by adopting the correct approach.

Attitude

Be polite and open with patients. Try to establish a good rapport. Be as honest as possible in explaining delays/errors.

Consent (see General Medical Council guidance)

Use the consent form liberally for anything that is complex, risky, or involves sedation or general anaesthetic (GA). Ensure that the patient understands what is involved in the procedure, together with its potential benefits and risks. Whenever possible, attempt to obtain consent from parent/guardian in minors, but do not delay life-saving treatment in order to obtain consent.

Documentation (📖 Note keeping, p.4)

Good notes imply good practice. Keep careful notes, using simple, clear, unambiguous language. Write your name legibly and document the time that you saw the patient. Remember that successful defence of a medical negligence claim may depend upon accurate, legible, comprehensive, contemporaneous notes. Try to avoid abbreviations, particularly where there is room for confusion. In particular, name the digits of the hand (thumb, index, middle, ring, and little fingers) and specify right or left by writing it in full.

Be meticulous in documenting the nature, size, and position of any wounds (📖 p.402). Write down a diagnosis, together with a full interpretation of any investigations. Ensure that all attached documents (nursing observations, blood results, ECG) are labelled. Document all instructions and advice given to the patient, together with any follow-up arrangements made.

Referral (📖 Discharge, referral, and handover, p.8)

Always seek senior help or refer those patients with problems beyond your knowledge or expertise. Record any referral made, together with the name and grade of the doctor referred to, the time it was made, and a summary of the facts communicated. After referral, be cautious about accepting telephone advice alone—an expert cannot usually provide an accurate opinion without seeing the patient.

Return visits

Take special care with any patient who returns to ED with the same presenting complaint, because it is no better, has deteriorated, or the patient is simply dissatisfied. Do not automatically rely upon previous diagnosis and X-ray interpretations as being correct—treat the patient as if they were attending for the first time. Try to involve the consultant in these cases.

Discharge against advice

Always attempt to persuade the patient to accept the treatment offered, but if this is refused, or the patient leaves before being seen, ask the patient to sign an appropriate form. Patients not deemed competent (see Mental Capacity Act below) to make this decision may need to be held against their wishes—seek senior help with this. Write full notes explaining what happened.

Mental Capacity Act (📖 p.629)

The Mental Capacity Act 2005 outlines how a person is unable to make a decision for himself if he/she is unable to:

- Understand the information relevant to the decision.
- Retain the information.
- Use or weight that information as part of the process of making the decision.
- Communicate his/her decision.

A patient lacks capacity if at the time he/she is unable to make a decision for himself/herself in relation to the matter because of an impairment or a disturbance in the functioning of the mind or brain.

Access to records

All ED staff should bear in mind that patients may gain access to their medical records and read what has been written about them. Patients in the UK have a statutory right of access to information about themselves (set out in the Data Protection Act 1998) and this includes medical records. Competent patients may apply for access to, and copies of, their own records. Applications are usually made in writing via the hospital's legal department.

Medical defence organization

Join a medical defence organization. The Medical Defence Union (MDU), MDDUS, and Medical Protection Society provide professional indemnity cover for emergencies outside hospital, and advice and support for all sorts of medicolegal matters that are not necessarily covered by NHS trusts, eg statements to the Coroner or Procurator Fiscal, support at inquests or fatal accident inquiries, allegations of negligence, legal actions, and problems with the GMC. They also provide members with useful information and booklets about consent, confidentiality and other issues.

Further information
www.the-mdu.com/hospital

www.mddus.com

www.medicalprotection.org

Medicolegal aspects: the law

Confidentiality

Medical information about every patient is confidential and should not be disclosed without the patient's consent. In the UK the police do not have routine access to clinical information, but some information may be divulged in certain specific circumstances:

- The Road Traffic Act (1972) places a duty on any person to provide the police, if requested, with information that might lead to the identification of a vehicle driver who is suspected of an offence under the Act. The doctor is obliged to supply the person's name and address, but not clinical information.
- Suspicion of terrorist activity.
- Gunshot wounds (see www.gmc-uk.org).
- Disclosure in the public interest. The General Medical Council advises that this might include situations where someone may be exposed to death or serious injury (eg murder, rape, armed robbery, child abuse). Although this may provide ethical permission for the doctor to reveal details without consent, it does not place him/her under any legal duty to do so. Discuss these cases with your consultant and/or your medical defence organization. (General Medical Council (GMC) advice: www.gmc-uk.org).

Ability to drive

A patient's ability to drive may be impaired by injury (especially limb or eye), by drugs (eg after GA, opiates, alcohol) or medical conditions (eg TIAs, epilepsy, arrhythmias). In each case, warn the patient not to drive and ensure that this warning is documented in the notes. It may be prudent to provide this warning in the presence of a close relative.

For further information on medical aspects of fitness to drive see: www.dft.gov.uk/dvla/medical/ataglance.aspx

Police requests for blood alcohol

In the UK, the police may request a blood or urine sample under Section 5 of the Road Traffic Act (1988) from a patient they suspect to have been in charge of a motor vehicle with an illegal blood alcohol level (>80mg/100mL). In such circumstances, specimens should only be taken if they do not prejudice the proper care and treatment of the patient. The relevant specimens should only be taken by a police surgeon (clinical forensic physician) and with the patient's consent.

A change in the law (Police Reform Act 2002) also allows a police surgeon to take a blood sample from an unconscious patient who is suspected of having been the driver of a motor vehicle while under the influence of alcohol and/or drugs. The blood sample is retained and tested later, depending upon the patient later giving consent. Again, only permit the police surgeon access to the patient if this will not delay or prejudice proper care and treatment of the patient.

Reporting deaths to the Coroner (or Procurator Fiscal)

Many deaths that occur in (or in transit to) the ED are sudden and unexpected, and/or follow trauma. The exact cause of death is seldom immediately apparent. Accordingly, do not be tempted to sign death certificates. Instead, report all deaths to the Coroner (the Procurator Fiscal in Scotland). See 📖 p.26 for details of the information required.

Police statements

Do not provide information to the police until patient consent has been obtained. Writing a police statement requires thought and care. Write the statement yourself. Keep statements brief and try to avoid hearsay, conjecture, or opinion on the likely outcome. List injuries using both medical and non-medical language, explaining terminology in detail as necessary. State the investigations and treatment provided as accurately as possible (eg what sutures and how many were used). Having written the statement, ask your consultant to read it and comment on it. Get the statement typed (a friendly ED secretary may help if you cannot type yourself, and will also know how you can claim the relevant fee). Having checked it, sign and date the statement, and give it to the officer concerned. Always keep a copy of the statement and the ED notes, so that they are easily available if you are called to court.

Court appearances

In advance Discuss the case with your consultant, and review the notes, the questions that you might be asked, and the likely court procedures. Get a good copy of the notes and any investigations. Ask whether you should take the original records to court.

On the day Dress smartly, arrive early, and behave professionally. Be prepared for a long wait, so take a book to read. Turn off your mobile phone. Once in court, you have the option of taking an oath before God or affirming without religious connotation. You are equally bound to tell the truth whichever you choose. Use the same form of address that others have already used (eg 'My Lord', 'Your Honour'). Answer directly and simply. Use comprehensible language, free of medical jargon. Remember that you are a professional witness, not an expert. Therefore, confine the expression of opinion to within the limits of your knowledge and experience—if asked something outside this, say so!

Inquest/fatal accident inquiry If you are called to give evidence at an inquest (in Scotland, a fatal accident inquiry), discuss the case with your consultant and also with your medical defence society.

Further information and advice about reports and appearing in court The medical defence organizations (📖 p.29) have useful advice sheets for their members about writing reports and appearing in court.

Infection control and prevention

Staff in the ED have an important role in preventing and controlling infection, which can be a serious risk to patients, relatives, and staff.

Organisms such as *Staph. aureus*, including MRSA (📖 p.235), can readily be transmitted by contaminated hands or equipment, causing infection of wounds, fractures, and in-dwelling devices (eg catheters or chest drains). Infected blood can transmit many infections, including hepatitis B and C (📖 p.239) and human immunodeficiency virus (HIV; 📖 p.242). Viral gastroenteritis is usually spread by the faecal-oral route, but vomiting may cause widespread viral contamination of the surroundings and equipment, with a risk of transmission to other patients and staff.

Coughing and sneezing produces small droplets of infected secretions, which could involve viruses such as influenza (📖 Influenza pandemics, avian flu, and swine flu, p.252), severe acute respiratory syndrome (SARS; 📖 p.251), and respiratory syncytial virus (RSV; 📖 p.682). A nebulizer used on an infected patient may spread respiratory viruses widely, as occurred in the outbreak of SARS in Hong Kong in 2003 which involved many ED staff.

Standard precautions for preventing infection

Standard precautions (also known as 'universal precautions') should be used at all times and with all patients to reduce the risks of infection. Blood and body fluids from all patients should be treated as infected. These standard precautions include:

- *Hand hygiene* Essential, but often neglected. Decontaminate your hands before and after every patient contact, and after any activity that might contaminate hands, including removing gloves. Hands that are visibly dirty or possibly grossly contaminated must be washed with soap and water, and dried thoroughly. Alcohol hand gel can be used if the hands look clean. Cover broken skin with a waterproof dressing.
- *Personal protective equipment (PPE)* Wear suitable disposable *gloves* for any contact with blood, body fluids, mucous membranes, or non-intact skin. Latex gloves are widely used, but cause allergic reactions in some patients and staff, who need special nitrile gloves. Use a *disposable plastic apron* if there is a risk of blood or body fluids contaminating clothing. After use, dispose of it and wash your hands. *Impervious gowns* are needed if there is a high risk of contamination. Use a *mask, face shield,* and *eye protection* if blood or body fluids might splash in your eyes or mouth. Protection against respiratory viruses, eg SARS or influenza requires special *masks* or *respirators* (eg FFP3), which must be fitted and used properly. *Powered air-purifying respirators* should be used for high-risk procedures such as intubating patients with serious viral infections.
- *Safe handling and disposal of sharps* Avoid handling needles directly or using hand-held needles. Never re-sheathe needles. Place used needles and blades immediately into a 'sharps bin'. If possible, use safety needles and cannulae, which reduce the risk of needlestick injury. If, despite all precautions, a *needlestick injury* does occur follow local approved

procedures to minimize the risk of infection and look after the people involved (see 📖 Needlestick injury, p.418).

• *Managing blood and bodily fluids* Samples of blood or other body fluids must be handled safely, with care not to contaminate request forms or the outside of the container. Follow local approved procedures for dealing with spillages of blood or body fluids: wear suitable PPE (usually a disposable apron and gloves) and disinfect the spillage with an appropriate agent such as diluted bleach.

Planning for outbreaks of infectious diseases

Planning to cope with an outbreak of a serious infectious disease such as SARS or pandemic flu (📖 p.252) is a considerable challenge for ED staff and for the whole community. The ED must be organized so that patients can be assessed properly with a minimum risk of infecting staff or other patients. If possible, patients with serious airborne diseases should be treated in negative pressure isolation rooms by staff in appropriate PPE who are fully trained to minimize the risks of spreading and acquiring the infection. In high risk situations a 'buddy' system for staff may be helpful, with each doctor or nurse being watched closely by another person to check that full safety precautions are maintained.

Assessment of febrile patients

Hospitals in Hong Kong with experience of SARS use the *FTOCC* criteria when assessing febrile patients for potentially serious infectious diseases:
• F—fever (>38°C).
• T—travel history.
• O—occupational history.
• C—clustering of cases.
• C—contact history (eg someone with SARS or avian flu).

Similar criteria are used in the UK Health Protection Agency's algorithm: www.hpa.org.uk/Topics/InfectiousDiseases/InfectionsAZ/AvianInfluenza/

Further information

Standard precautions
www.rcn.org.uk/downloads/publications/public_pub/002725.pdf

Masks and respirators
www.hpa.org.uk/Topics/InfectiousDiseases/InfectionsAZ/SevereAcute RespiratorySyndrome/Guidelines/sars040Facemasksand respiratorsFAQ/

Pandemic influenza/avian flu
📖 Influenza pandemic, avian flu, and swine flu, p.252.

SARS
📖 SARS, p.251.

What to carry in your car

If you are interested in out of hospital work, join the British Association for Immediate Care (BASICS: www.basics.org.uk), which is a valuable source of information and expertise. It can give advice on clothing, medical and protective equipment and their suppliers, and Immediate Care courses.

The equipment that could be carried is extensive. In the UK, except in the most remote situations, it is likely that an ambulance will be on scene quickly. Emergency ambulances carry many items of equipment, eg for intubation, volume infusion and splintage, and also some drugs. There is a risk of carrying too much equipment in your car and getting diverted from the primary aims of pre-hospital care, which are to perform only relevant life-saving techniques, and to transfer the patient rapidly and safely to the nearest appropriate hospital.

The equipment listed below is a personal choice based on experience attending out-of-hospital calls over the past 20 years:

Personal equipment
- High quality wind/waterproof reflective jacket and over-trousers. If your finances do not run to this, at least have a reflective 'Doctor' tabard.
- Protective helmet.
- Protective footwear—leather boots with steel toecaps are ideal.
- 2 pairs of latex gloves.
- 1 pair of protective gloves (eg leather gardening gloves).

General equipment
- Reflective warning triangle.
- Fire extinguisher.
- Heavy-duty waterproof torch.
- Clothes-cutting scissors.
- Mobile phone.

Medical equipment

The equipment listed is only of value if you know how to use it, it is secure (ie locked in a case in a locked vehicle), and it is in date:

- Stethoscope.
- Hand-held suction device + Yankauer and soft flexible suckers.
- Laryngoscope, adult curved blade, spare batteries, and bulb.
- Selection of tracheal tubes of varying sizes + syringe to inflate cuff.
- Magill's forceps.
- Selection of oropharyngeal and nasopharyngeal airways.
- Laerdal pocket mask.
- Venous tourniquet.
- Selection of IV cannulae (2 each of 14G and 16G) and syringes.
- 2 × IV-giving sets.
- 2 × 1000mL 0.9% saline bags.
- 1 roll of 1-inch zinc oxide tape.
- 1 roll of 3-inch Elastoplast.
- Small selection of dressings and bandages.
- Cervical collar.
- Cricothyrotomy kit.
- Intercostal chest drain set.
- 2 × 0/0 silk suture on a hand-held cutting needle.
- Local anaesthetic, eg lidocaine 1% (for nerve blocks).
- Splints for IV cannulation sites.

At the roadside

Priorities

It is easy in an emergency to forget the simplest, most life-saving procedures. At worst, an individual trying to help can aggravate the situation, slow the process of care, and even become a casualty themselves.

If you arrive first at the scene of a collision, the initial priority is to ensure your own safety and that of other rescuers.

- Park safely so your car will not obstruct other vehicles (including emergency vehicles), preferably where its presence will alert other road users to the collision. Put your hazard warning lights on. If you have a warning beacon, put it on the roof of the car and switch it on.
- If you have a mobile phone, dial '999' and request ambulance, fire, and police to attend. Remember to give the exact location, a brief description of the incident, and number of casualties. Tell the emergency service operator who you are, as well as the number of your mobile phone.
- Switch off the engine of your car and of any other vehicles.
- Ensure that no-one is smoking or displays a naked flame.
- Events involving electricity or chemicals have specific hazards. Involvement of overhead or underground electric cables poses risks, compounded if water is involved or sparks produced. The risk from high tension cables extends for several metres. Phone the power company to ensure that the source is turned off before approaching. Electrified rail lines may be short-circuited by a trained individual using a special bar carried in the guard's compartment.

Chemical incidents

Do not approach a chemical incident until declared safe by the Fire Service. Lorries carrying hazardous chemicals must display a 'Hazchem' board (see Fig. 1.2). This has:

- Information on whether the area should be evacuated, what protective equipment should be worn, aspects relating to fire-fighting, and if the chemical can be safely washed down storm drains (top left). A white plate means that the load is non-toxic.
- A 4-digit UN product identification number (middle left).
- A pictorial hazard diamond warning (top right).
- An emergency contact number (bottom).

The European 'Kemler' plate contains only the UN product number (bottom) and a numerical hazard code (top)—a repeated number means intensified hazard. Mixed loads <500kg may only be identified by a plain orange square at the front and rear of the vehicle.

The transport emergency card (TREM card) carried in the driver's cab gives information about the chemical for use at the scene of a crash. The fire tender may be equipped with CHEMDATA—a direct link with the National Chemical Information Centre at Harwell. Alternatively, contact a Poisons Information Centre or the transport company.

Helicopters

If helicopters are used for transport/evacuation, remember:

- Communications in or near helicopters are difficult because of the noise.
- Ensure any loose objects are secured to prevent them being blown away.

- Never enter the landing space area during landing or take-off.
- Never enter or leave the rotor disc area without the pilot's permission.
- Duck down in the rotor disc area and only approach in full view of the pilot.
- If the helicopter cannot land and the winch is used, do not touch the cable before it has touched the ground to earth any static electrical charge.

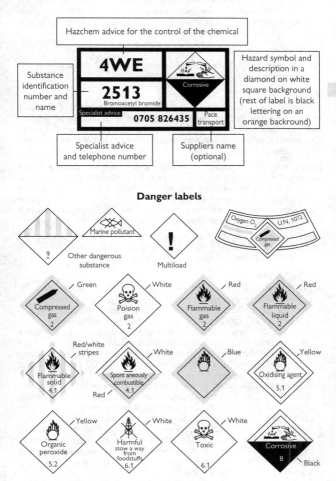

Danger labels

Fig. 1.2 Hazchem advice and danger labels.

Major incidents

A major incident involves a lot of people. The casualties may have multiple injuries, minor injuries/burns, or other emergencies such as food poisoning or chemical inhalation. Every hospital accepting emergencies has a Major Incident plan to use when the normal resources are unable to cope and special arrangements are needed. There will be action cards for key staff detailing their duties. All staff need to familiarize themselves with their roles in advance.

Call-in lists must be up to date and available at all times.

Major incident practices must be held regularly to check arrangements and contact details and to remind staff what they should do.

Alert

The ambulance service or the police should warn the hospital of a possible or definite major incident. Initial messages are often inaccurate because they are based on confused and incomplete information from the scene. Occasionally, patients arrive without warning from a major incident near the hospital.

Ensure that the *ED consultant* on duty is informed immediately of any suspected major incident, enabling them to participate in the decision to start the major incident procedure. Senior medical, nursing, and administrative staff will set up the hospital's *Control Centre* and prepare for action. If the major incident is confirmed, the full hospital response is initiated, following the procedures in the plan.

Communications are vital, but switchboards rapidly become overloaded. Staff should therefore be called in using non-switchboard phones if possible. All staff should wear their identification badges.

Action in the ED

- Check that the ED consultant and hospital switchboard know about the incident and that the major incident procedure has been started.
- Inform all ED staff on duty (doctors, nurses, receptionists, porters).
- Call in other ED staff in accordance with the Major Incident plan.
- Clear the ED of any patients who are not seriously ill or injured. Prepare the department to receive patients from the incident.
- Doctors and nurses arriving to help should be given appropriate action cards. Staff should have labels or tabards so that ED staff and other specialties (eg anaesthetists) can be identified easily.
- Prepare a triage point at the ambulance entrance. This should be staffed by a senior doctor and nurse who direct patients to the most appropriate area of the department. If possible, a nurse should stay with each patient until he/she is discharged or admitted to a ward.
- All patients should be labelled immediately with a unique Major Incident number, which is used on all notes, forms, blood samples, property bags, and lists of patients. Collect names, addresses, and other details as soon as possible, but this must not delay triage or emergency treatment. Keep lists of anyone leaving the ED.
- Ensure that the hospital *Control Centre* is regularly updated regarding the situation in the ED.

Wards and theatres

Beds must be cleared to receive patients, preferably on 1 or 2 wards, rather than many different wards. A senior surgeon should triage patients needing operations and co-ordinate theatre work.

Relatives and friends

Relatives and friends of casualties should be looked after by social workers and chaplaincy staff in an area near to, but separate from, the ED, perhaps in the outpatient department. Keep relatives informed as soon and as much as possible. *Security staff* at each entrance to the ED should direct relatives and friends of casualties to the appropriate area and not allow them into the ED.

Press

Journalists and television crews will arrive rapidly after a major incident. Keep them out of the ED—direct them to a pre-arranged room to be briefed by a press officer and senior staff.

Arrangements at the site of a major incident

The police are in overall command. The fire service take control of the immediate area if there is a fire or chemical risk. The police, fire, and ambulance services will each have a control vehicle, with an *Incident Officer* to co-ordinate their staff and the rescue work.

There may be a *Medical Incident Officer* (MIO) and also a *Mobile Medical Team* of doctors and nurses, who should if possible be sent from a supporting hospital, rather than the hospital receiving the first casualties. These staff must be properly clothed (yellow and green high-visibility jacket marked 'Doctor' or 'Nurse', over trousers, green helmet with visor and chin strap, safety boots, gloves, knee pads, torch, ID badge), and must be trained and equipped with suitable medical supplies and action cards.

The mobile medical team must report to the MIO, who is in charge of all medical and nursing staff on site and works closely with the *Ambulance Incident Officer* (AIO). The MIO should record the names of the mobile medical team and brief them about their duties and the site hazards and safety arrangements. The MIO is responsible for supervising the team, arranging any necessary equipment and supplies, and making sure that the team are relieved when necessary. The MIO and AIO relay information to the hospitals and distribute casualties appropriately.

Debriefing staff

Debriefing is important after a major incident, so that staff can discuss what happened and express their feelings. Mutual support of the team is essential. Counselling may be required. Senior staff should prepare a report on the incident and review the major incident plan.

Further information
NHS Emergency Planning guidance
www.dh.gov.uk/en/Managingyourorganisation/Emergencyplanning/index.htm

CBRN (Chemical, Biological, Radiological and Nuclear) incidents
📖 Decontamination of patients, p.211.

Life-threatening emergencies

Life-threatening emergencies in children are considered in
Chapter 15, Paediatric emergencies *631*

Anaphylaxis

(*Anaphylaxis in children* is covered in 📖 p.650)

Anaphylaxis is a generalized immunological condition of sudden onset, which develops after exposure to a foreign substance. The mechanism may:

- Involve an IgE-mediated reaction to a foreign protein (stings, foods, streptokinase), or to a protein–hapten conjugate (antibiotics) to which the patient has previously been exposed.
- Be complement mediated (human proteins eg γ-globulin, blood products).
- Be unknown (aspirin, 'idiopathic').

Irrespective of the mechanism, mast cells and basophils release mediators (eg histamine, prostaglandins, thromboxanes, platelet activating factors, leukotrienes) producing clinical manifestations. Angio-oedema caused by ACE inhibitors and hereditary angio-oedema may present in a similar way to anaphylaxis. Hereditary angio-oedema is not usually accompanied by urticaria and is treated with C1 esterase inhibitor.

Common causes

- Drugs and vaccines (eg antibiotics, streptokinase, suxamethonium, aspirin, non-steroidal anti-inflammatory drugs (NSAIDs), intravenous (IV) contrast agents).
- *Hymenoptera* (bee/wasp) stings.
- Foods (nuts, shellfish, strawberries, wheat).
- Latex.

Clinical features

The speed of onset and severity vary with the nature and amount of the stimulus, but the onset is usually in minutes/hours. A prodromal aura or a feeling of impending death may be present. Patients on β-blockers or with a history of ischaemic heart disease (IHD) or asthma may have especially severe features. Usually two or more systems are involved:

Respiratory Swelling of lips, tongue, pharynx, and epiglottis may lead to complete upper airway occlusion. Lower airway involvement is similar to acute severe asthma—dyspnoea, wheeze, chest tightness, hypoxia, and hypercapnia.

Skin Pruritus, erythema, urticarial, and angio-oedema.

Cardiovascular Peripheral vasodilation and ↑ vascular permeability cause plasma leakage from the circulation, with ↓ intravascular volume, hypotension, and shock. Arrhythmias, ischaemic chest pain, and electrocardiogram (ECG) changes may be present.

GI tract Nausea, vomiting, diarrhoea, abdominal cramps.

Treatment
- Discontinue further administration of suspected factor (eg drug). Remove stings by scraping them carefully away from skin.
- Give 100% oxygen (O_2).
- Open and maintain airway. If upper airway oedema is present, get specialist senior help immediately. Emergency intubation or a surgical airway and ventilation may be required.
- In patients with shock, airway swelling, or respiratory difficulty give 0.5mg (0.5mL of 1:1000 solution) adrenaline intramuscular (IM). Repeat after 5min if there is no improvement. In adults treated with an adrenaline auto-injector (eg EpiPen®) the 300mcg dose is usually sufficient, but additional doses may be required. Give only 50% of the usual dose of adrenaline to patients taking tricyclic antidepressants, MAOIs, or β–blockers.
- In profound shock or *immediately life-threatening* situations, give CPR/ALS as necessary, and consider *slow* IV adrenaline 1:10,000 or 1:100,000 solution. This is recommended only for experienced clinicians who can also obtain immediate IV access. Note the different strength of adrenaline required for IV use. If there is no response to adrenaline, consider glucagon 1–2mg IM/IV every 5min (especially in patients taking β-blockers).
- Give a $β_2$-agonist (eg salbutamol 5mg) nebulized with O_2 for bronchospasm, possibly with the addition of nebulized ipratropium bromide 500mcg.
- Give IV fluid if hypotension does not rapidly respond to adrenaline. Rapid infusion of 1–2L IV 0.9% saline may be required, with further infusion according to the clinical state.
- Antihistamine H_1 blockers (eg chlorphenamine 10–20mg slow IV) and H_2 blockers (eg ranitidine 50mg IV) are commonly given. They are second line drugs that, with hydrocortisone 100–200mg slow IV, may reduce the severity/duration of symptoms.
- Admit/observe after initial treatment: prolonged reactions and biphasic responses may occur. Observe for at least 4–6hr after all symptoms have settled.

Report anaphylactic reactions related to drugs/vaccines to the Committee on Safety of Medicines. Further investigation of the cause (and possibly desensitization) may be indicated. Where identified, the patient and GP must be informed and the hospital records appropriately labelled. Medic-Alert bracelets are useful.

Notes on treatment algorithm on 📖 p.44
1 An inhaled $β_2$-agonist such as salbutamol may be used as an adjunctive measure if bronchospasm is severe and does not respond rapidly to other treatment.
2 If profound shock judged *immediately* life-threatening give CPR/ALS if necessary. Consider slow IV adrenaline (epinephrine) 1:10,000 solution. This is *hazardous* and is recommended only for an experienced practitioner who can also obtain IV access without delay. Note the different strength of adrenaline (epinephrine) that may be required for IV use.
3 If adults are treated with an EpiPen® the 300mcg will usually be sufficient. A second dose may be required. Half doses of adrenaline (epinephrine) may be safer for patients on amitriptyline, imipramine, or β-blocker.
4 A crystalloid may be safer than a colloid.

Treatment algorithm for adults with anaphylaxis[1]

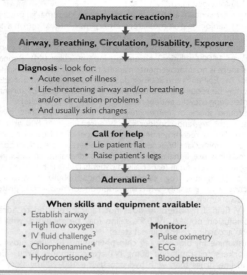

Anaphylactic reaction?

Airway, **B**reathing, **C**irculation, **D**isability, **E**xposure

Diagnosis - look for:
* Acute onset of illness
* Life-threatening airway and/or breathing and/or circulation problems[1]
* And usually skin changes

Call for help
* Lie patient flat
* Raise patient's legs

Adrenaline[2]

When skills and equipment available:
* Establish airway
* High flow oxygen
* IV fluid challenge[3]
* Chlorphenamine[4]
* Hydrocortisone[5]

Monitor:
* Pulse oximetry
* ECG
* Blood pressure

---

1 Life-threatening problems:
Airway:	Swelling, hoarseness, stridor
Breathing:	Rapid breathing, wheeze, fatigue, cyanosis, SpO_2 < 92%, confusion
Circulation:	Pale, clammy, low blood pressure, faintness, drowsy/coma

2 Adrenaline *(give IM unless experienced with IV adrenaline)*
IM doses of 1:1000 adrenaline (repeat after 5 min if no better)
* Adult: 500 micrograms IM (0.5 mL)
* Child more than 12 years: 500 micrograms IM (0.5 mL)
* Child 6–12 years: 300 micrograms IM (0.3 mL)
* Child less than 6 years: 150 micrograms IM (0.15 mL)

Adrenaline IV to be given **only by experienced specialists**
Titrate: Adults 50 micrograms; Children 1 microgram/kg

3 IV fluid challenge:
Adult - 500–1000 mL
Child - crystalloid 20 mL/kg

Stop IV colloid
if this might be the cause of anaphylaxis

	4 Chlorphenamine (IM or slow IV)	5 Hydrocortisone (IM or slow IV)
Adult or child more than 12 years	10 mg	200 mg
Child 6–12 years	5 mg	100 mg
Child 6 months to 6 years	2.5 mg	50 mg
Child less than 6 months	250 micrograms/kg	25 mg

See also: ► Anaphylactic reactions – Initial treatment

Fig. 2.1 Anaphylaxis algorithm.

---

1 Resuscitation Council (UK) guidelines, 2008. See: www.resus.org.uk

Choking

The management of choking is rightly taught as part of first aid. Recognition of the problem is the key to success. Clues include a person experiencing a sudden airway problem whilst eating, possibly combined with them clutching their neck.

Severity of airway obstruction
Victims with severe airway obstruction may be unable to speak or breathe and become unconscious (see Fig. 2.2).

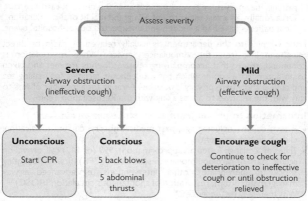

Fig. 2.2 Adult choking algorithm.[1]

1 Resuscitation Council (UK) guidelines, 2010 (www.resus.org.uk)

Cardiac arrest

Clinical features and recognition

Follow resuscitation algorithm (www.resus.org.uk) shown opposite. Cardiac arrest is a *clinical* diagnosis:

- Suspect cardiac arrest in any patient who is unconscious and who does not have signs of life. If you check a pulse, examine only for a major (carotid or femoral) one and take no longer than 10sec. Other 'confirmatory' clinical features (eg colour, pupil size/response) waste time and do not help. Note that some respiratory efforts, such as gasping, may persist for several minutes after the onset of cardiac arrest. Occasionally, an arrest may present as a grand mal fit of short duration.
- Most patients have had a sudden and unexpected out-of-hospital event.

Prior warning to the department is usually relayed by radio or direct telephone link from the Ambulance Service. While resuscitation is continued, ensure that accompanying relatives/friends are met and taken to an appropriate room, which has a telephone, facilities for making tea and coffee, and where privacy is possible. Arrange for a member of staff to stay with the relatives to act as a link with the Resuscitation Team.

Information to obtain from ambulance crew/relatives

- *Patient details:* including age, past medical history, current medication, chest pain before event
- *Times of:* collapse (often an approximation), 999 (or 112) call, arrival on scene, start of cardiopulmonary resuscitation (CPR), first defibrillating shock (if appropriate), other interventions (eg advanced airway management, drugs), restoration of spontaneous circulation (ROSC)
- *Was there any bystander CPR?*

Where a patient in cardiac arrest is brought to hospital by ambulance, the cardiac arrest team (ED staff, the hospital team, or a combination of both) should already be present in the resuscitation room with all equipment ready to receive the patient.

The team leader

The team leader controls, co-ordinates, organizes the team and makes treatment decisions. 4–6 team members are optimal. Each should know their role. Perform resuscitation in a calm, quiet, confident manner with minimal interruption to the performance of basic life support (BLS) or defibrillation.

Start the following procedures *simultaneously:*

- Continue BLS.
- Remove/cut clothing from the upper body to allow defibrillation, ECG monitoring, chest compression, and IV access.
- Obtain the ECG trace (through defibrillator pads or monitor leads). If already attached to an ECG monitor, note (print out if possible) the rhythm. Beware movement artefact, disconnected leads, electrical interference, etc.
- Follow the ALS algorithm (🔲 p.52).
- Do not interrupt CPR except to perform defibrillation.

In-hospital resuscitation algorithm[1]

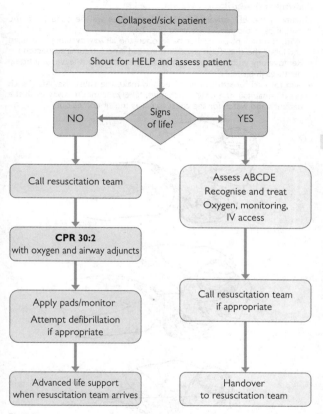

Fig. 2.3

---

1 Resuscitation Council (UK) guidelines, 2010 (www.resus.org.uk).

Adult basic life support

Airway and ventilation

Usually in the ED, advanced airway techniques will be used from the outset. If basic techniques are used (Fig. 2.4):

- With the patient on his/her back, open the airway by tilting the head and lifting the chin. (Use jaw thrust instead if neck trauma suspected.)
- Remove any visible obstructions from the mouth, but leave well-fitting dentures in place.
- Aim for each breath to last ≈1sec and make the chest rise. After each breath, maintain the head tilt/chin lift, take your mouth away from the patient's and watch for the chest to fall as the air comes out.

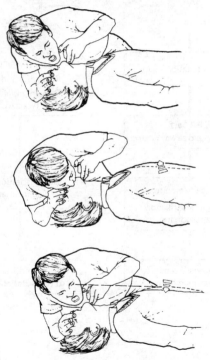

Fig. 2.4 Mouth to mouth ventilation.[1]

1 Colquhoun MC *et al.* (1999). *ABC of Resuscitation*, 4th edition. BMJ Books, London.

Technique for chest compression (Fig. 2.5)

- Place the heel of one hand over the middle of the lower half of the patient's sternum, with the other hand on top. Extend or interlock the fingers of both hands and lift them to avoid applying pressure to the patient's ribs.
- Positioned above the patient's chest and with arms straight, press down to depress the sternum 5–6cm.
- Release all the pressure and repeat at a rate of 100–120/min.
- Compression and release phases should take the same time.
- Use a ratio of 30 chest compressions to 2 ventilations (30:2).
- Aim to change the person providing chest compressions every 2 min, but ensure that this is achieved without causing significant pauses.

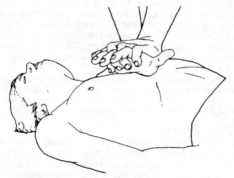

Fig. 2.5 Chest compressions.[1]

---

1 Colquhoun MC et al. (1999). *ABC of Resuscitation*, 4th edition. BMJ Books, London.

Cardiac arrest management

Defibrillation

- Most survivors have an initial rhythm of VF/VT. The treatment for this is defibrillation. With time, the chances of successful defibrillation and survival ↓ dramatically. Adhesive defibrillator pads have replaced manual paddles in most hospitals. Place one pad to the right of the upper sternum below the clavicle, the other in mid-axillary line level with V_6 ECG electrode position. Avoid placement over the female breast. To avoid problems with pacemakers, keep pads >15cm away from them.
- With biphasic defibrillators, use shock energy of 150J, for (mostly older) monophasic defibrillators, select 360J energy.
- Plan for chest compressions to be as continuous as possible, with minimal delays. Having paused briefly to assess the rhythm, recommence compressions until the defibrillator is charged. Pause briefly to deliver a shock (removing O_2 sources and transdermal glycerol trinitrate (GTN) patches), then immediately restart CPR with 30:2 compressions: ventilation, and continue for 2min before reassessing the rhythm or feeling for a pulse.
- In monitored patients with pulseless ventricular tachycardia/fibrillation (VT/VF) where defibrillation is not immediately available, give a single *precordial thump*. With a tightly clenched fist, deliver one direct blow from a height of ≈20cm to the lower half of the sternum.

Airway management

Techniques for securing the airway, providing oxygenation and ventilation are covered in 📖 Airway obstruction: basic measures, p.324. Although tracheal intubation has long been considered to be the gold standard definitive airway, only attempt this if suitably experienced. *Laryngeal mask airway* is a readily available, rapid alternative, which is easy to insert. Whatever method is used, aim to ventilate (preferably with 100% O_2) using an inspiratory time of 1sec, a volume sufficient to produce a normal rise of the chest, at a rate of 10/min. For patients with tracheal tubes or laryngeal mask airways, ventilate without interrupting chest compressions, which should be continuous (except for defibrillation or pulse checks as appropriate).

End-tidal CO_2 monitoring is very useful to confirm correct tracheal tube placement and indirectly measure cardiac output during CPR.

Drugs

There is little evidence that *any* drug improves outcome. Central venous cannulation is difficult, has risks and interrupts CPR. Peripheral access is easy and quick. Having given a peripheral IV drug, give a 20mL saline bolus and elevate the limb for 10–20sec. If IV access is impossible, consider intraosseous route (📖 p.640). It is no longer recommended for any drugs to be given by tracheal tube. Similarly, do not attempt intracardiac injections.

The first drug used in cardiac arrest (after oxygen) is adrenaline. In the case of VF/VT, administer adrenaline after three shocks, whereas in asystole/PEA, give it as soon as possible (see 📖 Adult life support algorithm, p.52).

Non-shockable rhythms: PEA and asystole

Pulseless electrical activity (*PEA*) is the clinical situation of cardiac arrest with an ECG trace compatible with cardiac output. PEA may be caused by:

- Failure of the normal cardiac pumping mechanism (eg massive MI, drugs such as β-blockers, Ca^{2+} antagonists or electrolyte disturbance, eg hypokalaemia, hyperkalaemia).
- Obstruction to cardiac filling or output (eg tension pneumothorax, pericardial tamponade, myocardial rupture, pulmonary embolism (PE), prosthetic heart valve occlusion, and hypovolaemia).

Prompt and appropriate correction of these can result in survival. Remember potentially reversible causes as the 4H's and 4T's (see Table 2.1).

Table 2.1

4H's	4T's
Hypoxia	Tension pneumothorax
Hypovolaemia	Tamponade (cardiac)
Hyper/hypokalaemia/metabolic disorders	Toxic substances (eg overdose)
Hypothermia	Thromboembolic/mechanical obstruction

Asystole is the absence of cardiac (particularly ventricular) electrical activity. If unsure if the rhythm is asystole or fine VF, continue chest compressions and ventilation in an attempt to increase the amplitude and frequency of VF, and make it more susceptible to defibrillation.

Length of resuscitation

The duration of the resuscitation attempt depends upon the nature of the event, the time since the onset, and the estimated prospects for a successful outcome. In general, continue resuscitation while VF/pulseless VT persists, always provided that it was initially appropriate to commence resuscitation. If VF persists despite repeated defibrillation, try changing pad position or defibrillator.

Asystole unresponsive to treatment and arrests which last >1hr are rarely associated with survival. However, exceptions occur—particularly in younger patients, hypothermia, near drowning, and drug overdose.

Mechanical CPR

There are several devices available that can provide mechanical CPR. These include the 'AutoPulse' circumferential load-distributing band chest compression device (comprising a pneumatically actuated constricting band and backboard) and the 'LUCAS' gas-driven sternal compression device (with accompanying suction cup to provide active decompression). Widespread use of these devices may develop if early encouraging results are confirmed by larger studies. Mechanical CPR is potentially very useful in situations where the resuscitation attempt is prolonged (eg cardiac arrest associated with hypothermia, poisoning or following fibrinolytic treatment for PE), ensuring consistent CPR over a long period of time and freeing up an additional member of the team.

Advanced life support algorithm[1]

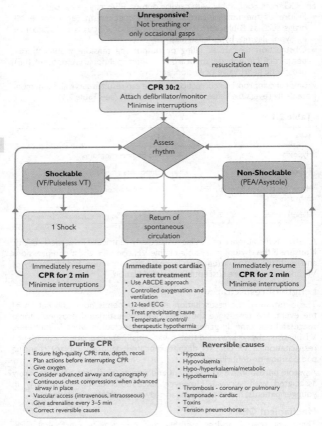

Unresponsive?
Not breathing or
only occasional gasps

Call
resuscitation team

CPR 30:2
Attach defibrillator/monitor
Minimise interruptions

Assess
rhythm

Shockable
(VF/Pulseless VT)

Non-Shockable
(PEA/Asystole)

1 Shock

Return of
spontaneous
circulation

Immediately resume
CPR for 2 min
Minimise interruptions

**Immediate post cardiac
arrest treatment**
• Use ABCDE approach
• Controlled oxygenation and
  ventilation
• 12-lead ECG
• Treat precipitating cause
• Temperature control/
  therapeutic hypothermia

Immediately resume
CPR for 2 min
Minimise interruptions

During CPR
• Ensure high-quality CPR: rate, depth, recoil
• Plan actions before interrupting CPR
• Give oxygen
• Consider advanced airway and capnography
• Continuous chest compressions when advanced
  airway in place
• Vascular access (intravenous, intraosseous)
• Give adrenaline every 3–5 min
• Correct reversible causes

Reversible causes
• Hypoxia
• Hypovolaemia
• Hypo-/hyperkalaemia/metabolic
• Hypothermia

• Thrombosis - coronary or pulmonary
• Tamponade - cardiac
• Toxins
• Tension pneumothorax

Fig. 2.6

1 Resuscitation Council (UK) guidelines, 2010 (www.resus.org.uk).

Notes on using the advanced life support algorithm

- Establish the underlying cardiac rhythm as quickly as possible in order to determine which 'loop' to follow to provide appropriate treatment—for VF/pulseless VT, the initial focus is defibrillation and good CPR; for asystole/PEA, the initial focus is good CPR, IV adrenaline, and searching for potentially reversible causes.
- Do not interrupt CPR except to perform defibrillation.
- Search for and correct potentially reversible causes of the arrest.
- Give IV adrenaline 1mg and amiodarone 300mg for VF/pulseless VT refractory to three shocks, followed by 1mg adrenaline every 3–5min. A further dose of 150mg IV amiodarone may be given for recurrent or refractory VF/VT. Lidocaine (1mg/kg) IV is an alternative to amiodarone, but do not give it if amiodarone has already been given.
- For torsade de pointes, and refractory VF in patients with suspected digoxin toxicity or hypomagnesaemia (eg on K^+ losing diuretics), give IV magnesium sulphate 2g (= 8mmol = 4mL of 50% solution).
- In asystole and PEA, give IV 1mg adrenaline as soon as possible and thereafter every 3–5min.
- Exercise caution before using adrenaline in arrests associated with cocaine or other sympathomimetic drugs.
- Atropine is no longer routinely recommended in asystole or slow PEA.
- In PEA arrests associated with hyperkalaemia, hypocalcaemia, or Ca^{2+} channel blocking drug or magnesium overdose, give 10mL 10% IV calcium chloride (6.8mmol).
- With good quality CPR, acidosis develops slowly. Do not 'routinely' give an alkali. Give 50mL of sodium bicarbonate 8.4% solution (50mmol) if arrest is associated with tricyclic overdose (📖 p.194) or hyperkalaemia and consider it in patients with severe acidosis (arterial pH<7.1, base excess less than −10). Allow further administration to be guided by repeated arterial blood gas (ABG) results.
- Follow loops of the algorithm for as long as it is considered appropriate for the resuscitation to continue. Provided that the attempt was commenced appropriately, it should not normally be stopped if the rhythm is still VF.

Pacing and external cardiac percussion

Pacing may be of value in patients with extreme bradyarrhythmias, but its value in asystole is unproven (except for rare cases of trifascicular block with P waves present). If there is a delay before pacing can be performed, external cardiac percussion can provide a cardiac output and 'buy time'. Perform *external cardiac percussion* using a clenched fist:

- Over the heart at a rate of 100/min.
- With a blow more gentle than a precordial thump.
- Each blow should generate a QRS complex. If this, and a detectable output, is not achieved restart conventional CPR.

Post-resuscitation care

Features such as coma or pupil reflexes are unreliable prognostic indicators in the early post-resuscitation phase. Accurate prognostication in an individual patient is rarely possible before 24–72hr. Involve the intensive care unit/critical care unit (ICU/CCU) team early.

Pending this and following ROSC

- Ensure that the airway is protected (📖 p.324).
- Maintain oxygenation and ventilation. Correct hypoxia and prevent hypercapnoea under ABG guidance (may require IPPV). Use pulse oximetry to monitor SpO_2 non-invasively, titrating inspired oxygen concentration to achieve SpO_2 of 94–98%.
- In intubated patients, insert an oro- or nasogastric tube to decompress the stomach.
- Obtain a 12-lead ECG and a CXR (check position of tracheal tube, central lines and presence of pneumothorax etc.).
- *Optimize cardiac output:* inotropes, vasodilators, fluids and/or diuretics may be needed under haemodynamic monitoring guidance. If the arrest is associated with an acute coronary syndrome, consider immediate thrombolysis and/or coronary revascularization.
- Cerebral blood flow autoregulation is deficient post-arrest. Maintaining arterial pressures 'normal' for the patient may prevent hypotensive hypoperfusion. ↑ BP above the normal for the patient may worsen cerebral oedema.
- Seizures aggravate brain injury by ↑ ICP and cerebral metabolic requirements. Treat with appropriate anticonvulsants (as 📖 p.149) and ensure adequate oxygenation and ventilation.
- Measure U&E, Ca^{2+}, Mg^{2+}, and correct abnormalities appropriately.
- Obtain full blood count (FBC) to exclude anaemia contributing to myocardial ischaemia and to provide an admission baseline.
- Both hypo- and hyperglycaemia compromise neurological outcome. Monitor plasma glucose concentration regularly and aim to avoid both hypo- and hyperglycaemia (keep the level ≤10mmol/L).
- No drug has been shown to improve cerebral outcome following cardiac arrest. The routine use of steroids, mannitol, Ca^{2+} channel blockers, etc., is unwarranted.
- When any drug is used, remember that pharmacokinetic profiles are often impaired post-resuscitation. Dose adjustment and careful monitoring are needed.
- Avoid/treat hyperthermia with antipyretic or active cooling.
- There is compelling data to support the early induction of mild *therapeutic hypothermia* (32–34°C) in patients who are comatose following out of hospital VF arrest. Mild hypothermia is believed to be neuroprotective in this situation (and pending more data, may be of benefit in other situations as well, eg other arrest rhythms, in-hospital arrests, paediatric patients). Cooling may be initiated by external techniques (cooling blankets, water or air circulating blankets) or internally by an infusion of 30mL/kg of 4°C 0.9% saline—liaise with ICU. Mild hypothermia is typically maintained for 12–24hr.

Training

Theoretical knowledge is important, but many of the skills required during the management of a cardiac arrest need expert teaching and supervised practice. Attend an approved Resuscitation Council (UK) *Advanced Life Support* course (see www.resus.org.uk)—preferably before starting in the ED.

Central venous access

Indications

Central venous access may be required for:
- Administration of emergency drugs.
- Central venous pressure measurement.
- Administration of IV fluids, especially when peripheral veins are collapsed or thrombosed. *Note:* other routes (eg femoral vein) are generally preferable for giving large volumes rapidly.
- Transvenous cardiac pacing.

Choice of vein

The external jugular vein is often readily visible and can be cannulated easily with a standard IV cannula.

The internal jugular and subclavian veins are generally used for central venous access in the ED. Subclavian vein cannulation has a relatively high risk of pneumothorax, so the internal jugular vein is usually preferable, via a 'high' approach. When possible, use ultrasound (USS) guidance and the right side of the neck (↓ risk of thoracic duct damage). If, however, a chest drain is already in situ, use the same side for central venous cannulation.

The femoral vein is useful for temporary access in severe trauma, burns, and in drug addicts with many thrombosed veins.

Seldinger technique for central venous access

The method of choice, because the relatively fine needle ↓ risk of complications such as pneumothorax. The technique involves inserting a hollow metal needle into the vein. A flexible guidewire is threaded through the needle, which is then removed. A tapered dilator and plastic cannula are inserted over the guidewire and advanced into the vein. The guidewire and dilator are removed, and the cannula secured. Once the cannula is in place, check that venous blood can be freely aspirated and secure the cannula.

Precautions and problems

Central venous access is a specialized technique with potentially life-threatening complications, including: pneumothorax, haemothorax, arterial puncture, thoracic duct damage, air embolism, and infection.
- Expert supervision is essential. Cannulation is particularly difficult and hazardous in hypovolaemic, shocked, or agitated patients. In such situations, consider whether it is possible to defer the procedure.
- *USS* has become widely available and is increasingly used by suitably trained ED specialists. It ↓ complications and failure rates by clarifying the relative positions of needle, vein, and surrounding structures. Variant anatomy and vein patency can also be assessed by USS.
- Bleeding dyscrasias and anticoagulant treatment are contraindications to internal jugular and subclavian vein access.
- Severe pulmonary disease is a relative contraindication to central venous access, especially by the subclavian route, because a pneumothorax would be particularly dangerous.

Methods

Use aseptic technique. If possible, tilt the trolley 10° head down to fill the internal jugular and subclavian veins and ↓ risk of air embolus. After successful or attempted subclavian or internal jugular cannulation, take a chest X-ray (CXR) to check for pneumothorax and the position of the cannula.

External jugular vein

The vein can be seen and felt as it crosses superficially over the sternomastoid muscle and runs obliquely towards the clavicle. Gentle pressure on the lower end of the vein will distend it. A standard IV cannula can easily be inserted into the external jugular vein, but passing a catheter centrally may be difficult because of valves and the angle at which the vein joins the subclavian vein.

Internal jugular vein

The internal jugular vein runs antero-laterally in the carotid sheath, parallel to the carotid artery, and deep to the sternocleidomastoid muscle. The high approach described has less risk of pneumothorax than lower approaches (Fig. 2.7).

- Turn the patient's head away from the side to be cannulated.
- Identify the carotid pulse at the level of the thyroid cartilage.
- Insert the needle 0.5cm lateral to the artery, at the medial border of sternomastoid muscle.
- Advance the needle at an angle of 45° parallel to the sagittal plane, pointing towards the ipsilateral nipple. The vein should be entered at a depth of 2–4cm and blood aspirated freely. If it is not, try again slightly more laterally.

Subclavian vein (infraclavicular approach)

- Turn the patient's head away from the side of cannulation.
- Identify the mid-clavicular point and the sternal notch.
- Insert the needle 1cm below the mid-clavicular point and advance it horizontally below and behind the clavicle, aiming at a finger in the suprasternal notch. The vein is usually entered at a depth of 4–6cm (Fig. 2.8).

Femoral vein

Insert the needle ≈1cm medial to the femoral artery and just below the inguinal ligament, pointing slightly medially and with the needle at 20–30° to the skin.

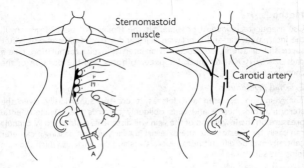

Fig. 2.7 Internal jugular cannulation.[1]

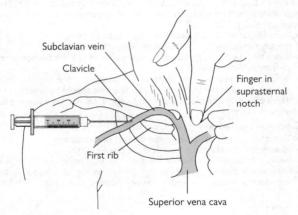

Fig. 2.8 Subclavian vein cannulation.[2]

1 Rosen M et al. Handbook of Percutaneous Central Venous Catheterization. W.B. Saunders, London.
2 Cosgriff JH. An Atlas of Diagnostic and Therapeutic Procedures for Emergency Personnel. J.B. Lippincott, Philadelphia.

Severe sepsis and septic shock

Septic patients have a systemic inflammatory response syndrome (SIRS) as a consequence of infection. Severe sepsis refers to septic patients with evidence of organ hypoperfusion. Septic shock is present when septic patients exhibit hypotension unresponsive to intravenous fluid resuscitation.

Systemic inflammatory response syndrome

This requires 2 or more of:
- Body temperature of >38°C or <36°C
- Heart rate >90/min
- Respiratory rate >20 breaths/min or $PaCO_2$ < 4.3kPa
- WCC >12 × 10^9/L or <4 × 10^9/L or >10% immature (band) forms

Management

Severely septic patients have SIRS with evidence of hypoperfusion (eg systolic BP <90mmHg and/or lactate >3mmol/L). Obtain senior/ICU help early. Intensive therapy of severely septic patients focuses upon certain *therapeutic goals:*
- CVP of 8–12mmHg.
- mean arterial pressure >65mmHg.
- urine output >0.5mL/kg/hr.
- central venous saturation >65%.

Adopt the following approach:
- Obtain senior/ICU assistance now.
- Assess and manage airway, breathing, circulation (ABC)—in particular, provide high flow oxygen, secure good IV access and give an initial IV fluid bolus of 20mL/kg of 0.9% saline. Some patients may require early tracheal intubation and IPPV.
- Look for obvious sources of infection.
- Check BMG (and treat if hypoglycaemic).
- Take blood cultures before starting antibiotics (the choice of antibiotics will depend upon the likely cause and is considered on p.60).
- Patients who remain hypotensive and/or have a lactate >3mmol/L require central venous and arterial catheterization in an intensive care/resuscitation setting, with IVI noradrenaline to maintain mean arterial pressure >65mmHg and IV 0.9% saline 500mL boluses every 20mins to achieve CVP 8–12mmHg (12–15mmHg in mechanically ventilated patients).

Shock

Shock is a clinical condition characterized by failure to adequately perfuse and oxygenate vital organs. Clinically, shock is recognized by:

- *Hypotension* Generally considered to be systolic BP <90mmHg (in adults), but values may be higher in young, fit or previously hypertensive patients. Associated *tachycardia* (>100/min) is common, but may not be present in patients with cardiac or neurological causes or in those taking β-blockers. A few patients with haemorrhagic shock have a paradoxical bradycardia.
- *Altered consciousness* and/or fainting (especially on standing or sitting up) may result from ↓ cerebral perfusion.
- *Poor peripheral perfusion* Cool peripheries, clammy/sweaty skin, pallor, ↓ capillary return, but note that in the early phase of endotoxic septic shock there may be vasodilatation with warm peripheries.
- *Oliguria* ↓ renal perfusion with urine output <50mL/hr (in adults).
- *Tachypnoea*.

Classification of shock

Traditional classification of types of shock is artificial—mixed aetiologies are common.

Hypovolaemic shock

- *Blood loss*: trauma, gastrointestinal (GI) bleed (haematemesis, melaena), ruptured abdominal aortic aneurysm, ruptured ectopic pregnancy.
- *Fluid loss/redistribution* ('third spacing'): burns, GI losses (vomiting, diarrhoea), pancreatitis, sepsis.

Cardiogenic shock

- *Primary*: myocardial infarction (MI), arrhythmias, valve dysfunction, myocarditis.
- *Secondary*: cardiac tamponade, massive pulmonary embolus, tension pneumothorax.

Septic shock (see 🔲 p.59)

More common at the extremes of age, in patients with diabetes mellitus, renal/hepatic failure and the immunocompromised (eg HIV infection, underlying malignancy, post-splenectomy, steroid therapy). Note that fever, rigors and ↑ white cell count (WCC) may not be present.

- *Organisms responsible* include Gram +ve and –ve, especially *Staph. aureus*, *Strep. pneumoniae*, *N meningitidis*, coliforms including enterococci and *Bacteroides* (especially in patients with intra-abdominal emergencies, such as ruptured diverticular abscess). In the immunocompromised, *Pseudomonas*, viruses, and fungi may cause septic shock.

Anaphylactic shock: see 🔲 p.42.

Neurogenic shock: see 🔲 p.382.

Other causes

These include poisoning (🔲 p.183) and Addison's disease (🔲 p.155).

Management of shock

Investigation and treatment should occur simultaneously. Get senior help immediately.

- Address the priorities—ABC.
- Give high flow O_2 by mask.
- Secure adequate venous access and take blood for FBC, U&E, glucose, liver function tests (LFTs), lactate, coagulation screen, and if appropriate, blood cultures.
- Monitor vital signs, including pulse, BP, SpO_2, respiratory rate.
- Check ABG.
- Monitor ECG and obtain 12 lead ECG and CXR.
- Insert a urinary catheter and monitor urine output hourly.
- For shock associated with ↓ effective circulating blood volume, give IV crystalloid (0.9% saline) 20mL/kg as bolus. Give further IV fluids including colloid ± blood (aim for haematocrit (Hct) >30%) according to aetiology and clinical response (and in particular, pulse, BP, central venous pressure (CVP), and urine output). Use caution with IV fluid infusion in shock related to cardiogenic causes, and in ruptured or dissecting aortic aneurysm.
- Look for, and treat specifically, the cause(s) of the shock. Echocardiography, USS, CT, and/or surgical intervention may be required. Specific treatments include:
  - *Laparotomy*: ruptured abdominal aortic aneurysm, splenic and/or liver trauma, ruptured ectopic pregnancy, intra-abdominal sepsis.
  - *Thrombolysis/angioplasty*: MI.
  - *Thrombolysis*: PE.
  - *Pericardiocentesis/cardiac surgery*: cardiac tamponade, aortic valve dysfunction.
  - *Antidotes*: for certain poisons.
  - *Antibiotics*: sepsis. The choice of antibiotic will depend upon the perceived cause and local policies (eg ceftriaxone for meningococcal disease). Where there is no obvious source, empirical combination therapy is advised (eg co-amoxiclav + gentamicin + metronidazole). Obtain specialist microbiological advice early, especially in neutropaenic/immunocompromised patients.
- Inotropic and vasoactive therapy, assisted ventilation, and invasive monitoring (including arterial and CVP lines) are often needed as part of goal directed therapy. Get specialist ICU help early.

Chapter 3

Medicine

Medicine

Electrocardiogram interpretation

The electrocardiogram (ECG) is normally recorded so that a deflection of 10mm = 1mV. The recording rate is 25mm/sec, 1mm = 0.04sec, 1 large square = 0.2sec. There is an ECG ruler on the inside back cover. Follow a systematic approach.

Rate Calculate the rate by dividing 300 by the number of large squares in one R–R interval.

Frontal plane axis Normally lies between −30° and +90° (see Fig. 3.1). With a normal axis, QRS complexes in I and II are both +ve. An axis more −ve than −30° (I +ve, aVF and II −ve) is *left axis deviation* (causes: left anterior hemiblock, inferior myocardial infarction (MI), ventricular tachycardia (VT), Wolf Parkinson White (WPW) syndrome). An axis more +ve than +90° (I −ve, aVF +ve) is *right axis deviation* (causes: pulmonary embolism (PE), cor pulmonale, lateral MI, left posterior hemiblock).

P wave Normally <0.12sec wide and <2.5mm tall. They are best seen in leads II and V_1 which are chosen for rhythm strips or monitoring. A tall peaked P wave in II may reflect right atrial hypertrophy; a widened bifid P wave left atrial hypertrophy. P waves are absent in atrial fibrillation (AF).

PR interval Normally 0.12–0.2sec (<5 small squares). A short PR interval (abnormally fast conduction between atria and ventricles) implies an accessory pathway (eg Wolf Parkinson White syndrome).

A prolonged PR interval occurs in heart block (first, second or third degree, see 📖 Bradyarrhythmias, p.80).

QRS width Normally 0.05–0.11sec (<3 small squares). Prolonged QRS complexes may be due to: right bundle branch block (RBBB) (RsR' or M shape in V_1), left bundle branch block (LBBB) (QS or W shape in V_1 with RsR' or M shape in V_6), tricyclic antidepressant poisoning (📖 p.194), hypothermia, ventricular rhythms, and ectopics.

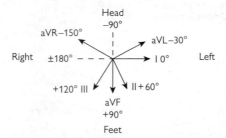

Fig. 3.1 Diagram of the ECG frontal axis.

QRS amplitude The QRS amplitude can indicate left ventricular hypertrophy (LVH). Signs of LVH are: (S in V_2 + R in V_5) > 35mm; R in I > 15mm; R in aV_L > 11mm.

Q waves May be normal in III, aV_R, and V_1, but are abnormal in other leads if >0.04sec or > ½ of the height of the subsequent R wave.

ST segment elevation is caused by: acute MI, pericarditis (concave up), ventricular aneurysm, Prinzmetal's angina, LVH, Brugada syndrome, hypertrophic cardiomyopathy, benign early repolarization.

ST segment depression is caused by: ischaemia, digoxin, LVH with strain.

QT interval = start of Q wave to end of T wave.

$QT_c = QT/\sqrt{R-R}$ (Bazett's formula). Normal QT_c is <440msec.

At rates of 60–100/min, QT should be <1/2 R–R interval.

A *prolonged* QT_c predisposes to 'torsades de pointes' (□ Broad complex tachyarrhythmias, p.87) and is caused by acute MI, hypothermia, hypocalcaemia, drugs (quinidine, tricyclic antidepressants), certain congenital diseases (eg Romano–Ward syndrome).

T waves Abnormal if inverted in V_{4-6}. Peaked T waves are seen in early acute MI and hyperkalaemia (□ p.162). Flattened T waves (sometimes with prominent U waves) occur in hypokalaemia.

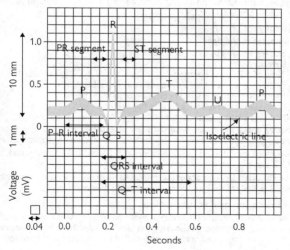

Fig. 3.2

Chest pain

Always take chest pain seriously. It may reflect life-threatening illness. Triage patients with chest pain as 'urgent' and ensure that they are seen within a few minutes. Ischaemic heart disease is understandably the first diagnosis to spring to mind in the middle-aged or elderly, but chest pain may have a variety of other disease processes, many of which are also potentially life-threatening (Table 3.1).

Table 3.1 The differential diagnosis of chest pain

Common causes	Less common causes
Musculoskeletal (eg costochondritis)	Aortic dissection*
Acute coronary syndrome*	Cholecystitis
Pneumothorax*	Herpes zoster
Oesophagitis	Oesophageal rupture*
Pneumonia	Pancreatitis*
Pulmonary embolism*	Vertebral collapse
Obscure origin (eg precordial catch)	Tabes dorsalis (very rare)

*Potentially rapidly fatal.

Reaching the correct conclusion requires accurate interpretation of the history, examination and investigations, bearing in mind recognized patterns of disease presentations.

History

Characterize the pain
- Site (eg central, bilateral or unilateral).
- Severity.
- Time of onset and duration.
- Character (eg 'stabbing', 'tight/gripping', or 'dull/aching').
- Radiation (eg to arms and neck in myocardial ischaemia).
- Precipitating and relieving factors (eg exercise/rest/GTN spray).
- Previous similar pains.

Enquire about associated symptoms Breathlessness, nausea, and vomiting, sweating, cough, haemoptysis, palpitations, dizziness, loss of consciousness.

Document past history, drug history, and allergies. Old notes and old ECGs are invaluable—request them at an early stage.

Quickly consider contacting cardiologists if acute coronary syndrome (ACS) is likely (ST segment elevation MI: treatment, p.76).

Examination and resuscitation

Evaluate Airway, Breathing, Circulation (ABC) and resuscitate (O_2, venous access, IV analgesia) as appropriate. Listen to both lung fields and check for tension pneumothorax and severe left ventricular failure (LVF). Complete full examination.

Investigations

These depend upon the presentation and likely diagnosis, but an ECG and CXR are usually required. Remember that these may initially be normal in MI, PE and aortic dissection. Ensure that all patients receive ECG monitoring in an area where a defibrillator is readily available.

Angina

Angina is defined as discomfort in the chest, arm, neck, or adjacent areas due to myocardial ischaemia. It can be brought on by exertion, cold weather and emotion. It occurs when coronary artery blood flow fails to meet the O_2 demand of the myocardium (eg during exercise, coronary artery spasm or anaemia). Ischaemia may produce ST depression or inversion, which resolves on recovery.

First presentation of angina

Patients may come to the ED with angina as a first presentation of ischaemic heart disease (IHD). Always consider the possibility of MI. In particular, suspect myocardial cell death with any pain lasting >10min (even if relieved by glyceryl trinitrate (GTN)). *A normal examination, normal ECG and normal baseline cardiac markers do not exclude MI. If in any doubt, admit the patient.* If considering discharge, discuss with senior ED/medical staff.

Atypical cardiac chest pain

Patients with acute MI are occasionally sent home from the ED inadvertently. Cardiac chest pain may be poorly localized, and may present with musculoskeletal features or gastrointestinal (GI) upset. In particular, patients with acute coronary syndromes commonly have chest wall tenderness. Some patients understandably play down symptoms in order to avoid admission to hospital. If the clinical history is suspicious of cardiac pain (especially in a patient with risk factors, such as family history of IHD, hypertension, smoking), then refer for admission. Do not be fooled by a normal ECG, normal examination, or the fact that the patient is <30 years old. Remember that oesophageal pain may improve with GTN and true cardiac pain may appear to improve with antacids. The decision whether or not to refer the patient for admission and investigation depends upon an assessment of the risk of MI. In general, exclude an MI where chest pain lasting >15min has some features of IHD. Also refer patients who look unwell, even if the chest pain lasts <15min.

Acute coronary syndromes

Coronary artery plaque rupture can result in a variety of ischaemic conditions which fall under the overall term of 'acute coronary syndrome' and include unstable angina, non-ST segment elevation MI (NSTEMI) and ST segment elevation MI (STEMI). Patients labelled as having acute coronary syndrome, but without initial ST elevation, comprise a relatively heterogenous group—some later proving (on the basis of elevated blood troponin levels) to have suffered an NSTEMI.

The patient presenting with unstable angina or NSTEMI

Unstable angina can occur as worsening angina or a single episode of 'crescendo' angina, with a high risk of infarction. Features include angina at rest, ↑ frequency, ↑ duration, and severity of pain (including response to GTN). It may be difficult to distinguish between unstable angina and NSTEMI in the ED.

- Provide O_2 to maintain SpO_2 94–98% and attach cardiac monitor.
- Administer IV opioid analgesia (± antiemetic) as required.
- Give aspirin 300mg PO and clopidogrel 300mg PO.
- Start low molecular weight heparin (LMWH), eg dalteparin 120units/kg SC every 12hr (max 10,000U) or enoxaparin 1mg/kg SC every 12hr. Synthetic pentasaccharide fondaparinux 2.5mg SC may be used instead. Follow local guidelines.
- If pain is unrelieved, commence GTN intravenous infusion (IVI; start at 0.6mg/hr and ↑ as necessary), provided systolic BP is >90mmHg.
- Glycoprotein IIb/IIIa inhibitors (eg eptifibatide and tirofiban) are going out of favour for patients at risk of NSTEMI or high TIMI risk score (see Table 3.2).
- If high risk of NSTEMI, haemodynamically stable and no contraindications, consider atenolol (5mg IV slowly over 5mins repeated once after 15mins), according to local policy. Contraindications include: hypotension, bradycardia, second or third degree heart block, heart failure and severe reactive airways disease.
- Refer for admission, repeat ECGs and blood troponin testing 12hr after pain onset.
- Discuss with cardiology all patients at high risk of NSTEMI or with TIMI score >3. They may benefit from early revascularization procedures.

Table 3.2 TIMI risk score: increasing score predicts mortality or adverse event

Risk factor	Points
Age >65	1
3+ risk factors for coronary artery disease	1
Family history of IHD, hypertension, hypercholesterolemia, diabetes, or smoker	
Known coronary artery disease with stenosis ≥50%	1
Aspirin use in last 7 days	1
Recent episode of angina prior to this event	1
Raised troponin levels (or other cardiac marker)	1
ST segment deviation ≥0.5mm on ECG	1

Normal lead II (Fig. 3.3)

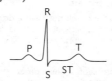

Fig. 3.3

Ischaemic changes in lead II (Fig. 3.4)

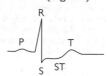

Fig. 3.4

Prinzmetal's or 'variant' angina

Angina associated with ST elevation may be due to coronary artery vasospasm. This may occur with or without a fixed coronary abnormality and may be indistinguishable from an acute MI until changes resolve rapidly with GTN as pain is relieved.

ST segment elevation MI

IHD is the leading cause of death in the Western world. Mortality from acute MI is believed to be 45%, with 70% of these deaths occurring before reaching medical care. Contributory risk factors for MI include smoking, hypertension, age, male sex, diabetes, hyperlipidaemia, and family history.

MI pathology

MI mostly affects the left ventricle. It usually results from sudden occlusion of a coronary artery or one of its branches by thrombosis over a pre-existing atheromatous plaque. Patients with IHD are at risk of sustaining an MI if additional stresses are placed upon their already critically impaired myocardial circulation (eg a high level of carboxyhaemoglobin (COHb) following smoke inhalation). MI may also occur in vasculitic processes, eg cranial arteritis (p.132) and Kawasaki disease.

MI diagnosis

The diagnosis of acute MI requires 2 out of the following 3 features:
* A history of cardiac-type ischaemic chest pain.
* Evolutionary changes on serial ECGs.
* A rise in serum cardiac markers.

Note that 50–60% of patients will not have a diagnostic ECG on arrival and up to 17% will have an entirely normal initial ECG. Late presentation does not improve diagnostic accuracy of the ECG.

History

The classic presentation is of sudden onset, severe, constant central chest pain, which radiates to the arms, neck, or jaw. This may be similar to previous angina pectoris, but is much more severe and unrelieved by GTN. The pain is usually accompanied by one or more associated symptoms: sweating, nausea, vomiting, breathlessness.

Atypical presentation is common. Have a high level of suspicion. Many patients describe atypical pain, some attributing it to indigestion (be wary of new onset 'dyspeptic' pain). Up to a third of patients with acute MI do not report any chest pain. These patients tend to be older, are more likely to be female, have a history of diabetes or heart failure, and have a higher mortality.

These patients may present with:
* LVF.
* Collapse or syncope (often with associated injuries eg head injury).
* Confusion.
* Stroke.
* An incidental ECG finding at a later date.

In a patient who presents with possible MI, enquire about past medical history (IHD, hypertension, diabetes, hyperlipidaemia) and contraindications to thrombolysis. Ask about drug history, including drugs of abuse (particularly cocaine p.215).

Examination

Examination and initial resuscitation (maintain SpO_2 in normal range, IV cannula, analgesia) go hand in hand. The patient may be pale, sweaty, and distressed. Examination is usually normal unless complications have supervened (eg arrhythmias, LVF). Direct initial examination towards searching for these complications and excluding alternative diagnoses:

- Check pulse, BP and monitor trace (?arrhythmia or cardiogenic shock).
- Listen to the heart (?murmurs or 3rd heart sound).
- Listen to the lung fields (?LVF, pneumonia, pneumothorax).
- Check peripheral pulses (?aortic dissection).
- Check legs for evidence of deep vein thrombosis (?PE).
- Palpate for abdominal tenderness or masses (?cholecystitis, pancreatitis, perforated peptic ulcer, ruptured aortic aneurysm).

Investigations

The diagnosis of ST segment elevation myocardial infarction within the first few hours is based upon history and ECG changes (serum cardiac markers may take several hours to rise—see below).

- Record an ECG as soon as possible, ideally within a few minutes of arrival at hospital. Sometimes patients arrive at hospital with ECGs of diagnostic quality already recorded by paramedics. If the initial ECG is normal, but symptoms are suspicious, repeat the ECG every 15min and re-evaluate.
- Request old notes (these may contain previous ECGs for comparison).
- Ensure continuous cardiac monitoring and pulse oximetry.
- Monitor BP and respiratory rate.
- Obtain venous access and send blood for cardiac markers, U&E, glucose, FBC, lipids.
- Obtain a CXR if there is suspicion of LVF or aortic dissection.

Cardiac markers

Troponins are now universally used. Troponin T (cTnT) and Troponin I (cTnI) are proteins virtually exclusive to cardiac myocytes. They are highly specific and sensitive, but are only maximally accurate after 12hr. Troponin T and I cannot be used to rule out MI in the first few hours. In addition, cardiac cells may release troponin into the blood when cardiac muscle is damaged by pericarditis, pulmonary embolism with a large clot burden, or sepsis. Renal failure reduces excretion of troponin.

Chest pain assessment units

These units are becoming established in some EDs. A combination of ECGs, ST segment monitoring, cardiac markers, and exercise testing is used to allow discharge of low to moderate risk patients within 6–12hr. However, simply excluding an acute coronary syndrome is only part of the assessment of chest pain.

Myocardial infarction: ECG changes 1

Infarction of cardiac muscle results in ECG changes that evolve over hours, days, and weeks in a relatively predictable fashion.

Hyperacute changes

Frequently ignored, although often subtle, some or all of the following may be observed within minutes of infarction:

- ↑ *Ventricular activation time*, since the infarcting myocardium is slower to conduct electrical impulses. The interval between the start of the QRS and apex of the R wave may be prolonged >0.045sec.
- ↑ *Height of R wave* may be seen initially in inferior leads in inferior MI.
- *Upward-sloping ST segment*—having lost normal upward concavity, the ST segment straightens, then slopes upwards, before becoming elevated.
- *Tall, widened T waves.*

Evolving acute changes

In isolation, none of these changes are specific to MI. In combination, and with an appropriate history, they can diagnose MI:

- *ST elevation*: the most important ECG change. ST segments become concave down and are significant if elevated >1mm in 2 limb leads, or >2mm in 2 adjacent chest leads.
- *Reciprocal ST depression* may occur on the 'opposite side' of the heart.
- *Pathological Q waves* (defined on 📖 p.65) reflect electrically inert necrotic myocardium. ECG leads over a large transmural infarct show deep QS waves. Leads directed towards the periphery of a large infarct or over a smaller infarct may show a QR complex or a *loss of R wave amplitude*.
- *T wave inversion*: typically deeply inverted, symmetrical and pointed.
- *Conduction problems* may develop. LBBB in a patient with acute cardiac chest pain makes interpretation of the ECG very difficult. LBBB does not have to be new to be significant. Do not delay intervention in patients with a good clinical history of MI in order to obtain old ECGs.

Sgarbossa criteria for diagnosing ACS in the presence of LBBB

- ST segment elevation >1mm in leads with positive QRS complexes.
- ST segment depression in leads V1, V2, or V3.
- ST segment elevation >5mm in lead with negative QRS complexes.

If all 3 are present, MI is likely.

Chronic changes

In the months following an MI, ECG changes resolve to a variable extent. ST segments become isoelectric, unless a ventricular aneurysm develops. T waves gradually become +ve again. Q waves usually remain, indicating MI at some time in the past.

Electrocardiogram changes following myocardial infarction (Fig. 3.5)

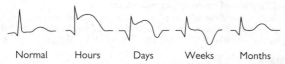

| Normal | Hours | Days | Weeks | Months |

Fig. 3.5

Electrocardiograms after myocardial infarction (Figs 3.6 and 3.7)

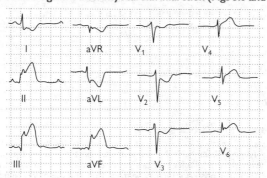

Fig. 3.6 Acute inferolateral infarction with 'reciprocal' ST changes in I, aVL, and V_2–V_3.

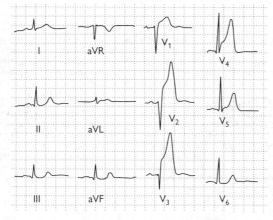

Fig. 3.7 Acute anteroseptal infarction with minimal 'reciprocal' ST changes in III and aVF.

Myocardial infarction: ECG changes 2

Localization of myocardial infarction

MI usually affects the left ventricle (LV), occasionally the right ventricle (RV), but virtually never the atria. The part of myocardium affected is implied by which leads show changes (Table 3.3).

Table 3.3

ECG leads	Location of MI
V_{1-3}	Anteroseptal
V_{5-6}, aV_L	Anterolateral
V_{2-4}	Anterior
V_{1-6}	Extensive anterior
I, II, aV_L, V_6	Lateral
II, III, aV_F	Inferior
V_1, V_4R	Right ventricle

Posterior myocardial infarction

Posterior MI nearly always occurs as part of inferior (postero-inferior) or lateral (postero-lateral) MI. No conventional electrode views the posterior heart, since intervening tissues result in an attenuated signal. ECG diagnosis of true posterior MI may be made from the use of V_{7-9} and from reciprocal changes seen in leads V_{1-3}: tall, slightly widened R (reciprocal of Q), concave up ST depression (reciprocal of ST elevation), upright tall widened T (reciprocal of inverted T).

Right ventricular infarct

This occurs most often as part of an inferior MI. In the presence of changes of acute MI in the inferior leads, ST elevation in V_1 suggests right ventricular involvement. In this case, record an ECG trace from lead V_4R. The diagnosis of RV infarct helps determine treatment of ensuing cardiac failure. Treat RV failure with IV fluids to maintain adequate filling pressure and exercise caution if considering use of nitrates.

Blood supply to the heart and coronary artery dominance

The left anterior descending artery supplies the anterior and septal cardiac areas (Fig. 3.9). The circumflex branch supplies the anterolateral aspect of the heart. The right coronary artery supplies the right ventricle. In most people the right coronary artery also supplies the sino-atrial node, the inferior wall of the left ventricle and the ventricular septum. In 15% of individuals, the inferior wall is supplied by the circumflex branch of the left coronary artery (left dominance).

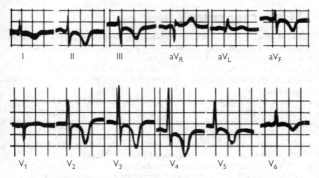

Fig. 3.8 ECG of subendocardial infarct.

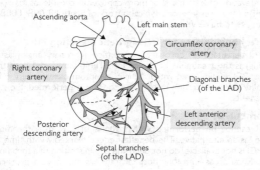

Fig. 3.9

STEMI: treatment

Speed is crucial—time is muscle. Ambulance control may alert the ED in advance of a patient with cardiac-type chest pain. Work efficiently as a team to ensure treatment is not delayed.

- Give O_2 to maintain SpO_2 94–98% and attach cardiac monitor.
- Obtain IV access and take samples for U&E, glucose, FBC, cardiac markers.
- Provide small increments of IV opioid analgesia titrated to effect.
- Ensure the patient has had 300mg aspirin and 300mg clopidogrel PO.
- Contact cardiology for primary percutaneous coronary intervention (PCI). Arrange transport to the cath lab.
- For patients undergoing PCI, consider IV glycoprotein IIb/IIIa receptor antagonist as an adjuvant. Be guided by local protocol.
- If PCI is not available, consider thrombolysis and monitor carefully. Start LMWH, heparin, or fondaparinux, according to local protocols.
- If pain continues, give IVI GTN (start at 0.6mg/hr and ↑ as necessary), provided systolic BP is >90mmHg.
- Consider atenolol (5mg slowly IV over 5min, repeated once after 15min), or metoprolol, unless contraindicated (eg uncontrolled heart failure, hypotension, bradyarrhythmias, COPD).

Indications for PCI or thrombolysis
- ST elevation of >1mm in 2 limb leads, or
- ST elevation of ≥2mm in 2 or more contiguous chest leads, or
- LBBB in the presence of a typical history of acute MI (NB: LBBB does not have to be new).

Primary angioplasty for ST segment elevation MI

Primary percutaneous coronary intervention (coronary angioplasty and stenting) is the treatment of choice for STEMI. Compared with thrombolysis, PCI administered within 12hr of symptom onset results in lower mortality and re-infarction rates. The sooner it is performed, the greater the benefits.

Thrombolysis

If PCI cannot be performed within 90min of diagnosis, thrombolytic therapy is an alternative. The benefits reduce markedly with time delay, so if PCI is not available, do not delay the administration of a thrombolytic agent. Rural areas with long hospital transfers may have a protocol for ambulance administered thrombolysis, aided by telemedicine advice from the ED or cardiology. Patients presenting >12hr after symptom onset will not benefit from thrombolysis.

Strokes, intracranial haemorrhage and major bleeds are more common in patients given thrombolysis. Intracranial bleeding is more common in older patients, those with hypertension on admission and those given tPA. Prior to administering thrombolysis, always explain the benefits and risks to the patient. Obtain verbal consent to give the medication and record this in the notes.

Contraindications to thrombolysis

Most are relative, but discuss any contraindications with the patient and cardiology:

- Head injury, recent stroke, previous neurosurgery or cerebral tumour.
- Recent GI or GU bleeding, menstruation, or coagulopathy/warfarin.
- Severe hypertension (eg systolic BP >200mmHg, diastolic BP>120mmHg), aortic dissection or pericarditis.
- Puncture of non-compressible vessel (eg subclavian vein), traumatic CPR, ↓ GCS post-arrest.
- Major surgery within recent weeks.
- Pregnancy.

Choice of thrombolytic agents

Tissue plasminogen activator (tPA), rather than streptokinase, is the agent of choice. Always use tPA if streptokinase was given >5 days ago or in anterior MI in a patient <75 years old and <4hr of onset of symptoms, or if hypotensive (systolic BP <90mmHg).

Alteplase (recombinant tPA (rtPA)) is most effective given by an accelerated regimen, eg 15mg IV bolus, followed by 0.75mg/kg (max 50mg) IVI for 30min, then 0.5mg/kg (max 35mg) IVI over 60min. Give LMWH (eg enoxaparin 1mg/kg stat) or heparin concomitantly through a separate IV line (5000unit IV bolus, then 1000units/hr IV), according to local protocols.

Reteplase (modified tPA) can be given as two IV boluses of 10units each exactly 30min apart. Give LMWH/heparin as for alteplase.

Tenecteplase (modified tPA) is given as a single IV bolus over 10sec. Dose according to weight (<60kg = 30mg; 60–69kg = 35mg; 70–79kg = 40mg; 80–89kg = 45mg; >90kg = 50mg). Give LMWH/heparin as for alteplase.

Streptokinase Given as 1.5mega-units by continuous IVI over 1hr. Streptokinase is allergenic (may require slow IV chlorphenamine 10mg and IV hydrocortisone 100mg) and frequently causes hypotension (↓ IVI rate and tilt the bed head down—treatment rarely needs to be discontinued). After a recent streptococcal infection, streptokinase may be ineffective due to the antibodies produced.

Further management

Arrhythmias Occur commonly after MI. Occasional ventricular ectopics or transient AF (lasting <30sec) require no treatment. Watch for sudden VT/VF and treat as in 📖 Cardiac arrest, p.46.

Hypokalaemia Treat if K$^+$<4mmol/L.

Pulmonary oedema Treat as described on 📖 p.101.

Cardiogenic shock ↓ cardiac output with tissue hypoxia, which does not improve with correction of intravascular volume. Mortality is 50–80%. Contact ICU and cardiologist. Echocardiography may be required to exclude conditions requiring urgent surgical repair (mitral regurgitation from papillary muscle rupture, aortic dissection, ventricular septum rupture, cardiac tamponade from ventricular wall rupture) or massive PE. If these are excluded, emergency coronary intervention may ↑ survival.

Pericarditis

Acute inflammation of the pericardium characteristically produces chest pain, low grade fever, and a pericardial friction rub. Pericarditis and myocarditis commonly co-exist.

Causes

- Myocardial infarction (including Dressler's syndrome—see 📖 p.79).
- Viral (Coxsackie A9, B1-4, Echo 8, mumps, EBV, CMV, varicella, HIV, rubella, Parvo B19).
- Bacterial (pneumococcus, meningococcus, *Chlamydia*, gonorrhoea, *Haemophilus*).
- Tuberculosis (TB; especially in patients with HIV)—see 📖 p.232.
- Locally invasive carcinoma (eg bronchus or breast).
- Rheumatic fever—see 📖 Acute arthritis, p.497.
- Uraemia.
- Collagen vascular disease (SLE, polyarteritis nodosa, rheumatoid arthritis).
- After cardiac surgery or radiotherapy.
- Drugs (hydralazine, procainamide, methyldopa, minoxidil).

Diagnosis

Classical features of acute pericarditis are pericardial pain, a friction rub and concordant ST elevation on ECG. The characteristic combination of clinical presentation and ECG changes often results in a definite diagnosis.

Chest pain is typically sharp, central, retrosternal, and worse on deep inspiration, change in position, exercise, and swallowing. A large pericardial effusion may cause dysphagia by compressing the oesophagus.

A pericardial friction rub is often intermittent, positional, and elusive. It tends to be louder during inspiration, and may be heard in both systole and diastole. Low grade fever is common.

Appropriate investigations include: ECG, chest X-ray, FBC, erythrocyte sedimentation rate (ESR), C-reactive protein (CRP), U&E, and troponin. Obtain blood cultures if there is evidence of sepsis or suspicion of a bacterial cause (eg spread of intrathoracic infection). A pericardial effusion is most quickly and easily demonstrated by echocardiography or FAST scanning: clinical evidence of cardiac tamponade is rare.

ECG changes

In *acute pericarditis* ECG changes result from associated epicardial inflammation (see Fig. 3.10). Sinus tachycardia is usual, but AF, atrial flutter or atrial ectopics may occur. ST elevation is concave up (unlike MI, 📖 p.72), and present in at least 2 limb leads and all chest leads (most marked in V_{3-6}). T waves are initially prominent, upright, and peaked, becoming flattened or inverted over several days. PR depression (reflecting atrial inflammation) may occur in the same leads as ST elevation (this PR–ST discordance is characteristic). Pathological Q waves are not present.

Pericardial effusion causes ↓ QRS amplitude in all leads. Electrical alternans is diagnostic, but rare.

Management

Refer to the medical team for echocardiography and treatment. The appropriate treatment depends on the underlying cause.

Idiopathic pericarditis or viral pericarditis in young patients is usually benign and self-limiting, responding to symptomatic treatment (high dose NSAID ± PPI cover). Occasionally, it follows a relapsing course before 'burning itself out'.

Dressler's syndrome (autoimmune pericarditis ± effusion 2–14 weeks after 3% of MIs) requires cardiology specialist care.

Pericardial effusion may occur with any type of pericarditis. It is relatively common in acute bacterial, tuberculous, and malignant pericarditis. Acute tamponade may occur following cardiac rupture with MI, aortic dissection, or after cardiac surgery. Summon senior help and arrange immediate echocardiography for patients with signs of tamponade, with pericardiocentesis under ultrasound guidance, and then a definitive drainage procedure. Emergency 'blind' pericardiocentesis is described on p.343.

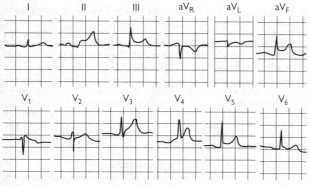

Fig. 3.10 ECG of pericarditis.

Bradyarrhythmias

Bradycardia is a ventricular rate of <60/min in the adult. It usually reflects influences on or disease of the sino-atrial (SA) node, or atrioventricular (AV) block. Intraventricular conduction disturbances may progress to AV block. Sinus bradycardia may be physiological (eg athletes), due to drugs (β-blockers), or pathological (hypothyroidism, hypothermia, hypoxia, ↑ICP, sick sinus syndrome, MI, myocardial ischaemia). Bradycardia also occurs in up to 1/3 of patients with hypovolaemia (eg GI bleed, ectopic pregnancy).

Sick sinus syndrome (or 'sinus node disease') is usually the result of ischaemia or degeneration of SA node. It is characterized by sinus pauses (>2sec) or sinus arrest. Junctional or other escape beats may occur and occasionally a tachyarrhythmia may emerge ('tachy-brady' syndrome). Patients may present with dizziness, collapse, loss of consciousness or palpitations. A continuous 24hr ECG tape may demonstrate arrhythmias.

AV block may be caused by IHD, drugs (eg excess digoxin) or cardiac surgery.

First degree AV block Conduction from atria to ventricles occurs every time, but is delayed. The PR interval is >0.2sec (5 small squares on standard ECG) (Fig. 3.11).

Second degree AV block Only a proportion of P waves are conducted to the ventricles. There are two types:
- *Mobitz type I block (Wenckebach):* the PR interval becomes increasingly lengthened until a P wave fails to conduct (Fig. 3.12).
- *Mobitz type II block:* failure to conduct P waves may occur regularly (eg 3:1) or irregularly, but the PR interval remains constant (Fig. 3.13).

Third degree (complete) heart block Atrial activity is not conducted to ventricles. With a proximal block (eg at the AV node), a proximal escape pacemaker in the AV node or bundle of His may take over, producing narrow QRS complexes at a rate of ≈50/min. With distal AV block, a more distal escape pacemaker results in broad bizarre complexes at a rate of ≈30/min. Ventricular asystole may occur if the escape pacemaker stops discharging, unless a subsidiary pacemaker takes over (Fig. 3.14).

Intraventricular conduction disturbances

The intraventricular conducting system commences as the bundle of His and divides into right and left bundle branches—the latter subdivides further into antero-superior and postero-superior divisions. These two divisions and the right bundle branch are referred to as the 'fascicles'. Blockage of 2 out of 3 fascicles = *bifascicular block*.
- RBBB + left anterior hemiblock causes left axis deviation and RBBB pattern on ECG.
- RBBB + left posterior hemiblock causes right axis deviation and RBBB pattern on ECG.

Trifascicular block is present when bifasicular block is accompanied by a prolonged PR interval. Note that true blockage of all 3 fascicles would cause complete heart block, so 'trifasciular block' represents impending progression to complete heart block.

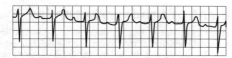

Fig. 3.11 ECG of first degree heart block.

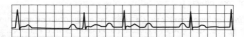

Fig. 3.12 ECG of Mobitz type I AV block.

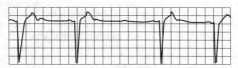

Fig. 3.13 ECG of Mobitz type II AV block.

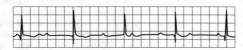

Fig. 3.14 ECG of complete AV block.

Treatment of bradyarrhythmias

The emergency treatment of bradycardia depends upon two important factors: the clinical condition of the patient and the risk of asystole. Give O$_2$, insert an IV cannula and follow the 2010 European Resuscitation Council Guidelines shown opposite (www.resus.org.uk).

Atropine is the first-line drug. The standard dose is 500mcg IV, which may be repeated to a total of 3mg. Further doses are not effective and may result in toxic effects (eg psychosis, urinary retention).

Adrenaline (epinephrine) can be used as a temporizing measure prior to transvenous pacing if an external pacemaker is not available. Give by controlled infusion at 2–10mcg/min, titrating up according to response (6mg adrenaline in 500mL 0.9% saline infused at 10–50mL/hr).

External transcutaneous pacing is available on most defibrillators. It allows a pacing current to be passed between 2 adhesive electrodes placed over the front of the chest and the back. Select external demand pacing mode at a rate of 70/min, then gradually ↑ the pacing current from zero until capture is shown on the monitor. Clinically, capture results in a palpable peripheral pulse at the paced rate and clinical improvement in the patient's condition. Provide small doses of IV opioid ± sedation if the patient finds external pacing very uncomfortable.

Transvenous cardiac pacing is the treatment of choice for bradycardic patients who are at risk of asystole. The technique should only be performed by an experienced doctor. The preferred route of access is the internal jugular or subclavian vein. However, if thrombolysis has recently been given or is contemplated, or if the patient is taking anticoagulants, use the right femoral vein instead. Obtain a CXR to exclude complications. A correctly functioning ventricular pacemaker results in a pacing spike followed by a widened and bizarre QRS (Fig. 3.15).

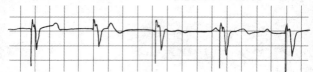

Fig. 3.15 Paced rhythm.

Permanent pacemakers and implantable defibrillators

Increasingly sophisticated implantable devices are being used to manage arrhythmias. Occasionally, a patient will present to the ED with a malfunctioning pacemaker. Get urgent specialist advice. External transcutaneous pacing will provide temporary support whilst the problem is resolved. A special magnet may be needed to inactivate an implantable defibrillator which fires repeatedly.

Algorithm for the management of bradycardia (Fig. 3.16)

See www.resus.org.uk

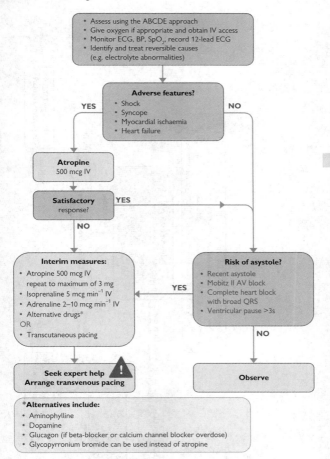

Fig. 3.16 Algorithm for the management of bradycardia.

Tachycardia algorithm—with pulse

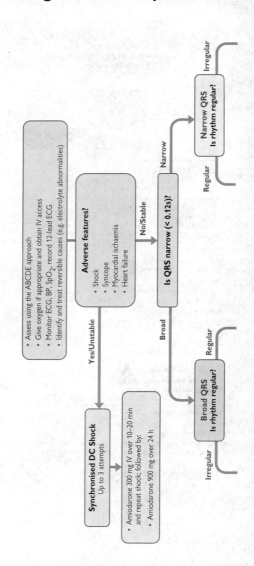

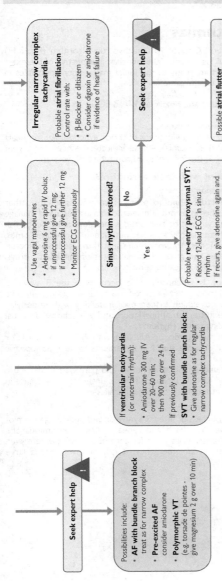

Irregular narrow complex tachycardia

Probable **atrial fibrillation**
Control rate with:
• β-Blocker or diltiazem
• Consider digoxin or amiodarone if evidence of heart failure

Seek expert help

Possible **atrial flutter**
• Control rate (e.g. β-Blocker)

• Use vagal manoeuvres
• Adenosine 6 mg rapid IV bolus; if unsuccessful give 12 mg; if unsuccessful give further 12 mg
• Monitor ECG continuously

Sinus rhythm restored?

No

Yes

Probable **re-entry paroxysmal SVT**:
• Record 12-lead ECG in sinus rhythm
• If recurs, give adenosine again and consider choice of anti-arrhythmic prophylaxis

If **ventricular tachycardia** (or uncertain rhythm):
• Amiodarone 300 mg IV over 20–60 min; then 900 mg over 24 h
If previously confirmed
SVT with bundle branch block:
• Give adenosine as for regular narrow complex tachycardia

Seek expert help

Possibilities include:
• **AF with bundle branch block** treat as for narrow complex
• **Pre-excited AF** consider amiodarone
• **Polymorphic VT** (e.g. torsade de pointes - give magnesium 2 g over 10 min)

Fig. 3.17 Tachycardia algorithm with pulse (www.resus.org.uk).

Tachyarrhythmias

The single Resuscitation Council 2010 tachycardia algorithm (Fig. 3.17) (see www.resus.org.uk) is based on the fact that, irrespective of the exact underlying cardiac rhythm, many of the initial management principles in the peri-arrest setting are the same:

- Rapidly assess ABC.
- Monitor cardiac rhythm and record a 12-lead ECG.
- Provide O_2.
- Identify and treat reversible causes.
- Assess for evidence of instability (signs of shock, syncope, signs of heart failure, or myocardial ischaemia)—these indicate the need for urgent intervention, initially in the form of synchronized cardioversion.

The unstable patient with tachyarrhythmia

Synchronized cardioversion

This requires two doctors—one to perform cardioversion, the other (experienced in anaesthesia) to provide sedation/anaesthesia and manage the airway. The patient will not be fasted and is therefore at particular risk of aspiration. The arrhythmia may ↓ cardiac output and ↑ circulation times, so IV drugs take much longer to work than usual. If the 'sedation doctor' does not appreciate this and gives additional doses of anaesthetic drugs, hypotension and prolonged anaesthesia may result.

Electrical cardioversion is synchronized to occur with the R wave to minimize the risk of inducing VF. Synchronized cardioversion is effective in treating patients who exhibit evidence of instability with underlying rhythms of SVT, atrial flutter, atrial fibrillation, and VT—choose an initial level of energy according to the rhythm:

- For broad complex tachycardia or AF, start with 200J monophasic or 120–150J biphasic. If unsuccessful, ↑ in increments to 360J monophasic or 150J biphasic.
- Start with a lower energy for atrial flutter and paroxysmal SVT—use 100J monophasic or 70–120J biphasic. If this is unsuccessful, increase in increments to 360J monophasic or 150J biphasic.

Amiodarone

If cardioversion is unsuccessful after 3 synchronized shocks, give amiodarone 300mg IV over 10–20min and repeat shock. Give amiodarone by central vein when possible as it causes thrombophlebitis when given peripherally. However, in an emergency, it can be given into a large peripheral vein.

Broad complex tachyarrhythmias

May be caused by VT, or rarely by SVT with aberrant conduction. The default position should be that broad complex tachycardia is VT. Provide O_2 as appropriate, insert an IV cannula and follow the Resuscitation Council guidelines (Fig. 3.17) and (www.resus.org.uk).

The priorities in broad complex arrhythmias associated with tricyclic overdose are airway management, oxygenation, ventilation and correction of metabolic disorders: give IV bicarbonate, but avoid anti-arrhythmic drugs (📖 Tricyclic antidepressant poisoning, p.194).

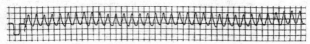

Fig. 3.18

Evaluating ECGs: is it VT or SVT with aberrant conduction?

VT is much more likely as a cause of the broad complex tachycardia if:

- The patient is >60 years.
- The patient has a history of IHD or cardiomyopathy.
- There is clinical evidence of AV dissociation (intermittent cannon 'a' waves seen on jugular venous pressure (JVP), first heart sound of variable intensity).
- Inverted P waves in lead II.
- The frontal plane axis is bizarre (−90° to −180°).
- The QRS is >0.13sec.
- There are 'capture' or 'fusion' beats.
- The QRS is bizarre, not resembling a bundle branch block pattern
- All chest leads ($V_{1–6}$) are concordant (QRS complexes point the same way).
- R>R′ (or r′) in V_1.
- There is a deep S wave (either QS, rS or RS) in V_6.

Torsades de pointes

This is a rare form of polymorphic VT, associated with hypomagnesaemia, hypokalaemia, long QT interval (congenital or drug related, eg sotalol, antipsychotics, antihistamines, antidepressants). A constantly changing electrical axis results in QRS complexes of undulating amplitude. Usually paroxysmal, it may degenerate to VF. Get expert help and treat with IV magnesium sulphate (2g over 10min = 8mmol or 4mL 50% magnesium). Refractory cases may require overdrive pacing.

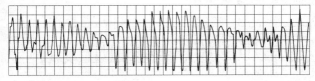

Fig. 3.19

Narrow complex tachyarrhythmias

These are almost always of supraventricular origin. Underlying rhythms include:

- Sinus tachycardia.
- Paroxysmal AV re-entrant tachycardia (often referred to as 'SVT').
- AF with fast ventricular response.
- Atrial flutter.
- Atrial tachycardia.
- Junctional tachycardia.

Give O_2, insert an IV cannula, and follow the algorithm in Fig. 3.17 (www.resus.org.uk). Determine if the rhythm is regular. Treat irregular rhythms (AF) as outlined in Fig. 3.17. If the ventricular rate is exactly 150/min, atrial flutter with 2:1 block is likely (Fig. 3.20).

The compromised patient with shock, syncope, acute cardiac failure, or cardiac ischaemia should be treated with emergency electrical cardioversion. It is reasonable to give IV adenosine while arranging the cardioversion, as long as this does not delay the procedure.

For stable patients consider

Vagal stimulation The most effective way is a Valsalva manoeuvre while supine or tilted head down. Instruct the patient to attempt to blow the plunger out of a 50mL bladder tip syringe. If unsuccessful, in the young patient, massage the carotid sinus for 15sec (1 side only), by gently rubbing in a circular action lateral to the upper border of the thyroid cartilage. Carotid sinus massage may be dangerous (especially if there is a carotid bruit or previous stroke/TIA).

Adenosine This temporarily blocks conduction through the AV node. It has a very short half-life (10–15sec). Adenosine can successfully terminate re-entrant tachycardias and may 'unmask' other conditions (eg atrial flutter) by temporarily producing a conduction block. It is contraindicated in 2° or 3° AV block, patients with WPW and asthmatics. The effects are blocked by theophylline and potentiated markedly (and dangerously) in the presence of dipyridamole, carbamazepine or in a denervated heart—seek advice. Warn the patient about transient flushing and chest discomfort. Give adenosine by fast bolus 6mg IV injection into an IV cannula in the antecubital fossa and flush with 0.9% saline (Fig. 3.17) while recording a rhythm strip. If unsuccessful, repeat with 12mg, then 12mg.

If adenosine is contra-indicated, consider IV *verapamil* 2.5–5mg over 2min. Avoid verapamil in patients with cardiac failure, hypotension, concomitant β-blocker therapy, or WPW.

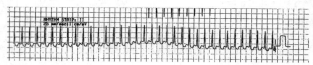

Fig. 3.20 Narrow complex tachycardia.

Atrial fibrillation

Atrial fibrillation is rapid, irregular, uncoordinated atrial activity, and is associated with an irregular ventricular response.

Causes

Acute AF may be associated with: IHD (33%), heart failure (24%), hypertension (26%), and valvular heart disease (7%). *Other cardiac causes* are sick sinus syndrome, pericarditis, infiltrative heart disease, cardiomyopathy, myocarditis, congenital heart disease, and post-cardiac surgery.

Non-cardiac causes include: sepsis, PE, thyrotoxicosis, electrocution, lung or pleural disease, chest trauma, hypokalaemia, hypovolaemia, hypothermia, drug abuse (eg cocaine). Paroxysmal AF sometimes occurs in fit athletes.

Holiday heart: binge drinking or occasionally alcohol withdrawal may cause acute AF in patients with no other predisposing factors. AF usually resolves spontaneously within 48hr. The diagnosis of 'holiday heart' is one of exclusion after cardiac disease and other causes have been ruled out.

Clinical features

AF ↓ cardiac output by 10–20%, irrespective of underlying ventricular rate. Clinical presentation varies according to the cause and effect of the AF. Some patients are asymptomatic; others suffer life-threatening complications (heart failure, angina). Patients with underlying IHD may develop ischaemia during periods of rapid ventricular rate.

Treatment

Patients in AF can be treated with cardioversion or rate control. If signs of shock, syncope, acute cardiac failure, or ischaemia are present, consider electrical cardioversion under sedation. Patients may also be chemically cardioverted with flecainide 50–150mg IV (contraindicated in patients with cardiac disease) or amiodarone 300mg IV (safer in patients with cardiac disease). Both drugs may cause hypotension. If the patient has had symptoms for longer than 48hr, they are at risk of cardiac thromboembolism and stroke when cardioverted, so instead, give rate control medications and commence IV or low molecular weight heparin. Rate control drugs include metoprolol 5mg IV and diltiazem (IV form not available in UK). Digoxin 500mcg IV is the drug of choice in patients with CCF. See 2006 NICE guidelines (www.nice.org.uk).

Atrial fibrillation in Wolff Parkinson White syndrome

This may result in an irregular, broad complex tachycardia. Impulses are conducted from the atria via the AV node and an accessory pathway. Do not give AV-blocking drugs (digoxin, verapamil, or adenosine) as this can result in acceleration of conduction through the accessory pathway, leading to cardiovascular collapse or VF. Seek expert help.

Atrial flutter

The typical atrial rate is 300/min, so a regular 2:1 block will give a QRS rate of 150/min. Variable block may result in an irregular rate. Consult with an expert to discuss treatment.

Hypertensive problems

Bear the following points in mind when managing a hypertensive patient in the ED:
- Most patients with hypertension are asymptomatic.
- Hypertension is an important risk factor for cardiovascular disease and stroke.
- Most patients found to be hypertensive in the ED do not require any immediate intervention or treatment, but do require careful follow-up—usually by their GP.
- Never intervene on the basis of a single raised BP measurement in the absence of any associated symptoms and signs.

Approach

Approach patients found to be hypertensive as follows:
- Those with no previous history of hypertension, and no other concerns or history of other conditions (eg diabetes, peripheral vascular disease, IHD, or stroke)—arrange follow-up and monitoring with GP.
- Those known to be hypertensive already on treatment—arrange follow-up and monitoring with GP.
- Those displaying evidence of end organ damage (eg LV hypertrophy, retinal changes, renal impairment)—refer to the medical team.
- Those with hypertension associated with pain, vasoconstriction (eg acute pulmonary oedema) or stroke—treat underlying cause where possible. Do not intervene in stroke associated hypertension except under the direction of a neurologist or stroke specialist.
- Those with hypertension directly associated with symptoms or signs—contact the medical team and consider whether intervention is appropriate (see below).

Mild/moderate hypertension (diastolic 100–125mmHg)

Ascertain if the patient has a past history of hypertension and is taking drug therapy for this. Examine for retinal changes and evidence of hypertensive encephalopathy. Investigate as appropriate (U&E, urinalysis, CXR, ECG). Further management will depend upon the BP and the exact circumstances. If the BP is moderately elevated (ie diastolic BP: 110–125mmHg) and the patient is symptomatic, refer to the medical team. If the patient is asymptomatic with normal examination and renal function, he/she may be suitable for GP follow up.

Severe hypertension (diastolic >125mmHg)

Patients with a diastolic BP >125mmHg require urgent assessment. Search for evidence of *hypertensive encephalopathy*: headache, nausea, vomiting, confusion, retinal changes (haemorrhages, exudates, papilloedema), fits, focal neurological signs, ↓ conscious level. Ask about recent drug ingestion (eg ecstasy or cocaine—🕮 pp. 214 & 215).

Investigations

Insert an IV cannula and send blood for U&E, creatinine, and glucose. Obtain a CXR and ECG, and perform urinalysis. If there is ↓ conscious level, focal signs, or other clinical suspicion that the hypertension may be secondary to stroke or intracranial haemorrhage, arrange an emergency CT scan.

Management

- Refer patients with a diastolic pressure >125mmHg or evidence of hypertensive encephalopathy to the medical team. Resist commencing emergency treatment until consultation with an expert. There is a significant risk of complications (stroke or MI) if the BP is reduced rapidly. It may be appropriate to commence oral antihypertensive therapy using a β-blocker (eg atenolol or labetalol) or calcium channel blocker (eg nifedipine).
- If treatment is appropriate, commence an IVI of sodium nitroprusside, labetalol or GTN with continuous BP monitoring via an arterial line and admit to high dependency unit (HDU) or ICU. Sodium nitroprusside has a very short half-life (≈1–2min) and acts as a vasodilator of both arterioles and veins. IV labetolol may be preferred if aortic dissection (🕮 p.92) or phaeochromocytoma are suspected.
- Beta-blockers are contraindicated in hypertension caused by cocaine, amphetamine or related sympathomimetic drugs (🕮 p.215), since β-blockade may cause unopposed α-adrenergic activity with paradoxical hypertension and ↓ coronary blood flow.

Hypertension in pregnancy

Hypertension may be part of pre-eclampsia or eclampsia (see 🕮 p.592). Pre-eclampsia is diagnosed with 2 or more of: hypertension (>140/90), proteinuria and oedema. This can be associated with haemolysis, elevated liver function tests (LFTs), low platelets (HELLP syndrome). Check urine for protein and check blood for FBC, LFT, platelets, and coagulation screen. Call for senior obstetric help. Eclampsia is diagnosed with the onset of grand mal seizures after 20 weeks gestation, and carries a significant mortality rate.

Aortic dissection

Remember: hypertensive patients with sudden, severe chest, and/or back pain may have acute aortic dissection.

Pathology

Aortic dissection is longitudinal splitting of the muscular aortic media by a column of blood. The dissection may spread proximally (possibly resulting in aortic incompetence, coronary artery blockage, cardiac tamponade), distally (possibly involving the origin of various arteries), or rupture internally back into the aortic lumen, or externally (eg into the mediastinum, resulting in rapid exsanguination).

More than 70% of patients have a history of hypertension. It occurs more frequently in those with bicuspid aortic valve, Marfan's syndrome or Ehlers–Danlos syndrome. Up to 20% follow recent cardiac surgery or recent angiography/angioplasty.

Dissection may be classified Stanford type 'A' or 'B', according to whether the ascending aorta is involved or not, respectively. Overall mortality is 30% (35% type A and 15% type B).

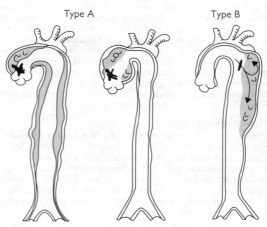

Fig. 3.21

History

Aortic dissection may mimic the presentation of an MI, requiring a high index of suspicion. It typically presents with abrupt onset sharp, tearing or ripping pain (maximal at onset) in anterior or posterior chest. Migration of the pain may reflect extension of the dissection. Syncope occurs in ≈10% of patients, sometimes in the absence of any pain. Occasionally, patients can present with neurological deficit associated with chest pain.

Examination

The patient is usually apprehensive and distressed, with pain which is difficult to alleviate, even using IV opioid. Clues to the diagnosis include:
- An aortic regurgitation murmur (30%).
- Asymmetry or absence of peripheral pulses or a pulse deficit (15–20%).
- Hypertension.
- Hypotension with features of tamponade or neurological signs in association with pain (eg secondary to spinal/carotid artery involvement).

Investigations

- Send blood for U&E, glucose, FBC, coagulation, and cross-matching.
- Obtain an ECG and CXR.

Thoracic aortic dissection usually results in an abnormal CXR. One or more of the following changes may be seen:
- A widened or abnormal mediastinum (present in ≈75%).
- A 'double knuckle' aorta.
- Left pleural effusion (≈20%).
- Deviation of the trachea or nasogastric (NG) tube to the right.
- Separation of two parts of the wall of a calcified aorta by >5mm (the 'calcium sign').

The ECG may demonstrate MI, LVH. or ischaemia.

Note that ≈12% of patients with aortic dissection have a normal CXR and ≈30% have a normal ECG.

CT angiography or formal angiography will provide the definitive diagnosis. In a haemodynamically unstable patient, trans-oesophageal echo in theatre may be the investigation of choice.

Management

On suspicion of aortic dissection:
- Provide O_2 by face mask as appropriate.
- Insert 2 large-bore (14G) IV cannulae and cross-match for 6U (inform blood bank of suspected diagnosis).
- Give IV morphine and titrate according to response (± anti-emetic).
- Call cardiothoracic team and cardiologist at an early stage.
- Insert an arterial line (preferably right radial artery) and discuss with specialist teams how to control the BP (eg labetalol infusion).
- Arrange further investigation based upon specialist advice and available resources (eg aortography, echocardiography, CT scan, MRI).

Type A dissections are usually treated surgically; type B lesions are usually treated medically.

Haemoptysis

Haemoptysis may be the chief or sole complaint of patients presenting to the ED. It always warrants investigation.

Causes of haemoptysis

Respiratory	• Infection (URTI, pneumonia, TB, lung abscess) • Carcinoma (bronchial or laryngeal) • Bronchiectasis
Cardiovascular	• Pulmonary oedema • PE • Ruptured aortic aneurysm (aorto-bronchial fistula)
Coagulation disorder	• Drugs (eg warfarin, heparin) • Inherited (eg Haemophilia, Christmas disease)
Trauma	• Penetrating or blunt
Other	• Goodpasture's, Wegener's granulomatosis

Presentation

Ascertain the exact nature and volume (eg 'bright red streaks' or 'dark brown granules'). Patients sometimes have surprising difficulty distinguishing vomited blood from that coughed up. Enquire about weight loss, and take a drug history and smoking history.

Investigation

- Send blood for FBC, coagulation screen, U&E, LFTs.
- Request Group and Save if evidence of significant haemorrhage.
- If SpO_2 <94% on air, or the patient has COPD, check ABG.
- Obtain CXR and ECG.
- Perform urinalysis—if shocked, insert catheter and monitor output.
- Collect sputum samples. Send for microscopy, culture, and sensitivity.
- Initiate further investigations according to the likely diagnosis.

Treatment

- *Airway*: clear and secure (coughing/suction). Put on a face mask and shield if maintaining the airway or intubating. Ensure nearby high flow suction. Massive haemorrhage may require tracheal intubation. Whilst preparing for this, tilt trolley so that the patient is head-down.
- *Breathing*: provide O_2 to maintain saturations at 94–98%. If ventilation is inadequate, assist with bag and mask or tracheal tube.
- *Circulation*: insert a large bore (14G) IV cannula (use 2 if hypovolaemic). Give IV fluids/blood/clotting factors as clinically indicated (p.172).

Further treatment

Commence specific treatment measures aimed at life-threatening underlying cause (eg LVF, PE, infection, coagulopathy). In cases of large haemoptysis, it is appropriate to admit for further investigation and treatment. If the patient is stable and has only had a small amount of blood stained sputum, urgent outpatient investigation may be appropriate.

Oxygen

Oxygen is the most commonly administered hospital therapy. In recent years, high flow oxygen was widely used in the treatment of medical and surgical emergencies, and initial resuscitation. There is now a move towards safer treatment with controlled oxygen therapy.

Common problems
- Failure to prescribe oxygen.
- Failure to check ABG in patients requiring oxygen therapy.
- Failure to monitor or review patients on oxygen therapy.
- Inadvertent administration of another gas other than oxygen.
- Inadvertent disconnection from the oxygen supply.
- Depletion of an oxygen tank during transfer (www.nrls.npsa.nhs.uk).

Oxygen cylinders
When administering oxygen in the ED, always use piped oxygen from the wall outlet. Only use an oxygen cylinder when transporting the patient to the radiology department or ward. Oxygen is highly flammable. Do not take a cylinder out of its support cage and never let it fall. In the UK, oxygen cylinders are colour-coded white. The commonest small cylinder is B (or M-6), which holds 170L oxygen. The commonest large cylinder is E (or M-24), holding 680L. Before a patient leaves the ED, always check that the cylinder is full. If the patient is being transferred to another hospital, check there is enough oxygen for the journey. The formula is:

Volume of cylinder in L/flow rate = minutes cylinder will last

Oxygen requirements
The aim of oxygen therapy is to optimize tissue oxygen delivery. Use pulse oximetry to guide whether the patient requires supplemental oxygen. In previously healthy patients, aim for SpO_2 94–98%, but in patients with known COPD or type II respiratory failure, aim for SpO_2 88–92%. Always take an ABG in patients with chronic lung disease, to assess their optimal oxygen treatment (see 📖 p.98 on ABG interpretation). Repeat the ABG within 30 min after changing the inspired oxygen concentration. When assessing a critically ill patient, it is appropriate to give high flow oxygen and to titrate the inspired oxygen concentration (FiO_2) down according to the ABG results.

Oxygen delivery
- Use a high concentration oxygen reservoir mask (non-rebreathing mask) in hypoxic patients without chronic lung disease.
- Use a simple face mask for patients with a mild hypoxia, without chronic lung disease.
- Use a 28% Venturi mask for patients with COPD or known type II respiratory failure.
- Use a tracheostomy mask for patients with tracheostomy.

Prescribing oxygen
The oxygen prescription should include the target SpO_2, the oxygen mask type and oxygen flow rate. In an emergency, it is appropriate to administer oxygen prior to prescribing, but do not forget to prescribe the oxygen after resuscitation. See www.brit-thoracic.org.uk.

The dyspnoeic patient

The normal adult respiratory rate is 11–18/min, with a tidal volume of 400–800mL. Acute dyspnoea is a common presenting symptom.

Common causes of acute dyspnoea

Cardiac
- Cardiogenic pulmonary oedema (📖 p.100).
- MI (📖 p.68).
- PE (📖 p.120).
- Arrhythmias (📖 p.80).

Respiratory
- Asthma (📖 p.104) or exacerbation of COPD (📖 p.108).
- Pneumonia (📖 p.110).
- Pleural effusion (📖 p.103).
- Pneumothorax (📖 p.114).

Trauma
- Aspiration of FB or vomit (📖 p.112).
- Pneumothorax/haemothorax (📖 p.334).
- Flail chest (📖 p.332).
- Drowning incident (📖 p.258).

Other
- Hypovolaemia or fever from any cause.
- Hyperventilation syndrome (📖 p.97).
- Respiratory compensation for metabolic acidosis (DKA, salicylate overdose).

Approach

Follow the ABC approach and resuscitate as necessary. The main aim of treatment is to correct life-threatening hypoxia. Enquire about speed of onset of dyspnoea, past medical history and associated symptoms (cough, haemoptysis, fever, wheezing, chest pain). Examine carefully, paying attention to the respiratory rate, depth, and pattern. Apply a pulse oximeter.

Pulse oximetry

This is simple, rapid, safe, and non-invasive, but it does *not* provide information about ventilation or arterial partial pressure of carbon dioxide (pCO_2). A normal oxygen saturation does not exclude significant lung pathology (eg PE). Pulse oximetry may be inaccurate or misleading in:
- Poor peripheral perfusion/shock.
- Methaemoglobinaemia.
- Hypothermia.
- CO poisoning (see 📖 p.208). SpO_2 values may be falsely high as COHb reads as oxyhaemoglobin. COHb can be measured on venous blood gas testing or COHb pulse oximeter.
- Nail varnish/synthetic fingernails (if a finger probe is used).
- Excessive movement.

Correlate readings with clinical findings: a non-pulsatile trace (or heart rate different from that on cardiac monitor) suggests the saturation reading is probably inaccurate.

Hyperventilation

Hyperventilation is breathing which occurs more deeply and/or more rapidly than normal. CO_2 is 'blown off ', so that pCO_2 ↓. Hyperventilation may be primary ('psychogenic') or secondary. A classical secondary cause is DKA—Kussmaul's respiration represents respiratory compensation for a metabolic acidosis.

Secondary causes of hyperventilation

- Metabolic acidosis (eg DKA, uraemia, sepsis, hepatic failure).
- Poisoning (eg aspirin, methanol, CO, cyanide, ethylene glycol).
- Pain/hypoxia.
- Hypovolaemia.
- Respiratory disorders (eg PE, asthma, pneumothorax).

Primary (psychogenic or inappropriate) hyperventilation

Typically, the patient is agitated and distressed with a past history of panic attacks or episodes of hyperventilation. They may complain of dizziness, circumoral paraesthesia, carpopedal spasm, and occasionally sharp or stabbing chest pain. Initial examination reveals tachypnoea with equal air entry over both lung fields, and no wheeze or evidence of airway obstruction. It is important to consider secondary causes (such as PE or DKA). Therefore, perform the following investigations:

- SpO_2.
- ECG.
- ABG if SpO_2 ↓, or if symptoms do not completely settle in a few minutes.
- BMG.

If symptoms do not completely settle in a few minutes, obtain:

- CXR.
- U&E, blood glucose, FBC.

Treatment

Do not sedate a patient who is hyperventilating. Once serious diagnoses have been excluded, use this information to help reassure the patient with primary hyperventilation. Often this is all that is required, but it may be helpful to try simple breathing exercises (breathe in through nose—count of 8, out through mouth—count of 8, hold for count of 4 and repeat). Discharge the patient with arrangements for GP follow-up. If these simple measures fail, reconsider the diagnosis and refer the patient to the medical team for subsequent observation and treatment.

Arterial blood gases

Blood gas sampling is useful in assessing breathless patients, septic patients, diabetic patients in ketoacidosis, those who are critically ill and patients who have ingested poisons. This enables rapid measurement of blood pH, bicarbonate, O_2 and CO_2. Most ED blood gas analysers will also measure blood glucose, K^+, Hb, and lactate, so arterial or venous blood gas sampling will also test for anaemia, hyperkalaemia, and hypoglycaemia.

Assessing respiratory function

Arterial sampling helps in the assessment of a patient with low SpO_2, or in patients with known lung disease (especially if they are receiving supplemental oxygen). If possible (caution required), take the first sample with the patient breathing room air. If this is not possible, document the inspired oxygen concentration. Look specifically for:

- Hypoxia, (pO_2 <10.6kPa on air).
- Hypercarbia, (pCO_2 >6.0kPa).
- Bicarbonate retention (HCO_3^- >28mmol/L).
- Acidosis (pH <7.35).

Differentiating between type I and type II respiratory failure

In type I failure there is hypoxia with normal or ↓ pCO_2. In type II failure, there is hypoxia with ↑ pCO_2, and frequently an ↑ HCO_3^-. In type II failure, the patient may develop life-threatening respiratory failure if administered high concentrations of oxygen. Aim to maintain SpO_2 at 88–92%, and recheck ABGs in 30min.

Differentiating between acute and chronic type II respiratory failure

Patients who normally have a slightly ↑ pCO_2 will also show ↑ HCO_3^- on ABG. The kidneys adapt over a period of days to retain bicarbonate, in attempt to buffer the respiratory acidosis (see nomogram inside front cover). Respiratory acidosis in a patient with chronic type II respiratory failure (↑ pCO_2, ↑ HCO_3^- and pH <7.35) indicates life-threatening impairment of lung function.

In acute respiratory failure, the lungs are unable to eliminate CO_2 (caused by ↓ GCS or hypoventilation from any cause), which results in ↑ pCO_2 and a respiratory acidosis. Patients may require ventilatory support.

A venous blood sample will give accurate readings for K^+, lactate, glucose, HCO_3^-, Hb and COHb. In addition, a normal venous pCO_2 will exclude hypercarbia.

Other blood gas results

Blood gas analysers calculate the base excess from the HCO_3^- concentration and pH. Levels <−2mmol/L indicate that the patient has a metabolic acidosis. Levels >2mmol/L indicate a metabolic alkalosis (for example, as a result of chronic bicarbonate retention in type II respiratory failure).

Metabolic acidosis

The usual pattern of results in metabolic acidosis is pH<7.35, HCO_3^- <24mmol/L and BE <−2mmol/L. There may be compensatory hypocarbia (pCO_2<4.5kPa). Metabolic acidosis has many possible causes:

- ↑ Acid load (lactic acidosis, ketoacidosis, or ingestion of salicylates, methanol, ethylene glycol, or metformin.
- ↓ Removal of acid (renal failure or renal tubular acidosis types 1 and 4).
- Loss of bicarbonate from the body (diarrhoea, pancreatic, or intestinal fistulas, acetazolamide, or renal tubular acidosis type 2).

The anion gap

The anion gap is the quantity of anions not balanced out by cations, (a measurement of negatively charged plasma proteins). The normal value is 12–16mmol/L. It is measured by:

$$(Na^+ + K^+) - (Cl^- + HCO_3^-) \text{ all measured in mmol/L}$$

Measuring the anion gap helps distinguish the cause of a metabolic acidosis. A high anion gap indicates that there is excess H^+ in the body. The commonest cause of a high anion gap metabolic acidosis is lactic acidosis. Most blood gas analysers will measure lactate (normal <2.0mmol/L).

Causes of a lactic acidosis

- Tissue hypoperfusion (trauma with major haemorrhage, septic shock).
- Tissue hypoxia (hypoxaemia, carbon monoxide or cyanide poisoning).
- Hepatic failure.
- Renal failure.
- Ethylene glycol or methanol poisoning (📖 p.203; 📖 p.202).
- Cocaine or amphetamines (📖 p.215).
- Salicylate poisoning (📖 p.189) or iron poisoning (📖 p.201).
- Biguanides (metformin).
- Isoniazid.
- Strenuous exercise.

The other causes of a high anion gap metabolic acidosis are *ketoacidosis* (diabetic or alcohol induced) and renal failure.

Causes of a normal anion gap metabolic acidosis are chronic diarrhoea, pancreatic or intestinal fistulas, acetazolamide, or renal tubular acidosis.

The osmolal gap

This is the difference between calculated serum osmolarity and laboratory measured serum osmolality. Serum osmolarity can be calculated by:

$$(2 \times Na^+) + urea + glucose \text{ (all measured in mmol/L)}$$

Subtract the calculated result from the laboratory measured osmolality to give the osmolal gap. Normally this is <10mOsm/kg.

An elevated osmolal gap can be caused by alcohol, methanol, ethylene glycol or acetone ingestion, mannitol, or sorbitol.

Cardiogenic pulmonary oedema

Left heart failure results in ↑ left ventricular end-diastolic pressure, causing ↑ pulmonary capillary hydrostatic pressure. Fluid collects in extravascular pulmonary tissues faster than the lymphatics clear it.

Causes of cardiogenic pulmonary oedema

Often an acute complication of MI and IHD, or exacerbation of pre-existing cardiac disease (eg hypertension, aortic/mitral valve disease). Other causes are:
- Arrhythmias.
- Failure of prosthetic heart valve.
- Ventricular septal defect.
- Cardiomyopathy.
- Negatively inotropic drugs (eg β-blockers).
- Acute myocarditis.
- Left atrial (LA) myxoma (may produce syncope, fever, ↑ ESR, but is very rare).
- Pericardial disease.

The history is frequently dramatic. Dyspnoea and distress may prevent a full history from being taken. Find out the length of the history and whether there is any chest pain. Check current drug therapy/allergies and establish what emergency prehospital treatment has been administered.

Examination usually reveals a tachypnoeic, tachycardic, and anxious patient. If the pulmonary oedema is severe, the patient may be cyanosed, coughing up frothy pink sputum and unable to talk. Check pulse and BP, auscultate the heart for murmurs, and 3rd/4th heart sounds of gallop rhythm. Look for ↑ JVP (also a feature of PE and cardiac tamponade). Listen to the lung fields—fine inspiratory crepitations (crackles) may be limited to the bases or be widespread. Wheeze may be more prominent than crepitations. Cardiogenic pulmonary oedema is associated with evidence of ↓ cardiac output (sweaty, peripherally cool, and pale). Consider other diagnoses (eg sepsis) in patients with warm, flushed extremities.

Investigation

Commence treatment before completing investigations:
- Attach a cardiac monitor and check SpO_2 with pulse oximeter.
- Obtain ECG. Check for arrhythmias, LAD, LVH, LBBB, recent or evolving MI.
- Send blood for U&E, glucose, FBC, troponin.
- If severely ill or SpO_2<94% in air obtain ABG.
- Request old hospital notes/ECGs.
- Obtain a CXR and look for features of cardiogenic pulmonary oedema:
  - upper lobe diversion (distension of upper pulmonary veins)
  - cardiomegaly (LV and/or LA dilatation)
  - Kerley A, B, or C septal lines
  - fluid in interlobar fissures
  - peribronchial/perivascular cuffing and micronodules
  - pleural effusions
  - bat's wing hilar shadows.

Treat urgently. Provide the following within the first few minutes:
- Check that the airway is clear.
- Raise the back of the trolley to sit the patient up and support with pillows if necessary.
- Provide high flow O_2 by tight-fitting face mask.
- If systolic BP >90mmHg, give 2 puffs of GTN SL (800mcg) and commence GTN IVI, starting at 10mcg/min, ↑ every few minutes according to clinical response (monitor BP closely; take special care to avoid hypotension). Alternatively try buccal GTN (3–5mg).
- Give IV furosemide 50mg. Larger doses may be needed in patients already taking oral furosemide.
- If the patient has chest pain or is distressed, give very small titrated increments of IV opioid (with anti-emetic). Do not give opioids to patients who are drowsy, confused. or exhausted as this may precipitate respiratory arrest.
- Consider inserting a urinary catheter and monitor urine output.
- Treat underlying cause and associated problems (arrhythmias, MI, cardiogenic shock, acute prosthetic valve failure).

Monitor the SpO_2 and the clinical response to this initial treatment. Rapid improvement may occur, due to venodilatation and reduction of preload. If the patient does not improve, recheck ABG and consider:
- Non-invasive ventilation (continuous positive airway pressure (CPAP) or bilevel positive airway pressure (BiPAP). Non-invasive ventilation (NIV) appears safe in acute cardiogenic pulmonary oedema and may avoid the need for intubation.
- If hypotensive refer to ICU for treatment of cardiogenic shock (📖 p.77). An intra-arterial line, Swan–Ganz catheter and inotropic support (dobutamine) are likely to be required. Echocardiography may help to exclude valve or septal rupture and guide treatment.
- Rapid sequence intubation in the presence of cardiogenic pulmonary oedema may be associated with cardiovascular collapse. Stop nitrates prior to administering anaesthesia and be ready to give pressors ± fluids immediately post-induction.

Prosthetic valve failure

Always consider valve failure in patients with prosthetic valves, of which a large variety are in common use. All are associated with some risks (eg embolism, failure, obstruction, infection, haemorrhage from associated anticoagulation), which vary according to design. Acute failure of a prosthetic aortic or mitral valve results in dramatic acute onset pulmonary oedema with loud murmurs. The patient may deteriorate rapidly and not respond to standard drug treatment. Resuscitate as described above. CXR will show a prosthetic heart valve ± pulmonary oedema. Call urgently for expert help (ICU team, cardiologist, and cardiothoracic surgeon). Emergency transthoracic or transoesophageal echocardiography confirms the diagnosis. Immediate valve replacement is required.

Non-cardiogenic pulmonary oedema

Pulmonary oedema may occur in the absence of ↑ pulmonary venous pressure. The following mechanisms may be responsible:
- ↑ Capillary permeability.
- ↓ Plasma oncotic pressure.
- ↑ Lymphatic pressure.

Changes in capillary permeability, secondary to a variety of triggers, is the mechanism most frequently implicated in non-cardiogenic pulmonary oedema, when it occurs as the Adult Respiratory Distress Syndrome (ARDS). Since the mechanisms producing cardiogenic and non-cardiogenic pulmonary oedema differ, so the approach to treatment differs.

Causes of non-cardiogenic pulmonary oedema
- ARDS (sequel to sepsis, trauma, pancreatitis).
- Intracranial (especially subarachnoid) haemorrhage.
- IV fluid overload.
- Hypoalbuminaemia (liver failure, nephrotic syndrome).
- Drugs/poisons/chemical inhalation.
- Lymphangitis carcinomatosis.
- Smoke inhalation.
- Near drowning incidents.
- High altitude mountain sickness.

Approach

Distinguishing non-cardiogenic from cardiogenic pulmonary oedema is usually apparent from the history. Evaluate the patient and resuscitate according to ABCs. Direct treatment towards the underlying cause and according to the physiological disturbance. To estimate the latter, invasive monitoring may be required (urinary, intra-arterial, central venous and pulmonary artery catheters). Involve ICU early and provide appropriate IV fluids, inotropes, tracheal intubation, IPPV and positive end expiratory pressure (PEEP) as required.

Pleural effusion

Under normal circumstances, each pleural cavity contains <20mL fluid.

Causes

An exudate is diagnosed if the pleural fluid:serum protein >0.5, fluid:serum LDH >0.6, or fluid LDH >2/3 the upper limits of laboratory normal value for serum LDH.

Exudates
- Pneumonia (bacterial, viral, mycoplasma).
- Malignancy (bronchial carcinoma, mesothelioma, lymphoma).
- TB.
- PE with pulmonary infarction.
- Collagen vascular disease (SLE, rheumatoid arthritis).
- Subphrenic abscess.
- Amoebic liver abscess.
- Pancreatitis.
- Chylothorax (thoracic duct injury—rare).

Transudates
- Cardiac failure.
- Nephrotic syndrome.
- Hepatic failure.
- Ovarian hyperstimulation.
- Ovarian fibroma (Meig's syndrome—rare).
- Peritoneal dialysis.

Clinical presentation

Symptoms are usually due to the underlying disease process. A mild dull ache and dyspnoea (initially on exercise, later at rest) may occur if the effusion is large. A history of vomiting followed by chest pain points to a ruptured oesophagus—a surgical emergency.

Signs of an effusion are not apparent until >500mL are present. Dyspnoea, stony dullness to percussion, with absent breath sounds over the effusion are characteristic. Bronchial breathing may be heard just above the effusion. Very large unilateral effusions may produce evidence of mediastinal shift (away from the collection of fluid).

Investigations

CXR can demonstrate pleural effusions as small as 250mL, as blunting of the costophrenic angle. Other investigations depend on likely cause.

Treatment

Provide O_2 and resuscitate as necessary, according to the underlying pathology. Emergency therapeutic pleural aspiration is rarely required in the ED, except where haemothorax is suspected. Refer to the medical team for further investigation (including ultrasound guided diagnostic pleural aspiration).

Acute asthma: assessment

Follow the British Thoracic Society guidelines (www.brit-thoracic.org.uk) to assess and manage adults presenting with asthma, 📖 p.106. The guidelines reflect continuing concern over asthma deaths. Patients with severe asthma and one or more adverse psychosocial factors (psychiatric illness, alcohol or drug abuse, unemployment) have ↑ mortality. Measure the peak expiratory flow rate and compare it against that expected (see Fig. 3.22). The peak flow acts as an immediate triage tool: remember that patients with life-threatening asthma may be too dyspnoeic to do this.

Make an initial assessment of the severity of acute asthma based upon a combination of clinical features, peak flow measurement and pulse oximetry as outlined below.

Moderate exacerbation of asthma
- Increasing symptoms.
- Peak flow 50–75% best or predicted.
- No features of acute severe asthma (below).

Acute severe asthma
Any 1 of:
- Inability to complete sentences in 1 breath.
- Respiratory rate ≥25/min.
- Heart rate ≥110/min.
- Peak flow 33–50% best or predicted.

Life-threatening asthma
A patient with severe asthma with any 1 of:
- Cyanosis.
- Exhaustion, confusion, coma.
- Feeble respiratory effort.
- SpO_2<92%.
- Silent chest.
- Bradycardia, arrhythmia, hypotension.
- pO_2<8kPa.
- Normal pCO_2 (4.6–6.0kPa).
- Peak flow <33% best or predicted.

Near fatal asthma
- ↑ pCO_2 and/or requiring mechanical ventilation with ↑ inflation pressures.

Other investigations
Obtain *ABG* if SpO_2<92% or if there are other features of life-threatening asthma.

Obtain a CXR (without delaying treatment) if there is:
- Suspected pneumomediastinum or pneumothorax.
- Suspected consolidation.
- Life-threatening asthma.
- Failure to respond to treatment satisfactorily.
- Requirement for ventilation.

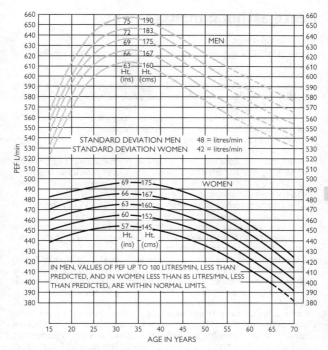

Fig. 3.22 Peak expiratory flow rates in normal adults.
Nunn AJ, Gregg I. (1989). New regression equations for predicting peak expiratory flow in adults. *Br Med J* **298**: 1068–70.

Acute asthma: management

Initial treatment

Follow BTS/SIGN guidelines (www.brit-thoracic.org.uk) summarized as follows:

- Provide high flow O_2.
- Put the trolley back and side rails up so the patient is sitting up and holding on to the side rails (to use pectoral muscles as accessory muscles of respiration).
- If the patient cannot talk, start treatment, but get senior ED and ICU help in case intubation and ventilation are required.
- Check trachea and chest signs for pneumothorax.
- Ask about previous admissions to ICU.
- Administer high dose nebulized β_2 agonist (eg salbutamol 5mg or terbutaline 10mg), or 10 puffs of salbutamol into spacer device and face mask. For severe asthma or asthma that reponds poorly to the initial nebulizer, consider continuous nebulization.
- Give a corticosteroid: either prednisolone 40–50mg PO or hydrocortisone (preferably as sodium succinate) 100mg IV.
- Add nebulized ipratropium bromide (500mcg) to β_2 agonist treatment for patients with acute severe or life-threatening asthma or those with a poor initial response to β_2 agonist therapy.
- Consider a single dose of IV magnesium sulphate (1.2–2g IVI over 20min) after consultation with senior medical staff, for patients with acute severe asthma without a good initial response to inhaled bronchodilator therapy or for those with life-threatening or near-fatal asthma.
- Use IV aminophylline only after consultation with senior medical staff. Some individual patients with near-fatal or life-threatening asthma with a poor response to initial therapy may gain additional benefit. The loading dose of IVI aminophylline is 5mg/kg over 20min unless on maintenance therapy, in which case check blood theophylline level and start IVI of aminophylline at 0.5–0.7mg/kg/hr.
- IV salbutamol is an alternative in severe asthma, after consultation with senior staff. Draw up 5mg salbutamol into 500mL 5% dextrose and run at a rate of 30–60mL/hr.
- A patient who cannot talk will be unable to drink fluids and may be dehydrated.
- Avoid 'routine' antibiotics.
- Repeat ABG within an hour.
- Hypokalaemia may be caused or exacerbated by β_2 agonist and/or steroid therapy.

Criteria for admission

Admit patients with any features of
• A life-threatening or near-fatal attack.
• Severe attack persisting after initial treatment.

Management of discharge

Consider for discharge those patients whose peak flow is >75% best or predicted 1hr after initial treatment. Prescribe a short course of oral prednisolone (eg 40–50mg for 5 days) if initial peak expiratory flow rate (PEFR) <50%, and ensure adequate supply of inhalers. If possible arrange for review by an asthma liaison nurse before discharge. At a minimum, inhaler technique and peak expiratory flow monitoring should be reviewed. Arrange/advise GP/asthma liaison nurse follow-up within 2 days. Fax or email the discharge summary to GP. Advise to return to hospital if symptoms worsen/recur.

Referral to intensive care unit

Refer any patient requiring ventilatory support or with acute severe or life-threatening asthma failing to respond to therapy, evidenced by:
• Drowsiness, confusion.
• Exhaustion, feeble respiration.
• Coma or respiratory arrest.
• Persisting or worsening hypoxia.
• Hypercapnoea.
• ABG showing ↓ pH.
• Deteriorating peak flow.

Cardiac arrest in acute asthma

The underlying rhythm is usually PEA. This may reflect one or more of the following: prolonged severe hypoxia (secondary to severe bronchospasm and mucous plugging), hypoxia-related arrhythmias or tension pneumothorax (may be bilateral). Give advanced life support according to the guidelines in 📖 Cardiac arrest, p.46 and treat tension pneumothorax if present (📖 p.328). Aim to achieve tracheal intubation early in view of the higher than normal required lung inflation pressures and the attendant risk of gastric inflation in the absence of a tracheal tube.

COPD

Chronic obstructive pulmonary disease (COPD) is characterized by chronic airflow limitation due to impedance to expiratory airflow, mucosal oedema, infection, bronchospasm and bronchoconstriction due to ↓ lung elasticity. Smoking is the main cause, but others are chronic asthma, α-1 antitrypsin deficiency and chronic infection (eg bronchiectasis).

History

Exertional dyspnoea, cough, and sputum are usual complaints. Ask about:

- Present treatment including inhalers, steroids, antibiotics, theophyllines, nebulizers, opiate analgesia, and home O_2 treatment.
- *Past history:* enquire about previous admissions and co-morbidity.
- *Exercise tolerance:* how far can they walk on the flat without stopping? How many stairs can they climb? Do they get out of the house?
- *Recent history:* ask about wheeze and dyspnoea, sputum volume and colour. Chest injuries, abdominal problems and other infections may cause respiratory decompensation.
- *Read the hospital notes:* have there been prior ICU assessments? Has the respiratory consultant advised whether ICU would be appropriate?

Examination

Examine for dyspnoea, tachypnoea, accessory muscle use, and lip-pursing. Look for hyperinflation ('barrel chest') and listen for wheeze or coarse crackles (large airway secretions). Cyanosis, plethora (due to secondary polycythaemia) and right heart failure (cor pulmonale) suggest advanced disease. Look for evidence of hypercapnia: tremor, bounding pulses, peripheral vasodilatation, drowsiness, or confusion.

Check for evidence of other causes of acute dyspnoea, particularly: asthma (📖 p.104), pulmonary oedema (📖 p.100), pneumothorax (📖 p.114), PE (📖 p.120). Remember that these conditions may co-exist with COPD.

Investigations

- SpO_2, respiratory rate, pulse rate, BP, $T°$, and peak flow (if possible).
- CXR (look for pneumothorax, hyperinflation, bullae, and pneumonia).
- ECG.
- ABG (or capillary blood gas), documenting the FiO_2. Use pCO_2 to guide O_2 therapy.
- FBC, U&E, glucose, theophylline levels and, if pneumonia is suspected and/or pyrexial, blood cultures, CRP, and pneumococcal antigen.
- Send sputum for microscopy and culture if purulent.

Treatment

Give O_2—remember that hypercapnoea with O_2 is multifactorial. The aim is to maintain SpO_2 88–92% without precipitating respiratory acidosis or worsening hypercapnoea (see 📖 Oxygen, p.95 and 📖 Arterial blood gases, p.98). If the patient is known to have COPD and is drowsy or has a documented history of previous hypercapnoeic respiratory failure, give FiO_2 of 28% via a Venturi mask and obtain ABG. Titrate up the FiO_2 with serial ABG sampling until the minimum FiO_2 that achieves SpO_2 88–92%. Reduce inhaled oxygen concentration if SpO_2 >92%.

Give bronchodilators and steroids
- Give nebulized salbutamol 5mg or terbutaline 5–10mg.
- Consider adding nebulized ipratropium 0.5mg.
- Use O_2 driven nebulizers unless the patient has hypercapnoeic, acidotic COPD, in which case use nebulizers driven by compressed air, supplemented by O_2 via nasal prongs at 1–4L/min.
- Give steroids (eg prednisolone 30mg PO stat or IV hydrocortisone 100mg).

Other drug treatments
- Give antibiotics (eg amoxicillin, tetracycline, or clarithromycin) if the patient reports ↑ purulent sputum, or there is clinical evidence of pneumonia and/or consolidation on CXR.
- Consider IV aminophylline or salbutamol if there is an inadequate response to nebulized bronchodilators.
- Consider naloxone if the patient is taking an opioid analgesic that may cause respiratory depression.

See NICE guideline on COPD, 2010 (www.nice.org.uk).

Non-invasive ventilation (NIV)

NIV is recommended as standard early therapy for hypercapnoeic ventilatory failure during exacerbations of COPD. NIV will improve the blood gas measurements in the ED, ↓ intubation rates, ↓ mortality, and length of hospital stay.

NIV takes two forms—CPAP and BiPAP, (which may be more suitable for treating type II respiratory failure in COPD). Both CPAP and BiPAP have been used to treat acute cardiogenic pulmonary oedema. Patients with sleep apnoea use CPAP at night. The positive airway pressure is delivered by a tightly adhered face mask, which is sized to fit the patient. The patient is awake, and must be compliant with wearing the mask.

Unlike tracheal intubation, NIV does not protect the airway. Therefore, contraindications include coma and vomiting. Absolute contraindications include apnoea and cardiac arrest. A pneumothorax will be converted into a tension pneuomthorax with NIV. Severe agitation may make effective NIV impossible.

The patient should always be cared for by staff who are familiar with the ventilator and mask, in the resuscitation room.

Start BiPAP at 10cmH$_2$O inspiratory positive airway pressure (IPAP)/ 5cmH$_2$O expiratory positive airway pressure (EPAP), and titrate upwards:
- To treat persistent hypercapnoea, increase IPAP by 2cm at a time.
- To treat persistent hypoxia, increase IPAP and EPAP by 2cm at a time.
- The maximum IPAP/EPAP is 25/15cmH$_2$O.
- For CPAP, commence treatment at 5–8cmH$_2$O.

Pneumonia

Pneumonia involves symptoms and signs of lower respiratory tract infection (breathlessness, productive cough, and fever) usually associated with CXR abnormalities. Pneumocystis pneumonia may occur with minimal or no CXR changes. Consider pneumonia in patients with septicaemia or acute confusional states.

Causes

Bacterial (80–90%) Streptococcus pneumoniae is the commonest cause of community-acquired pneumonia. Others include *Mycoplasma pneumoniae, Haemophilus influenzae, Legionella, Chlamydia psittaci, Staphylococcus aureus* (can cause fulminant pneumonia in patients with influenza). Gram –ve and anaerobic infections are rare. Always consider TB, particularly in chronic alcoholism, poor social circumstances, immigrants and those travelling to developing countries, or individuals not BCG vaccinated. Immunosuppressed patients (eg HIV, steroid therapy) are at ↑ risk of TB and *Pneumocystis jirovecii* pneumonia.

Viral (10–20%) Predominantly influenza A&B, respiratory synctal virus (RSV), rarely varicella and severe acute respiratory syndrome (SARS).

Rickettsial (1%) Rarely, *Coxiella burnetti*.

Signs and symptoms

Fever, cough, and production of sputum are common complaints. Breathlessness, pleuritic chest pain, myalgia, rigors, or haemoptysis may occur. Pneumonia can present without obvious chest signs: *Mycoplasma* pneumonia may present in children and young adults with sore throat, headache, nausea, abdominal pain and diarrhoea. *Legionella* can present with constitutional upset, diarrhoea or confusion, particularly in the elderly. *Pneumocystis* pneumonia in immunosuppressed patients may present with cough, dyspnoea, and marked hypoxia, with relatively few other findings.

Examination and investigation

- Check respiratory rate, pulse, and BP.
- Auscultation may reveal a patch of inspiratory crackles, signs of consolidation are present in <25%.
- Check BMG, SpO_2 (obtain ABG if <94%, or known to have COPD).
- Assess for signs of SIRS (2 or more of RR>20, HR>90, temp>38.3°C or <36.0°C, WCC<4 or >12 × 10^{12}/L, confusion, glucose >8.3mmol/L), which in combination with signs of pneumonia signify sepsis.
- Assess for signs of severe sepsis (sepsis + signs of organ dysfunction 📖 p.59). Oxygen dependence, poor urine output, systolic BP<90mmHg, blood lactate >3mmol/L. Commence fluid resuscitation immediately if present, take blood cultures and give IV antibiotics.
- Obtain CXR. Look for patchy or lobar opacification, mass lesions, or an air bronchogram. In early pneumonia the CXR may be normal.
- Obtain blood cultures, sputum cultures, and consider urinary pneumococcal and *Legionella* antigen testing.

Assessment: admit or discharge

Some patients with 'mild' illness, good social circumstances, and no significant co-morbidity may be safely discharged with appropriate antibiotics (eg amoxicillin 0.5–1g PO tds), simple analgesia for pleuritic pain to aid deep breathing/coughing and GP follow-up.

Patients with CURB-65 score ≥3 have severe pneumonia with a high risk of death; those who score 2 are at ↑ risk of death and should be considered for inpatient treatment or hospital-supervised outpatient care; patients with CURB-65 score 0 or 1 are at low risk of death and may be suitable for home treatment (www.brit-thoracic.org.uk; see Table 3.4).

Table 3.4

CURB-65 score for pneumonia	Score
Confusion	1
Urea >7mmol/L	1
Respiratory rate ≥30/min	1
Low BP (systolic <90mmHg or diastolic ≤60mmHg)	1
Age ≥65 years	1

Treatment

Patients deemed suitable for discharge

Provide simple analgesia, oral antibiotics, and GP follow-up.

Patients admitted, but not severely unwell

Start either oral or IV antibiotics, as follows:
- *Either* amoxicillin 0.5–1g PO tds + erythromycin 500mg PO qds (or clarithromycin 500mg bd).
- *Or* if IV therapy is needed: ampicillin 500mg IV qds + erythromycin 500mg IV qds (or clarithromycin 500mg bd). Local guidelines will apply.
- *Monitor* SpO$_2$ and provide O$_2$ accordingly.
- *Provide* simple analgesia.

Patients with sepsis or severe sepsis (see 📖 p.59)

Commence IV crystalloid fluids, take blood cultures and administer IV antibiotics (eg co-amoxiclav 1.2g IV tds + clarithromycin 500mg IV bd) immediately. Contact ICU and make preparations for arterial line, central line and urinary catheter insertion. Aim for CVP >8mmHg, MAP>65mmHg and urine output >0.5mg/kg/hr. See severe sepsis guidelines (www.survivingsepsis.org).

Differential diagnosis

Pneumonia-like presentations can occur with pulmonary oedema, pulmonary infarction, pulmonary vasculitis (eg SLE, PAN, Churg–Strauss and Wegener's), aspergillosis, allergic alveolitis, bronchial or alveolar cell carcinoma, acute pancreatitis, and subphrenic abscess.

Pulmonary aspiration

Aspiration of solid or liquid material into the upper and lower airways is likely when one or more of the following features are present:

- ↓ GCS: head injury, stroke, overdose, seizures, sedation, anaesthesia.
- ↓ Cough and/or gag reflexes: related to above factors and/or bulbar dysfunction, intubation/extubation, Guillain–Barré syndrome, multiple sclerosis, myasthenia gravis.
- Tendency to regurgitate/vomit: alcohol, full stomach, upper GI tract pathology (including hiatus hernia, oesophageal obstruction, pregnancy).
- May occur in infirm or elderly fed via nasogastric tube.

Clinical features

Large food particles sufficient to cause complete airway obstruction cause choking, inability to speak, ↑ respiratory effort, cyanosis, loss of consciousness, and death. Smaller particles may pass through the vocal cords causing coughing, stridor, tachypnoea, and wheeze. 80% of patients are aged <4 years, with peanuts being the classic inhaled objects. Delayed presentation with cough, wheeze, haemoptysis, unresolved pneumonia, abscess formation, or empyema occurs in ≈30% often days or weeks later.

Vomiting/regurgitation is often witnessed and pulmonary aspiration confirmed by seeing gastric contents in the oropharynx or trachea during intubation or following suction. Gastric content is a mixture of semi-solid and liquid material—aspiration leads to a sudden onset of severe dypsnoea, wheeze, and cyanosis. Its acid nature causes severe damage to the alveolar-capillary membrane, with denaturation of pulmonary surfactant, ↑ pulmonary permeability with oedema and atelectasis.

Hydrocarbons (eg petrol, paraffin) cause severe pulmonary toxicity if aspiration occurs during ingestion or following regurgitation/vomiting.

Investigations

ABG

These show hypoxaemia within minutes of acid aspiration. Initially, patients may hyperventilate with ↓ pCO_2 until pulmonary compliance ↑ work of breathing sufficient to result in hypoventilation.

CXR

Abnormalities develop in >90% of patients, but may take hours/days. Appearances depend on the nature of the aspirated material and the patient's position at the time of the episode (right lower lobe is most frequently and severely affected, followed by left lower lobe and right middle lobe). In severe aspiration, diffuse bilateral infiltrates and pulmonary oedema similar to ARDS appearances are present. Less severe episodes produce atelectasis followed by alveolar infiltration.

Intrapulmonary foreign body (including peanuts)

Rarely radio-opaque. Resulting collapse, hyperinflation, or consolidation is usually obvious and depends on whether obstruction is complete or partial and if supervening infection is present. If the history strongly suggests an inhaled FB, but CXR is normal, consider an expiratory CXR, which may show evidence of air trapping distal to the obstruction.

Prevention

Prevention is everything. Pay meticulous attention to airway protection. This may involve positioning (tilt head down on the right hand side), suction to the oropharynx (Yankauer catheter avoiding stimulation of the gag reflex) and if necessary, tracheal intubation. Tracheal intubation does not completely protect against aspiration of fluid into the lungs, but it is the best preventative measure. In at-risk patients, pass an NG tube to empty the stomach. However, NG tubes can also predispose to aspiration by preventing closure of the oesophageal sphincters and interfering with coughing and clearing the pharynx.

Treatment

Correct hypoxia and give nebulized salbutamol for associated bronchospasm. If particulate aspiration is present, refer for urgent bronchoscopy. Although secondary infection is common, the use of antibiotics or steroids is not routinely indicated.

Spontaneous pneumothorax

Primary spontaneous pneumothorax (PSP) may occur in previously healthy individuals. Secondary spontaneous pneumothorax (SSP) occurs in older patients with pre-existing chronic lung disease (like COPD or TB) and may also occur with asthma, bronchial carcinoma, Marfan's syndrome, infection, cystic fibrosis, and oesophageal rupture.

Presentation

Most patients present with unilateral pleuritic chest pain and dyspnoea. Classical physical signs may not be present (depending upon the size of the pneumothorax): tachypnoea, tachycardia, normal/hyper-resonant percussion note with ↓ air entry on the affected side. Rarely, there may be a clicking sound at the cardiac apex.

Severe symptoms (inability to speak, gasping, low SpO_2) should prompt rapid assessment for tension pneumothorax: tracheal deviation, tachypnoea, tachycardia, and hypotension. Treat tension with immediate decompression using a needle in the second intercostal space (just above the third rib) in the mid-clavicular line (📖 p.328). Severe symptoms are also found in patients with SSP (disproportionate to the pneumothorax size). In the absence of signs of tension pneumothorax, obtain an emergency portable CXR and involve an experienced doctor.

Investigation and treatment

- Monitor pulse, SpO_2, and BP. Ensure IV access.
- Administer high flow oxygen (aim SpO_2 90–92% in patients with COPD).
- When there are no signs of tension, an ABG will help assess patients with chronic lung disease, and guide oxygen therapy.

Erect CXR

- When using digital images, always use a picture archiving and communication system (PACS) workstation. The signs of pneumothorax may be subtle and difficult to spot.
- Look for a displacement of the pleural line.
- Do not mistake the scapular edge for the lung edge.
- Some patients with COPD have emphysematous bullae, which can mimic pneumothorax. If in doubt, ask for senior review prior to treating for pneumothorax.
- An air fluid level at the costophrenic angle may be present.

CT scan

Can be of use in the sub-acute setting for assessing bullous lung disease in a stable patient. CT is not a primary diagnostic modality.

Intervention

- Should be guided primarily by the patient's symptoms. If the patient is breathless, they should undergo an intervention.
- The size of the pneumothorax can be estimated on CXR by measuring from the chest wall to the lung edge at the level of the hilum. This is

only an estimate and assumes symmetrical lung collapse. The cut-off of 2cm is used to determine treatment.
- Intervention for PSP is needle aspiration. If unsuccessful, do not repeat aspiration. Instead insert a Seldinger chest drain.
- Treatment for symptomatic SSP is chest drain insertion and admission.
- Treatment for SSP without breathlessness is admission. Aspiration should be performed by an experienced doctor and may require CT.
- Always insert chest drains for bilateral pneumothoraces.
- Always insert a chest drain immediately following emergency needle decompression.
- Pleural aspiration and drain insertion should be performed by a doctor who has prior training and experience.
- Ensure the patient has IV access. Perform in a monitored environment with an assistant and appropriate supervision. Use aseptic technique.
- Always discuss the procedure with the patient and document that they have given their consent.
- If the patient is on anticoagulation or has a known coagulopathy disorder, discuss with a haemotologist first.

Aspiration technique

Confirm the side of the pneumothorax. Sit the patient upright. Infiltrate 1% lidocaine, then insert a 16G IV cannula just above the 3rd rib (in the 2nd intercostal space) in the mid-clavicular line. Alternatively, lay the patient on their side with the pneumothorax side upwards. Insert cannula in the 5th intercostal space, in the anterior axillary line. Remove the needle, attach a three-way tap, then aspirate air with a 50mL syringe. Continue aspiration until the patient coughs excessively, or until 2.5L of air is removed.

Seldinger chest drain insertion

Confirm the side of the pneumothorax. Keep the patient comfortable, ensure adequate analgesia (this may require 1mg increments of morphine IV), but avoid sedation. Sit the patient upright and rest their hand behind their head. Infiltrate 10mL 1% lidocaine at the anterior axillary line in the 5th intercostal space. Aspirate a small amount of pleural air during infiltration and note the depth of the pleural space. Locate the pleural space with the introducer needle (aspirate while advancing through chest wall), then advance the guidewire through the needle. Remove the introducer needle, make a small skin incision and gently pass the dilator over the guidewire using a twisting action. Do not push the dilator more than 1cm past the depth of the pleural space. Pass the chest drain over the guide wire to a depth of 10–12cm. Remove the guide wire, connect to an underwater seal drain and suture in pace. Check the drain is bubbling and swinging, and organize a CXR.

Discharge

Patients without breathlessness, with small PSP may be considered for discharge. Give the patient verbal and written instructions to return if their symptoms worsen and warn them not to fly. Ensure they have an appointment with a respiratory physician in the next week.

See http://www.brit-thoracic.org.uk

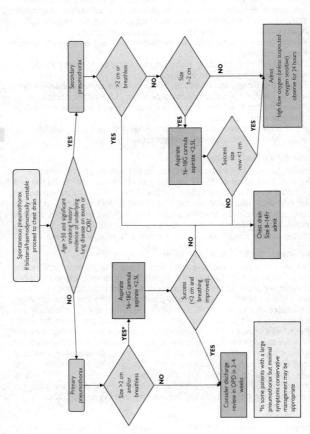

Fig. 3.23 Management of pneumothorax.[1]

Deep venous thrombosis

DVT and PE are manifestations of the same disease process whereby abnormal clotting occurs in the veins of the legs or pelvis. The clots may break from the vein wall and embolize to the lungs. Untreated DVTs are associated with a 1–2% mortality from PE. Around half of those with DVT will go on to develop post-thrombotic syndrome, with lifelong pain and swelling of the leg.

Risk factors

- Recent surgery (where a general anaesthetic was administered, especially orthopaedic, abdominal, spinal and obstetric).
- Recent admission to hospital.
- Current malignancy.
- Being bedbound.
- Sepsis.
- IV drug use (where patient injects in the femoral vein).
- Pregnancy/pelvic masses.
- Immobility such as recent fracture with crutches and plaster cast.
- Previous DVT/PE.
- Thrombophilia or family history of venous thromboembolism.

Clinical features

DVT classically produces leg pain with swelling, warmth, tenderness, and dilated superficial veins in the affected leg. These signs are non-specific and often not present. A small or partially occluding thrombus may be completely asymptomatic. History and clinical examination alone cannot safely exclude DVT—if a DVT is suspected, investigate further. Investigate for PE, rather than DVT if the patient has tachycardia, hypoxia, increased respiratory rate, or breathlessness (📖 Pulmonary embolus, p.120).

Differential diagnosis

- *Muscular tear:* typically acute onset.
- *Rupture of a Baker's cyst:* again, typically acute onset.
- Cellulitis or other infection.

Investigation and management

- Record pulse rate, RR, BP, SpO_2, and T° in all patients.
- Take a full history including concurrent illness, past history, recent operations, travel, and family history.
- Examine the affected leg for signs of plethora, deep vein tenderness, swelling (measure both legs, 10cm distal to tibial tuberosity), oedema and dilation of the skin veins.
- Perform full examination checking for signs of PE or occult carcinoma.
- Calculate the clinical probability assessment score. The Wells score (Table 3.5) is the most widely used clinical prediction score.
- Take FBC, U&E, CRP, glucose.
- Take D-dimer if Wells score indicates DVT is 'unlikely' (<3 points).
- If D-dimer normal *and* DVT 'unlikely', DVT has been ruled out.

Table 3.5 Wells clinical probability assessment score for DVT

Clinical feature	Score
Active cancer (treatment within 6 months or palliative care)	1
Paralysis, paresis, or recent POP immobilization of a leg	1
Recently bedridden for >3 days or major surgery <12 weeks	1
Localized tenderness along the distribution of the deep venous system	1
Entire leg swelling	1
Calf swelling >3cm compared with asymptomatic leg	1
Pitting oedema (greater in the symptomatic leg)	1
Dilated superficial veins (non-varicose)	1
Previously documented DVT	1
Another diagnosis more likely than DVT	-2

Total score < 3 means DVT is 'unlikely'. Score of 3 or more signifies DVT is 'likely'.

The Wells score was not developed with injecting drug users or pregnant women, both of whom are at higher risk of DVT. These patients should always undergo ultrasound scanning.

All patients investigated for DVT with a 'likely' Wells score (≥3) or an elevated D-dimer level require ultrasound scanning. A normal whole leg ultrasound scan (femoral, popliteal, and calf vein scan) will exclude DVT. If a thigh scan is performed (the femoral and popliteal veins), DVT can only be excluded by two normal thigh ultrasound scans, one week apart.

All patients with a 'likely' score should be anticoagulated with LMWH while awaiting an outpatient ultrasound scan.

Patients diagnosed with calf or thigh DVT should be treated with LMWH and discharged with a week's supply, an appointment for the anticoagulation services, and medical outpatient follow-up. Advise them to return immediately if they become breathless or have chest pain.

Upper limb DVT
Seen almost exclusively in patients with in-dwelling central or long lines, often for chemotherapy. May be associated with plethora and swelling of the arm or face. If suspected, request an ultrasound of the arm and neck veins, or a CT scan with contrast.

Superficial thrombophlebitis
Patients present with a painful, tender area of skin. The diagnosis is made clinically with a firm, tender superficial vein, and overlying erythema. This may co-exist with DVT and superficial thrombus may propagate into deep veins. If there is any doubt as to the presence of a DVT, investigate using the DVT protocol. Otherwise, treat with NSAID. Arrange follow up either in the ED, a medical clinic or with the GP.

Pulmonary embolism

The mortality of diagnosed and treated pulmonary embolism is 7%. Many more people die from undiagnosed PE. Venous thromboembolism develops in patients already suffering from sepsis, cancer, or COPD or in patients recovering from stroke, MI, surgery, and joint replacement. Pulmonary embolic disease can result in a variety of symptoms often misdiagnosed as asthma, anxiety, pneumonia and ACS.

History

Most patients with PE experience dyspnoea, commonly without other symptoms. Syncope with cyanosis, cardiac arrest or angina are signs of massive PE. A minority present with pleuritic chest pain, some with additional haemoptysis. Always consider PE in patients with unexplained hypoxia or breathlessness. Take a full history of concurrent illness, surgical procedures, recent hospital admission, past history including DVT and PE, travel and family history.

Examination

Examination may be normal.
- Tachycardia and tachypnoea are common.
- Pyrexia following lung infarction is common.
- 30% of all patients with PE have normal SpO_2.
- Always record BP. Hypotension indicates massive PE.
- Perform a full respiratory and cardiovascular examination.
- Always examine the legs for signs of DVT.

Table 3.6 Modified Wells clinical probability assessment score for PE

Clinical feature	Score
Signs of DVT (minimum of objective leg swelling and tenderness)	3.0
IV drug use	3.0
PE is the most likely diagnosis	3.0
HR >100	1.5
Prior PE or DVT diagnosis	1.5
Bed ridden for >3 days or surgery, within the past 4 weeks	1.5
Cancer (treated actively or with palliation within last 6 months)	1.0
Haemoptysis	1.0

Total score <2.0 = low risk PE, 2.0–6.0 = moderate risk PE, >6.0 = high risk PE.

Any patient scoring 2.0 or more on the Wells score, OR who has an elevated D-dimer, requires pulmonary imaging. Note that a normal D-dimer will not exclude PE in a patient with moderate or high probability of PE. Only a normal D-dimer *and* a low clinical probability will safely exclude PE.

Investigations for suspected pulmonary embolus

- If hypoxic, tachycardic, or hypotensive, insert an IV cannula.
- All patients should have blood taken for FBC and U&Es.
- Take a D-dimer test on any patient who scores <2.0 on the Wells score (Table 3.6). Normal D-dimer in a patient scoring <2.0 excludes PE.
- Arrange ECG (to look for MI or pericarditis) and CXR (to look for pneumothorax, pneumonia). Many patients with PE have a normal ECG and CXR.

Diagnostic imaging for pulmonary embolus

There are two forms of imaging for PE: CT pulmonary angiography (CTPA) and ventilation-perfusion (V/Q) scanning. CTPA uses a higher dose of radiation (not good for young patients or pregnant patients), but will give a definitive answer, as well as diagnose other conditions often confused with PE (like aortic dissection).

V/Q scanning uses a low dose of radiation (good for the young and pregnant), but may not give a definitive answer. V/Q scans are reported as low, intermediate and high probability of PE. The V/Q scan probability must concord with the clinical probability to diagnose or exclude PE (both low probability or both high probability). All other combinations are non-diagnostic and the patient must have a CTPA.

Pitfalls in diagnosis

- Investigating for PE because the patient has an elevated D-dimer. The D-dimer is irrelevant if there are no clinical symptoms or signs of PE.
- Deciding not to take the D-dimer because the patient is post-surgery, elderly, or has had recent trauma. If the Wells score is <2.0, a D-dimer test is rapid and may avoid admission for diagnostic imaging if normal.

Treatment of pulmonary embolus

Anticoagulate with LMWH and arrange to commence the patient on warfarin therapy. If the patient is ambulant, not hypoxic with a normal pulse rate and RR, many hospitals commence warfarin and follow-up as an outpatient. Admit patients who are hypoxic, hypotensive, tachycardic, tachypnoeic, or elderly for further management.

Suspected massive PE

- In patients with marked hypoxia and/or cardiovascular compromise, call for urgent ICU expert help.
- If available, an emergency echo will demonstrate a dilated right ventricle and right heart failure.
- Do not take unstable patients for a CT or V/Q.
- If suspicion of PE is high and the patient is haemodynamically unstable, administer thrombolytic therapy. Do not delay. Administer alteplase (rTPA) 100mg over 2 hr or 0.6mg/kg (max 50mg) over 15min as per European Cardiology guidelines (www.escardio.org).

Upper gastrointestinal bleeding

Causes of upper gastrointestinal bleeding

Common
- Peptic ulceration.
- Mucosal inflammation (oesophagitis, gastritis, or duodenitis).
- Oesophageal varices.
- Mallory–Weiss tear.
- Gastric carcinoma.
- Coagulation disorders (thrombocytopenia, warfarin).

Rare
- Aorto-enteric fistula (especially after aortic surgery).
- Benign tumours (eg leiomyomas, carcinoid tumours, angiomas).
- Congenital (eg Ehlers–Danlos, Osler–Weber–Rendu, pseudoxanthoma elasticum).

History

Take a detailed history, whilst resuscitating as necessary. Upper GI bleeding usually presents with haematemesis and/or melaena. Major upper GI bleeding may present with fresh PR bleeding.

Ask about the amount and duration of bleeding, any past history of GI bleeding or liver problems, and associated symptoms (abdominal pain, weight loss, anorexia). Syncope usually infers a significant bleed. Take a full drug history (ask about aspirin, NSAIDs, warfarin, iron) and enquire about alcohol consumption.

Examination

Check ABCs. Rapidly assess for evidence of hypovolaemic shock (pulse and respiratory rates, BP, GCS, skin colour/temperature, capillary refill). Look at any available vomit or faeces. Check for abdominal masses, tenderness or surgical scars (including aortic grafting). Look for stigmata of liver disease. Perform a PR examination and check for faecal occult blood (FOB).

Investigation and diagnosis

Request old hospital notes and send blood for FBC, clotting screen, U&E, blood glucose, Group and Save or cross-matching (according to clinical features). Urea may be ↑, but creatinine will be normal unless renal function is impaired. Check SpO_2 (obtain ABG if <94%) and consider CXR and ECG. Endoscopy is the investigation of choice to identify the source of the bleeding.

Risk of further bleeding and death

The risk of mortality and further complications increases with increasing age, co-morbidities (especially cancer and heart failure), liver disease, continued bleeding, elevated urea, and passage of PR blood.

Table 3.7 Initial Rockall Score for risk of death in upper GI bleeding

Points	0	1	2	3
Age	<60	60–79	>80	
Shock	HR<100	HR>100	Systolic BP<100mmHg	
	Systolic BP>100mmHg	Systolic BP>100mmHg		
Comorbidity			Cardiac failure, ischaemic heart disease or any major co-morbidity	Renal failure Liver failure Disseminated malignancy

Any score >0 signifies increased risk of mortality.

Only consider patients scoring 0 on the initial Rockall score (Table 3.7), with no further evidence of bleeding, for discharge home from the ED with follow-up. Any patient scoring >0 requires urgent endoscopy.

Treatment of moderate/severe haemorrhage
- Check airway and breathing. Provide O_2 to maintain SpO_2 94–98%. Insert 2 large (14G) IV cannulae, send FBC, U&E, clotting, cross-match.
- Start IV fluids followed by blood as necessary.
- Avoid omeprazole acutely unless the patient has known peptic ulcer disease (give 40mg diluted in 100mL saline as IVI over 30min).
- If the patient is anticoagulated, or has a clotting disorder (eg due to liver disease), discuss with a haematologist and give vitamin K/clotting factors/fresh frozen plasma (FFP) accordingly.
- Insert a urinary catheter and monitor the urine output.
- Ensure that patients with severe uncontrolled variceal bleeding, severe encephalopathy, hypoxia, acute agitation, or evidence of aspiration have their airways secured, if necessary by tracheal intubation.

Managing severe haemorrhage possibly due to varices
For unstable patients with a past history of varices or clinical features of hepatic failure, arrange emergency endoscopic treatment:
- Commence fluid rescucitation.
- Give terlipressin (2mg IV repeated every 4–6hr).
- Check International Normalized Ratio (INR) and give IV vitamin K if prolonged.
- Give prophylactic antibiotics eg ciprofloxacin or second/third generation cephalosporin which may ↓ mortality in severe haemorrhage.
- Consider ballon tamponade as a salvage procedure in a patient with massive haemorrhage, at risk of death. If experienced in the technique, insert a 4 lumen Sengstaken/Minnesota tube. Inflate the gastric balloon then the oesophageal balloon to a pressure of 30–40mmHg in order to tamponade the bleeding varices. Regularly aspirate both ports.

See http://www.sign.ac.uk

Lower gastrointestinal bleeding

The commonest cause of apparent lower GI bleeding is upper GI haemorrhage. ≈20% of acute GI haemorrhage is from the colon or rectum. Angiodysplasia and bleeding from diverticulae are the most frequent causes, but inflammatory bowel disease or, very rarely, aorto-enteric fistulae may be responsible. Lower GI haemorrhage often settles spontaneously: localization of the bleeding source may be difficult.

History

Nature of bleeding Melaena may occur following small bowel or proximal colon bleeding, as well as upper GI haemorrhage. Conversely, large volumes of fresh or 'plum-coloured' rectal bleeding may follow upper GI haemorrhage. Bloody diarrhoea suggests inflammatory bowel disease or infective colitis.

Associated symptoms Weight loss, anorexia, or a change in bowel habit raise suspicion of colonic carcinoma. Abdominal pain may be a feature of ischaemic colitis, inflammatory bowel disease, or carcinoma. Anal pain commonly occurs with anal fissure or complication of haemorrhoids.

Syncope or postural dizziness May indicate significant haemorrhage.

Past medical history Ask about inflammatory bowel disease, peptic ulceration, or other illnesses. Previous aortic surgery with graft insertion can rarely result in formation of an aorto-enteric fistula (symptoms include sporadic or fulminant bleeding, often with syncope).

Drug history Ask about salicylates, NSAIDs, corticosteroids, and anticoagulants.

Family and social history Note any family history of peptic ulcers, inflammatory bowel disease. Enquire about alcohol consumption.

Examination

First assess for signs of hypovolaemia and commence resuscitation if necessary. Document pulse, BP (comparing erect and supine, noting any postural drop), T° and SpO_2. Examine the abdomen and PR in all cases.

Investigations

Obtain blood for cross-matching (ask for 4–6U of type specific if urgent), FBC, U&E, glucose, and coagulation studies. Perform an ECG on any patient >50 years.

Risk of further bleeding and death

The risk of mortality and further complications increases with increasing age, co-morbidities, haemodynamic disturbance, and the use of NSAIDs or aspirin. Only consider discharge if the patient is young, otherwise healthy, has passed only a small amount of blood PR, and does not take NSAIDs or anticoagulants. Always arrange follow up for these patients.

Treatment

Patients with signs of hypovolaemia require immediate resuscitation:

- Give O_2.
- Attach monitoring (cardiac monitor, SpO_2, BP monitoring).
- Insert two large bore IV cannulae.
- Give 1L of 0.9% saline or Hartmann's solution IV stat and give further fluids according to response.
- Insert a NG tube.
- Insert a urinary catheter.
- Correct any coagulopathy.
- Consider the need for a central venous line.
- Contact the surgical team and ICU.

See http://www.sign.ac.uk

Headache

Headaches of non-traumatic origin account for ≈0.5% of ED attendances; 10–15% have serious underlying pathology. Patients typically present in one of three ways:
- Severe headache, unlike any previous one ('first severe' or 'worst ever').
- Headache with associated worrying features (altered mental status, fever, focal neurology).
- Chronic severe headache unresponsive to treatment.

Causes

Primary headaches
- Migraine.
- Tension headaches.
- Cluster headaches.
- Miscellaneous (benign cough headache, benign exertional headache, headache associated with sexual activity).

Secondary headaches
- Head injury.
- Vascular (stroke, intracranial haematoma, subarachnoid haemorrhage, unruptured arterio-venous malformation, venous thrombosis, hypertension).
- Non-vascular intracranial disorder (↑ cerebrospinal fluid (CSF) pressure, post-LP, intracranial tumour).
- Substance misuse or withdrawal (including analgesia withdrawal or rebound).
- Infection (encephalitis or meningitis).
- Metabolic (hypoxia, hypercapnoea, hypoglycaemia, carbon monoxide (CO) poisoning, dialysis).
- Craniofacial disorder (pathology of skull, neck, eyes, nose, ears, sinuses, teeth, mouth, temporomandibular joint dysfunction).
- Neuralgias (trigeminal, occipital and other cranial nerves).

Approach

Use a detailed history and examination (including vital signs and neurological examination) to search for potentially serious causes. Look particularly for the following (some typical features in brackets):
- Subarachnoid haemorrhage (sudden, severe onset, syncope)—📖 p.128.
- Meningitis or encephalitis (fever, neck rigidity)—📖 p.224.
- Head injury (history or signs of trauma)—📖 p.354.
- ↑ intracranial pressure (papilloedema, loss of retinal vein pulsation).
- Stroke (focal neurological signs)—📖 p.144.
- Acute glaucoma (painful red eye, ↓ VA, irregular semi-dilated pupil)—📖 p.542.
- Cranial arteritis (jaw pain, temporal artery tenderness)—📖 p.132.

History

Features suggesting possible serious pathology are:
- Sudden onset headache.
- Worst headache ever.
- Dramatic change in pattern of headache.
- Known HIV or malignancy.
- The presence of a ventriculo-peritoneal shunt.
- Headache coming on during exertion.
- New onset headache in those aged >50 years.

Ask about drugs and the possibility of toxins (eg CO).

Examination

Check GCS, pulse rate, respiratory rate, BP, T° and SpO_2:
- Feel the head for muscular tenderness, arterial tenderness, trigger points for neuralgia, and look for evidence of head injury.
- Examine the eyes for VA, pupil reactions, eye movements. Look at the fundi for papilloedema.
- Palpate the sinuses for tenderness.
- Look in the ears for haemotympanum or infection.
- Check the oral cavity for infection.
- Look for evidence of purpura/rash of meningococcal infection.
- Complete a full neurological examination (include cranial nerves, limb tone, power, sensation, co-ordination and reflexes).

Check for *Kernig's sign:* straightening the knee whilst the hip is flexed produces discomfort in the presence of meningeal irritation.

Management

Investigation and emergency treatment will be tailored according to the presentation of the patient, based upon the likely diagnosis.
- Check FBC, ESR, CRP, U&E, blood glucose.
- If pyrexial and no other obvious source of infection found, take blood cultures and consider IV cefotaxime 2g. Start IV fluids and admit.
- Give paracetamol (oral or IV if vomiting) and an NSAID.
- An effective treatment for headache is IV metoclopramide 10mg with IV fluids.
- Arrange an emergency CT brain for any patient with an acute severe headache, or with a history of seizure, or an abnormal neurological exam. Arrange a CT for any patient with HIV.
- If subarachnoid haemorrhage is suspected and CT normal, admit for lumbar puncture.

It may be safe to discharge home a patient with slow onset headache that has resolved following treatment, with normal examination and blood tests. Arrange GP follow up. Always advise to reattend if symptoms worsen.

Subarachnoid haemorrhage

Consider subarachnoid haemorrhage in any 'worst ever'
or sudden onset headache

Atraumatic subarachnoid haemorrhage can occur at any age and is an important cause of sudden collapse and death. Most bleeds follow rupture of saccular ('berry') aneurysms in the circle of Willis. Other bleeds may be due to arteriovenous malformations, tumours, or connective tissue disorders.

History

Up to 70% of patients with subarachnoid haemorrhage report rapid onset or 'worst ever' headache. This is classically described as 'like a blow to the back of the head', accompanied by neck pain, photophobia, and vomiting. In 25%, exertional activities precede the event. The patient may present after syncope or fits. Drowsiness and confusion are common. 'Warning headaches' may precede subarachnoid haemorrhage. Unilateral eye pain may occur.

Examination

Document pulse rate, BP, T°, and GCS. An unconscious patient with signs of Cushing's response signifies ↑ intracranial pressure. Perform full cranial and peripheral nerve examination. There may be focal motor and sensory signs due to intracerebral extension of the haemorrhage or vasospasm, subhyaloid haemorrhages (blotchy haemorrhages seen in the fundi) or cranial nerve palsies. Oculomotor nerve palsy is characteristic of a berry aneurysm involving the posterior communicating artery. Neck stiffness is often absent in ED presentations, either because meningeal irritation has not yet occurred or because the patient is deeply unconscious.

Investigation

This may need to proceed alongside resuscitation in seriously ill patients:
• Assess airway and breathing. If the patient is unconscious, open the airway and contact ICU. Consider urgent RSI, tracheal intubation and ventilation.
• Obtain venous access and check BMG, FBC, clotting screen, U&E.
• CXR may show changes of neurogenic pulmonary oedema.
• ECG may demonstrate ischaemic changes.
• Arrange emergency CT scan for all suspected cases (maximally sensitive within 12hr). Admit for lumbar puncture (LP) (done >12hr after headache onset) even if CT scan is normal.
• Involve the neurosurgical team early. It may be useful to use the Hunt and Hess score (see Table 3.8) when communicating severity by phone.

Table 3.8 Hunt and Hess scale for subarachnoid haemorrahage

Grade	
1	Asymptomatic, mild headache, slight nuchal rigidity
2	Moderate to severe headache, nuchal rigidity, no neurologic deficit other than cranial nerve palsy
3	Drowsiness/confusion, mild focal neurological deficit
4	Stupor, moderate-severe hemiparesis
5	Coma, decerebrate posturing

Treatment

Tailor this according to the presentation and the need for resuscitation:
- Maintain SpO_2 94–98%.
- Provide adequate analgesia and antiemetic. Codeine (30–60mg PO), paracetamol (1g PO) and/or NSAID may suffice. Some patients require more potent analgesics (eg morphine titrated in 1mg increments IV according to response)—proceed slowly to avoid drowsiness.
- If unconscious (GCS < 8), severely agitated or combative, tracheal intubation (with general anaesthetic (GA)) will allow IPPV and control of pCO_2 to within normal levels. Insert a urinary catheter and arterial line.

Contact neurosurgical team—further treatment options include:
- Nimodipine (60mg PO every 4hr or 1mg/hr IVI) to prevent and treat ischaemic neurological deficits secondary to vasospasm.
- Mannitol IV (eg 200mL of 10%) if there is evidence of ↑ ICP.

Migraine

Patients with recurrent migraine rarely attend the ED unless symptoms are different from usual—take care to avoid missing more serious conditions. The pathogenesis of migraine is not entirely clear, but there is initial vasoconstriction and subsequent vasodilatation of both intracranial and extracranial blood vessels.

Presentation

Precipitants include fatigue, alcohol, menstruation, oral contraceptive pill (OCP), hunger, chocolate, cheese, shellfish, and red wine.

A prodrome lasting 5–30min occurs in a third of patients, with blurred vision, photophobia, or scintillating scotomata (an area of blurred or absent vision surrounded by moving zig-zag lines), malaise, anorexia, and vomiting. A few experience hemiparaesthesiae, mild unilateral weakness, ataxia, or dysphasia. The following headache may last 4–72hr, and is usually 'throbbing' and unilateral, but may be generalized. Photophobia, nausea, or phonophobia is common.

Rare forms of migraine

Hemiplegic migraine Profound hemiplegia precedes the development of the headache by 30–60min. The weakness and other focal deficits usually resolve quickly. Occasionally, they may be slow or fail to resolve.

Basilar migraine Brainstem disturbances, with impaired consciousness, vertigo, dysarthria, diplopia, and limb weakness.

Ophthalmoplegic migraine Transient unilateral ophthalmoplegia and ptosis, which may last several days.

Acephalgic migraine Very occasionally, neurological defects may be present without headache.

Examination

Look for evidence of other serious diagnoses.

Treatment of acute attacks

- Give simple analgesia (eg paracetamol 1g PO PRN qds or NSAID) in combination with an anti-emetic (eg metoclopramide 10mg PO, or IV).
- Refer for admission patients who have neurological signs, altered mental status, or where there is diagnostic uncertainty (including change in severe headache pattern).
- Acute attacks that fail to respond to simple measures may respond to other drugs, but these are associated with significant adverse effects. $5HT_1$ agonist sumatriptan (6mg SC or 50mg PO or 20mg intranasally) is effective, but discuss with a senior first.

Sumatriptan causes vasoconstriction and is therefore contraindicated in IHD, uncontrolled hypertension, basilar, and hemiplegic migraine. Rebound headache may occur in up to 45%.

Ergotamine is best avoided (see *BNF*). It causes nausea, vomiting, abdominal pain, and muscular cramps. It is contraindicated in peripheral vascular disease, IHD, pregnancy, breast feeding, hemiplegic migraine, Raynaud's disease, liver and renal impairment, and hypertension.

Other causes of headache

Cluster headache

These are more common in men. Often there is a family history. Headache usually occurs at night, waking the patient. Sometimes alcohol may act as a precipitant. Headaches are typically 'clustered' into up to eight attacks per day each lasting between 15 and 180min. Pain is usually severe, centred upon the eye. Associated symptoms, often unilateral, include conjunctival injection, lacrimation, nasal congestion, rhinorrhoea, forehead, and facial sweating, miosis, ptosis.

Treatment High flow O_2 (12L/min via reservoir mask) for 15min sometimes provides relief. Otherwise, use paracetamol/NSAID. Consult before contemplating starting ergotamine or sumatriptan.

Trigeminal neuralgia

Characterized by stabbing unilateral pain within the distribution of the trigeminal nerves. Stimulation of the 'trigger area' (eg by touching, hair brushing, or even chewing) induces very severe pain. Treat with carbamezepine and oral analgesia. Admit if the pain is severe and unrelieved.

Tension headache

The diagnosis is only made after exclusion of more serious pathology.

The history may be described in a dramatic manner. The headache is usually continuous, pressing, or tight ('band-like') in nature. It is usually bitemporal or occipital. Usual features of migraine are absent and the headache does not worsen with exertion.

Examination often reveals pericranial muscle tenderness, but is otherwise normal.

Treat with simple analgesia (eg paracetamol 1g PO qds PRN) and advise GP follow-up. Reassure the patient that a thorough history and examination have not revealed any worrying features.

Cranial ('temporal' or 'giant cell') arteritis (see 📖 p.541)

Consider this in all patients >50 years with recent onset of headache or change in headache pattern. There may be weight loss, night sweats, low grade fever, jaw claudication, and ↓ vision (up to 10% present with acute visual loss), shoulder girdle stiffness, and muscular aches (polymyalgia). Involvement of carotid or vertebral arteries may lead to TIAs or stroke.

Examination: the temporal arteries may be tender, reddened, pulseless, or thickened. Fundoscopy is usually normal, but papilloedema can occur later in the disease.

Investigation: ↑ ESR >> 40mm/hr, often with a low grade anaemia and leucocytosis. A normal ESR does not exclude temporal arteritis.

Treatment: in view of the serious risk of rapidly progressive visual loss, if suspected give 200mg IV hydrocortisone (or 40mg prednisolone PO) immediately. Refer to the neurologist or ophthalmologist as an emergency—the diagnosis may be confirmed by temporal artery biopsy.

Space-occupying lesions

If the headache is always located on the same side, consider space occupying lesions and arteriovenous malformations. Headaches that are dull, aching, and made worse by lying down or straining are typical of space occupying lesions.

Malignant hypertension

Hypertension is an unusual cause of headaches, but is seen in patients with malignant hypertension and diastolic BP > 130mmHg (◻ p.90).

Ventricular shunts

Assume that any patient who presents with headaches associated with a ventricular shunt has infection/blockage and refer as an emergency. Associated drowsiness is a particular pointer to blockage.

Analgesic headache

Chronic use of simple analgesics, sympathomimetics, ergotamine, or cocaine is associated with headaches. Stopping or starting certain medications (eg OCP) can also cause headache, as can withdrawal from caffeine. Exclude serious causes and advise GP follow-up with advice on medication use.

Cerebral venous thrombosis

This is more common than was previously realized. It presents in similar fashion to subarachnoid or subdural haemorrhage: sudden onset headache with nausea and vomiting. It may be associated with sinus infections, pregnancy and the post-partum period. The diagnosis may be missed on CT, but a clue includes ↑ ICP at LP.

Meningitis (see ◻ p.224)

Encephalitis

Miscellaneous causes

Headaches may also result from:
- *Hypoxia and hypercapnoea.*
- *Poisons:* eg CO and solvents (◻ p.208).
- *Drugs:* eg nitrates, sildenafil.
- *Post-traumatic* (◻ p.368).

Acute confusional state (delirium)

Definition of delirium

Delirium is a form of organic brain syndrome characterized by:

- Disturbed conscious level and mood (overactivity, excitement, drowsiness or stupor).
- Global disturbance of cognition (memory, orientation, attention, speech, motor function).
- Rapid onset with fluctuating course (often worse at night, with reversal of usual sleep–wake cycle) and brief duration.
- Perceptual distortions and hallucinations (especially visual).

Causes of acute confusion

One or more of the following may be the underlying cause of an acute confusional state (several causes frequently co-exist):

- *Prescribed medication:* digoxin, cimetidine, steroids, analgesics, diuretics, anticholinergics, antiparkinsonian drugs.
- *Drugs of abuse:* opioids, benzodiazepines, ecstasy, amphetamines, hallucinogens.
- *Withdrawal:* from alcohol, opioids, hypnotics or anxiolytics.
- *Infection:* pneumonia, UTI, septicaemia, meningitis, encephalitis.
- *Metabolic:* hypoxia, hypercapnia, hypoglycaemia, acidosis, hyponatraemia, hypercalcaemia.
- *Cardiac:* acute MI, cardiac failure, endocarditis.
- *Neurological:* head injury, chronic subdural haematoma, meningitis, post-ictal state.
- *Organ failure:* respiratory, renal and hepatic failure.
- *Endocrine:* myxoedema, thyrotoxicosis, diabetes, Addison's disease.

Differential diagnosis

Delirium can occur at any age, but is much more common in the elderly. It is often misdiagnosed as schizophrenia, depression, or dementia (see opposite). Differentiation can be difficult, but the following are more suggestive of physical illness:

- Non-auditory hallucinations.
- Dysarthria.
- Ataxia.
- Gait disturbance.
- Incontinence.
- Focal neurological signs.

Approach

Search systematically for (and exclude) the physical causes of acute confusion outlined above.

Investigation of acute confusion

Perform a thorough, careful physical and mental state examination (see
📖 Mental state examination, p.606) on acutely confused patients. It may
be impossible to obtain an accurate history from the patient, so actively
seek other sources of information: relatives, carers, GP, and previous
medical records.

Look carefully for evidence of alcohol/drug intoxication or evidence of
withdrawal states. Examine for focal neurological signs and signs of acute
cardiac, respiratory, or abdominal abnormalities (including acute urinary
retention). Document basic vital signs (GCS, pulse, BP, respiratory rate
and T°) in all cases.

Mandatory basic investigations

- BMG.
- U&E, FBC, and blood glucose.
- Urinalysis.
- SpO_2 and ABG.
- ECG.
- CXR.

Adopt a low threshold for additional investigations based on clinical
suspicion—blood cultures, serum paracetamol and salicylate, CT brain
scan, and even LP may be indicated.

Be careful not to miss: hypoglycaemia, head injury, Wernicke's encephalopathy,
opioid intoxication, acute alcohol withdrawal, CO poisoning.

Dementia

Dementia is an acquired, progressive decline in intellect, behaviour, and
personality. It is irreversible and typically occurs with a normal level of
consciousness. Note that patients with dementia are at risk of delirium
resulting from an acute infective or metabolic origin—a clue to this may
be an acute deterioration in mental state.

The commonest causes of dementia are Alzheimer's disease, vascular
dementia, and Lewy body dementia.

The unconscious patient: 1

Common causes	Uncommon causes
• Hypoglycaemia	• Type 2 respiratory failure
• Drug overdose	• Cardiac failure
• Head injury	• Arrhythmias
• Stroke	• Hypovolaemic shock
• Subarachnoid haemorrhage	• Anaphylaxis
• Convulsions	• Hepatic/renal failure
• Alcohol intoxication	• Hypothermia/hyperthermia
	• Meningitis/encephalitis
	• Malaria
	• DKA/HHS
	• Non-convulsive status epilepticus
	• Wernicke's encephalopathy

Treatment may be needed before any diagnosis is made. Remember:
• *Airway*.
• *Breathing*.
• *Circulation*.

Initial resuscitation

Airway and cervical spine Whatever the cause of coma, a patient may die or suffer brain damage due to airway obstruction, respiratory depression, or circulatory failure. Clear and protect the airway immediately, and immobilize the cervical spine if trauma is suspected.

Breathing If breathing appears inadequate ventilate with O_2 using a self-inflating bag with an O_2 reservoir. An uninjured patient who seems to be breathing adequately can be examined supine, but nurse him/her in the recovery position to ↓ risk of airway obstruction. Record RR.

Circulation Measure pulse and BP. Observe and feel the skin for colour, sweating and T°. Obtain reliable venous access. Monitor ECG. Replace IV fluid if indicated.

Conscious level Assess level of consciousness using GCS (📖 Head injury: examination, p.360). Check the blood glucose (initially by BMG) and treat hypoglycaemia immediately (📖 p.150). Record pupil size. Give slow IV thiamine (ie 2 pairs of Pabrinex® ampoules in 100mL 5% glucose over 30min—see *BNF*) to patients with a history of alcoholism or who appear malnourished.

History

Obtain a history from the ambulance crew and the patient's relatives and friends. Ask:
- How was the patient found?
- When was he/she last seen?
- Is there any suggestion of trauma?
- Is there any history of fits?
- Has there been recent foreign travel?
- Previous symptoms and medical history (including depression).
- Note any drugs available.

Check previous ED records and hospital notes.

Examination

Examine thoroughly for illness and injury. Check clothes and possessions for tablets and cards/bracelets warning of pre-existing disease.

↑ **Respiratory rate** may reflect obstructed airway, aspiration, pneumonia, DKA, liver/renal failure, salicylate poisoning, methanol, or ethylene glycol.

Respiratory depression may be due to poisoning (eg barbiturates, opioids, tricyclics) or ↑ ICP. Brainstem compression or damage by stroke may cause rapid, irregular or intermittent (Cheyne–Stokes) breathing.

If bradycardic consider: hypoxia, complete heart block, ↑ ICP, digoxin or β-blocker poisoning (📖 p.198).

If tachycardic consider: airway obstruction, hypoxia, hypovolaemia, SVT, VT, or anticholinergic overdose.

AF may be associated with cerebral emboli.

Hypotension suggests hypoxia, shock (hypovolaemic, anaphylactic, septic), or poisoning.

Hypertension may be due to ↑ ICP.

Skin: look for pallor, cyanosis, jaundice, spider naevi, skin crease/scar pigmentation (Addison's disease), rashes (eg purpura in meningococcal infection or DIC), injection marks (drug addiction or medical treatment), and signs of trauma. Erythema or blistering over pressure points indicate the patient has been unconscious for some hours.

Measure rectal T° with a low-reading thermometer if the skin feels cold. Coma is common at <30°C (📖 Hypothermia: presentation, p.254).

The unconscious patient: 2

Neurological examination include GCS, limb strength, muscle tone and reflexes, optic fundi, ear drums, neck stiffness (except in neck injury), and palpation of the fontanelle in babies. Lateralizing signs, such as facial or limb weakness, may be caused by a stroke, intracranial bleeding or pre-existing problems (eg previous stroke or Bell's palsy). Ocular nerve palsy or divergent squint with coma can indicate Wernicke's encephalopathy, requiring IV thiamine or tricyclic poisoning. Look for subtle signs of seizure activity (eg twitching of ocular muscles or eyelids, unusual limb movements), which may indicate non-convulsive status epilepticus. Look at the fundi—spontaneous central retinal venous pulsations are rare with ↑ ICP. Subhyaloid haemorrhages (blotchy fundal haemorrhages) suggest subarachnoid haemorrhage.

Hypoglycaemia can cause localized weakness/coma and mimic stroke.

Coma without lateralizing signs is usually due to poisoning, a post-ictal state, brainstem stroke, or hepatic failure: extensor plantar reflexes are common in these conditions.

Tricyclic antidepressants often cause coma with dilated pupils, a divergent squint, ↑ muscle tone, jerky limb movements, and extensor plantars. In severe poisoning, there may be muscle flaccidity with respiratory depression and ↓ reflexes (p.194).

Coma with small pupils and respiratory depression suggests opioid poisoning (p.188). In unexplained coma, give a therapeutic trial of naloxone (0.4–0.8mg IV), observing for changes in conscious level, respiratory rate, and pupil size.

Investigations
- BMG and blood glucose. If BMG is low, do not wait for the laboratory result to confirm this before starting treatment.
- ABG (record FiO_2 and whether breathing spontaneously or IPPV).
- FBC, prothrombin time, U&E.
- Check paracetamol and salicylate levels if poisoning is suspected: para- cetamol alone does not cause coma (except in late cases with liver failure), but a mixture of drugs may have been taken. Drug screening for sedatives/hypnotics is not needed, but in unexplained coma keep blood for later analysis if necessary.
- ECG may show arrhythmias (Tricyclic antidepressant poisoning, p.194).
- CXR may show pneumonia, aspiration, trauma, or tumour.
- CT scan may be needed to diagnose subarachnoid haemorrhage, stroke, or head injury.

Psychogenic coma
Patients sometimes pretend to be unconscious. It can be difficult to be certain of this—exclude other causes first. Suspect psychogenic coma if serious pathology has been excluded and when the eyes are opened, only the sclera show as the eyes deviate upwards (Bell's phenomenon).

Collapse and syncope

Syncope is a sudden, transient loss of consciousness, with spontaneous recovery.

Priorities

- Identify serious or life-threatening problems and institute treatment.
- Decide which patients require admission.
- Decide which patients require follow-up.

History of syncopal episode

Was it a simple faint? Vasovagal or neurally-mediated syncope is a common response to an overwarm environment or prolonged standing, and can be precipitated by sudden fright or visual stimuli (eg the sight of blood). Other contributors are large meals, prolonged starvation or alcohol. There are usually premonitory symptoms of feeling unwell, nauseated, dizzy, or tired, with yawning, blurred or 'tunnel' vision, or altered hearing. If the fainter cannot get supine (eg bystanders keeping them upright), seizure-like twitching may occur (*convulsive syncope*). Vomiting and incontinence may occur and do not reliably discriminate seizures from faints.

Was it a seizure? Look at the ambulance records. An eyewitness account is crucial. Ask what the witnesses *actually saw* (do not assume they know what a 'fit' looks like). There should typically be no prodrome, there is often a cry followed by tonic/clonic movements. Cyanosis, saliva frothing from the mouth, heavy breathing, tongue biting, or incontinence suggest a generalized seizure. Post-ictal drowsiness or confusion is normal—very rapid recovery questions the diagnosis.

Was it a cardiac event? Cardiac syncopal events are also abrupt in onset (eg collapse due to hypertrophic cardiomyopathy) and may be accompanied by pallor and sweating. Recovery may be rapid with flushing and deep/sighing respiration in some cases (eg Stokes–Adams attacks). Nausea and vomiting are not usually associated with syncope from arrhythmias. Ask about previous episodes and chest pain, palpitations, history of cardiac disease, and family history of sudden death. Syncope associated with exertion is a worrying feature: possible causes include aortic or mitral stenosis, pulmonary hypertension, cardiomyopathy, or coronary artery disease.

Other causes Carotid sinus syncope is neurally mediated, and often occurs with shaving or turning the head. Syncope may be secondary to effects of medication (eg GTN, β-blockers, anti-hypertensive drugs). Syncope may also be the presenting feature of subarachnoid haemorrhage, ruptured ectopic pregnancy, aortic or carotid dissection, PE, or GI bleed. Syncope is rarely caused by a TIA.

Assessment and treatment

If a patient suddenly loses consciousness in the ED, assess responsiveness and check for a pulse. Keep the airway clear, give O_2, and monitor pulse and ECG. Note any neurological signs during the episode and obtain BP, SpO_2, and BMG.

Patients seen following syncope Obtain a detailed account from the patient and witnesses. Look for signs of tongue biting, incontinence, or other injuries, examine the CVS for murmurs, arrhythmias or abnormalities. Perform a neurological examination and look for focal signs. Do postural tests (supine and standing or sitting pulse and BP). A degree of postural hypotension is common, but postural symptoms (eg dizziness, weakness, etc.) are always significant (look for causes of hypovolaemia eg GI bleed, ectopic pregnancy). Check BMG to exclude hypoglycaemia and an ECG looking for arrhythmias, LVH, ischaemia, previous or acute MI, and QT prolongation. An abnormal ECG may be the only clue to an underlying hypertrophic cardiomyopathy (HCM) or Brugada syndrome.

Disposal

Admit patients for cardiology review within 24 hr if they present with:
- An ECG abnormality.
- Heart failure.
- Loss of consciousness on exertion.
- Family history of sudden death <40 year or inherited cardiac condition.
- Age >65 year with no prodromal symptoms.
- A heart murmur.

Refer patients for assessment by a specialist in epilepsy if they present with one or more of:
- A bitten tongue.
- Amnesia, unresponsiveness, unusual posturing, or prolonged limb jerking, head turning to one side.
- History of a prodrome.
- Post-ictal confusion.

It may be appropriate to discharge patients with full recovery, appropriate history for vasovagal syncope and a normal examination.

See www.nice.org.uk

Diagnoses not to be missed

- *GI bleed:* syncope (± postural symptoms) indicate significant blood loss and hypovolaemia. Perform PR examination to check for blood/melaena.
- *Ectopic pregnancy:* suspect this in women with syncope and abdominal pain or gynaecological symptoms. Do a pregnancy test.
- Ruptured abdominal aortic aneurysm.
- PE (📖 Pulmonary embolism, p.120). A witness may give a history of cyanosis. Indicative of massive thrombus.

Acute generalized weakness

Weakness may be a feature of common neurological problems (eg TIA/ stroke), or accompany many of the causes of collapse (see 📖 Collapse and syncope, p.140). Less commonly, generalized muscle weakness may be the presentation of a number of other diseases.

Guillain–Barré syndrome

Guillain–Barré follows a respiratory or GI viral infection and is characterized by progressive symmetrical weakness, spreading from distal muscles to involve proximal muscles. Symptoms and signs include muscle tenderness, back pain, loss of muscle reflexes, sensory symptoms (paraesthesiae of fingers and toes) and disturbance of the autonomic nervous system (hyper- or hypotension, tachy- or bradycardia, bladder atony). Beware respiratory failure, which can rapidly progress to respiratory arrest. Serial vital capacity measurements are advised. Refer to the medical team/ICU.

Multiple sclerosis

Multiple sclerosis (MS) is a demyelinating disease of the CNS. It is more common in females and usually presents between ages 20–50. The disease follows a relapsing and remitting course with sensory loss, stiffness, and weakness of legs, ataxia, autonomic impairment (bladder dysfunction), and diplopia. Patients may present with these symptoms during their first exacerbation or with optic neuritis (pain in one eye with visual blurring). Arrange admission under neurology. If patient has eye symptoms, arrange urgent ophthalmology review.

Polymyositis

Polymyositis is an inflammatory myopathy that presents with symmetrical proximal muscle weakness, arthritis and sometimes muscular tenderness. Patients report difficulty climbing stairs, standing from a low chair, or lifting arms to brush hair. Creatine kinase (CK) levels are raised. Refer to a rheumatologist for treatment.

Myasthenia gravis

This is a rare autoimmune disease, which results in painless weakness in which the muscles are fatiguable, but tendon reflexes and pupil responses are normal. Ptosis, diplopia, and blurred vision are the commonest presentations. Usually, cranial nerves are involved to a greater extent than limb muscles and the distribution is asymmetrical. Crises may present with severe muscle weakness in which the major concern relates to respiratory compromise—the patient may require emergency temporary ventilatory support.

If the diagnosis is suspected in a patient not known to have myasthenia gravis, refer to a specialist who may wish to perform an *edrophonium test*. Patients with known myasthenia gravis may present with weakness due to under-treatment, over-treatment (cholinergic crisis), or an adverse reaction to an unrelated drug. Refer to the medical team for investigation.

Periodic paralysis

This encompasses a family of hereditary diseases associated with defects in muscle ion channels. Episodes of weakness can be associated with fluctuations in serum potassium levels lasting a few hours to a week. Patients may develop myotonia between attacks and fixed proximal muscle weakness. Treatment tends only to be required for hypokalaemic periodic paralysis with oral potassium supplementation.

Wound botulism

Botulism has made a recent come back in the IV drug injecting community. Botulinum toxin inhibits the release of acetylcholine at neuromuscular junctions, sympathetic and parasympathetic synapses. Wound infection with *Clostridium botulinum* presents with diplopia, blurred vision, ptosis, and neck weakness, which can progress to respiratory failure. Treatment is with antitoxin, benzylpenicillin, and metronidazole, along with respiratory support.

It is worth remembering that generalized weakness may also be caused by:
- Spinal cord compression.
- Tetanus.
- Alcoholic myopathy.
- Diphtheria.
- Lead poisoning.

Stroke

A *stroke* is an acute onset of focal neurological deficit of vascular origin which lasts >24hr. The blood supply to the brain has two sources—the internal carotid and the basilar arteries. The internal carotids supply the anterior and middle cerebral arteries, known as the anterior circulation. The basilar artery supplies the posterior cerebral artery in 70% of people (the posterior circulation). Anterior and posterior communicating arteries in the circle of Willis provide collateral circulation in cases of carotid artery stenosis.

Pathogenesis

70% of strokes occur in those aged >70yrs, but they can occur at *any* age.

Cerebral infarction (80%)

Results from:
- Thrombosis secondary to atherosclerosis, hypertension and rarely arteritis.
- Cerebral embolism from AF, valve disease/replacement, post-MI, ventricular aneurysm, myxoma, endocarditis or cardiomyopathy.
- An episode of hypoperfusion.

Cerebral haemorrhage (20%)

Associated with:
- Hypertension (rupture of small arteries in the brain).
- Subarachnoid haemorrhage (see 📖 p.128).
- Bleeding disorders (including anticoagulants) and intracranial tumours.

Presentation

Stroke preceded by neck pain may indicate carotid/vertebral artery dissection or subarachnoid haemorrhage. Headache is an unusual presentation of stroke and may indicate cerebral haemorrhage. Be alert to the possibility of different pathology requiring urgent treatment (eg hypoglycaemia, Todd's paresis, hemiplegic migraine, meningitis, encephalitis, brain abscess, head injury, Bell's palsy, 'Saturday night palsy', tumours).

Undertake a thorough examination including:
- Assessment of mental status/GCS and signs of meningeal irritation.
- Evidence of head or neck injury.
- Examination of pupils, fundi, and cranial nerves.
- Assessment of motor function (tone, power, and reflexes).
- Assessment of sensory function (including speech and comprehension).
- Examination for cerebellar signs (co-ordination, speech).
- Check for sources of embolism (AF, murmurs, carotid bruits).

Localization on clinical grounds alone can be difficult, and differentiation between infarction and haemorrhage requires CT/MRI. NICE recommend the use of the ROSIER score to identify patients presenting with acute stroke (see Table 3.9). The ROSIER score will pick up the majority of patients who are having a stroke, but may not identify patients with posterior circulation infarcts.

Table 3.9 ROSIER score for stroke recognition

Criteria	Points
Facial weakness (asymmetrical)	1
Arm weakness (asymmetrical)	1
Leg weakness (asymmetrical)	1
Speech disturbance	1
Visual field defect	1
Loss of consciousness or syncope	−1
Seizure	−1

Stroke unlikely if score 0 or less.

Investigation

Examine and investigate firstly to exclude other conditions and secondly to confirm the diagnosis of stroke. As a minimum requirement: BMG, FBC, ESR, U&E, blood glucose, ECG, CXR. Monitor with pulse oximeter (if SpO_2 <94% obtain ABG) and cardiac monitor.

Emergency CT

Arrange emergency CT scan where:

- The patient presents with symptoms under 4hr of duration. They may be eligible for emergency thrombolysis treatment. Time is of the essence.
- The patient is on warfarin, heparin, or other anticoagulant.
- There is a known bleeding disorder.
- GCS <13.
- Unexplained progressive or fluctuating symptoms.
- Papilloedema, neck stiffness or fever.
- There was a severe headache at onset of symptoms.

Management

- Immediately correct hypoglycaemia if present (see 🕮 p.150).
- Hypertension and labile BP are common in the early post-stroke period. Do not attempt to reduce the BP on presentation.
- Give supplemental oxygen only if SpO_2 <95%.
- Screen the patient's ability to swallow (try a teaspoon of water).
- If intracranial haemorrhage has been excluded, all patients should receive aspirin 300mg as soon as possible. Give this rectally if unable to swallow. Give PPI if there is a history of dyspepsia. If allergic to aspirin, give alternative antiplatelet drug such as clopidogrel.
- Wherever possible, admit patients directly to units where they can be cared for by staff specializing in stroke treatment and rehabilitation.

Thrombolysis

If intracranial haemorrhage has been excluded within 4hr of onset of symptoms, alteplase may be administered by a trained and supported emergency physician, only where the patient is managed within a specialist acute stroke service. See local guidelines and http://www.nice.org.uk

Transient ischaemic attacks

A *TIA* is an episode of transient focal neurological deficit of vascular origin lasting <24hr. A TIA gives major warning for the development of stroke (5% within 48hr, up to 50% in 5 years). Even in patients with resolution of symptoms/signs, most have evidence of infarction on CT/MRI.

Presentation

Carotid territory involvement produces unilateral weakness or sensory changes, dysphasia, homonymous hemianopia, or amaurosis fugax.

Vertebrobasilar territory involvement produces blackouts, bilateral motor or sensory changes, vertigo, and ataxia.

Causes

Most TIAs result from thrombo-embolic disease involving either the heart (AF, mitral stenosis, artificial valves, post-MI) or extracranial vessels (carotid artery stenosis). Other causes include:
- Hypertension.
- Polycythaemia/anaemia.
- Vasculitis (temporal arteritis, polyarteritis nodosa, SLE).
- Sickle cell disease.
- Hypoglycaemia.
- Any cause of hypoperfusion (eg arrhythmia, hypovolaemia).
- Syphilis.

Assessment

To diagnose a TIA, the symptoms must have resolved within 24hr.

Document vital signs and perform a thorough neurological examination. Look for possible sources of emboli eg arrhythmias (especially AF), heart murmurs, carotid bruits, MI (mural thrombus).

Investigations
- Check BMG.
- Send blood for FBC, ESR, U&E, blood glucose, lipids (INR if on anti-coagulants).
- Record an ECG to search for MI, arrhythmia.

Management
- Calculate the $ABCD^2$ score (Table 3.10).
- Admit to a stroke unit patients scoring 4 or more points, or anyone with more than one TIA in the previous week.
- Patients scoring 3 or less points, or who present one week after symptoms have resolved, may be suitable for discharge with stroke team follow-up in the next week.
- Start the patient on daily aspirin 300mg immediately.
- Admit patients with continuing symptoms or residual deficit (by definition, not a TIA).

See http://www.nice.org.uk

Table 3.10 ABCD^2 score for TIAs

Criteria		Points
Age	Age 60 or over	1
BP at assessment	Systolic >140mmHg or diastolic >90mmHg at assessment	1
Clinical features	Speech disturbance	1
	Unilateral weakness	2
Duration of symptoms	10–59min	1
	60 min or more	2
Diabetes		1

Patients scoring >4 points are at increased risk.

Seizures and status epilepticus

First fit

A first fit has enormous consequences—do not diagnose without good evidence

A detailed history from both the patient and any witnesses is crucial to the diagnosis. The presence of jerking movements or incontinence does not necessarily reflect epilepsy. Carefully document what was seen, in order to avoid confusion with vasovagal syncope or other types of collapse. Full rapid recovery suggests a syncopal event. Always consider alcohol/drug use, withdrawal states, hypoglycaemia, arrhythmia, head injury, subarachnoid haemorrhage, stroke/TIA, infection (including meningitis) or metabolic disturbance.

As part of the general examination, carefully examine the CNS, documenting: GCS, confusion, focal abnormalities, findings on fundoscopy. Examine the cardiovascular system and check for signs of aspiration.

Todd's paresis may follow seizures—focal deficit or hemiparesis may persist for up to 24hr and indicates a high chance of structural lesion.

Investigations BMG, glucose, FBC, U&E, blood cultures if pyrexial, ECG, and if there are chest signs, a CXR. Check urine pregnancy test if of child-bearing age. All patients with new onset seizures need brain imaging at some stage: a significant number have structural CNS abnormalities.

Arrange emergency CT scan for patients with focal signs, head injury, known HIV, suspected intracranial infection, bleeding disorder (including anticoagulants), or where conscious level fails to improve as expected.

Disposal A patient presenting with a first seizure may be discharged home, accompanied by an adult, if they have normal neurological and cardiovascular examinations, the ECG and electrolytes are normal, and there is an appointment with an epilepsy specialist in the coming week. Admit any patient with more than one seizure that day or who does not fit the above criteria. Ensure clear documentation of follow-up arrangements, including booked clinic appointment. Meantime, advise the patient not to drive or use machinery and to take sensible precautions, with supervision when performing activities, such as swimming/bathing until reviewed. *Document this advice* in the notes.

Seizures in known epileptics

Ask about any change from the patient's normal seizure pattern. Possible causes of poor seizure control include: poor compliance with medication, intercurrent illness/infection, alcohol, or drug ingestion. Examine to exclude any injury occurring from the fit, especially to the head. Occult dislocations (eg shoulder) may occur. Check vital signs, BMG and anticonvulsant levels if toxicity or poor compliance is suspected. Refer patients with a significant change in seizure pattern to the medical team. Discharge to the care of a responsible adult those patients who are fully recovered with no injuries, symptoms or other concerns.

Status epilepticus

This is continuous generalized seizures lasting >30min or without intervening recovery. Cerebral damage ↑ with duration. Precipitants include cerebral infection, trauma, cerebrovascular disease, toxic/metabolic disturbances, childhood febrile seizures. Mortality is ≈10% (due to underlying pathology). Although seizures typically start as generalized, tonic/clonic, these features may gradually diminish, making diagnosis difficult (coma with virtually no motor evidence of seizure, eg minimal twitching of ocular muscles only). Complications include hypoglycaemia, pulmonary hypertension, pulmonary oedema and precipitous ↑ ICP can also occur.

Treatment of status epilepticus

- Establish a clear airway (a nasopharyngeal airway may help).
- Give high flow O₂.
- Monitor ECG, SpO₂, T°, pulse rate, and BP.
- Obtain IV access, check BMG and correct hypoglycaemia if present (50mL of 20% glucose IV).
- Give IV lorazepam 4mg slowly into a large vein (diazepam 10mg is an alternative). Repeat IV lorazepam 4mg slowly after 10min if seizures continue.
- Buccal midazolam 10mg (can be repeated once) or rectal diazepam solution 10–20mg (can be repeated up to total 30mg) are alternatives if there is no venous access.
- If alcohol abuse or malnutrition is suspected, give slow IVI thiamine in the form of Pabrinex® 2 pairs of ampoules in 100mL of 0.9% saline (this occasionally causes anaphylaxis; be prepared to treat—see *BNF*).
- Consider the possibility of pregnancy-related fits (eclampsia) in women of childbearing age and treat accordingly (with IV magnesium sulphate—as outlined on 🕮 p.592).
- Check ABG and save blood for cultures, FBC, U&E, glucose, calcium, magnesium, LFTs, clotting, drug levels (and toxicology screen if poisoning/overdose is suspected).
- Search for features of injury (especially head injury) and infection (look for a rash).
- If seizures continue despite above therapy, call ICU and consider the use of phenytoin (18mg/kg IV, 50mg/min) with ECG monitoring, or fosphenytoin (20mg/kg phenytoin equivalent IV, <150mg/min). A 70kg patient would require 1400mg phenytoin equivalent of fosphenytoin (28mL Pro-Epanutin®) diluted in 100mL 0.9% saline or 5% glucose, given over 10–15min.
- After 30min, contact ICU and proceed without delay to rapid sequence induction (ideally with thiopental), tracheal intubation, and continue anticonvulsant medication.

Hypoglycaemia

Hypoglycaemia can mimic any neurological presentation including coma, seizures, acute confusion, or isolated hemiparesis.

> *Always exclude hypoglycaemia in any patient with coma, altered behaviour, neurological symptoms, or signs*

Plasma glucose is normally maintained at 3.6–5.8mmol/L. Cognitive function deteriorates at levels <3.0mmol/L, but symptoms are uncommon >2.5mmol/L. In diabetics, however, the threshold for symptoms can be very variable. Hypoglycaemia is potentially fatal, and accounts for 2.4% of deaths in diabetics on insulin. Even mild episodes aggravate pre-existing microvascular complications and lead to cumulative brain damage.

Causes

In diabetics, the commonest cause is a relative imbalance of administered versus required insulin or oral hypoglycaemic drug. This may result from undue or unforeseen exertion, insufficient or delayed food intake, excessive insulin administration (due to time, dose or type of insulin). Other causes are:

- Alcohol (in addition to alcohol directly causing hypoglycaemia, the features of hypoglycaemia may be mistaken for alcohol intoxication or withdrawal).
- Addison's disease.
- Pituitary insufficiency.
- Post-gastric surgery.
- Liver failure.
- Malaria.
- Insulinomas.
- Extra-pancreatic tumours.
- Attempted suicide or homicide with large doses of insulin or oral hypoglycaemic drug.

Symptoms and signs

Common features: sweating, pallor, tachycardia, hunger, trembling, altered or loss of consciousness, irritability, irrational or violent behaviour, fitting, focal neurological deficit (eg hemiplegia). Look for Medic-Alert bracelet/chain.

Diagnosis

Check venous or capillary blood with glucose oxidase strip (BMG). If <3.0mmol/L, take a venous sample for a formal blood glucose level, but *give treatment* without waiting for the result. Take appropriate samples if overdose of insulin, oral hypoglycaemic agent, or other drugs is suspected.

Treatment

This depends upon the conscious state and degree of co-operation of the patient. Choose the appropriate option from the following:

- 5–15g of fast-acting oral carbohydrate (eg Lucozade®, sugar lumps, Dextrosol®, followed by biscuits and milk).
- *Glucagon 1mg:* SC, IM, or IV. Can be administered by relatives, ambulance crew and when venous access is difficult. Glucagon is not suitable for treatment of hypoglycaemia due to sulphonylurea drugs, liver failure or in chronic alcoholism (as there may be little liver glycogen available for mobilization).
- Glucose 10% solution 50mL IV, repeated at 1–2min intervals until the patient is fully conscious or 250mL (25 g) has been given.
- Glucose 50% solution (25–50mL IV) is hypertonic, liable to damage veins and no more effective than glucose 10%. If glucose 50% is used, give it into a large vein and follow with a saline flush.
- The time taken for return of consciousness and the incidence of nausea, vomiting and other adverse effects are similar for IV glucagon and glucose.

The persistence of an altered conscious level suggests another underlying pathology (eg stroke), or may reflect the development of cerebral oedema due to hypoglycaemia, which has a high mortality. Maintain plasma glucose at 7–11mmol/L, contact ICU and consider mannitol and/or dexamethasone. Arrange urgent investigation (eg CT scan) and search for other causes of altered consciousness.

Overdose Glucose infusions may be needed for 24hr or longer after poisoning with insulin or oral hypoglycaemic drug, depending upon exactly what and how much has been taken. Hypokalaemia may be a problem. Block excision of the injection site has been used as successful treatment for insulin overdose. Octreotide may be helpful in recurrent hypoglycaemia due to overdose of a sulphonylurea drug (📖 p.197).

Discharge

90% of patients fully recover in 20min. Provided that the cause for the episode has been identified and fully corrected, it is reasonable to discharge the patient after observation in the ED, with appropriate follow-up.

Arrange follow up having considered the following:

- Why did this episode occur?
- Has there been a recent change of regimen, other drugs, alcohol, etc.?
- Is the patient developing hypoglycaemic unawareness or autonomic dysfunction?

Hyperglycaemic crises

Diabetic keto-acidosis (DKA) is caused by absolute or relative ↓ insulin levels. Plasma glucose ↑ causes an osmotic diuresis, with Na^+ and water loss (up to 8–10L), hypotension, hypoperfusion, and shock. Normal compensatory hormonal mechanisms are overwhelmed and lead to ↑ lipolysis. In the absence of insulin this results in the production of non-esterified fatty acids, which are oxidized in the liver to ketones.

Younger undiagnosed diabetics often present with *DKA* developing over 1–3 days. Plasma glucose levels may not be grossly ↑; euglycaemic ketoacidosis can occur. Urinalysis demonstrates ketonuria.

Hyperosmolar hyperglycaemic state (HHS) is caused by intercurrent illness, inadequate diabetic therapy and dehydration. It develops over days/weeks, and is more common in the elderly. HHS is characterized by ↑ glucose levels (>30mmol/L), ↑ blood osmolality, and a lack of urinary ketones. Mortality is ≈5–10%, but may be even higher in the elderly.

Causes
Think of the four 'I's separately or (often) in combination:
- *Infection:* common primary foci are urinary tract, respiratory tract, skin.
- *Infarction:* myocardial, stroke, GI tract, peripheral vasculature.
- *Insufficient insulin.*
- *Intercurrent illness:* many underlying conditions precipitate or aggravate DKA and HHS.

Clinical features
Hyperglycaemic crisis may present in various ways. Some of the following are usually present:

Signs of dehydration thirst, polydipsia, polyuria, ↓ skin turgor, dry mouth, hypotension, tachycardia.

GI symptoms are common in DKA with nausea, vomiting, and abdominal pain. This can be severe and mimic an 'acute surgical abdomen'.

Hyperventilation (respiratory compensation for the metabolic acidosis) with deep rapid breathing (Kussmaul respiration) and the smell of acetone on the breath, is pathognomonic of DKA.

True coma is uncommon, but altered conscious states and/or focal neurological deficits (which may correct with treatment) are seen particularly in older patients with HHS.

Diagnosis and investigations
Aim to confirm the diagnosis and search for possible underlying cause(s):
- Check BMG and test the urine for glucose and ketones.
- Send blood for U&E, blood glucose, creatinine, osmolality (or calculate it): mOsm/L= $(2 \times Na^+)$ + glucose (mmol/L) + urea (mmol/L).
- Check ABG (look for metabolic acidosis ±respiratory compensation).
- FBC and CXR (to search for pneumonia).
- ECG and cardiac monitoring (look for evidence of hyper/hypokalaemia).
- Blood cultures and if appropriate, throat or wound swabs.
- Urine/sputum microscopy and culture.

Treatment

- If altered consciousness/coma is present, provide and maintain a patent airway.
- Give high FiO_2 by mask. Consider the possible need for GA and IPPV for coma ± severe shock.
- Commence *IV infusion* with 0.9% saline (if the lab result subsequently shows initial plasma Na^+ to be >150mmol/L, give 0.45% saline). Give 1000mL of 0.9% saline over 0.5–1hr, then 500mL/hr for next 2–3hr. Persistent hypotension may require ↑ in infusion rate and/or colloid administration. Avoid over-rapid infusion with the risks of pulmonary oedema and ARDS, especially in the elderly and patients with IHD.
- *Insulin:* start an infusion of soluble insulin using an IV pump or paediatric burette at 6U/hr. No loading dose is required. Check plasma glucose levels every hour initially. When plasma glucose <14mmol/L, ↓ insulin infusion rate to 4U/hr and replace the saline solution with 10% dextrose to help ketone clearance and acid-base state.
- *Electrolyte balance:* although total body K^+ is low, plasma K^+ may be normal, ↑ or ↓. With treatment, K^+ enters cells and plasma levels ↓: therefore unless initial K^+ levels are >5.5mmol/L, give 20mmol/hr of KCl, monitor ECG, and check K^+ levels hourly. Despite the presence of metabolic acidosis, do not give sodium bicarbonate. Other electrolytes such as Ca^{2+}, Mg^{2+}, and PO_4^{2-} are commonly disturbed, but rarely need emergency correction.
- Consider an NG tube to ↓ risk of gastric dilation and aspiration.
- Monitor urine output (most accurate with urinary catheter).
- Consider a central venous catheter to monitor CVP to guide treatment in the elderly or severe illness.
- Arrange admission to ICU, HDU, or acute medical admissions unit.

Other aspects of treatment

Signs of infection are often masked. T° is rarely ↑, and ↑ WCC may only reflect ketonaemia. If in doubt, treat with a broad-spectrum antibiotic.

Over-rapid fluid replacement can cause cardiac failure, cerebral oedema, and ARDS, especially in patients with underlying cardiac disease or the elderly. CVP monitoring may be needed.

Clotting Hyperglycaemia causes a hypercoagulable state: DVT or PE may occur. Administer prophylactic anticoagulation with LMWH in DKA or hyperosmolar states.

Sodium derangements

Abnormal sodium states can occur with hypervolaemia, euvolaemia, or hypovolaemia, depending on the underlying pathophysiological process.

Hypernatraemia

Causes include diabetes insipidus (lack of ADH or lack of renal response to ADH), diarrhoea, vomiting, diuretics, hypertonic saline, sodium bicarbonate administration, or Cushing's syndrome.

Treatment should not correct the Na concentration faster than 1mmol/L/hr. Use 0.9% saline to correct hypovolaemia (patients who have tachycardia, hypotension, or postural hypotension). Once the patient is euvolaemic, use an infusion of 0.45% saline, or 5% dextrose. The *free water deficit* can be calculated using the formula:

Free water deficit (in litres) = $0.6 \times$ weight (kg) $\times$ (serum Na/140−1)

and should be replaced over 48hr (in addition to normal maintenance fluids). Check serum Na^+ after 2–3hr to monitor correction rate.

Complications of hypernatraemia include seizures, subdural and intra-cerebral haemorrhages, ischaemic stroke, and dural sinus thrombosis. Rapid correction of sodium levels (particularly in chronic hypernatraemia) can cause cerebral oedema and further neurological complications.

Hyponatraemia

Causes include excessive fluid loss replaced by hypotonic fluids (diarrhoea, burns, prolonged exercise, such as marathon running), polydipsia, ecstasy ingestion, syndrome of inappropriate ADH secretion, nephrotic syndrome, renal impairment, hepatic cirrhosis, cardiac failure, and many prescription drugs (including diuretics, heparin, and ACE inhibitors).

Treatment of acute hyponatraemia (<24hr duration) Those with mild symptoms can be effectively treated by fluid restriction. Patients who present with seizures or signs of raised intracranial pressure are at risk of death and should be treated more aggressively. Serum Na^+ <120mmol/L is associated with risk of brain herniation. Give up to 200mL of 2.7% saline IV over 30min and recheck serum Na^+ levels.

Treatment of chronic hyponatraemia (>24hr duration) is associated with central pontine myelinolysis, particularly in patients with low K^+ levels or alcoholic patients. Chronic hyponatraemia should be corrected no faster than 10mmol/L in 24hr. Treat the underlying cause. This may be as simple as discontinuing a diuretic. Patients with cardiac failure, cirrhosis, or nephrotic syndrome (hypervolaemic patients) should be fluid restricted. Severe hyponatraemia in association with seizures or ↓ GCS may be cautiously treated with hypertonic saline (2.7% saline 200mL over 30min and recheck serum Na^+). Aim to increase serum Na^+ by no more than 5mmol/L using this method.

See www.gain-ni.org

Addisonian crisis

Acute adrenocortical insufficiency is rare and easily missed. The most common cause is sudden withdrawal of chronic steroid therapy (deliberately or inadvertently). An Addisonian crisis may also be precipitated in these patients by intercurrent injury, infection or stress—increasing steroid requirement. 80% of Addison's disease in the UK is idiopathic (autoimmune), and may be associated with Graves' disease, Hashimoto's thyroiditis, insulin dependent diabetes mellitus (IDDM), pernicious anaemia, hypoparathyroidism, and ovarian failure. Other causes include TB, fungal infections, metastatic disease, congenital adrenal hyperplasia, drugs (eg metyrapone or cytotoxic agents), haemorrhage into the adrenal glands occurring as a complication of anticoagulation or meningococcal septicaemia (Waterhouse–Friderichsen syndrome). Look for a Medic–Alert bracelet indicating that the patient is taking steroids.

Precipitating factors

Infection, trauma, MI, cerebral infarction, asthma, hypothermia, alcohol, pregnancy, exogenous steroid withdrawal or reduction.

Clinical features

Addison's disease frequently has an insidious onset with weakness, apathy, anorexia, weight loss, abdominal pain (which may be severe enough to mimic an acute abdomen), and oligomenorrhoea. In crisis, the main features may be shock (tachycardia, peripheral vasoconstriction, severe postural hypotension occasionally with syncope, oliguria, profound muscle weakness, confusion, altered consciousness leading to coma), and hypoglycaemia. Chronic features of Addison's disease are: areas of vitiligo and hyperpigmentation in the palmar creases, buccal mucosa, areolae, scars, and in the axillae.

Investigations

Hyperkalaemia, hyponatraemia, hypoglycaemia, uraemia, mild acidosis, hypercalcaemia, and eosinophilia may be present. If Addisonian crisis is suspected, take appropriate blood samples, but start treatment without waiting for results.

Management

- Obtain IV access.
- Take blood for cortisol (10mL in a heparinized tube) and ACTH if possible. Contact the biochemistry lab to warn them that these tests will be required.
- If features of haemodynamic compromise are present, commence volume replacement with IV 0.9% saline if shocked.
- Give hydrocortisone sodium succinate 100mg IV stat.
- Take blood, urine, and sputum for culture and sensitivity.
- Check BMG and blood glucose, and treat hypoglycaemia with 50mL of 10% glucose IV (repeated if necessary).
- If infection is suspected as a precipitating cause, consider giving broad spectrum antibiotics.
- Refer for admission.

Thyrotoxic crisis

A rare condition, occurring in 1–2% of patients with established hyperthyroidism (usually toxic diffuse goitre 'Graves' disease'). Mortality is significant (≈10%).

Causes

It is often precipitated by a physiological stressor:
- Premature or inappropriate cessation of anti-thyroid therapy.
- Recent surgery or radio-iodine treatment.
- Intercurrent infection (especially chest infection).
- Trauma.
- Emotional stress.
- DKA, hyperosmolar diabetic crisis, insulin-induced hypoglycaemia.
- Thyroid hormone overdose.
- Pre-eclampsia.

Clinical features

Onset may be sudden with features of hyperthyroidism and adrenergic overactivity. Fever, cardiovascular, and neurological symptoms are common. Weight loss, ↑ appetite, tremor, irritability, emotional lability, heat intolerance, sweating, itch, oligomenorrhoea, agitation, anxiety, confusion, coma, palpitations, tachycardia, AF (rarely, complete heart block). It may mimic an 'acute abdomen', with abdominal pain, diarrhea, and vomiting.

Differential diagnosis

Includes acute pulmonary oedema, neuroleptic malignant syndrome, septic shock, anticholinergic or sympathomimetic overdose, drug withdrawal, or acute anxiety states.

Investigations

- U&E, BMG, and blood glucose, Ca^{2+} (hypercalcaemia occurs in ≈10%).
- FBC, differential WCC, coagulation screen.
- *Screen for infection:* MSU, blood cultures, sputum.
- T_4 and T_3 (for later analysis), TSH.
- CXR (searching for pulmonary infection or congestive heart failure).
- ECG (looking for arrhythmias).

Treatment

- Manage the airway and give O_2 if indicated.
- Obtain IV access and commence IVI 0.9% saline (initially 500mL 4-hourly).
- Pass NG tube if vomiting.
- If sedation is required, give small titrated amounts of benzodiazepine (eg diazepam 5–20mg PO/IV) or haloperidol.
- Commence dexamethasone 4mg 6 hourly PO or give hydrocortisone 100mg IV.
- Give broad spectrum antibiotic if infection is suspected.
- Consider cooling measures in hyperthermia.
- Refer for admission (consider admission to ICU).
- Once admitted, propranolol (or esmolol) and carbimazole will normally be given together with iodine.
- Do not give aspirin (this can exacerbate the clinical problem by displacing thyroxine from thyroid binding globulin).

Urinary tract infection

The urinary tract is normally bacteriologically sterile. Urine infection is present if >10^5 colony-forming units are present per mL of urine. Except at the extremes of age, urinary tract infections (UTIs) are much more common in females due to the shorter urethral length. Most UTIs occur because of organisms invading the bladder via the urethra. Proximal invasion via the ureter may result in acute or chronic pyelonephritis, particularly if anatomical derangement exists with impaired ureteric or bladder emptying. In both sexes, underlying structural abnormality ↑ UTI risk. Blood-borne spread of infection to the urinary tract can occur, (eg in bacterial endocarditis or systemic Gram −ve infection). UTI is usually caused by a single organism. The commonest organism (90%) at all ages is *E. coli. Proteus, Klebsiella,* and saprophytic staphylococci account for most of the remainder in adults. Other organisms (eg *Pseudomonas*) more commonly cause UTI in hospitalized patients or following instrumentation.

Urinary tract infection: presentation

UTIs usually present to the ED in one of two ways

Lower UTI (cystitis) Dysuria, frequency, haematuria, suprapubic discomfort, urgency, burning, cloudy urine with an offensive smell. Patients with acute urethral syndrome have identical symptoms, but −ve urine culture.

Upper UTI (acute pyelonephritis) Often systemically unwell with malaise, fever, loin and/or back pain, vomiting, rigors and occasionally Gram −ve septicaemia.

Investigations

Reagent strip (dipstix) urinalysis may show haematuria, proteinuria, +ve nitrite, and leucocyte esterase tests. A patient with clear urine, −ve on dipstix testing, is extremely unlikely to have a UTI. False +ve results may be secondary to urinary tract tumours or excessive exercise. A false −ve nitrite test may reflect pathogens that do not convert dietary nitrates to nitrites.

Urine microscopy may show leucocytes (>100/mL correlates well with infection, but may be due to contamination or other urinary tract pathology). RBCs are commonly seen on microscopy, but in isolation have a low degree of sensitivity or specificity for UTI. Underlying renal pathology is suggested by finding urinary crystals, RBC, or granular casts.

MSU for culture and sensitivity. Transport the sample to the laboratory without delay to ensure that bacterial overgrowth does not artificially ↑ the count. Dipslides dipped into freshly passed urine and transported in a plastic container to the laboratory are an alternative.

Treatment

- It is usually reasonable to discharge female patients with uncomplicated lower UTIs with *antibiotics*. Commence a 3–6 day course of trimethoprim or nitrofurantoin. Provide *advice* regarding fluid intake, no 'holding on', and voiding after intercourse. Drinking barley water is as effective as attempts at urinary alkalinization with sodium bicarbonate. (*Note:* urinary alkalinization renders nitrofurantoin ineffective). Advise the patient to see her GP for review, MSU result, and repeat MSU.
- Elderly men and women with asymptomatic bacteriuria should not receive antibiotic treatment unless they show signs of being unwell.
- In pregnancy, both symptomatic and asymptomatic bacteriuria should be treated with an antibiotic such as amoxicillin.
- Given the difficulty in distinguishing prostatitis from simple UTI in men, they should receive a 2-week course of ciprofloxacin, trimethoprim, or co-amoxiclav. Arrange GP follow-up.
- Treat catheterized patients with symptoms or signs of UTI for 7 days with ciprofloxacin or co-amoxiclav. Treatment is more effective if the catheter is changed in the ED prior to commencing antibiotics.
- Do not treat catheterized patients with asymptomatic bacteriuria with antibiotics.

Refer for investigation and treatment all male patients and females with recurrent infections, pregnancy, GU malformation, immunosuppression, or renal impairment.

Patients with acute pyelonephritis usually require admission for parenteral antibiotics, fluid replacement, and analgesia. Assess and treat for severe sepsis (📖 Shock, p.60).

See http://www.sign.ac.uk

Chronic renal failure

Patients with established chronic renal failure (CRF) are likely to be very well known to the hospital. Obtain old notes and recent blood results, and liaise early with in-patient specialist teams.

Established chronic renal failure (not on dialysis)

Patients with mild CRF (glomerular infiltration rate (GFR) >40mL/min—100mL/min) are unlikely to have specific problems related to their underlying renal failure. With GFR <40mL/min, and especially if GFR <10mL/min, complications may influence presentation and treatment. These patients are prone to pathological fractures.

Secondary hyperparathyroidism and osteomalacia (lack of active vitamin D) occur in moderate GFR. In severe CRF, aluminium bone disease, and β_2-microglobulin related amyloidosis may be associated with pathological fractures.

'Pseudo-gout' due to high Ca^{2+}/PO_4^- production and twitching/tetany due to hypocalcaemia may occur.

Other problems include:

Defective regulation of extra-cellular fluid volume There is an ↑ risk of fluid depletion in moderate CRF and fluid retention in severe CRF. High dose diuretics may be required in severe disease: the combination of furosemide and metolazone may be effective even with very low GFRs.

Hyperkalaemia Most patients preserve potassium balance, but cannot deal with sudden K^+ loads (eg dietary, tissue damage/catabolism, GI bleed). Associated ↓ Ca^{2+} compounds the cardiac effects. Plasma K^+ may ↑ very quickly, so monitor ECG and check K^+ frequently.

Hypertension Often severe and resistant, with an ↑ incidence of accelerated phase. Ciclosporin and erythropoietin ↑ BP, and can precipitate hypertensive encephalopathy.

Drug effects Drugs may accumulate (eg opioids, acyclovir, some antibiotics), worsen renal failure (eg NSAIDs, ACE inhibitors, which ↓ renal perfusion), cause hyperkalaemia (eg K^+ sparing diuretics, ACE inhibitors, NSAIDs).

Infections Impaired WBC function, with ↑ risk of severe infection and features of infection (eg pain, fever) may be masked by the relative immuno-compromised state.

Bleeding Platelet function is impaired.

Pericarditis A sign of severe CRF, indicating the need for dialysis.

Neurological dysfunction Usually a sign of severe uraemia—convulsions and/or altered conscious state indicate a global metabolic disturbance.

Common emergency presentation in haemodialysis patients

Pulmonary oedema Usually occurs shortly before the next dialysis session and may reflect fluid overload due to non-compliance with diet and fluid restriction. Most are virtually anuric, so diuretics are ineffective. Get the patient on dialysis without delay. While this is being arranged give high flow O_2 and SL buccal or IV nitrates.

Pre-dialysis hyperkalaemia May present with neuromuscular symptoms (eg muscle spasms, weakness, paralysis, paraesthesiae) or arrhythmias, including cardiac arrest. Standard treatment (📖 p.162) can buy time while emergency dialysis is arranged. When giving glucose/insulin, give 6U of insulin at most (there is a risk of late hypoglycaemia, since insulin half-life will be ↑).

Complications of vascular access Arteriovenous fistulae are a dialysis patient's lifeline—never occlude limb with BP cuffs or tourniquets. Do not use for vascular access unless life-threatening emergency. Acute shunt thrombosis (loss of palpable thrill, often local pain/redness) is a vascular emergency. Arteriovenous fistulae and central lines are common infection sources (usually staphylococcal), often with no overt external abnormality, but presenting with acute 'viral illness' symptoms.

Continuous ambulatory peritoneal dialysis

Bacterial peritonitis Occurs every 12–18 patient-months. Features are cloudy drained dialysate bags, abdominal pain, and peritonism. Systemic sepsis is usually absent or minimal. Staphylococci are most common organisms. Suspect underlying surgical cause (most often diverticular abscess) if Gram –ve organisms or anaerobes present in drainage fluid, and particularly if >1 type of organism is found on microscopy or culture.

Diabetic patients on continuous ambulatory peritoneal dialysis can develop acute severe (usually non-ketotic) *hyperglycaemia*, related to high dialysate glucose concentrations (80–140mmol/L).

Hernias of all types, leakage of dialysate into the abdominal wall or the pleural cavity, and scrotal swelling (open processus vaginalis) may occur.

Transplant patients

Contact the transplant team whenever any transplant patient presents to the ED. They will know the patient well and will advise about drug therapy, intercurrent problems, and help with follow-up.

Acute rejection Signs include pain, tenderness, and swelling over graft, ↓ urine output, fever, systemic upset, biochemical deterioration. Often indistinguis\hable from acute bacterial infection: if in doubt treat for both, pending results of further testing by specialists (renal biopsy, blood, and urine cultures).

Infections May be opportunist, whilst 'conventional' infections are unduly severe, with response modulated by steroids.

Poor wound healing, avascular necrosis and pathological fractures May be caused by steroids.

Hyperkalaemia

Hyperkalaemia is classified as mild (K^+ 5.5–6.0mmol/L), moderate (K^+ 6.1–6.9mmol/L) or severe (K^+ >7.0mmol/L).

Causes

Spurious Sample haemolysed or taken from limb with IVI containing K^+.

↓ *Renal excretion* Acute kidney injury, patients with chronic renal failure or on dialysis with K^+ load, K^+ sparing diuretics (eg spironolactone, amiloride).

Cell injury Crush injury and other causes of rhabdomyolysis, burns, tumour cell necrosis, massive, or incompatible blood transfusion.

K^+ *cellular shifts* Acidosis from any cause (eg DKA), drugs (suxamethonium, β-blockers).

Hypoaldosteronism Addison's disease, drug-induced (NSAIDs, ACE inhibitors).

Clinical features

There may be muscle weakness/cramps, paraesthesiae, hypotonia, focal neurological deficits. Dangerous hyperkalaemia may be asymptomatic.

ECG changes

ECG changes typically progress as hyperkalaemia worsens as follows:
- Peaked T waves.
- Small, broad, or absent P waves.
- Widening QRS complex.
- Sinusoidal ('sine wave' pattern) QRST.
- AV dissociation or VT/VF.

Management of severe hyperkalaemia

Urgent treatment is needed if K^+ >6.5mmol/L, unless this is a spurious and incorrect result. If K^+ is reported as >6.5mmol/L obtain venous access, monitor and review the ECG. Start treatment immediately (as indicated below) if there are ECG changes of hyperkalaemia. If there are no ECG signs of hyperkalaemia take another blood sample for U&E, with care to avoid haemolysis, and a heparinized sample to measure K^+ on a blood gas machine:
- Give 10mL of 10% calcium chloride slowly IV (over 5min). This does not lower K^+, but antagonizes cardiac membrane excitability. Hypercalcaemia may possibly potentiate toxicity in patients on digoxin, so give as an IVI over 30min in these patients.
- Give 10U of short-acting human soluble insulin with 50mL of 50% glucose IV. This helps ↑ cellular uptake of K^+, lowering serum levels by up to 1mmol/L within 1hr.
- Give 5mg nebulized salbutamol, repeated once as necessary. This will lower K^+ in most patients, acting in ≈30min.
- Correct volume deficits/acidosis with IV fluids and isotonic (1.26%) sodium bicarbonate or aliquots (25–50mL) of 8.4%. Beware fluid overload/osmolar effects, especially in dialysis patients.
- Correct the underlying cause if possible (eg steroid therapy for Addison's disease).
- Contact the nephrology team urgently for patients with acute or chronic renal failure as emergency dialysis may be needed.

Hyperkalaemia in children—see 📖 Renal failure, p.694.

Management of hyperkalaemic cardiac arrest

If a patient in cardiac arrest is known to have hyperkalaemia, follow the standard ALS guidelines (📖 p.46), plus one or more of the following:
- Give 10mL of 10% calcium chloride IV by rapid bolus injection.
- Consider giving 10U of short-acting insulin + 100mL 50% glucose rapidly IV.
- If there is severe acidosis, give 50mL 8.4% sodium bicarbonate rapidly IV.
- Consider haemodialysis for cardiac arrest induced by hyperkalaemia which is resistant to medical treatment.

Management of moderate hyperkalaemia

Provided that the result is not spurious, a K^+ of 6–6.5mmol/L may be regarded as 'moderately' severe hyperkalaemia.
- Obtain venous access and monitor ECG.
- If there are ECG changes, treat as for severe elevation opposite.
- If there are no ECG changes, give 10U of short-acting human soluble insulin with 50mL of 50% glucose IV over 15–30min.
- Look for and treat the underlying cause and consider: diuretics (eg furosemide 1mg/kg IV slowly) and dialysis.

Management of mild hyperkalaemia

K^+ of 5.5–6mmol/L. Treat the underlying cause and treat any associated hypovolaemia. Discuss need for specific intervention (diuretic, dialysis) with the medical team.

Hypokalaemia

Defined as K^+ <3.5mmol/L, it is relatively common. Moderate hypokalaemia may result in lethargy, weakness, and leg cramps. In severe cases (K^+ <2.5mmol/L), rhabdomyolysis and respiratory difficulties may occur.

ECG changes include prominent U waves and flattened T waves.

Treatment In most instances, aim to replace potassium gradually. The maximum recommended IV infusion rate of potassium is 20mmol/hr. Restrict more rapid rates of IV infusion (eg 20mmol in 20–30min) to those patients who have unstable arrhythmias when cardiac arrest is imminent (obtain senior/expert advice). Ensure cardiac monitoring occurs during any potassium IVI.

Associated magnesium deficiency

Many patients with potassium deficiency are also magnesium deficient. Consider replacing magnesium in those patients who have severe hypokalaemia.

See also www.resus.org.uk

Porphyria

The porphyrias are haem biosynthesis disorders in which enzyme deficiencies cause accumulation of porphyrin and porphyrin precursors. Most cases are hereditary, but abnormal porphyrin metabolism may develop in iron deficiency, alcohol excess and lead poisoning. The acute porphyrias (acute intermittent porphyria, variegate porphyria and hereditary coproporphyria) affect ≈1 in 10,000 people in the UK. The non-acute porphyrias (eg porphyria cutanea tarda) do not produce acute attacks, but cause skin photosensitivity sometimes associated with liver disease.

Attacks of acute porphyria are often caused by drugs: barbiturates, oestrogens, progesterones, sulphonamides, methyldopa, carbamazepine, phenytoin, sulphonylureas, chloramphenicol, tetracyclines, danazol, some antihistamines. Other precipitants include: alcohol, smoking, dieting, emotional and physical stress, infection, substance misuse, pregnancy.

Clinical features of acute porphyria

- Abdominal pain is common and can be severe, with nausea, vomiting and constipation. Abdominal examination may be normal or there may be mild generalized tenderness.
- Peripheral neuropathy is usually motor, rather than sensory, and may progress to paralysis and respiratory failure.
- Tachycardia, hypertension, and postural hypotension.
- Psychiatric manifestations: agitation, depression, mania and hallucinations.
- Hyponatraemia due to inappropriate ADH secretion can cause fits or coma.

Investigation and management of acute porphyria

Look for a Medic-Alert bracelet. Obtain old medical notes.

If an acute attack is suspected, send a fresh urine sample (protected from light) to test for amino laevulinic acid and porphobilinogen. In an attack, urine goes dark red or brown, especially if left exposed to light (due to polymerization of porphobilinogen).

Treat acute attacks supportively (if necessary in ICU). Maintain carbohydrate intake (PO or IV). Control mild pain with paracetamol or aspirin; moderate/severe pain with morphine (± anti-emetic). Consider chlorpromazine for agitation; propranolol to control severe hypertension. Management of status epilepticus is difficult as many anticonvulsants are contraindicated: choose IV diazepam in the first instance. Haem arginate helps some patients with acute crises (take specialist advice).

Prescribing for patients with porphyria

Many drugs can precipitate attacks, so check with the patient and the *BNF*.

However, the safety of many drugs in porphyria is uncertain and effects vary between patients. If in doubt, obtain specialist advice. In addition to those mentioned earlier, safe drugs appear to be: ibuprofen, penicillin, ciprofloxacin, bupivicaine.

Data is also available on the internet at www.uq.edu.au/porphyria

Bleeding disorders: 1

> *Contact a haematologist whenever treating a patient with a known or suspected bleeding disorder*

Haemostasis requires co-ordination between the *vascular system, platelets and coagulation pathways* to limit blood loss from the circulation. Platelets interact with vascular subendothelium, forming a primary platelet plug, which is strengthened by cross-linked fibrin strands formed via the coagulation cascade to allow restoration of vascular integrity (see Fig. 3.24). The fibrinolytic systems prevent excess clot formation, and inappropriate local or generalized thrombosis, by promoting lysis of fibrin.

Recognition of bleeding

Bleeding is expected after trauma, but suspect a bleeding disorder if spontaneous or excess haemorrhage occurs from multiple or uninjured sites, into deep tissues, joints or delayed bleeding occurs (hr/day). Bleeding disorders may be congenital or acquired. Ask about previous bleeding after trauma, dentistry or surgery and the family history.

Congenital disorders Haemophilia A (Factor VIII deficiency), Haemophilia B (Factor IX deficiency), and von Willebrand's disease. Most adults with a congenital disorder know the nature of it and carry a National Haemophilia card or Medic-Alert bracelet giving details. Many haemophiliacs know more about their required treatment than you! They will be registered and known at a haemophilia centre.

Acquired disorders May be due to liver disease, uraemia, drug use (ask specifically about aspirin, NSAIDs, warfarin/anticoagulants, alcohol), or unrecognized conditions such as haematological malignancy.

Hypothermia (📖 p.254) from whatever cause aggravates any bleeding tendency. For example, an INR assay performed at 32°C will be prolonged to the same extent as would occur with a Factor IX level of 2.5% of normal. The severity of this may not be recognized merely from standard tests as these are performed at 37°C.

The site of bleeding can give a clue as to the abnormality. Platelet problems (usually thrombocytopenia) often present with mucocutaneous bleeding (eg epistaxis, GI, GU, or heavy menstrual bleeding, bruising, purpura, and petechial haemorrhages). Bleeding into joints or potential spaces (eg retroperitoneal) and delayed bleeding is more often due to coagulation factor deficiencies. Patients with mucocutaneous bleeding and haemorrhage into deep spaces may have a combined platelet and coagulation factor abnormality (eg disseminated intravascular coagulation (DIC)).

Investigations

FBC Remember that in acute bleeds, Hb and Hct values fail to demonstrate the severity of red cell loss as haemodilution takes time. Platelet counts <100 × 10^9/L indicate thrombocytopenia, and <20 × 10^9/L are associated with a risk of spontaneous bleeding. Bleeding because of platelet problems can occur with 'normal' counts if platelet function is abnormal (eg with aspirin or clopidogrel).

Prothrombin time (INR) Used to monitor anticoagulant control in patients on coumarin drugs and may be prolonged in liver disease.

Activated partial thromboplastin time (APTT) Tests components of intrinsic and common coagulation pathways (essentially all factors except VII and XIII).

Individual factor levels Can be determined by specific assays together with inhibitor screening tests for antibodies that can prolong normal plasma clotting.

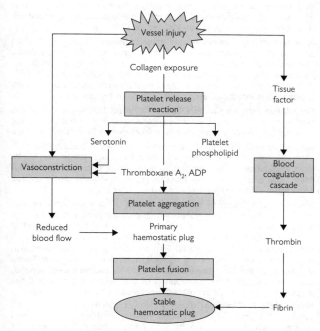

Fig. 3.24 Reactions involved in haemostasis.

Bleeding disorders: 2

General aspects of treatment

- Perform routine wound/fracture management of patients with bleeding disorders, but consider need for prior or simultaneous administration of factor concentrates/platelets under haematological guidance.
- Spontaneous or traumatic bleeding into the neck or pharynx may cause rapid airway compromise.
- Always consider intracranial haemorrhage in a patient with headache, neurological symptoms or minor head trauma. Consult to consider need for commencing treatment before specific investigation (eg CT).
- Never give IM injections.
- Do not attempt central line placement except in extremis, since life-threatening, uncontrollable bleeding can result.
- Before giving any drug, check whether it may aggravate the condition or interfere with intercurrent therapy.

Specific conditions

Vascular lesions May be inherited (Ehlers–Danlos syndrome, pseudo-xanthoma elasticum, osteogenesis imperfecta, haemorrhagic telangiectasia) or acquired (eg due to steroids, infection e.g. meningococcaemia, thrombotic thrombocytopenic purpura, vasculitis, scurvy).

Platelet disorders Capillary-related mucocutaneous bleeding is common and may occur immediately after injury/surgery (eg dental extractions). The platelet count may be normal or ↓. Acquired thrombocytopenia may be due to drugs, toxins, infections, autoimmune conditions (eg ITP), DIC, or to massive blood transfusion. Abnormal platelet function occurs with uraemia, myeloproliferative disorders, and drugs (eg aspirin).

Coagulation pathway disorders Congenital coagulation pathway disorders predominate in males. They cause intramuscular or deep soft tissue haematomas. Bleeding onset after injury/surgery may be delayed 2–3 days.

von Willebrand's Disease The commonest congenital bleeding disorder, with VW Factor and Factor VIII deficiency, and abnormal platelet function. Clinically, the condition is similar to a platelet disorder, but milder. Bleeding is commonly mucosal (eg epistaxis) and usually treated with Factor VIII concentrate (which includes VW Factor).

Haemophilia A Caused by a lack of functional factor VIII which is needed for clot formation. Often presents with bleeding into deep muscles, large joints or urinary tract. Intracranial bleeding is a major cause of death at all ages. Anticipate bleeding up to 3 days after trauma.

In UK, haemophilia A associated with bleeding or potential bleeding is normally treated by Factor VIII concentrate (some patients have 'home supplies' and may bring them to hospital). The volume (dose) depends upon the severity of the haemophilia of the individual patient and the purpose of treatment (ie prophylaxis or therapy for current bleeding).

Haemophilia B (Christmas disease) Involves a deficiency of Factor IX activity and is genetically and clinically indistinguishable from haemophilia A, but much less common. It is normally treated with factor IX concentrate.

Disseminated intravascular coagulation (DIC)

Patients may present with DIC due to infection (especially Gram −ve sepsis), trauma, malignancy, pregnancy (amniotic fluid embolism, placental abruption, toxaemia, retained products), any cause of shock, incompatible blood transfusion or massive volume replacement. Following triggering of the coagulation process, consumption of platelets, and coagulation factors (particularly fibrinogen, V, VIII, and XIII) occurs with thrombin formation overwhelming the normal inhibition system, resulting in systemic fibrin deposition (Fig. 3.25). Activation of the fibrinolytic system results in dissolution of fibrin and release of fibrin degradation products.

Investigations Platelet count is usually ↓, INR ↑ and APTT ↑, fibrinogen level ↓, fibrin degradation products ↑.

Treatment Is complex and requires control of the primary cause of the DIC to avoid total depletion of clotting factors. Obtain expert advice about replacement therapy with platelets, FFP, prothrombin complex concentrate, heparin and blood (particularly required if the patient is actively bleeding).

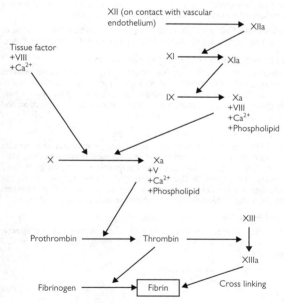

Fig. 3.25 Coagulation cascade.

Patients on anticoagulants

The commonest oral anticoagulant is warfarin sodium, a vitamin K antagonist. This inhibits the production of Factors II (prothrombin), VII, IX and X and ↓ plasma levels of these factors. Patients, or their relatives, who are able to give a history will usually know if they are taking warfarin, and their most recent prothrombin time or INR test result, together with any changes in treatment.

If this history is not available, suspect patients with prosthetic heart valves, mitral valve disease, AF, a past history of DVT/PE or TIAs to be on anticoagulants. Intercurrent illness, liver disease and changes in diet, and/or alcohol consumption may affect anticoagulant control. Concurrent drug administration with unrecognized potential for interaction is the commonest cause for acute changes in anticoagulant control.

These patients usually present with one of three problems.

Acute haemorrhage

Spontaneous bleeding in patients on warfarin most commonly affects the GI tract, GU tract, joints, or muscles. After injury, expect excessive or continuing bleeding. Anticipate the ↑ risks of occult or unrecognized bleeding (eg intraperitoneally or intracranially) after even minor trauma and maintain a high index of suspicion as to these possibilities.

Check INR and FBC in all patients. Other investigations (eg CT scan of head/abdomen, USS) will be dictated by the nature of the acute problem.

Patients with life-threatening haemorrhage

For patients with life-threatening haemorrhage, commence volume replacement and blood transfusion as appropriate (see 📖 Blood transfusion 1, p.172). Contact haematology for specialist advice which may include phytomenadione (vitamin K_1) up to 10mg by slow IV injection and provision of prothrombin complex concentrate.

Patients with less severe haemorrhage

Patients with muscle haematomas, haematuria, or epistaxis also require hospital admission for observation and specific local treatment. Stop warfarin therapy for one or more days. Phytomenadione 0.5–2mg by slow IV injection may be advised by the haematologists. Note that vitamin K_1 can interfere with warfarinization for several days, so take expert advice when the patient is also at high risk of thrombosis (prosthetic heart valve).

INR levels within the therapeutic range

Patients who develop bleeding with INR levels within the therapeutic range require investigation of a possible underlying cause (eg GI or GU tract pathology).

See http://www.bcshguidelines.com

Check of control of anticoagulation

The therapeutic range for the INR may vary according to the indication for anticoagulation. An INR of 2.0–3.0 is usually appropriate for DVT prophylaxis and 3.0–4.0 for patients with mechanical prosthetic heart valves.

For patients who have INR 4.0–7.0 without haemorrhage, withhold warfarin therapy for 1 or 2 days, and arrange review by appropriate specialist team or GP. For patients with INR >7.0 without haemorrhage, withhold warfarin and obtain specialist consultation before considering phytomenadione (vitamin K_1) 5mg by slow IV injection or orally.

Interactions with other prescribed or proprietary medicines

Many drugs can interfere with anticoagulant control. Before giving or stopping any drug in a patient taking warfarin or other anticoagulant, check the potential for interaction—Appendix I in the *BNF*.

Particular groups of drugs, likely to be prescribed in the ED, which may cause problems include analgesics (especially NSAIDs), antibacterials and anti-epileptics. Always *LOOK IT UP*.

Other oral anticoagulants

Dabigatran (a direct thrombin inhibitor) and rivaroxaban (a Factor Xa inhibitor) are among a group of new oral anticoagulants which may be prescribed instead of warfarin or low molecular weight heparin, in certain conditions. They do not require routine blood monitoring. To date, there are no guidelines for measuring their effect in patients who are bleeding, and there is no proven way to reverse their effect. Always discuss bleeding patients on new oral anticoagulants with a haematologist. Attempts at reversal may include FFP or prothrombin complex concentrate.

Blood transfusion 1

> *It is better to stop bleeding than to have to replace blood loss*

General aspects

Correctly documenting and labelling blood tubes and forms, combined with checking blood products prior to administration, is crucial for safe patient care. If a patient's name(s), date of birth, clinical details and address are unknown or uncertain, identify them for transfusion purposes by a unique number (usually their unique ED number) and inform the blood transfusion laboratory.

To avoid confusion, the doctor taking the blood sample must label and sign the tube at the patient's bedside, complete the form, and contact the transfusion service. Only take blood from one patient at a time. Label tubes immediately to minimize the risk of mislabelling. Blood banks may refuse to handle incorrectly labelled forms/tubes.

If you knowingly give a blood product (or animal product e.g. gelatin) to a patient whom you know would not accept this (eg a Jehovah's Witness) you are likely to face an indefensible medicolegal claim.

What to send

10mL clotted blood is usually adequate for adults. Where it is obvious that massive transfusion may be required, send two 10mL samples. On the request form, indicate how much blood is needed, when and where the blood is to be sent. Date and sign the form.

What to request

The amount of blood to be delivered and to be kept available at the transfusion centre for immediate dispatch depends on the patient's clinical state and assessment of future blood losses. Assessment of a patient with hypovolaemic shock is complex and includes recognition of the clinical situation, the potential blood loss, together with a current assessment of the patient and investigations. Hb and Hct values may be misleading. It may take hours for their values to equilibrate to those indicating the degree of blood loss.

Group and screen The patient's ABO and Rhesus D group is determined and the serum tested for unexpected red cell antibodies. Subsequently, if required, blood can be provided within 10–15min, assuming the antibody screen is clear. Request 'Group and screen' where a patient does not need transfusion in the ED, but may require it later.

Cross-match Full blood compatibility testing may take up to 1hr. If blood is required more urgently, ABO and Rh compatible units can usually be provided within 15min, including an 'immediate spin cross-match' as a final check on ABO compatibility. In exsanguinating haemorrhage, uncross-matched group O Rhesus –ve blood can be issued immediately.

Blood products

The UK uses blood component therapy. There appears to be no specific advantage in using 'whole' blood as opposed to red cells plus a volume expander.

Red cells (additive solution) Each pack (volume 300mL) is from a single donor and has a Hct of 0.65–0.75 (0.55–0.65 for RBCs in additive solution). A transfusion of 4mL/kg will ↑ circulating Hb by ≈1g/dL.

Whole blood A 'unit' contains 530mL (470mL of blood from a single donor + 63mL preservative solution), with a Hct of 0.35–0.45.

Platelet concentrate either pooled or from a single donor by platelet pheresis.

Fresh frozen plasma contains clotting factors and fibrinogen.

Cryoprecipitate is derived from FFP when it is thawed. It is rich in factor VIII, fibrinogen, and von Willebrand Factor.

Prothrombin complex concentrate is a combination of vitamin K dependent Factors II, VII, IX and X. Use PCC to reverse warfarin.

Transfusion precautions (UK Blood Safety & Quality Regulations 2005)

- 2 practitioners must confirm all the following steps before commencing transfusion. If there is *ANY* discrepancy, *DO NOT* transfuse.
- Confirm the details on the traceability label on the blood component match the patient's full name, date of birth, and hospital number (wrist band if unconscious).
- Check that the traceability label is attached to the blood bag.
- Ensure the donation number, the patient's blood group/RhD type all match and that any special requirements are covered.
- Check every component before starting transfusion for signs of discolouration, leaks, clots etc. and the expiry date.
- If all checks are satisfactory, the 2 practitioners should ensure that the component has been prescribed (prescription form and/or fluid balance chart) and sign the front of the traceability label before commencing the transfusion.
- Infuse all components through a giving set with integral filter to trap large aggregates. Microaggregate filters are not routinely required.
- Never add any drug to a blood component infusion.
- Do not use giving-sets which previously contained glucose or gelatin.
- Red cell concentrates may be diluted with 0.9% saline using a Y giving-set to improve flow rates. Never add any other solution.
- Use a blood warmer, especially for large and/or rapid transfusions.
- Once the transfusion has started, peel off the portion of the signed label and attach to the appropriate place in the fluid balance sheet.
- Sign the prescription form to confirm the patient identity checks.
- Complete and sign the label and return it to the laboratory.

See: www.transfusionguidelines.org.uk

Blood transfusion 2

Massive transfusion

Loss of 50% of circulating blood volume within 3hr is perhaps the most relevant ED definition. Resuscitation requires an interdisciplinary team and clear organization.

In the event of massive blood loss

- Protect the airway and give high flow O_2.
- Get help—two nurses and a senior doctor.
- Insert two large bore cannulae and start IV warm saline 1000mL stat.
- Take FBC, U&E, LFTs, coagulation, and cross-match. Label the blood tubes and ensure they are sent directly to the laboratory. Do not leave them unlabelled or lying around in the resuscitation room.
- Telephone the haematology laboratory to warn of potential massive transfusion. Request ABO group-specific red cells if the patient is peri-arrest. This will take only 10min in the laboratory. Otherwise, request full cross-match and give number of units required.
- Accurate patient ID is essential, even if the patient is unknown.
- Call appropriate senior surgeon—to stop bleeding as soon as possible.
- Start blood transfusion if the patient remains tachycardic and/or hypotensive despite crystalloid resuscitation.
- Repeat all bloods, including FBC, clotting, U&Es, calcium, and magnesium levels, every hour.
- Start platelet transfusion if platelet count falls below 75×10^9/L.
- Anticipate the requirement for FFP and consider giving early during the resuscitation. FFP will replace clotting factors and fibrinogen. Aim to maintain fibrinogen >1.0g/L and the INR and APTT <1.5 normal. Cryoprecipitate may also be used.
- Recombinant Factor VIIa might be used as a 'last ditch attempt' to control bleeding in young patients where surgical control of bleeding is not possible, and the above has already been corrected. If the drug is available it is usually ordered by a haematologist.

Massive transfusion complications

Rapid infusion of blood products may lead to:

Hypothermia Blood products are normally stored at 2–6°C. Rapid infusion can cause significant hypothermia. Use blood warmers routinely for rapid transfusions (eg >50mL/kg/hr or 15mL/kg/hr in children). Never warm a blood product by putting a pack into hot water, on a radiator or any other heat source.

Electrolyte disturbances With massive transfusion, the citrate anticoagulant may cause significant toxicity, ↓ plasma Ca^{2+} (impairing cardiac function) and acid–base balance disturbance. This is aggravated in patients with underlying liver disease, hypotension or hypothermia. Citrate may also bind Mg^{2+}, causing arrhythmias. Prophylactic or routine administration of IV calcium salts is not recommended. Monitor ECG and measure ionized plasma Ca^{2+} levels during massive transfusion. K^+ levels ↑ in stored blood and hyperkalaemia may follow massive infusion. Routinely monitor the ECG and check plasma K^+ levels. Transient hypokalaemia may follow 24hr after large volume transfusion

Blood product administration

Blood transfusion is not a panacea. An improvement in O_2 delivery cannot be assumed. RBC function deteriorates during storage and changes in O_2 affinity occur with ↓ 2,3-DPG levels, while ↓ ATP levels alter RBC membrane deformability causing ↑ cell stiffness and micro-circulatory problems. UK donations are routinely screened for hepatitis B, HIV, HTLV, syphilis, and where necessary, CMV. However, blood cannot be sterilized: small but definite risks of infection transmission exist.

Transfusion reactions

Monitor the patient closely for the first 5–10min of the infusion of each unit of blood to detect early clinical evidence of acute reactions. If the patient develops a temperature, shortness of breath, chest or abdominal pain or hypotension, suspect a transfusion reaction. Treat allergic reactions including itching, urticaria, bronchospasm and fever conventionally (see 🕮 Anaphylaxis treatment, p.43).

Mismatched transfusion By far the commonest cause is a clerical error when labelling, ordering or administering blood. Transfusion of ABO incompatible blood causes acute severe haemolysis and circulatory collapse. In a hypovolaemic, shocked, or anaesthetized patient these features may be obscured and missed.

If a transfusion reaction is suspected:

ABO incompatability, haemolytic reaction, bacterial infection, severe allergic reaction, or transfusion-related acute lung injury:
- Stop the transfusion.
- Keep the IV line open with 0.9% saline.
- Record all observations, give supplemental oxygen.
- Double-check the blood unit label with the patient's wrist identity band and other identifiers.
- Send the unit of blood product and the giving set to the blood bank.
- Take 40mL of blood. Send it as follows:
  - 5mL anticoagulated and 5mL clotted blood to blood bank;
  - 10mL for U&E;
  - 10mL for coagulation screening;
  - 10mL for blood cultures.
- Contact the blood bank directly by phone.
- Contact haematologist directly.
- Give broad spectrum antibiotic if infection suspected.
- Monitor fluid balance and urinary output.

Sickle cell disease

Sickle cell disease occurs in African, Indian, Middle Eastern, Caribbean, USA, and Mediterranean populations. It is caused by a genetic mutation in one of the chains of the Hb molecule. The normal adult Hb genotype AA produces HbA. In heterozygotes (sickle cell trait) one gene is abnormal (HbAS) and about 40% of the patient's Hb will be HbS. In homozygotes (sickle cell anaemia), both genes are abnormal (SS) and >80% of the Hb will be HbS. **HbS molecules** polymerize in deoxygenated or acidotic conditions, causing RBC sickling. Sickle cells are rigid and fragile. They may haemolyse, or block small vessels leading to tissue ischaemia, infarction and further sickling (see Fig. 3.26). Sickling also occurs with genes coding other analogous amino acid substitutions (eg HbSC and SD diseases).

Clinical features

Sickle cell trait causes no disability except during conditions of severe hypoxia (eg sudden depressurization in aircraft, or cardiac arrest).

Patients with **sickle cell anaemia** have chronic anaemia (Hb 8–10g/dL) with alternating good health and acute crises. Later, chronic ill health supervenes with renal failure, bone necrosis (evident in 50% of patients by age 35 years), osteomyelitis, leg ulcers and iron overload as a consequence of transfusions. There is predisposition to infection, especially *Staphylococcus, Pneumococcus,* and *Haemophilus.*

Sickle cell crises can occur de novo or follow infection, cold, dehydration, or any situation where tissue hypoxia/ischaemia occurs. The crisis may involve thrombosis, haemolysis, marrow aplasia, or acute splenic/liver sequestration (especially in children aged <5 years). Any acute medical or surgical emergency may be mimicked (eg acute abdomen, PE, stroke). Severe aching bony pain and low-grade fever (even in the absence of infection) is common. Cerebral sickling may present with bizarre behaviour, psychosis, fits, TIAs, stroke, or other focal neurological signs. Priapism, jaundice, and painful swelling of hands and feet may occur.

Acute chest syndrome

The leading cause of death in sickle cell anaemia. It presents as chest pain, hypoxia and pulmonary infiltrates. There may be cough, tachypnoea, and wheezing. Poorly understood, but infection may be a precipitant.

Acute splenic sequestration

Sudden trapping of large numbers of RBCs in the spleen results in severe anaemia, an enlarging spleen, hypovolaemia, and thrombocytopenia. It occurs most commonly in young children—those with sickle cell disease have a 30% chance of having acute splenic sequestration by the age of 5 years. It may present with shock and splenomegaly, with a mortality of >15%.

Osteomyelitis and septic arthritis

Osteomyelitis and septic arthritis occur more commonly in sickle cell disease. Be suspicious if a patient presents with high fever, soft tissue swelling, or pain in a different pattern to normal. *Salmonella* is frequently implicated.

Investigations

No specific tests can detect a sickle cell crisis:

- All patients in the at-risk groups require a sickle test before any anaesthetic procedure (including regional anaesthesia, Bier's block).
- Sickle testing (using an oxidizing agent) will detect sickling in homo- and heterozygote forms. Hb electrophoresis can then distinguish between HbSS, HbAS and other Hb variants.
- FBC typically shows anaemia (Hb 6–8g/dL, but Hb may be much lower if acute haemolysis, sequestration or aplasia is present). Post-splenectomy features may be seen on blood film. WCC may be ↑ (20–60 × 10^9/L) in the absence of infection and platelet count is also usually ↑.
- Infection screen, including blood cultures, midstream specimen of urine (MSU) and CXR.
- Joint aspiration for culture if septic arthritis is suspected.
- U&E, ABG, ECG.
- Arrange CT brain scan if there are neurological symptoms or signs.

Management of crises

Provide supportive therapy, directed to the patient's symptoms:

- Get expert help!
- Keep the patient warm, rested and give O_2 if any obvious symptoms or SpO$_2$ <94%.
- Opioids (given IV and titrated to the response) are often required for pain. Consider morphine IVI or patient analgesia pump.
- Commence rehydration with oral or IV fluids, but take care not to pre-cipitate heart failure.
- Transfusion may be required if severe anaemia from acute haemolysis, sequestration or aplasia occurs, or if there are central nervous system (CNS) or lung complications.

Empirical antibiotic therapy may be required if infection is thought to be the trigger for the sickling crisis.

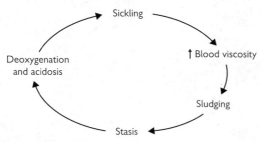

Fig. 3.26 Sickling cycle.

Toxicology

Poisons: general principles

Emergency treatment

Clear and maintain the *Airway*.

If *Breathing* appears inadequate ventilate with oxygen using a bag and mask or ET tube (not mouth-to-mouth in poisoned patients). Give naloxone for respiratory depression due to opioids (📖 p. 188).

Circulation Check pulse. If unconscious and pulseless, start CPR.

Types of poisoning

Unintentional or 'accidental' poisoning is most common in inquisitive small children (1–4 years) who eat tablets, household chemicals, and plants. Older children and adults may be poisoned by chemicals at school or work, or by drinking toxic fluids decanted into drinks bottles. Poisoning by drugs may result from miscalculation or confusion of doses or by taking the same drug under different names. Drug smugglers who swallow drugs wrapped in condoms or polythene, or stuff them in the rectum or vagina, may suffer poisoning if the packages leak (📖 p.217).

Deliberate self-poisoning is the commonest form of poisoning in adults and may occur in children as young as 6yrs (usually with a family history of self-poisoning). Drugs or poisons are often taken impulsively, sometimes to manipulate relatives or friends. Suicidal intent is relatively uncommon, but assess all patients for this (📖 p.612). A few patients leave suicide notes, and conceal the drugs or poison to evade detection.

Non-accidental poisoning of children is a form of fabricated or induced illness (previously known as Munchausen's syndrome by proxy—📖 p.733), in which a parent deliberately poisons a child. Homicidal poisoning is rare and may involve acute or chronic poisoning with chemicals such as arsenic or thallium.

Chemical plant incidents and terrorism are potential threats to large numbers of people.

Information about poisons

Tablets may be identified from *MIMS Colour Index* and descriptions in the *BNF*. Drug Information Centres and Poisons Information Services (see opposite) have access to *TICTAC*, a computer-aided tablet and capsule identification system (www.tictac.org.uk).

Martindale[1] gives information on many drugs and poisons, and detailed constituents of non-prescription drugs.

Identification of *plants* and *fungi* from reference books may be difficult, especially if only vague descriptions or chewed fragments are available. The CD-ROM computer software *Poisonous Plants and Fungi in Britain and Ireland*[2] helps with identification and details of toxicity. Local botanic gardens may provide additional help. See also 📖 p.212.

---

1 Sweetman SC (ed). (2009) *Martindale: The Complete Drug Reference*, 36th edn. Pharmaceutical Press, London.
2 Dauncey EA et al. (2002) *Poisonous Plants and Fungi in Britain and Ireland* (interactive identification system on CD-ROM), 2nd edn. Kew Publishing, Kew, www.kewbooks.com.

Poisons Information Centres in the UK

TOXBASE, the UK National Poisons Information Service's database on clinical toxicology, is on the internet (www.toxbase.org) with a backup site at www.toxbasebackup.org. It includes information about poisoning with drugs, household products, plants and fungi, as well as industrial and agricultural chemicals and agents which might be deliberately released by terrorists. Access to TOXBASE is password protected and is restricted to NHS professional staff in the UK and also hospitals in Ireland.

TOXBASE or reference books provide sufficient information for most cases of poisoning. More detailed information and specialist advice is available from Poisons Information Centres and is especially useful for complex cases or severe poisoning.

The UK National Poisons Information Service has four centres, with a single telephone number 0844 892 0111 which directs the call to the nearest centre, or to the on-call centre out of hours. In Ireland advice is available from the National Poisons Information Centre, Dublin, telephone (01) 809 2566.

Enquiries to Poisons Information Centres are usually answered initially by an information officer using TOXBASE and other reference sources. Medical staff with specialist toxicology experience are available for advice about seriously poisoned patients. Poisons Information Centres can also advise about sources of supply of antidotes that are needed only occasionally, and about laboratory analyses that may be helpful in managing some patients.

Admission and psychiatric assessment after poisoning

Adults

Patients who are seriously poisoned need admission to a medical ward, or if appropriate, to ICU. However, most patients who take overdoses suffer no serious ill effects and may be treated satisfactorily on an ED observation ward or a Clinical Decisions Unit. Even if there is no risk of toxicity, admission overnight provides a 'cooling off' period for the patient to get away from the situation that precipitated the overdose. This should allow a more rational appraisal of the problems and may reduce the risk of further self-poisoning.

Look for the causes of every episode of deliberate self-harm. A patient who seems suicidal (see 📖 p.612) must be observed carefully in the ED and on the ward, because of the risk of further self-harm.

Children with poisoning

Serious poisoning is uncommon in children. Many children appear well but have been exposed to an unknown amount of a compound which could be toxic. Admit such children to a paediatric ward for observation: they can be discharged after a few hours if no toxic effects occur. A child may be discharged home directly from the ED if the substance taken is known to be non-toxic. The health visitor may usefully visit the home to advise about poisoning prevention. In children >6 years, consider the possibility of deliberate self-harm and the need for assessment by a child psychiatrist.

Diagnosis of poisoning

The patient or relatives/friends may state what drugs or poison have been taken, but this information is not always accurate. Self-poisoning is often an impulsive act whilst under the influence of alcohol: the patient may not know which tablets he/she took. The amount involved is often unclear. Check any bottles or packets for the names and quantities of drugs or poisons that were available. If a patient is unconscious or severely poisoned, look in hospital notes for details of previous overdoses, and find out from the GP what drugs had been prescribed. Record the time of ingestion of the drug or poison. Examine the patient all over for signs of poisoning, injection marks or self-injury. Exclude other diverse processes mimicking poisoning (eg head injury, meningitis). In the Far East, and in EDs where Asian people present with non-specific symptoms, hepatitis, or suspected poisoning, remember that traditional Chinese medicines or herbs can cause significant toxicity.

Toxidromes: features suggesting a particular poison

- Coma with dilated pupils, divergent squint, tachycardia, ↑ muscle tone, ↑ reflexes and extensor plantars suggests tricyclic antidepressant or orphenadrine poisoning (📖 p.194).
- Coma with hypotension, respiratory depression and ↓ muscle tone suggests barbiturates, clomethiazole (📖 p.196), benzodiazepines with alcohol, or severe tricyclic antidepressant poisoning (📖 p.194).
- Coma with slow respiration and pinpoint pupils is typical of opioid poisoning (give naloxone, 📖 p.188).
- Tinnitus, deafness, hyperventilation, sweating, nausea and tachycardia are typical of salicylate poisoning (📖 p.189).
- Agitation, tremor, dilated pupils, tachycardia, suggest amphetamines, ecstasy, cocaine, sympathomimetics (📖 p.214), tricyclic antidepressants (📖 p.194), or selective serotonin re-uptake inhibitors (📖 p.216).

Assessment and monitoring

- Assess and record conscious level (📖 p.361). Observe frequently.
- Check blood glucose in patients with confusion, coma or fits.
- Monitor breathing and record respiratory rate. Use a pulse oximeter, but note that SpO_2 may be misleadingly high in carbon monoxide (CO) poisoning—see 📖 p.208).
- Check ABG if patient is deeply unconscious or breathing abnormally.
- Record and monitor the ECG if a patient is unconscious, has tachy- or bradycardia or has taken drugs or poisons with risk of arrhythmias.
- Record BP and temperature.

Investigations in poisoned patients

The most useful investigations are paracetamol and salicylate levels, blood glucose, ABG, and urea & electrolytes (U&E). Measure paracetamol if there is any possibility of paracetamol poisoning (this includes all unconscious patients). Record the time of the sample on the bottle, and in the notes. Many labs can measure salicylate, iron and lithium and also check for paraquat if necessary. Comprehensive drug screening is rarely needed and is only available in specialist centres (ask Poisons Information Service, 📖 p.181).

Poisons: supportive care

Protect the airway
In an unconscious patient use a cuffed ET tube if there is no gag reflex. If an oral or nasal airway is used, nurse in the recovery position to minimize risk of aspiration should vomiting or regurgitation occur.

Monitor breathing and ventilate if necessary
Hypoxia and CO_2 retention are common in deep coma.

Hypotension
This may result from relative hypovolaemia, arrhythmias and cardio-depressive effects of drugs. Treat according to the cause. Elevate the foot of the trolley. If BP <90mmHg, consider giving saline or a plasma expander such as gelatin 500mL IV. Monitor CVP in patients who are elderly or have cardiac disease. Inotropes such as dopamine (2–5micrograms/kg/min), dob-utamine (2.5–10micrograms/kg/min), glucagon (📖 p.198) or insulin therapy (📖 p.187) are occasionally needed, under expert guidance.

Cardiac arrhythmias
Generally rare in poisoned patients. The most likely drugs responsible are tricyclic antidepressants, beta-blockers, chloral hydrate, digoxin, potassium, bronchodilators, verapamil, and amphetamines. Look for and correct hypoxia, respiratory depression, metabolic acidosis and electrolyte abnormalities. Anti-arrhythmic drugs are very rarely needed: consult a poisons expert first.

Convulsions
Dangerous because they cause hypoxia and acidosis, and may precipi-tate cardiac arrest. Drugs responsible include tricyclic antidepressants, mefenamic acid, and theophylline. Check for and correct hypoxia and hypoglycaemia. Do not give anticonvulsants if fits are single and brief, but if fits are repeated or prolonged give IV lorazepam 4mg (or PR diazepam or buccal midazolam if venous access is not available).

Hypothermia
May occur with any drug causing coma, especially barbiturates, clomethiazole, and phenothiazines. Check rectal T° with a low-reading thermometer. Insulation and passive rewarming are usually adequate.

Hyperthermia (📖 p.264)
May occur with amphetamines, cocaine, ecstasy, monoamine oxidase inhibitors, sympathomimetics, and theophylline. Convulsions and rhab-domyolysis are common. Active cooling, chlorpromazine and possibly dantrolene are needed. Get expert help.

Complications of immobility
Prolonged immobility (eg due to tricyclics and barbiturates) risks pressure areas. Treat blisters like minor burns. Immobility may cause rhabdomyolysis (leading to renal failure), nerve palsies, and compartment syndrome: if this is suspected check CK, test urine for myoglobinuria, and get urgent ortho-paedic advice about measuring compartment pressures.

Urinary retention
Common in coma, especially after tricyclic poisoning. Suprapubic pressure often stimulates reflex bladder emptying. Catheterization may be needed to empty the bladder or to measure urine output.

Reducing absorption of poison

Background information

If a poison has been swallowed it is logical to try to remove it and reduce absorption from the gut. Possible measures include gastric lavage, induced emesis (eg with ipecacuanha), oral adsorbents (especially activated charcoal) and whole-bowel irrigation. None of these can be recommended routinely. They may cause significant morbidity and there is very little evidence that they improve outcomes.

Gastric lavage

This does not empty the stomach of solids and may force gastric contents through the pylorus into the small bowel. It may cause hypoxia, aspiration pneumonia and occasionally oesophageal perforation. Gastric lavage >1hr after overdose is ineffective in ↓ absorption of poisons. Gastric lavage does not reduce mortality from poisoning, and it does not deter patients from taking repeated overdoses.

Practical advice on use of gastric lavage

Only consider this if the patient has taken a life-threatening amount of poison within the previous 1 hour or is deeply unconscious because of poisoning. Only consider performing it if there is a strong cough reflex or the airway is protected by a cuffed ET tube. Do not use lavage for poisoning with corrosives (risk of perforation) or with petrol/paraffin compounds (risk of pneumonitis), except rarely in severe poisoning on specialist advice.

- Before starting gastric lavage, check that powerful suction is immediately available.
- Elevate the foot of the trolley and place the patient in the left lateral position.
- Give O_2 via nasal cannulae. Monitor ECG.
- Lubricate large disposable stomach tube (36 or 40 French Gauge-FG) and pass it through the mouth into the stomach. Confirm position by aspirating gastric contents or blowing air down the tube while listening over the stomach.
- Aspirate gastric contents and keep labelled sample for later analysis if necessary.
- Perform lavage by pouring 300mL aliquots of tepid tap water down the tube and siphoning it back, while massaging over stomach to help dislodge tablet debris.
- Continue until the effluent is clear.
- Consider leaving activated charcoal (50g) in the stomach.
- While withdrawing the tube, occlude it between the fingers to prevent aspiration of fluid from the tube.

Induced emesis

Never use emetics. *Ipecacuanha* was once used frequently, but it may cause prolonged vomiting, drowsiness and aspiration pneumonia, and it does not reduce drug absorption. There is no indication for using ipecac. *Salt solutions* may cause fatal hypernatraemia and must never be used as an emetic.

Activated charcoal

Given within 1hr, this ↓ absorption of therapeutic doses of many drugs, but there is little evidence of clinical benefit after overdose. Charcoal ↓ the half-life of some drugs (eg digoxin), which undergo entero-hepatic recycling. However, charcoal is messy, unpleasant to take and often causes vomiting. Aspiration into the lungs can result in fatal pneumonitis. Various formulations of activated charcoal are available. *Actidose Aqua Advance*® is less unpalatable than some of the other formulations. *Carbomix*® may cause severe constipation, especially if given in repeated doses.

Do not give activated charcoal for substances which do not bind to it. These include: iron, lithium, boric acid, cyanide, ethanol, ethylene glycol, methanol, organophosphates, petroleum distillates and strong acids and alkalis. Charcoal is most likely to be useful for poisons which are toxic in small quantities (eg tricyclic antidepressants and theophylline derivatives). If a dangerous overdose has been taken in the previous 1hr, give charcoal (PO or via an orogastric tube: adult 50g; child 1g/kg, max 50g). Charcoal may be effective for >1hr for sustained release formulations or drugs that delay gastric emptying (eg tricyclic antidepressants and opioids). Obtain expert advice before giving charcoal in repeated doses, which are only helpful in life-threatening poisoning with a few drugs (eg carbamazepine, dapsone, digoxin, phenobarbital, quinine, theophylline, and salicylate, and a few other drugs rarely taken in overdose).

Whole-bowel irrigation

Whole-bowel irrigation is rarely needed and should only be used on expert advice. The aim of whole-bowel irrigation is to empty the bowel rapidly of solid contents by giving fluid down a nasogastric (NG) tube until the rectal effluent becomes clear. The value of this is uncertain. It may be useful for poisoning with sustained-release drug formulations or for poisons such as iron or lithium, which are not absorbed by activated charcoal. It has also been used to remove packets of cocaine from body packers and button batteries from children.

Bowel cleansing solutions of polyethylene glycol and electrolytes (eg Klean-Prep®) should be used for whole-bowel irrigation: 2L/hr in adults (500mL/hr in small children) for 2hr, or occasionally longer. Do not use normal saline since it may cause fluid overload and hypokalaemia.

Activated charcoal may be given by NG tube, if appropriate, before whole-bowel irrigation is started. Continue the irrigation until the rectal effluent is clear. Nausea, vomiting, abdominal pain and electrolyte disturbances may occur. Monitor ECG, U&E and urine output.

Antidotes for poisons

The provision of supportive care is essential in all patients. Antidotes are available for only a few drugs and poisons (Table 4.1), and are not always necessary. More information is available from reference books, TOXBASE and Poisons Information Centres (📖 p.181).

Table 4.1

Poison	Antidote	Notes
Beta-blockers	Glucagon, atropine	📖 p.198
Carbon monoxide	Oxygen	📖 p.208
Cyanide	Sodium nitrite, sodium thiosulphate, dicobalt edetate, hydroxocobalamin	📖 p.207
Digoxin	Digoxin antibodies (Digibind)[†]	📖 p.199
Ethylene glycol	Ethanol, fomepizole[†]	📖 p.203
Iron salts	Desferrioxamine	📖 p.201
Local anaesthetics	Lipid emulsion (Intralipid®)	📖 p.187, 📖 p.284
Methanol	Ethanol, fomepizole[†]	📖 p.202
Opioids	Naloxone	📖 p.188
Organophosphates	Atropine, pralidoxime[†]	📖 p.206
Paracetamol	Acetylcysteine, methionine	📖 p.190
Sulphonylureas	Glucose, octreotide	📖 p.197
Tricyclic antidepressants	Sodium bicarbonate, Intralipid®	📖 p.187, 📖 p.194
Warfarin	Vitamin K, clotting factors, FFP	📖 p.170
Adder bites	Zagreb antivenom	📖 p.417
Foreign snakes	Antivenoms[†]	Expert advice 📖 p.181

Antidotes are also available for arsenic, lead, mercury, thallium, and other metals. Specialist advice is essential.

Some antidotes (marked[†]) are very rarely needed: get expert advice (📖 p.181) about when and how to use these antidotes and where to obtain them.

Increasing elimination of poisons

The vast majority of poisoned patients recover with supportive care, plus appropriate antidotes if necessary. Active removal of absorbed poison is only needed in special circumstances. Alkalinization of the urine is useful in salicylate poisoning (📖 p.189), but forced alkaline diuresis is no longer recommended. Haemodialysis is occasionally helpful for severe poisoning with salicylates, ethylene glycol, methanol, lithium, phenobarbital, and chlorates. Haemoperfusion is rarely needed, but might be helpful in severe poisoning with barbiturates, chloral hydrate or theophylline: specialist advice is essential.

Lipid emulsion (Intralipid®) therapy for drug toxicity

IV lipid emulsion is rarely needed but can be lifesaving in overdoses of local anaesthetics such as lidocaine or bupivacaine (📖 p.284).[1,2,3] It may be useful in cardiac arrest caused by some other drugs: the indications are unclear but case reports record dramatic recovery from cardiac arrests due to haloperidol, verapamil, and a mixed overdose of bupropion and lamotrigine.[1,2] In animals,[2] lipid emulsion was effective in poisoning from verapamil (but not nifedipine) and clomipramine (but not amitriptyline). Consider lipid emulsion in drug-induced cardiac arrest unresponsive to standard treatment (📖 p.50). EDs, theatres, and ICU should stock lipid emulsion for this emergency.

Lipid emulsion acts as a 'lipid sink', binding lipophilic drugs and reducing the amount of active free drug. It may also affect myocardial metabolism. Lipid emulsion is not licensed for use in drug overdose and the safety of rapid infusion is unknown. Lipid interferes with analysis of blood samples, so if possible take these before starting lipid emulsion, including blood for later measurement of drug concentrations.

Give Intralipid® 20% 1.5mL/kg IV over 1min, then 15mL/kg/hr by intravenous infusion (IVI) (for a 70kg patient give 100mL over 1min, then 500mL over 30min). Continue CPR. If the circulation is still inadequate after 5min repeat IV bolus of Intralipid® 1.5mL/kg twice at 5min intervals and increase IVI to 30mL/kg/hr (500mL in 15min for 70kg). The maximum recommended total dose of Intralipid® 20% is 12mL/kg (840mL for a 70kg patient).[3]

Report cases in which lipid emulsion is used to the Poisons Information Service (📖 p.181) or the Lipid Registry (http://www.lipidregistry.org).

Insulin therapy in poisoning

Poisoning with cardiac drugs such as calcium channel blockers (📖 p.198) and β-blockers (📖 p.198) may cause severe hypotension. If standard treatments are ineffective, seek expert advice (📖 p.181) and consider using insulin therapy, which may improve myocardial carbohydrate metabolism and ↑ BP and cardiac output. Some case reports and animal studies of severe calcium channel blocker and β-blocker poisoning have shown benefits from high dose insulin, but the optimum dosage is unclear.[4,5]

Continuous monitoring is needed, with invasive BP monitoring. Check blood glucose and potassium at least hourly and give glucose 10% and potassium (max 20mmol/hr) as needed. Give an IV bolus of short-acting insulin 1 unit/kg, then 0.5–2units/kg/hr IVI, titrated to keep systolic BP > 90mmHg and heart rate >60/min. In extreme cases, consider increasing insulin dosage to 5–10units/kg/hr, titrated according to response.

1 http://lipidrescue.squarespace.com

2 Jamaty C et al. (2010) Lipid emulsions in the treatment of acute poisoning: a systematic review of human and animal studies. Clin Toxicol **48**: 1–27.

3 Association of Anaesthetists of Great Britain and Ireland (2010) Management of Severe Local Anaesthetic Toxicity. Available at: http://www.aagbi.org/publications/guidelines.htm

4 Lheureux PER et al. (2006) Bench-to-bedside review: Hyperinsulinaemia/euglycaemia therapy in the management of overdose of calcium-channel blockers. Critical Care **10**: 212. Available at: http://ccforum.com/content/10/3/212

5 Nickson CP, Little M (2009) Early use of high-dose insulin euglycaemic therapy for verapamil toxicity. Med J Aust **191**(6): 350–2.

Opioid poisoning

The opioids include morphine, diamorphine (heroin), pethidine, codeine, buprenorphine, nalbuphine, methadone, diphenoxylate, and related drugs. These are used as analgesics (sometimes combined with paracetamol, as in co-codamol and co-proxamol), cough suppressants and anti-diarrhoeal agents. Acute opioid poisoning often occurs in addicts (who may have needle marks and thrombosed veins and a high risk of HIV and hepatitis).

Clinical features

Opioid poisoning causes coma, ↓ respiratory rate, pinpoint pupils, and sometimes cyanosis, apnoea, convulsions and hypotension. Hypertension may occur in pentazocine poisoning. Non-cardiogenic pulmonary oedema may result from 'main-lining' heroin or other opioids.

Respiratory depression may cause death within 1hr of an opioid overdose. However, delayed respiratory depression can occur in poisoning with co-phenotrope (diphenoxylate and atropine), in which the opioid effects usually predominate over atropine toxicity. Delayed toxicity may occur with slow-release formulations of drugs, and also with methadone, which has a very long duration of action (half-life 25–50hr).

Treatment

Clear and maintain the airway. If breathing appears inadequate, ventilate on O_2 with a bag and mask or ET tube. Naloxone is a specific antagonist for opioids and reverses coma and respiratory depression if given in sufficient dosage. Naloxone may be used as a therapeutic trial in suspected opioid poisoning: record coma level, pupil size and respiratory rate and check for any response. The usual initial dose of naloxone for adults is 0.8mg IV, repeated at 2–3min intervals if necessary. However, in known or suspected drug addicts it is best to avoid reversing the opioid completely, so start with 0.1mg IV (or intranasal, if there is no venous access) and repeat this at 2–3min intervals until the patient is breathing adequately, but still drowsy. For children, give 10 micrograms/kg (IV, IM or IN), repeated as necessary. Intranasal naloxone is given by dripping or spraying the IV solution into the nose, where it is absorbed rapidly.

Naloxone has a much shorter duration of action than most opioids and so coma and respiratory depression often recur when naloxone wears off. The mean half-life of naloxone is 62min, but in some patients the half-life is >5hr. Careful observation is essential. More naloxone is often needed, given IV, by IVI or IM, the dose adjusted depending on the response (occasionally as much as 75mg in 24hr in methadone poisoning). Observation is needed for 6hr after the last dose of naloxone. Patients at risk of respiratory depression should not be allowed to leave hospital: rather than reversing an opioid fully it is better to keep a patient sedated but safe by constant observation and titration of naloxone. A patient who insists on leaving should be given naloxone IM, but will still be at risk of fatal respiratory depression. In opioid addicts, naloxone may precipitate a **withdrawal syndrome** with abdominal cramps, nausea and diarrhoea, but these usually settle within 2hr. Ventricular tachyarrhythmias occur occasionally.

Salicylate poisoning

Standard aspirin tablets contain 300mg acetylsalicylic acid. Ingestion of 150mg/kg body weight usually produces mild toxicity; 500mg/kg will cause severe and possibly fatal poisoning. Poisoning can result from absorption of salicylate ointment through the skin.

Clinical features

Commonly vomiting, tinnitus, deafness, sweating, vasodilatation, hyperventilation, and dehydration. Hypokalaemia may occur.

Severe poisoning may produce confusion, coma, and convulsions.

Children are prone to develop hyperpyrexia and hypoglycaemia.

Rare features include non-cardiogenic pulmonary oedema, cerebral oedema, and renal failure.

Metabolic and acid-base disturbances

These may be complex: adults usually have a mixed metabolic acidosis and respiratory alkalosis, but the respiratory effects predominate. In small children and a few adults, acidosis predominates, and is often associated with confusion or coma.

Management

Consider gastric lavage if a patient has ingested >500mg/kg body weight in the previous 1hr. After ingestion of >4.5g (or 2g in a child) give 50g activated charcoal (25g in a child) to ↓ absorption and ↑ elimination of salicylate. Measure plasma salicylate concentration (and repeat after a few hours if further symptoms occur, since salicylate level may ↑ due to continuing absorption). Check U&E, glucose, and ABG if there are CNS features or signs of severe poisoning. A second dose of charcoal may be useful if the plasma salicylate increases, suggesting delayed gastric emptying, or if enteric-coated tablets have been taken.

Mild poisoning Children with plasma salicylate <350mg/L (2.5mmol/L) and adults with <450mg/L (3.3mmol/L) usually need only ↑ oral fluids.

Moderate poisoning Children with salicylate >350mg/L and adults with >450mg/L need IV fluids to correct dehydration and ↑ elimination of salicylate: sodium bicarbonate 1.26% (adults 500mL hourly for 3hr) alkalinizes the urine (which is much more effective than a massive diuresis in ↑ salicylate excretion). Urine pH should be >7.5, ideally 8.0–8.5. Repeat salicylate level, check U&E and add K^+ as necessary.

Severe poisoning CNS features, acidosis or salicylate >700mg/L (5.1mmol/L) are associated with significant mortality. Get expert advice (📖 p.181) and consider urgent referral for haemodialysis. Correct acidosis and give repeated activated charcoal via a NG tube. In life-threatening poisoning with coma and extreme hyperventilation, paralysis and IPPV may help, while haemodialysis removes salicylate and corrects the electrolyte disturbances. Give glucose IV, since brain glucose levels may be low despite normal blood glucose concentrations. Do not use forced diuresis, which is ineffective and may cause pulmonary oedema.

Paracetamol poisoning

Paracetamol ('acetaminophen' in USA) may cause severe liver damage if 12g (24 tablets) or >150mg paracetamol/kg body weight are taken. Some patients have risk factors for enhanced toxicity (see below) and may be at risk if >75mg/kg has been taken.

In obese patients (>110kg) calculate the toxic dose in mg/kg, and the dose of acetylcysteine, using a weight of 110kg, rather than the patient's actual weight.

A metabolite of paracetamol (N-acetyl-p-benzoquinoneimine, NAPQI) binds glutathione in the liver and causes hepatic necrosis when stores of glutathione are exhausted. Renal failure from acute tubular necrosis occurs occasionally, but renal failure without liver failure is rare.

Risk factors for paracetamol toxicity
Alcoholics and patients on drugs that induce hepatic enzymes are at greater risk of toxicity, because of ↑ production of the toxic metabolite of paracetamol. The relevant drugs are anticonvulsants, rifampicin, and St John's wort.

Patients with malnutrition, anorexia, cachexia, HIV infection or cystic fibrosis may have ↓ glutathione stores and be at ↑ risk of liver damage.

Clinical features

Nausea, vomiting and abdominal discomfort are common within a few hours. In untreated patients developing liver damage, vomiting continues beyond 12hr and there is pain and tenderness over the liver (from 24hr), jaundice (at 2–4 days), and sometimes coma from hypoglycaemia (at 1–3 days) and hepatic encephalopathy (onset at 3–5 days). Loin pain, haematuria and proteinuria suggest incipient renal failure. Hepatic failure causes bleeding from coagulation abnormalities and hyperventilation from metabolic acidosis. In fatal cases cerebral oedema, septicaemia and DIC are common. However, many patients survive severe liver damage and recover completely.

LFTs are normal until >18hr after the overdose. The most sensitive lab evidence of liver damage is often a prolonged INR (from 24hr after overdose). Liver enzymes (ALT and AST) may reach >10,000units/L at 3–4 days. Bilirubin rises more slowly (max at about 5 days).

Paracetamol antidotes

Acetylcysteine (Parvolex®; previously called N-acetylcysteine) is given by IV infusion in 5% glucose. Initial dose is 150mg/kg body weight in 200mL glucose over 15min, 50mg/kg in 500mL over 4hr, then 100mg/kg in 1L over 16hr. Acetylcysteine can cause side effects (which are more likely if the plasma paracetamol level is low)—erythema and urticaria around the infusion site or more generalized rashes, itching, nausea, angioedema, bronchospasm, and rarely hypotension or hypertension. Side effects are dose related and usually start in the first hour of treatment. If they occur, stop the infusion and give an antihistamine (eg chlorphenamine 10mg IV over 1min). When symptoms have settled, acetylcysteine can usually be resumed at the lowest infusion rate (100mg/kg body weight over 16hr).

Methionine is rarely needed but may be useful in patients who refuse IV treatment or if acetylcsteine is not available. Methionine is given orally as capsules or tablets, 2.5g every 4hr to a total of 10g. Methionine has no significant adverse effects. It is less effective than acetylcysteine in patients who are vomiting or who present >8hr after ingestion. Methionine may be ineffective in patients treated with activated charcoal.

Children

Serious paracetamol poisoning is rare in children. Young children rarely take large amounts of paracetamol, and they metabolize it differently from adults and may have less risk of hepatotoxicity. However, there is no data for assessing the risk in children, so use the same treatment guidelines as for adults.

If it is certain that <150mg/kg has been taken (or <75mg/kg if there are risk factors for toxicity: see 🕮 p.190, then no investigation or treatment is needed and the child may be discharged.

Treatment with acetylcysteine is rarely needed in children. Doses are as for adults (opposite), but with smaller volumes of fluid for IV infusion.

Pregnancy

Assess the risk of toxicity and treat as for non-pregnant patients. Acetylcysteine and methionine do not seem to carry any risk to the fetus, and may protect the fetal liver from damage. Paracetamol overdose does not appear to cause teratogenic effects.

Staggered overdoses

If the patient took two or more paracetamol overdoses in a day assess the risk by plotting on the treatment graph the time interval since the first dose. For overdoses taken over several days the graph cannot be used. If the patient has symptoms of toxicity or the amount taken was >150mg/kg (75mg/kg in high risk groups) take blood for INR, LFTs, U&E and paracetamol (which may confirm that some was taken, even if the treatment graph cannot be used), and treat with acetylcysteine. If in doubt start treatment and get expert advice.

Outcome of treatment

Treatment with acetylcysteine or methionine within 8hr of an overdose is very effective in preventing liver and renal damage. Later treatment is less effective, but still worthwhile.

Late presentation after paracetamol poisoning

Patients who present late are more likely to be severely poisoned than those who present soon after ingestion. Late presenters often have continuing vomiting and abdominal pain, which are symptoms of liver damage. The treatment graph (🕮 p.193) may be unreliable at >15hr, because of insufficient data on untreated patients.

Liver transplantation

Liver transplantation is occasionally needed for hepatic failure due to paracetamol overdose in patients who presented or were treated late. Appropriate patients must be identified and referred to a liver transplant unit as soon as possible. Transplant criteria include arterial pH <7.30 (H^+ >50nmol/L) after resuscitation, or PT >100 seconds (INR >6.7) and creatinine >300micromol/L in patients with grade 3 or 4 hepatic encephalopathy.

Management of paracetamol poisoning

The time since ingestion is crucial in interpreting paracetamol concentrations and assessing the need for specific treatment. Record the time of ingestion as accurately as possible. When taking blood for paracetamol levels record the precise time in the notes and on blood bottles and forms. Start treatment immediately if the time of ingestion is unknown.

Management within 4 hours of ingestion

Consider activated charcoal (📖 p.185) if >12g or 150mg/kg paracetamol has been taken in the previous 1hr. Take blood at 4 hr from ingestion and use graph (Fig. 4.1) to assess risk of liver damage: use line A for most patients; line B for high risk patients. If the result is above the relevant line, give IV acetylcysteine or oral methionine (see 📖 p.190).

Management at 4–8 hours from ingestion

Measure paracetamol and use the graph to assess risk of liver damage: for most patients use line A, for high risk patients use line B. If above the relevant line, or only just below it, give IV acetylcysteine or oral methionine (for doses see 📖 p.190). Treatment is most effective if started before 8 hours: start it at once if paracetamol level is not available by this time and >150mg/kg has been taken. Patients treated with acetylcysteine or methionine within 8 hours of an overdose should be medically fit for discharge at the end of the treatment course.

Management at 8–15 hours from ingestion

Urgent action is needed: start treatment with IV acetylcysteine immediately if >150mg/kg or 12g paracetamol have been taken. Measure plasma paracetamol and use the graph to assess the risk of liver damage: for most patients use line A; for high risk patients use line B. If the paracetamol level is well below the line and patient is asymptomatic, stop acetylcysteine treatment. Continue acetylcysteine if level is above the relevant line, if there is doubt about the time of ingestion or if the patient has nausea or vomiting. At the end of acetylcysteine treatment check INR and plasma creatinine: if these are normal and the patient asymptomatic he/she is medically fit for discharge.

Management at 15–24 hours from ingestion

Urgent action is needed: give IV acetylcysteine immediately if >150mg/kg or >12g paracetamol have been taken. Measure plasma paracetamol, creatinine and INR. If at 24hr after ingestion a patient is asymptomatic, with normal INR, normal creatinine, and plasma paracetamol <10mg/L he/she may be discharged. Other patients need continuing monitoring and possibly further treatment with acetylcysteine.

Management at >24 hours from ingestion

Measure paracetamol, LFTs, U&E, creatinine, INR, and ABG. Start treatment with IV acetylcysteine if >150mg/kg or 12g paracetamol have been taken, investigations are abnormal or patient is symptomatic. Seek expert advice from Poisons Information Service (📖 p.181) or liver unit.

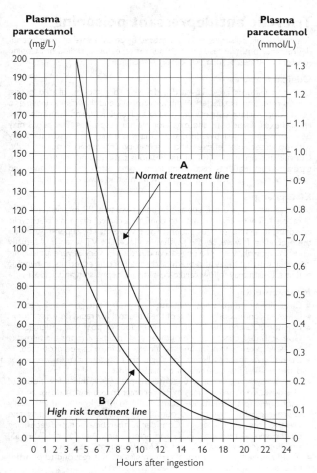

Fig. 4.1 Paracetamol treatment graph.

Normal treatment line A for most patients.

High risk treatment line B for patients with chronic alcoholism, malnutrition, anorexia, cachexia, HIV infection, or cystic fibrosis, or taking anticonvulsants, rifampicin or St John's wort.

Note Check whether the laboratory reports paracetamol in mg/L or mmol/L. Start treatment at once if in doubt about the time of the overdose, or if the plasma paracetamol is only just below the relevant treatment line.

Tricyclic antidepressant poisoning

Anticholinergic poisoning is usually caused by an overdose of tricyclic antidepressants, but may result from other drugs, eg procyclidine or atropine (present in *Atropa belladonna*, 'deadly nightshade').

Clinical features

Common features are tachycardia, dry skin, dry mouth, dilated pupils, urinary retention, ataxia, jerky limb movements, and drowsiness leading to coma. Unconscious patients often have a divergent squint, ↑ muscle tone and reflexes, myoclonus and extensor plantar responses. The pupils may be dilated and unreactive. In deep coma there may be muscle flaccidity with no detectable reflexes and respiratory depression requiring IPPV. Convulsions occur in ≈10% of unconscious patients and may precipitate cardiac arrest. Patients recovering from coma often suffer delirium and hallucinations and have jerky limb movements and severe dysarthria.

ECG changes

Sinus tachycardia is usual, but as poisoning worsens PR interval and QRS duration ↑. These changes help to confirm a clinical diagnosis of tricyclic poisoning in an unconscious patient. The P wave may be superimposed on the preceding T wave, so the rhythm can look like VT when it is actually sinus tachycardia with prolonged conduction. In very severe poisoning, ventricular arrhythmias and bradycardia may occur, especially in hypoxic patients. Death may follow cardio-respiratory depression and acidosis.

Management

- Clear airway, intubate and ventilate if necessary, and give nursing care.
- Observe continuously, in view of the potential for rapid deterioration.
- Monitor ECG and check ABG in unconscious or post-ictal patients.
- Give activated charcoal by mouth or gastric tube if more than 4mg/kg has been taken within 1hr and the airway is safe or can be protected.
- Do not give anticonvulsants for single brief fits, but give lorazepam or diazepam IV if fits are frequent or prolonged.
- Most arrhythmias occur in unconscious patients within a few hours of overdose. Treat arrhythmias by correcting hypoxia and acidosis. *Sodium bicarbonate* (8.4%, adult: 50–100mL IV; child: 1mL/kg) may dramatically improve cardiac rhythm and output (by altering protein binding and ↓ active free tricyclic drug). Consider further bicarbonate, depending on the clinical response, ECG and arterial pH. Aim for pH 7.5–7.55, avoiding excessive alkalosis (pH > 7.65), which may be fatal.
- Avoid anti-arrhythmic drugs. If arrhythmias do not respond to bicarbonate, discuss with a poisons specialist (📖 p.181).
- Correct hypotension by elevating the foot of the trolley and giving IV fluids. Glucagon may help in severe hypotension (📖 p.198). Dopamine (2–10micrograms/kg/min) is occasionally indicated for unresponsive hypotension on specialist advice.
- Consider Intralipid® (📖 p.187) for severe arrhythmias or cardiac arrest.
- Do not use physostigmine or flumazenil (risk of precipitating fits).
- Unconscious patients usually improve over about 12hr and regain consciousness within 36hr. Delirium and hallucinations may persist for 2–3 days and require sedation with oral diazepam in large doses (sometimes 20–30mg PO every 2hr initially).

ECG changes in tricyclic antidepressant poisoning

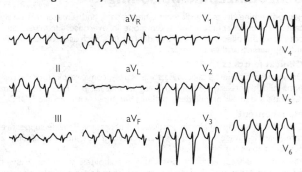

Fig. 4.2 ECG in tricyclic antidepressant poisoning, showing sinus tachycardia with prolonged conduction, which may be mistaken for VT.

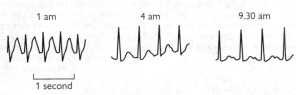

Fig. 4.3 Serial ECG rhythm strips in amitriptyline poisoning, showing spontaneous recovery with supportive care.

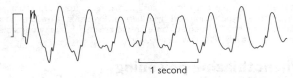

Fig. 4.4 ECG trace in very severe tricyclic antidepressant poisoning. The patient was unconscious, GCS 3, and was intubated and ventilated, with BP 70/50.

Benzodiazepine poisoning

Benzodiazepine drugs (eg diazepam, nitrazepam, and temazepam) rarely cause serious poisoning when taken alone in overdose. However, they potentiate the effects of other CNS depressants, such as alcohol, tricyclic antidepressants and barbiturates.

Clinical features

Drowsiness, dizziness, ataxia, dysarthria. Rarely, coma, respiratory depression, mild hypotension. Fatal poisoning is unusual, but may occur from respiratory depression in elderly patients and those with chronic COPD.

Management

Clear the airway and maintain ventilation if necessary. Provide supportive care. Gastric lavage and activated charcoal are not indicated if only a benzodiazepine has been taken.

Many benzodiazepines have long-acting metabolites, which may affect driving and other motor skills for several days or even weeks after an overdose. Give appropriate warnings about this.

Flumazenil is a specific benzodiazepine antagonist, but is not licensed in the UK for treating overdosage. It reverses the effects of benzodiazepines within 1min, but has a short duration of action (<1hr)—as a result, toxic effects often recur. Flumazenil can cause convulsions and cardiac arrhythmias and may precipitate a withdrawal syndrome in patients who are dependent on benzodiazepines. It is particularly dangerous in patients with combined benzodiazepine and tricyclic antidepressant poisoning, in whom it may cause convulsions and cardiac arrest. Flumazenil may occasionally be used by experts managing very severe benzodiazepine poisoning, but there is no place for its use by the non-specialist.

Clomethiazole poisoning

Clomethiazole overdosage may cause coma, respiratory depression, ↓ muscle tone, hypotension and hypothermia. Excessive salivation and a characteristic smell of clomethiazole on the breath are often noticeable. Treat supportively. IPPV may be necessary.

Phenothiazine poisoning

The phenothiazines (eg chlorpromazine), butyrophenones (eg haloperidol), and related drugs are used as antipsychotics and anti-emetics. In overdosage they may cause drowsiness, coma, hypotension, and hypothermia. Deep coma and respiratory depression are uncommon. Some conscious patients suffer *dystonic reactions* with oculogyric crises and muscle spasms causing torticollis or opisthotonus. Convulsions may occur. ECG changes of prolonged PR, QRS, and ST intervals, and arrhythmias are seen particularly with thioridazine poisoning.

Treat supportively. Activated charcoal may help. If cardiac arrhythmias occur, correct hypoxia, acidosis and electrolyte abnormalities before giving any anti-arrhythmic drug. Treat dystonic reactions with procyclidine (5mg IV or 5–10mg IM), repeated if symptoms recur.

Barbiturate poisoning

Now uncommon, except in drug addicts. Overdosage with phenobarbitone is seen occasionally. Barbiturate poisoning may cause coma, respiratory depression, hypotension and hypothermia. There are no specific neurological signs. Skin blisters and rhabdomyolysis may result from prolonged immobility. Treat supportively, with IPPV if necessary. Repeated doses of activated charcoal may help to remove barbiturates. Very rarely, charcoal haemoperfusion is indicated in some patients with deep and prolonged coma and respiratory complications.

Lithium poisoning

Clinical features Often due to therapeutic overdosage or drug interactions (eg with diuretics or NSAIDs), rather than deliberate self-harm. Symptoms may start up to 24hr after an overdose, especially with slow-release tablets. Nausea, vomiting and diarrhoea are followed by tremor, ataxia, confusion, increased muscle tone and clonus. In severe cases there may be convulsions, coma and renal failure. Lithium-induced nephrogenic diabetes insipidus may complicate treatment.

Investigations Measure U&E and lithium (plain tube, not lithium heparin). Therapeutic lithium levels are <1.2mmol/L. Toxic effects are often seen at >1.5mmol/L. Soon after a large overdose, higher levels may occur with little clinical effects, before lithium is distributed to tissues.

Management Activated charcoal does not absorb lithium. Gastric lavage is indicated within 1hr of a single large overdose, except for slow-release tablets, which are too large to pass up a gastric tube. Whole-bowel irrigation (📖 p.185) may be considered for slow-release tablets: discuss this with a poisons specialist (📖 p.181). Use standard supportive measures and control convulsions with diazepam. Observe all patients for >24 hours. Give oral fluids in conscious patients. Forced diuresis is contraindicated. Haemodialysis is the best treatment in severe poisoning, but often has to be repeated because of rebound release of lithium from tissue stores.

Sulphonylurea poisoning

Sulphonylurea drugs are used to treat non-insulin-dependent diabetes. Accidental or deliberate overdosage causes hypoglycaemia, which may recur over several days after long-acting drugs, such as chlorpropamide or glibenclamide. In the Far East, sulphonylurea contamination of illicit drugs used for erectile dysfunction has caused several cases of hypoglycaemia.

Check blood glucose and U&E. Correct hypoglycaemia with oral or IV glucose (📖 p.150). Observe for at least 24hr (72hr for long-acting drugs) and check BMG hourly. To prevent recurrent hypoglycaemia give 10% glucose IV infusion; in severe cases 20% glucose may be needed, via central line because of venous irritation. Hypokalaemia may occur. Check U&E and add potassium as needed. In severe poisoning, get expert advice (📖 p.181) and consider octreotide (unlicensed indication) which blocks pancreatic insulin release: initial dose for adults 50micrograms subcutaneous (SC) or IV.

Beta-blocker poisoning

Clinical features

Overdosage with β-blockers (propranolol, oxprenolol, atenolol, labetolol, sotalol) may cause rapid and severe toxicity with hypotension and cardiogenic shock. There is usually a sinus bradycardia, but sometimes the heart rate remains normal. Coma, convulsions, and cardiac arrest may occur. ECG changes include marked QRS prolongation, and ST and T wave abnormalities. Propranolol may cause bronchospasm in asthmatics and hypoglycaemia in children. Sotalol can cause prolonged QTc and VT, with torsades de pointes.

Management

Monitor ECG, heart rate, and BP. Obtain reliable venous access. Check U&E and blood glucose. Consider activated charcoal (🕮 p.185). Bradycardia and hypotension may respond to atropine (1–2mg for adult; 0.02mg/kg for child), but this is often ineffective.

Glucagon is the best treatment for severe cardiotoxicity and seems to work by activating myocardial adenylcyclase in a way not blocked by β-blockade. Glucagon 5–10mg IV (50–150micrograms/kg for a child) usually produces a dramatic improvement in pulse and BP, with return of cardiac output and consciousness. Glucagon often causes sudden vomiting—anticipate this and position the patient appropriately. In severe poisoning glucagon has a transient effect on cardiac output and further doses or an infusion are needed (4mg/hr, sometimes up to 15mg/hr, reducing gradually). Some patients need a total of 50–75mg of glucagon, which is reconstituted from 1mg vials of dry powder. If glucagon is unavailable or ineffective, give adrenaline (5–10micrograms/min) or dobutamine (2.5–10micrograms/kg/min), increasing the dose if necessary. Get expert advice (🕮 p.181) in severe poisoning.

Cardiac pacing may be tried for bradycardia, but is often ineffective. Occasionally, circulatory support has to be provided by prolonged chest compressions or extracorporeal cardiac bypass while more glucagon is obtained or the β-blocker is metabolized. Consider insulin therapy (🕮 p.187) for severe hypotension, and Intralipid® (🕮 p.187) in cardiac arrest.

Calcium antagonist poisoning

Poisoning with verapamil, nifedipine, diltiazem or other calcium-channel blockers is rare, but may be fatal. Nausea, vomiting, dizziness and confusion may occur. Bradycardia and AV block may lead to AV dissociation, with hypotension and cardiac arrest (especially in patients taking β-adrenergic blockers). Metabolic acidosis, hyperkalaemia and hyperglycaemia may occur.

Provide supportive treatment. Monitor ECG and BP. Obtain venous access. Consider activated charcoal. Check U&E, glucose, calcium. Give atropine (1–2mg, child 0.02mg/kg) for symptomatic bradycardia. Get expert help. Pacing may be needed. Calcium gluconate (10–20mL of 10% slowly IV, observing ECG) may ↓ prolonged intra-cardiac conduction. Glucagon may help, as in β-blocker poisoning (see above). Inotropic support with dobutamine, adrenaline or high dose insulin therapy (🕮 p.187) may be needed to maintain cardiac output. In severe poisoning or cardiac arrest consider Intralipid (🕮 p.187).

Digoxin poisoning

Toxicity from the therapeutic use of digoxin is relatively common. Acute poisoning is rare, but may be fatal. Similar effects occur with digitoxin and very rarely with plants containing cardiac glycosides (foxglove, oleander and yew).

Clinical features

Nausea, vomiting, malaise, delirium, xanthopsia (yellow flashes or discolouration of vision). Acute poisoning usually causes bradycardia with PR and QRS prolongation. There may be AV block, AV dissociation and escape rhythms, sometimes with ventricular ectopics or VT. Hyperkalaemia occurs, and in severe cases metabolic acidosis due to hypotension and ↓ tissue perfusion.

Management

Provide supportive treatment. Monitor ECG and BP. Obtain venous access. Give activated charcoal to ↓ absorption and prevent entero-hepatic recycling of digoxin (📖 p.185). Measure U&E, plasma digoxin, and ABG in severe poisoning. Get expert help for patients who are severely poisoned. Correct severe metabolic acidosis with sodium bicarbonate. Treat hyperkalaemia >6mmol/L (📖 p.162). Bradycardia and AV block often respond to atropine IV total 1–2mg (child 0.02mg/kg). Cardiac pacing is not always effective and a high voltage is often needed for capture. VT may respond to lidocaine or a β-blocker. Treat severe poisoning with digoxin antibodies (Digibind®), which rapidly correct arrhythmias and hyperkalaemia. Digibind® is expensive and rarely needed, so is not stocked in many hospitals: Poisons Information Services (📖 p.181) can advise about emergency supplies and the dose required for the patient's body weight and plasma digoxin concentration or the quantity taken.

ACE inhibitor poisoning

Overdosage with angiotensin converting enzyme (ACE) inhibitors (eg captopril, enalapril, lisinopril) may cause drowsiness, hypotension, hyperkalaemia and rarely, renal failure. Monitor BP and ECG. Give IV 0.9% saline if BP is low. Check U&E. Consider activated charcoal (📖 p.185).

Theophylline poisoning

Theophylline and aminophylline can cause fatal poisoning. Many preparations are slow-release and may not produce serious toxicity until 12–24 hours after ingestion, so careful observation is essential.

Features

Nausea, vomiting (often severe and not helped by anti-emetics), abdominal pain, haematemesis, restlessness, ↑ muscle tone, ↑ reflexes, headache, convulsions. Coma, hyperventilation, hyperpyrexia and rhabdomyolysis may occur. Sinus tachycardia may be followed by supraventricular and ventricular arrhythmias and VF. BP may initially ↑, but later ↓ in severe poisoning. Complex metabolic disturbances include a respiratory alkalosis followed by metabolic acidosis, hyperglycaemia, and severe hypokalaemia.

Management

- Treat supportively.
- Monitor ECG, heart rate and BP.
- Obtain venous access and measure U&E, glucose, ABG, plasma theophylline (repeated after a few hours). Repeat K^+ hourly if patient is symptomatic, since early correction of hypokalaemia may prevent dangerous arrhythmias. Correct hypokalaemia with K^+ (large amounts may be needed, but no faster than 20mmol/hr).
- Perform gastric lavage if <1hr since ingestion. Give repeated activated charcoal (📖 p.185), by NG tube if necessary.
- Intractable vomiting may respond to ondansetron (8mg slowly IV in adult).
- GI bleeding may require transfusion and ranitidine (but not cimetidine, which slows metabolism of theophylline).
- Tachycardia with an adequate cardiac output should be observed, but not treated. Non-selective β-blockers (eg propranolol) may help severe tachyarrhythmias and hypokalaemia, but cause bronchospasm in asthmatics. Lidocaine and mexiletine may precipitate fits, so disopyramide is preferable for ventricular arrhythmias.
- Control convulsions with diazepam or lorazepam. Paralyse, intubate, and provide IPPV if the airway is at risk from coma, fits and vomiting.
- Charcoal haemoperfusion may be needed in severe poisoning, especially if oral or NG activated charcoal is impracticable because of vomiting. Serious hyperkalaemia may occur during recovery from theophylline poisoning if large amounts of K^+ were given earlier.

Salbutamol poisoning

Poisoning with β_2-agonists (eg salbutamol, terbutaline) may cause vomiting, agitation, tremor, tachycardia, palpitations, hypokalaemia and hypertension. Rarely, there may be hallucinations, hyperglycaemia, ventricular tachyarrhythmias, myocardial ischaemia, and convulsions.

Treat supportively:
- Correct hypokalaemia by infusion of K^+ (max 20 mmol/hour).
- Monitor ECG and BP.
- Activated charcoal may ↓ drug absorption.
- Do not treat tachycardia if there is an adequate cardiac output. Propranolol may help severe tachyarrhythmias and hypokalaemia, but can precipitate bronchospasm in asthmatics.

Iron poisoning

Small children often eat iron tablets, many of which resemble sweets. Serious poisoning is uncommon, but fatalities can occur. Note that iron is present in some weed/seed preparations.

Different preparations contain the equivalent of 35–110mg of elemental iron per tablet, sometimes in slow-release form.

Serious toxicity is unlikely unless >60mg elemental iron/kg body weight has been taken. The estimated lethal dose is about 150–300mg/kg.

Features

In the first few hours after ingestion nausea, vomiting, diarrhoea and abdominal pain are common. Vomit and stools are often grey or black and may contain blood. Hyperglycaemia and ↑ WCC may occur. Most patients do not develop further features.

In severe poisoning, early effects include haematemesis, drowsiness, convulsions, coma, metabolic acidosis and shock.

Early symptoms settle after 6–12hr, but a few patients then deteriorate 24–48hr after ingestion, with shock, hypoglycaemia, jaundice, metabolic acidosis, hepatic encephalopathy, renal failure, and occasionally bowel infarction. Survivors may develop gastric strictures or pyloric obstruction 2–5 weeks after the overdose.

Management

- Check serum iron, FBC, glucose, and also ABG in severe poisoning.
- Perform gastric lavage if >20mg elemental iron/kg body weight has been taken in the previous 1hr. Do not give charcoal, which does not absorb iron. Iron tablets are radio-opaque and can be counted on a plain abdominal X-ray film. Whole-bowel irrigation (📖 p.185) may be useful if many tablets remain in the gut, especially with slow-release formulations.
- Use supportive measures if required.
- Obtain expert advice in serious poisoning. Coma and shock indicate severe poisoning needing immediate treatment with *desferrioxamine* by IV infusion (15mg/kg/hr, max 80mg/kg in 24hr). Desferrioxamine should also be given if the serum iron exceeds the expected total iron binding capacity (about 54–75mmol/L): measurement of total iron binding capacity may give misleading results after iron poisoning. Desferrioxamine causes hypotension if infused too rapidly and can produce rashes and rarely, anaphylaxis, pulmonary oedema or ARDS. The iron-desferrioxamine complex makes the urine orange or red, which confirms that free iron has been bound and that desferrioxamine was required. Reduce desferrioxamine dosage when there is clinical improvement and serum iron is less than the expected total iron binding capacity.
- Patients who still have no symptoms 6 hours after an iron overdose have probably not ingested toxic amounts and may be discharged, with advice to return if symptoms develop.
- Pregnancy does not alter the treatment needed for iron poisoning; use desferrioxamine if indicated.

Ethanol poisoning

Features

Overdosage of ethanol (ethyl alcohol or 'alcohol') is very common. Alcohol potentiates the CNS depressant effects of many drugs. It initially causes disinhibition and later ataxia, dizziness, dysarthria and drowsiness.

In severe poisoning there may be coma with respiratory depression, hypotension, hypothermia and a metabolic acidosis. Hypoglycaemia is a particular problem in children and may occur after some hours. Death may result from respiratory failure or aspiration of vomit.

For an adult, the *fatal dose of ethanol* alone is ≈300–500mL of absolute alcohol: whisky and gin usually contain 40–50% ethanol. Do not assume that ↓ GCS is due to alcohol until other causes have been excluded.

Rarely, alcohol causes lactic acidosis (especially in patients with liver disease or taking biguanide hypoglycaemic drugs) or ketoacidosis (due to dehydration and hypoglycaemia in alcoholics)—see 🔲 p.622.

Treatment

- Maintain a clear airway and adequate ventilation.
- Check blood glucose every 1–2 hours in severe poisoning.
- Correct hypoglycaemia with glucose, not with glucagon.
- Look for signs of injury, especially head injury.
- Emergency measurement of blood ethanol rarely alters management.
- Gastric lavage and activated charcoal are ineffective in ethanol intoxication.

Methanol poisoning

Methanol is used as a solvent and in antifreeze. Ingestion of 10mL of pure methanol may cause blindness and 30mL can be fatal, the toxic effects being due to the metabolites formaldehyde and formic acid.

Methylated spirits is a mixture of ethanol and water with about 5% methanol: toxicity is almost entirely due to ethanol.

Clinical features

Methanol initially causes only mild transient drowsiness. Serious toxicity develops after a latent period of 12–24 hours with vomiting, abdominal pain, headache, dizziness, blurring of vision, and drowsiness leading to coma. There is a severe metabolic acidosis, hyperglycaemia and ↑ serum amylase. Survivors may be blind from optic nerve damage and develop Parkinsonian problems.

Management

- Consider gastric lavage if <1hr since ingestion. Do not give charcoal.
- Measure ABG, U&E, Cl^-, HCO_3^-, glucose, FBC, LFTs and osmolality, and plasma methanol if possible. Calculate osmolal gap and anion gap.
- Read Toxbase advice (🔲 p.181). Discuss with Poisons Information Service.
- Observe for at least 6hr after ingestion, even if asymptomatic.
- Early use of fomepizole or ethanol (as for ethylene glycol, 🔲 p.203) minimizes methanol toxicity and should be started if poisoning is likely, especially if there is a high anion gap metabolic acidosis.
- Use sodium bicarbonate to correct metabolic acidosis (aim for pH 7.5). Large amounts may be needed and hypernatraemia may occur.
- Give folinic acid (1mg/kg, max 50mg, IV every 6hr for 48hr).
- In severe poisoning, refer to ICU for haemodialysis and possibly IPPV.

Ethylene glycol poisoning

Ethylene glycol is used mainly as antifreeze. Fatal dose for an adult is about 100g (90mL of pure ethylene glycol). Toxic effects are due to metabolites glycolaldehyde, glycolic acid and oxalic acid. Fomepizole or ethanol block ethylene glycol metabolism, preventing toxicity.

Clinical features

In the first 12hr after ingestion the patient looks drunk, but does not smell of alcohol. Ataxia, dysarthria, nausea, vomiting, and sometimes haematemesis occur, followed by convulsions, coma and severe metabolic acidosis.

From 12–24hr after ingestion hyperventilation, pulmonary oedema, tachycardia, cardiac arrhythmias and cardiac failure may develop. Hypocalcaemia may be severe. Acute tubular necrosis and renal failure occur at 24–72hr. Cranial nerve palsies may develop.

Urine microscopy shows calcium oxalate monohydrate crystals which are diagnostic of ethylene glycol poisoning. Some makes of antifreeze contain fluorescein, which makes urine fluoresce in ultraviolet light (eg a Wood's lamp from a dermatology department). This helps to confirm ethylene glycol poisoning, but the absence of fluorescence does not exclude poisoning.

Management

- Consider gastric lavage if <1hr since ingestion. Do not give charcoal.
- Measure ABG, U&E, Cl⁻, HCO₃⁻, glucose, FBC, LFTs, osmolality, and plasma ethylene glycol if possible. Calculate osmolal gap and anion gap.
- Read Toxbase advice (📖 p.181). Discuss with Poisons Information Service.
- Observe for at least 6hr after ingestion, even if asymptomatic.
- Monitor ECG, pulse, blood pressure, respiratory rate, and urine output.
- Early use of fomepizole or ethanol minimizes toxicity and should be started if poisoning is likely.
- High anion gap metabolic acidosis (📖 p.99) occurs in ethylene glycol poisoning (and also methanol poisoning, diabetic ketoacidosis, alcoholic ketoacidosis, and renal failure), but acidosis only develops after some ethylene glycol has been metabolized.
- Consider fomepizole: discuss with Poisons Information Service (📖 p.181) about indications, dosage, and where to obtain it.
- If fomepizole is not available give ethanol orally as whisky, gin or vodka (adult 125–150mL, child 2mL/kg) followed by IVI of ethanol, preferably as 5% solution in glucose. Initial IV adult dose is 12g ethanol/hr, ↑ for alcoholics and during haemodialysis and adjusted to maintain blood ethanol at ≈1g/L (discuss dose with Poisons Information Service).
- Use sodium bicarbonate to correct metabolic acidosis (aim for pH 7.5). Large amounts may be needed and hypernatraemia may occur.
- Correct severe hypocalcaemia with calcium gluconate (10mL of 10% slowly IV).
- Haemodialysis may be required in severe poisoning, with frequent measurements of blood ethylene glycol concentrations (and ethanol if this is used). Intensive care and ventilation may be needed.

Paraquat poisoning

Paraquat is an effective weedkiller which is very toxic if ingested: death is likely after 10mL of liquid paraquat (100 or 200g/L). Paraquat poisoning is now rare in the UK, where paraquat is no longer approved for sale or use, but accidental or deliberate poisoning still occurs in many developing countries.

Inhalation of dilute paraquat spray may cause sore throat and epistaxis, but not systemic poisoning. No specific treatment is needed and symptoms resolve in a few days. Prolonged contact of paraquat with the skin causes erythema and sometimes ulceration, but absorption is rarely sufficient to cause systemic toxicity. Remove soiled clothing and wash the skin thoroughly with water.

Splashes in the eyes cause pain and corneal ulceration. Immediately irrigate with water and refer for ophthalmological review.

Clinical features of paraquat ingestion

Paraquat is corrosive and causes immediate burning pain in the mouth and throat, nausea and vomiting, followed by abdominal pain and diarrhoea.

Large amounts (>6g) of paraquat result in rapid deterioration with shock, pulmonary oedema, metabolic acidosis, coma, convulsions, and death within 24hr.

Smaller quantities (3–6g) do not produce shock. After 24hr, chemical burns of the mouth and throat cause pain and difficulty in swallowing and speaking. The burns look white until the surface sloughs after about 3 days, leaving painful raw areas.

Renal failure occurs at 1–2 days and there is mild jaundice.

Paraquat lung usually develops by 5–7 days, with pulmonary oedema and fibrosis causing breathlessness and cyanosis. Lung shadowing is seen on CXR. Death from hypoxia occurs 7–14 days after poisoning. 1.5–2g of paraquat may produce slower respiratory failure, with gradual deterioration until death up to 6 weeks after ingestion. Survival with lung damage is uncommon.

Management

- Do not give O_2, which increases pulmonary toxicity of paraquat.
- Consider gastric lavage if <1hr since ingestion.
- Give oral activated charcoal immediately, with IV analgesia and anti-emetics.
- Send urine (and gastric fluid if available) for the laboratory to test for paraquat, which can be done very quickly using sodium dithionite. A negative test within 4 hours of suspected ingestion excludes significant poisoning. If paraquat is present, measure the plasma concentration if possible, since it helps assessment of the prognosis: the Poisons Information Services (📖 p.181) can advise about paraquat measurement and the interpretation of results.
- Unfortunately, no treatment improves the outcome of paraquat poisoning.
- Keep patients who are likely to die as comfortable as possible.

Petrol and paraffin poisoning

Petrol, paraffin (kerosene), and other petroleum distillates are used as fuels and solvents. They contain mixtures of hydrocarbons, often with small quantities of other chemicals. Unintentional poisoning occurs after liquids have been stored in inappropriate and unlabelled containers. The major problem is pneumonitis caused by aspiration of hydrocarbons into the lungs.

Clinical features

In many cases no symptoms occur. There may be nausea, vomiting, and occasionally diarrhoea. Aspiration into the lungs causes choking, coughing, wheeze, breathlessness, cyanosis and fever. X-ray changes of pneumonitis (shadowing in the mid or lower zones) may occur without respiratory symptoms or signs. Occasionally, pleural effusions or pneumatoceles develop. In severe cases, there may be pulmonary oedema, drowsiness, convulsions or coma. Rare problems include renal failure and intravascular haemolysis.

Management

Many patients remain well and need no treatment.

Avoid gastric lavage unless very large quantities have been taken or there is serious concern about another poison: in these rare cases lavage may be done on specialist advice if the patient has a good cough reflex or the airway is protected by a cuffed ET tube. Obtain a CXR and observe for respiratory problems. Patients with a normal initial CXR who have no symptoms or signs 6 hours after ingestion may be discharged with advice to return if symptoms develop.

If symptoms occur, treat supportively with O_2 and bronchodilators as necessary. Steroids and prophylactic antibiotics are unhelpful. IPPV is occasionally needed because of severe pulmonary oedema.

Organophosphate poisoning

Organophosphates are widely used as insecticides. Poisoning with these chemicals is rare in the UK, but common in many developing countries. Organophosphates are absorbed through the skin, bronchial mucosa and gut, and inhibit cholinesterases, causing accumulation of acetylcholine at nerve endings and neuromuscular junctions. The speed of onset, severity and duration of toxicity vary between different compounds. Irreversible binding of cholinesterase ('ageing') develops after some minutes or hours. Pralidoxime reactivates cholinesterase if given promptly, before ageing occurs.

Organophosphate nerve gas agents such as sarin may be released deliberately by terrorists. Information is available from Toxbase (📖 p.181).

Carbamate insecticides act similarly to organophosphates, but poisoning with carbamates is generally less severe and pralidoxime is not needed.

Clinical features

Minor exposure to organophosphates may cause subclinical poisoning with ↓ cholinesterase levels, but no symptoms or signs. Symptoms may be delayed by 12–24hr after skin exposure.

Early features of toxicity include anxiety, restlessness, insomnia, tiredness, headache, nausea, vomiting, abdominal colic, diarrhoea, sweating, hypersalivation, and miosis. Muscle weakness and fasciculation may develop.

In severe poisoning there is widespread paralysis with respiratory failure, pulmonary oedema, profuse bronchial secretions, bronchospasm, convulsions and coma. Hyperglycaemia and cardiac arrhythmias may occur. Occasionally, delayed effects of poisoning develop 1–4 days after acute poisoning, with cranial nerve palsies, muscle weakness and respiratory failure which resolve after 2–3 weeks. A peripheral neuropathy may develop after 2 weeks, usually involving the legs.

Management[1]

- Wear protective clothing and avoid getting contaminated yourself.
- Give supportive treatment as needed.
- Clear the airway and remove secretions. Give O_2 and IPPV if needed.
- Insert two IV cannulae. Take blood for cholinesterase.
- If there are profuse bronchial secretions or bronchospasm, give atropine IV (adult 2mg, child 0.02mg/kg), repeated every 5min with the dose doubled each time until the chest sounds clear, systolic BP >80mmHg and pulse >80. Some patients need >100mg of atropine.
- Give diazepam to treat agitation and control convulsions.
- In moderate or severe poisoning give pralidoxime mesylate (also called P2S). The dose of pralidoxime is 30mg/kg IV over 5–10min, repeated if necessary every 4hr. Improvement is usually apparent within 30min.
- Poisons Information Services can advise on pralidoxime supply and use: in the UK the Blood Transfusion Service will supply pralidoxime if there are multiple casualties with organophosphate poisoning.

---

1 Eddleston M et al. (2008) Management of acute organophosphorus pesticide poisoning. *Lancet.* **371**: 597–607.

Cyanide poisoning

Cyanide compounds are widely used in industry and may be ingested or inhaled inadvertently or deliberately. Cyanides produced by burning polyurethane foam ↑ mortality from smoke inhalation: if there is severe acidosis consider cyanide toxicity. Cyanide poisoning may be caused by the drug sodium nitroprusside or ingestion of amygdalin (laetrile) from the kernels of apricots, cherries and other fruits. Solutions for removing artificial fingernails may contain acetonitrile (methyl cyanide).

Cyanides inhibit cytochrome oxidase, blocking the tricarboxylic acid cycle and stopping cellular respiration. This process is reversible. Inhalation of hydrogen cyanide often causes death within minutes. Ingestion of cyanides can produce rapid poisoning, but food in the stomach may delay absorption and the onset of symptoms. Delayed poisoning may follow absorption of cyanides through the skin. Ingested cyanide compounds react with gastric acid to form hydrogen cyanide, which could poison first-aiders giving mouth to mouth resuscitation.

Clinical features

Acute poisoning causes dizziness, anxiety, headache, palpitations, breathlessness, and drowsiness. In severe cases, there may be coma, convulsions, paralysis, pulmonary oedema, cardiac arrhythmias and cardiorespiratory failure, with metabolic acidosis. Most of the clinical features result from severe hypoxia, but cyanosis is uncommon. Classically, there is a smell of bitter almonds on the breath, but many people cannot detect this.

Management

- Avoid getting contaminated yourself.
- Provide supportive measures: give 100% O_2 and monitor ECG.
- Remove contaminated clothing and wash exposed skin.
- Consider activated charcoal or gastric lavage within 1hr of ingestion.
- In mild poisoning, reassurance, O_2 and observation may be all that is required. Exposure to cyanide causes great anxiety and it may be difficult to distinguish between fear of poisoning and early symptoms of toxicity.
- *Specific antidotes* should be available, but are not always needed.

Some specific antidotes to cyanide are dangerous in the absence of cyanide—only give if poisoning is moderate or severe (eg coma). In severe cyanide poisoning, give *dicobalt edetate* (Kelocyanor®) 300mg IV over 1min, repeated if there is no improvement after 1min. In the absence of cyanide, dicobalt edetate may cause cobalt poisoning with facial, laryngeal and pulmonary oedema, vomiting, tachycardia and hypotension. Alternative treatment is *sodium thiosulphate* (adult dose 25mL of 50% solution IV over 10min; child 400mg/kg) with *sodium nitrite* (adult dose 10mL of 3% solution IV over 5–20min; child dose 0.13–0.33mL/kg of 3% solution/kg, ie 4–10mg/kg). Sodium thiosulphate often causes vomiting. Sodium nitrite may cause hypotension. High doses of *hydroxocobalamin* (5–10g, Cyanokit®) are useful and relatively safe in cyanide poisoning, especially in victims of smoke inhalation.

Carbon monoxide poisoning

Carbon monoxide (CO) is a tasteless and odourless gas produced by incomplete combustion. Poisoning may occur from car exhausts, fires and faulty gas heaters. CO is also produced by metabolism of methylene chloride (used in paint strippers and as an industrial solvent). CO ↓ the O_2-carrying capacity of the blood by binding haemoglobin (Hb) to form carboxyhaemoglobin (COHb). This impairs O_2 delivery from blood to the tissues and also inhibits cytochrome oxidase, blocking O_2 utilization. These effects combine to cause severe tissue hypoxia.

The elimination half-life of CO is about 4hr on breathing air, 1hr on 100% O_2, and 23min on O_2 at 3 atmospheres pressure.

Clinical features

Early features are headache, malaise, nausea and vomiting (sometimes misdiagnosed as a viral illness or gastroenteritis, especially if several members of a family are affected).

In severe poisoning, there is coma with hyperventilation, hypotension, ↑ muscle tone, ↑ reflexes, extensor plantars and convulsions. Cherry-red colouring of the skin may be seen in fatal CO poisoning, but is rare in live patients. Skin blisters and rhabdomyolysis may occur after prolonged immobility. Pulmonary oedema, MI and cerebral oedema can occur. Neurological and psychiatric problems sometimes develop some weeks after CO poisoning, but usually improve over the following year.

Management

- Remove from exposure.
- Clear the airway and maintain ventilation with as high a concentration of O_2 as possible. For a conscious patient use a tight-fitting mask with an O_2 reservoir, but if unconscious intubate and provide IPPV on 100% O_2.
- Record ECG and monitor heart rhythm: look for arrhythmias and signs of acute MI.
- Check ABG—SpO_2 measurements are misleading in CO poisoning, as are p_aO_2 values, but acidosis indicates tissue hypoxia.
- Check COHb levels (in blood or with a special pulse oximeter): although these correlate poorly with clinical features, COHb >15% after arrival at hospital suggests serious poisoning. COHb may be up to 8% in smokers without CO poisoning. A nomogram (📖 p.395) can help to estimate COHb at the time of exposure.
- Correct metabolic acidosis by ventilation and O_2: try to avoid bicarbonate, which may worsen tissue hypoxia.
- Consider mannitol if cerebral oedema is suspected.
- *Hyperbaric O_2* therapy is logical, but of no proven benefit for CO poisoning. Transfer to a hyperbaric chamber and pressurization may take hours and so hyperbaric treatment may be no more effective than ventilation on 100% normobaric O_2. Caring for a critically ill patient in a small pressure chamber may be impracticable. Discuss with a Poisons Information Service (📖 p.181) and consider hyperbaric treatment if a patient has been unconscious at any time, has COHb >20%, is pregnant, or has cardiac complications or neurological or psychiatric features. The Poisons Information Service can advise on the location and telephone numbers of hyperbaric chambers. Some details are in Table 6.1, 📖 p.261.

Chlorine poisoning

Chlorine gas causes lacrimation, conjunctivitis, coughing, wheezing, breathlessness, and chest pain. Laryngeal and pulmonary oedema may develop within a few hours.

- Remove from exposure and give O_2, with bronchodilators if necessary. If there is laryngeal or pulmonary oedema, consult an expert and give prednisolone in high dosage (adult 60–80mg/day initially). In severe cases, IPPV in ICU may be needed.
- If the eyes are painful, irrigate with water or saline, and examine with fluorescein for corneal damage.
- Casualties with minor exposure to chlorine but no symptoms may be allowed home with advice to rest and return if symptoms develop.
- Patients with symptoms when seen in hospital usually need admission for at least 12 hours for observation. Record serial peak expiratory flow rates, which may warn of deterioration.

CS gas (tear gas)

CS (orthochlorobenzylidene malononitrile) is used for riot control, police self-protection, and sometimes as a weapon in assaults. It is an aerosol or smoke, rather than a gas. Exposure to CS causes immediate blepharospasm and lacrimation, uncontrollable sneezing and coughing, a burning sensation in the skin and throat, and tightness of the chest. Vomiting may occur. These symptoms usually disappear within 10min in fresh air, but conjunctivitis may persist for 30min. Exposure in a confined space may cause symptoms for some hours and is particularly dangerous in people with pre-existing lung disease. Redness or blistering of the skin may develop, due to the solvent in the spray.

Treat patients exposed to CS gas in a well-ventilated area. Ensure that staff wear gloves and close-fitting goggles. Remove contaminated clothes and wash affected skin thoroughly. Give O_2 and bronchodilators if necessary. Reassure the patient that the symptoms will resolve.

If the eyes are painful, blow dry air on them with a fan to vaporize any remaining CS gas. The irritation should disappear in a few minutes. Alternatively, irrigate the eyes with saline (although this may cause a transient worsening of symptoms). When symptoms have settled, record visual acuity and examine the corneas using fluorescein. Refer to an ophthalmologist if symptoms persist.

CN gas (chloroacetophenone) is used in some countries for riot control and in personal defence devices. CN has similar effects to CS, but is more toxic.

Chemical incidents

Chemical incidents involving single or multiple casualties may result from accidents (eg release of chlorine gas) or deliberate release of chemicals (by terrorists or others). CBRN (Chemical, Biological, Radiological and Nuclear) incidents have many features in common.

If you know or suspect that a patient has been involved in a chemical incident:

• Inform senior ED staff.
• Avoid contaminating other staff or patients.
• Ensure that you are wearing suitable personal protective equipment (PPE), unless the patient has already been decontaminated.
• Decontaminate the patient according to departmental guidelines if this has not been done already (see 📖 p.211).
• Resuscitate as necessary: airway, breathing, and circulation.
• Assess the clinical features and toxic agent.
• Give antidotes if appropriate, and reassess the patient.
• Enquire whether other patients are expected.
• Inform the local Health Protection Team.
• Get expert advice from Toxbase, Poisons Information Service (📖 p.181) or HPA Chemical Hazards and Poisons Division (ChaPD tel. 0870 606 4444).
• If deliberate release is suspected inform the Police and involve other agencies and the press officer.

Chemical agents which might cause a chemical incident include:
• Chlorine—see 📖 p.209.
• CS gas (tear gas)—see 📖 CS gas (tear gas), p.209.
• Cyanide—see 📖 p.207.
• Organophosphates—see 📖 p.206.

Information about chemical incidents
• Health Protection Agency advice on CBRN and chemical incidents: www.hpa.org.uk/emergency/CBRN.htm
• TOXBASE (see 📖 p.181) section on Deliberate Release gives details of toxicity and antidotes, with medical, public health and public briefing documents about 60 chemicals that might be deliberately released.
• Home Office guidance on decontamination after CBRN incidents: http://www.cabinetoffice.gov.uk/ukresilience/emergencies/cbrn.aspx

Infection control and prevention: see 📖 p.32.

Major incidents: see 📖 p.38.

Radiation incidents: see 📖 p.268.

Decontamination of patients

Decontamination after exposure to a chemical, biological, or radiation hazard is intended to reduce the risks to the patient and to other people.

Casualties should be decontaminated at the scene after a CBRN incident, but some contaminated patients are likely to arrive at EDs without warning. Many people will be worried about contamination, but not actually at risk. Patients injured by industrial incidents, road traffic collisions, bombs, or other incidents may also be contaminated.

Even with advance planning it will be challenging to organize the ED, keep 'clean' areas clean, maintain order, and communicate between the 'decon' team (in PPE) and other ED staff.

Equipment for decontamination

- Scissors. Buckets. Sponges, soft brushes, wash cloths. Liquid soap.
- Disposable towels. Disposable gowns and slippers. Blankets.
- Plastic bags (large for clothing, small for valuables).
- ID labels and waterproof marking pens (for patients and property bags).
- Plastic bins with polythene liners (for used decontamination equipment).
- Warm or tepid water (hot water might increase chemical absorption).
- 0.9% saline and drip sets for eye and wound irrigation. LA eye drops.

Decontaminating non-ambulant patients

- Keep contaminated patients outside the ED.
- Clear, prepare, and secure the decontamination area.
- Protect yourself with appropriate PPE and use it properly.
- Work in teams of 2–4 people. Look after each other.
- Tell the team what to look for and what to do.
- In severe poisoning resuscitation, antidote administration, and decontamination may have to be done simultaneously.
- Tell casualties what you are doing.
- Record patient's name and number on wrist band and property bags.
- Remove or cut off clothing (which removes 80–90% of contamination). Do not pull clothing off over the head.
- Fold clothing outside-in and put it in property bags.
- Put valuables in a separate bag. Wash glasses and keep with patient.
- Clean face (protecting airway), open wounds, and sites for IV access, then from head to toes, front and back (log roll) including skin creases.
- Rinse affected areas with soapy water (saline for wounds and eyes).
- Wipe affected areas gently with a sponge to remove chemicals.
- Rinse with clean water.
- Dry patient. Cover in gown and blanket. Transfer to 'clean' trolley.
- Move patient to 'clean' area for further assessment and treatment.
- Put contaminated equipment in appropriate containers.
- Contain waste water if possible; if not, inform water/sewage agency.
- Rest and rotate staff as needed.
- Ensure staff are decontaminated before leaving the 'dirty' area.
- Record names of staff involved in decontamination.
- Warn staff of possible symptoms and check for signs of poisoning.
- Debrief staff and record events.

Plants, berries and mushrooms

Plants and berries

Many children eat plant leaves or brightly-coloured berries, but serious poisoning from plants is very rare. Identify the plant if possible, using reference books[1,2,3] or the CD-ROM computer software *Poisonous plants and fungi in Britain and Ireland* (📖 p.180). Advice on toxicity and any necessary treatment is available from Poisons Information Services. Many garden and house plants are non-toxic and no treatment is needed after ingestion.

Serious poisoning from *laburnum* is very rare, with only one death recorded in the UK in 50 years. No treatment needs to be provided for children who eat laburnum seeds, except for the very few with symptoms (nausea, salivation, vomiting, headache, rarely convulsions).

Mushroom poisoning

Serious poisoning from mushrooms or fungi is rare. Most deaths are due to *Amanita phalloides* (death cap mushroom). Reference books[1,4] are useful, but identification of mushrooms from the description or fragments available is often uncertain. Advice on toxicity and treatment is available from Poisons Information Services (📖 p.181).

Mushrooms found in gardens are unlikely to produce severe poisoning, but may cause vomiting and occasionally hallucinations, usually within 2hr of ingestion. Mushrooms which cause symptoms within 6hr are unlikely to be seriously toxic. Delayed toxicity occurs with *Amanita phalloides* and some other species, which grow throughout the UK.

Amanita phalloides poisoning causes vomiting and profuse watery diarrhoea after a latent period of 6–12hr, followed by hepatic and renal failure. The interval between ingestion and the onset of symptoms is crucial in distinguishing between non-serious and potentially fatal poisoning.

Try to ascertain if:
- More than one variety of mushroom was eaten (since poisonous and edible mushrooms often grow together).
- Whether the mushrooms were cooked (since some toxins are inactivated by heat).
- Whether alcohol was taken (since disulfiram-like effects may occur with *Coprinus* species, ink cap mushrooms).

For most toxic mushrooms only symptomatic treatment is required. Activated charcoal may ↓ absorption if given within 1hr. Get expert advice immediately if *Amanita* poisoning is suspected (📖 p.181).

1 Cooper MR, Johnson AW, Dauncey EA (2003) *Poisonous Plants and Fungi, An Illustrated Guide*, 2nd edn. TSO, London.
2 Dauncey EA (2010) *Poisonous Plants: A Guide for Childcare Providers*. Royal Botanic Gardens, Kew.
3 Frohne D, Pfänder HJ (2004) *Poisonous Plants*, 2nd edn. Manson Publishing Ltd, London.
4 Bresinsky A, Besl H (1990). *A Colour Atlas of Poisonous Fungi*. CRC Press, London.

Button batteries

Small children often swallow button or disc batteries intended for toys, watches, hearing aids, and other electrical equipment. The larger batteries may become stuck in the oesophagus, causing perforation or later stenosis. Most batteries that reach the stomach pass through the gut without any problem. Corrosive damage could occur from electrical discharge, but toxicity from battery contents is rare. Mercury poisoning is very unlikely since mercuric oxide batteries are no longer sold. The Poisons Information Service may identify the type of battery involved from the reference number, if this is available on the packet or on a similar battery to that ingested.

Management

X-ray the chest and abdomen or use a metal detector to find the battery. A battery stuck in the oesophagus should be removed immediately by endoscopy (which allows inspection for oesophageal damage and so is preferable to a magnet or Foley catheter).

An asymptomatic child with a battery in the stomach or bowel can be sent home with advice to return if any symptoms develop. If the battery has not been passed after 2 or 3 days, and is causing concern use a metal detector or repeat X-ray to look for the battery. If it is still in the stomach (which is rare) consider removal by endoscopy to avoid any risk of perforation or absorption of battery contents.

Batteries in the small or large bowel almost always pass spontaneously and should be left to do so, unless they cause symptoms. If abdominal pain, vomiting, diarrhoea or rectal bleeding occur an abdominal X-ray is needed to localize the battery, which may require removal by endoscopy or surgery.

Batteries in the nose

Button batteries lodged in the nose may cause corrosive burns and bleeding, sometimes with septal perforation after a few weeks. Liaise with an ENT specialist to remove batteries from the nose as soon as possible.

Illicit drugs

Many drugs are used illegally as stimulants or for mood-altering effects. Toxicity is often seen from heroin (📖 p.188), cocaine, ecstasy, and related drugs. Street names for drugs vary and may be confusing. The Street Terms database (http://www.whitehousedrugpolicy.gov/streetterms) and Toxbase (📖 p.181) have lists of slang names about drugs.

Illicit drugs vary in strength and are often mixed with other drugs or chemicals, which may cause unexpected effects. Drugs may be smoked, sniffed ('snorted'), swallowed or injected. Injecting drug users are at increased risk of hepatitis (📖 p.239), HIV (📖 p.242), necrotizing fasciitis (📖 p.234), botulism (📖 p.237), anthrax (📖 p.233) and endocarditis (📖 p.234).

Ecstasy (MDMA)

'Ecstasy' (3,4-methylenedioxymetamphetamine, MDMA) is an amphetamine derivative used as an illegal stimulant drug. The name 'ecstasy' is also used for benzylpiperazine (BZP), another illegal drug. 'Liquid ecstasy' is GHB (📖 p.215). MDMA is taken orally as tablets or powder, often at raves or parties. Some people who have previously tolerated the drug have idiosyncratic reactions, with severe toxicity from a single MDMA tablet.

MDMA causes release of serotonin, catecholamines and other hormones. Inappropriate ADH secretion, abnormal thirst, and excessive water intake may result in hyponatraemia and cerebral oedema, especially in women.

Clinical features Euphoria, agitation, sweating, dilated pupils, ataxia, teeth grinding, headache, tachycardia, hypertension. Severe poisoning can cause hyperpyrexia, muscle rigidity, rhabdomyolysis, convulsions, coma, cardiac arrhythmias, renal failure, hepatic failure, cerebral haemorrhage, and DIC. Metabolic acidosis is common. Features of serotonin syndrome may occur as may hypoglycaemia, severe hyponatraemia and hyperkalaemia.

Treatment Consider activated charcoal (📖 p.185) if <1hr since ingestion. Observe asymptomatic patients for at least 4hr. Monitor ECG, pulse, BP and temperature. Record ECG, check U&E, creatinine, glucose, LFTs and CK. Test urine for blood. In severe cases, check ABG and coagulation.

Supportively treat airway, breathing, and circulation. Get expert advice (📖 p.181) and ICU help in severe poisoning. Rapid sequence intubation may be needed because of trismus and fits: use rocuronium, rather than succinylcholine which may cause hyperkalaemia. Control agitation with oral or IV diazepam or lorazepam: large doses may be needed. For severe hypertension, give IV diazepam and GTN. Avoid β-blockers, which may cause unopposed α-adrenergic stimulation with ↑ BP and ↓ coronary blood flow. Do not treat single short fits, but give diazepam or lorazepam for repeated or prolonged fits.

Correct metabolic acidosis (possibly with sodium bicarbonate), checking ABG and U&E. Treat hyperkalaemia (📖 p.162). Treat mild hyponatraemia by fluid restriction. IV saline may be needed for severe hyponatraemia: rapid correction of chronic hyponatraemia can cause brain injury (central pontine myelinolysis), but this is less likely with acute hyponatraemia caused by MDMA. Cool as for heat stroke (📖 p.264) if hyperpyrexial. If rectal T >40°C, consider dantrolene 1mg/kg IV (up to 10mg/kg in 24hr). See also serotonin syndrome—📖 p.216.

Amphetamine

These sympathomimetic stimulants can be swallowed, snorted, smoked or injected. Body packers may suffer severe poisoning. Toxic features are euphoria, agitation, psychosis, sweating, dilated pupils, tachycardia, hypertension, vomiting, abdominal pain, fits, hyperpyrexia and metabolic acidosis. Severe poisoning may cause stroke, MI, rhabdomyolysis, renal failure and DIC. Cardiac arrest can occur in violent agitated patients who need physical restraint. Treat amphetamine poisoning as for MDMA (📖 p.214).

Mephedrone, methedrone, M-cat

Synthetic cathinone compounds, sold as 'plant food' (now illegal in the UK), are snorted or swallowed as stimulants. Toxic effects are similar to amphetamines: agitation, sweating, tachycardia, palpitations, hypertension. Some have nausea, hallucinations, fits, muscle spasms, nausea, peripheral vasoconstriction and myocardial ischaemia. Nasal irritation and epistaxis may occur after snorting these drugs. Treat as for MDMA/amphetamines.

Cocaine

Cocaine base ('crack') is usually smoked. Cocaine salt ('coke') is snorted, eaten or injected. Body packers may be poisoned if packages leak. Toxic effects (due to catecholamines, serotonin and amino acid stimulation and sodium channel blockade) are euphoria, agitation, delirium, ataxia, dilated pupils, sweating, vomiting, fits, tachycardia, arrhythmias and hypertension. Chest pain may be due to myocardial ischaemia or MI (from ↑ catecholamines, ↑ O_2 demand, coronary vasospasm and thrombosis), aortic dissection or pneumothorax. Cerebral haemorrhage, hyperpyrexia, rhabdomyolysis, renal failure, gut ischaemia and serotonin syndrome may occur. Cocaine is a local anaesthetic, so hot air from smoking crack can cause airway burns.

Treat as for MDMA (📖 p.214). Give diazepam for agitation (5–10mg IV, repeated at 5min intervals if needed, sometimes up to 100mg). Treat chest pain with diazepam, GTN, O_2 and aspirin. GTN, calcium blockers and phentolamine may ↓ BP and ↑ coronary blood flow. Avoid β-blockers, which may cause paradoxical hypertension and ↑ coronary vasoconstriction. If ECG suggests acute MI, consider angioplasty or thrombolysis.

Gammahydroxybutyrate (GHB, GBH, 'liquid ecstasy')

GHB is used illegally as a body-building agent and psychedelic drug. It is ingested or injected. Intoxication may cause vomiting, diarrhoea, drowsiness, confusion, ataxia, and agitation. Severe poisoning results in coma, respiratory depression, fits, bradycardia, and hypotension.

Treatment Consider activated charcoal (📖 p.185) if <1hr since ingestion. Observe for at least 4hr and monitor pulse rate, BP and breathing. Provide supportive treatment as needed. Control agitation and convulsions with diazepam. Naloxone may reverse some effects of GHB.

LSD (lysergic acid diethylamide)

Causes visual hallucinations, agitation, excitement, tachycardia and dilated pupils. Hypertension and pyrexia may occur. Paranoid delusions may require sedation. Massive overdose of LSD is rare, but may cause coma, respiratory arrest and coagulation disturbances. Treat supportively.

Serotonin syndrome

Background
The clinical picture of serotonin syndrome is increasingly recognized amongst those taking selective serotonin reuptake inhibitors (SSRIs). The syndrome can occur in patients who have taken therapeutic doses of SSRIs, and this is especially likely if they have recently started on the medication or if it is taken in combination with other drugs which increase production, availability or release of serotonin (eg cocaine, MDMA, amphetamines) or reduce metabolism (eg MAOIs). Serotonin syndrome can also occur after an acute overdose. Numerous drugs have been implicated—in addition to those mentioned above, they include: tricyclic antidepressants, venlafaxine, tramadol, pethidine, buprenorphine, St John's wort, olanzapine and lithium.

Clinical features
Altered mental status
Confusion, hallucinations, and agitation may occur, with drowsiness and reduced conscious level in severe cases.

Neuromuscular features
Rigidity, shivering/tremor, teeth grinding, ataxia, and hyper-reflexia (especially affecting the lower limbs) may occur.

Autonomic effects
These include tachycardia, hypertension (or hypotension), flushing, diarrhoea, vomiting and hyperthermia.

Severe cases can result in fits, rhabdomyolysis, renal failure and coagulopathy.

Differential diagnosis
This includes neuroleptic malignant syndrome, malignant hyperthermia, severe infection (eg encephalitis), other direct effects of drug overdose or withdrawal.

Investigations
Check U&E, glucose, LFTs, CK, FBC, urinalysis, ABG, ECG ± CXR.

Treatment
Provide supportive measures and obtain expert advice (see 📖 p.181). Agitation, hyperthermia, myoclonic jerking and fits may benefit from diazepam therapy. Treat rhabdomyolyis with IV fluids and urine alkalinization.

Cyproheptadine (dose 4–8mg orally) is a serotonin receptor antagonist. Although data are lacking, there is a good theoretical basis for its use in serotonin syndrome.

Body packers

Body packers try to smuggle drugs such as cocaine or heroin by ingesting multiple packages of drugs wrapped in condoms or latex. Packages may also be hidden in the rectum or vagina (individuals who do this are sometimes referred to as '*body pushers*'). Serious or even fatal poisoning may occur if any packages leak and the drugs are absorbed.

Risk factors

Risk factors for complications occurring when an individual has concealed drugs include:

- Vomiting, abdominal pain, abnormal vital signs.
- Clinical evidence of poisoning.
- Home made or improvised packaging.
- Large size and/or large number of packets.
- Delayed passage of the packets (beyond 48hr).
- Fragments of packets in the stool.
- Poisoning in a cotransporter.
- Previous abdominal surgery (↑ risk of obstruction due to adhesions).
- Concomitant drug use (especially constipating agents).

Management

Suspected body packers need careful assessment and observation. Check for rectal and vaginal packages if the patient consents: get senior advice if there is any problem or uncertainty about consent. Try to determine the drug involved, and the number of packages and type of packaging used. Observe for at least 8hr for toxic effects, monitoring heart rate, BP, ECG and SpO_2. Urine toxicology screening may detect heroin or cocaine.

Give activated charcoal (▢ p.185). Consider a naloxone infusion (▢ p.188) for heroin body packers. Abdominal CT or X-ray may show packets of drugs, which can be removed by whole bowel irrigation (▢ p.185). Surgery may be needed for bowel obstruction or to remove leaking packages. Avoid endoscopic removal which may damage packaging and increase drug leakage. Advice is available from Poisons Information Centres (▢ p.181).

Body stuffers

This term is sometimes applied to individuals who swallow drugs immediately prior to being apprehended by the police. The quantity of drugs ingested in this way may be less than by body packers or pushers. However, any packaging is likely to be much less robust than that used by body packers or pushers, thereby increasing the risk of the packages leaking.

Infectious diseases

Incubation periods

Incubation period usually <1 week

Staphylococcal enteritis	1–6 hours
Salmonella enteritis	6–48 hours (usually 12–24 hours)
Bacillary dysentery (*Shigella*)	1–7 days (usually 1–3 days)
Botulism	12–96 hours (usually 18–36 hours)
Cholera	12 hours–6 days (usually 1–3 days)
Dengue	4–7 days
Diphtheria	2–5 days
Gas gangrene	6 hours–4 days
Legionnaires' disease	2–10 days (usually 7 days)
Meningococcaemia	1–7 days (usually 3 days)
Scarlet fever	1–4 days
Yellow fever	3–6 days

Incubation period usually 1–3 weeks

Brucellosis	7–21 days (occasionally some months)
Chickenpox	10–20 days (usually about 14 days)
Lassa fever	6–21 days
Leptospirosis	2–26 days (usually 7–12 days)
Malaria (falciparum)	7–14 days (occasionally longer)
Malaria (vivax, malariae, ovale)	12–40 days (occasionally >1 year)
Measles	10–18 days (rash usually 14–18 days)
Mumps	14–18 days
Pertussis (whooping cough)	5–14 days (usually 7–10 days)
Poliomyelitis	3–21 days (usually 7–10 days)
Rubella	14–21 days
Tetanus	1 day–3 months (usually 4–14 days)
Typhoid	3–60 days (usually 7–14 days)
Typhus	7–14 days

Incubation period usually >3 weeks

Amoebiasis	2 weeks–many months
Hepatitis A	2–6 weeks (usually 4 weeks)
Hepatitis B, hepatitis C	6 weeks–6 months
HIV	2 weeks–3 months (anti-HIV appears)
Infectious mononucleosis	4–7 weeks
Rabies	4 days–2 years (usually 3–12 weeks)
Syphilis	10 days–10 weeks (usually 3 weeks)

Duration of infectivity of infectious diseases

Chickenpox	3 days before rash until last vesicle crusts
Hepatitis A	2 weeks before until 1 week after jaundice starts
Measles	4 days before rash until 5 days after rash appears
Mumps	3 days before to 1 week after salivary swelling
Pertussis	3 days before to 3 weeks after start of symptoms (5 days if on appropriate antibiotic)
Rubella	1 week before to 1 week after onset of rash
Scarlet fever	10–21 days from onset of rash (1 day if on penicillin)

Notifiable infectious diseases

In Britain certain infectious diseases are 'notifiable'. A doctor who knows or suspects that a patient has one of these diseases is obliged to notify the local Health Protection department. Use the special notification form if available. Telephone the consultant in Communicable Disease Control if investigation or control of an outbreak may be needed.

HIV and AIDS are not notifiable diseases, but may be reported in strict confidence in the same way.

Notifiable infectious diseases in Britain (ND)

Anthrax
Botulism
Brucellosis
Cholera
Diphtheria
Encephalitis (acute)*
Erysipelas**
Food poisoning*
Haemolytic uraemic syndrome (HUS)
Haemophilus influenzae type b (Hib)**
Infectious bloody diarrhoea (*E. coli* O157 infection**)
Infectious hepatitis (acute)*
Invasive group A streptococcal disease and scarlet fever*
Legionnaires' disease*
Leprosy*
Malaria*
Measles
Meningitis (acute)*
Meningococcal septicaemia*/meningococcal disease**
Mumps
Necrotizing fasciitis**
Paratyphoid
Pertussis (whooping cough)
Plague
Poliomyelitis
Rabies
Rubella
Severe acute respiratory syndrome (SARS)
Smallpox
Tetanus
Tuberculosis
Tularaemia**
Typhoid
Typhus*
Viral haemorrhagic fever (VHF)
West Nile fever**
Yellow fever

* Notifiable only in England and Wales.
** Notifiable only in Scotland.

Childhood infectious diseases

Children at risk

Unimmunized children are at risk of infections which would be prevented by the standard immunization schedule. Always ask about vaccination status in any febrile, unwell child. The common infectious diseases of childhood can be very serious in children with *immune deficiency* or those on *immunosuppressant drugs*. Refer such children for specialist advice if they develop an infectious disease or have been in contact with one. Children with cystic fibrosis can become very ill with measles, whooping cough or chickenpox—refer these also. Neonates rarely develop the common exanthems of childhood, but require referral if these occur. Chickenpox can be particularly serious in this age group.

Measles[ND]

A virus infection spread by airborne droplets.

Incubation period =10–18 days. Infectious from just before the onset of symptoms until 5 days after the rash appears.

Initial features (lasting ≈3 days) are fever, malaise, coryza, conjunctivitis and cough. Koplik's spots (small white spots like grains of salt) appear inside the cheeks. 1–2 days later a red maculopapular rash starts behind the ears, and spreads to the face and down the body.

Treatment is symptomatic unless there are complications (eg otitis media or bacterial pneumonia). Febrile convulsions may occur. Encephalitis is rare, but can be fatal. Hospital admission is rarely needed unless the child is very ill or has pre-existing disease. In the tropics many malnourished children die from measles, but in the UK the mortality is very low.

Mumps[ND]

Mumps is a virus infection spread by saliva and respiratory droplets. Infectivity is greatest at the onset of symptoms, but many sub-clinical cases also spread infection.

Incubation period = 14–18 days.

Typical features are fever with pain and swelling in one or both parotid glands. Aseptic meningitis may occur. Orchitis affects 10–15% of post-pubertal males, but rarely causes sterility. The pain of orchitis may be relieved by analgesia and a short course of steroids. Orchitis is uncommon before puberty, so consider torsion of the testis if a child presents with testicular pain and swelling (□ p.700).

Rubella (German measles)[ND]

Rubella is usually a mild disease, but infection during pregnancy may cause severe congenital disorders, particularly eye defects, heart defects and deafness. Guidance on the management of, and exposure to, rubella in pregnancy is available from the Health Protection Agency based in London (www.hpa.org.uk/infections). The virus is spread mainly by the airborne route, with an incubation period of 2–3 weeks and infectivity from 1 week before symptoms until 1 week after the rash appears. A macular rash occurs on the face and trunk, with mild fever, occipital lymphadenopathy and sometimes transient arthralgia. Rare complications are encephalitis and thrombocytopenia.

Treatment is generally symptomatic. The clinical diagnosis of rubella is unreliable: similar rashes may occur with enterovirus and parvovirus infections. If there is concern about rubella infection in pregnancy take blood for viral antibody levels and arrange urgent follow-up by the GP or obstetrician.

Whooping cough

see p.684.

Meningitis

Causative organisms

Meningitis may be *bacterial, viral,* or occasionally *fungal.* Bacterial causes of meningitis include meningococci, pneumococci, *Haemophilus influenzae, Listeria,* and tuberculosis (TB). Other bacteria may also cause meningitis in neonates, the elderly, and immunosuppressed patients.

Clinical features of bacterial meningitis

Some patients with meningitis have the classic features of headache, neck stiffness, photophobia, fever and drowsiness. However, the clinical diagnosis of meningitis may be very difficult in early cases. Neonates may present with anorexia, apnoea, or fits. Meningitis may start as a 'flu-like' illness, especially in the immunosuppressed or elderly. Consider meningitis in any febrile patient with headache, neurological signs, neck stiffness, or ↓ conscious level.

Meningococcal meningitis^ND is caused by *Neisseria meningitidis.* It can result in septicaemia, coma, and death within a few hours of the first symptoms. Skin rashes occur in 50% of patients, often starting as a maculopapular rash before the characteristic petechial rash develops. There may be DIC and adrenal haemorrhage (Waterhouse–Friderichsen). Meningococcal septicaemia (🕮 p.666) may occur without meningitis.

Management

Resuscitate if necessary, give oxygen and obtain venous access.

Start antibiotics *immediately* (without waiting for investigations) if the patient is shocked or deteriorating or there is any suspicion of meningococcal infection (especially a petechial or purpuric rash): give IV ceftriaxone or cefotaxime (adult 2g; child 80mg/kg). Chloramphenicol is an alternative if there is a history of anaphylaxis to cephalosporins (see *BNF*). In adults >55 years add ampicillin 2g qds to cover *Listeria.* Give vancomycin ± rifampicin if penicillin-resistant pneumococcal infection is suspected. Give IV dexamethasone (0.15mg/kg, max 10mg, qds for 4 days) starting with or just before the first dose of antibiotics, especially if pneumococcal meningitis is suspected.

Initial investigations are FBC, U&E, glucose, clotting screen, ABG, CRP, blood cultures, EDTA sample for PCR, and clotted blood for serology. LP is needed if meningitis is suspected, unless there is a coagulopathy or ↑ ICP: do CT scan if there is suspicion of ↑ ICP (confusion/coma, hypertension, bradycardia or papilloedema) or focal neurological signs.

Provide supportive treatment including:
• IV fluids.
• Pressure area care.
• Monitor conscious level, T°, BP, ECG, SpO₂, and fluid balance.

Get expert help promptly and organize ICU care.

For the latest advice and algorithms see www.meningitis.org and www.nice.org.uk/guidance/CG102/quickrefguide

For meningitis and LP in children see 🕮 p.666.

Prophylaxis of meningococcal infection

While intubating a patient with suspected meningococcal infection wear a suitable mask (eg FFP3) and a face shield to reduce the risk of infection.

Meningococcal infection is spread by droplets from the nose of an infected carrier, who may be well. Notify the consultant in Communicable Disease Control (📖 p.221) immediately about any suspected meningococcal infection and obtain advice about antibiotic prophylaxis. Prophylactic antibiotics (rifampicin, ciprofloxacin or ceftriaxone) are needed for the patient's family and close contacts. Hospital and ambulance staff do not need prophylaxis unless they have given mouth to mouth ventilation or intubated the patient without using protective equipment.

Rifampicin is given 12 hourly for 2 days (5mg/kg for child aged <1 year; 10mg/kg at 1–12 years; 600mg at age >12 years. It makes the urine orange or brown, discolours soft contact lenses, and ↓ effectiveness of OCP for ≈4 weeks (see *BNF*)—give appropriate warnings and record this in the notes.

Ciprofloxacin is given as a single oral dose of 500mg (adults), 250mg (child 5–12 years) or 125mg (child 2–5 years), although it is not licensed for chemoprophylaxis of meningitis.

Ceftriaxone is given as a single IM dose of 250mg (adults and children >12 years) or 125mg (children <12 years).

Tell contacts of meningococcal patients to report to a doctor at once if they develop symptoms.

TB meningitis

Often gradual onset, with malaise, anorexia, vomiting, headache and eventually signs of meningitis. Cranial nerve palsies, spastic paraplegia and coma can occur. Meningitis may be part of miliary TB (📖 p.232), which may be apparent on chest X-ray. Ophthalmoscopy may show choroidal tubercles and papilloedema, which is found more commonly than in other forms of meningitis. Refer for specialist investigation and treatment.

Viral meningitis

Viral causes of meningitis include coxsackie, mumps, and echoviruses. Viral meningitis produces similar clinical features to bacterial infection, but the illness is often less severe. The initial management is the same as for suspected bacterial meningitis. Refer for admission and investigation.

Fungal meningitis

Fungal meningitis is usually part of disseminated infection in immuno-suppressed patients, (eg those with AIDS (📖 p.242), lymphoma, or on steroid therapy). *Cryptococcus neoformans* is the commonest organism. Symptoms usually develop slowly, as with TB meningitis. There may be papilloedema and focal neurological signs. Admit for specialist investigation and treatment.

Gastroenteritis/food poisoning[ND]: 1

Diarrhoea is the usual presenting symptom of gastroenteritis, but it may also occur in many other conditions as diverse as otitis media, appendicitis and ulcerative colitis. Antibiotics often cause diarrhoea. Constipation may present as diarrhoea if there is overflow around an obstructing stool. A rectal tumour may present similarly.

A baby's parents may seek advice about diarrhoea when in fact the stools are normal. Breast-fed babies almost always have loose stools, which may be yellow or green and very frequent, often after every feed. However, gastroenteritis is very rare in fully breast-fed babies. In children aged >6 months, normal stool frequency ranges from 1 stool on alternate days to 3 stools daily.

Diarrhoea and vomiting may be caused by many types of bacteria and viruses, and also by some toxins and poisons. Many episodes of gastroenteritis result from contaminated food, usually meat, milk or egg products, which have been cooked inadequately or left in warm conditions. The specific cause is often not identified. Some infections are spread by faecal contamination of water (eg cryptosporidiosis from sheep faeces). *Rotavirus* infection (common in children) may be transmitted by the respiratory route. Severe illness with bloody diarrhoea, haemolysis and renal failure may result from infection with verocytotoxin producing *E. coli* (VTEC O157).

Stool microscopy and culture are unnecessary in most cases of gastro-enteritis, but obtain them if the patient has been abroad, is severely ill, has prolonged symptoms, comes from an institution or works as a food-handler.

Food poisoning is a notifiable disease (□ p.221). Immediate notification by telephone is mandatory if an outbreak is suspected. The food eaten, symptoms and incubation period may suggest the organism or toxin involved (see Table 5.1). Carbon monoxide poisoning (□ p.208) may cause malaise and vomiting in several members of a family and be misdiagnosed as food poisoning.

History

Record the duration of symptoms and the frequency and description of stools and vomit. Document other symptoms (eg abdominal pain, fever), food and fluid ingested and drugs taken. Enquire about affected contacts, foreign travel and occupation (especially relevant if a food-handler).

Examination

Look for abdominal tenderness, fever and other signs of infection. Record the patient's weight and compare this with any previous records. Assess the *degree of dehydration*—this is traditionally classified as mild (<5%), moderate (5–10%), or severe (>10%), as outlined opposite.

Clinical evidence of mild dehydration (<5%)
- Thirst.
- ↓ urinary output (in a baby <4 wet nappies in 24hr).
- Dry mouth.

Clinical evidence of moderate dehydration (5–10%)
- Sunken fontanelle in infants.
- Sunken eyes.
- Tachypnoea due to metabolic acidosis.
- Tachycardia.

Clinical evidence of severe dehydration (>10%)
- ↓ skin turgor on pinching the skin.
- Drowsiness/irritability.

Table 5.1 Food poisoning characteristics

Cause	Incubation	Food	Symptoms*
Staph. aureus	1–6 hours	Meat, milk	D, V, P, shock
Bacillus cereus	1–16 hours	Rice	D, V, P
Salmonella	6–48 hours	Meat, eggs	D, V, P
Escherichia coli	1–2 days	Any food	D, V, P
E. coli VTEC 0157	1–2 days	Meat, milk	D, V, P
Campylobacter	1–3 days	Meat, milk	Fever, P, D
Shigella	1–3 days	Any food	Bloody D, V, fever
Vibrio parahaem	2–3 days	Seafood	Watery D
Cholera	12hr–6 days	Water, seafood	D (watery), shock
Rotavirus	1–7 days		D, V, fever, cough
Botulism	12–96 hours	Preserved food	V, paralysis
Histamine fish poisoning (scombrotoxin)	<1 hour	Fish	Flushing, headache, D, V, P (📖 p.229)
Ciguatera fish poisoning	1–6 hours (rarely 30 hours)	Fish from tropical coral reef	D, V, P, paraesthesiae, muscle weakness (📖 p.229)
Paralytic shellfish poisoning	30 min– 10 hours	Shellfish	Dizziness, paraesthesiae, weakness, respiratory failure (📖 p.229)
Chemicals	<2 hours	Food, water	Various
Mushrooms	<24 hours	Mushrooms	D, V, P, hallucinations (📖 p.212)

*D = diarrhoea, V = vomiting, P = abdominal pain.

Gastroenteritis/food poisoning[ND]: 2

Treatment

Most cases are self-limiting, but careful attention is needed to ensure adequate fluid replacement and also to prevent cross-infection (📖 p.32).

Hospital treatment is needed if the patient looks seriously ill, dehydration is >5%, there is a high fever or the family are unlikely to cope with the patient at home. Babies aged <3 months may be difficult to assess and can deteriorate rapidly—refer for admission. Severely dehydrated (>10%) children need immediate IV fluids, initially 0.9% saline (10–20mL/kg over 5min, repeated as necessary).

Oral rehydration therapy (ORT) is effective in most patients with gastroenteritis (<5% dehydration). Standard ORT products (eg Dioralyte®) contain glucose, sodium, potassium, chloride and citrate (details in *BNF*). Glucose is important to enhance absorption of sodium and water.

Usual dose of ORT: infant 1–1½ times usual feed volume.
child 200mL after each loose stool.
adults 200–400mL after each loose stool.

Extra ORT can be given if the patient is still thirsty. Frequent small sips are usually tolerated better than a large drink. Check that the patient (or parent/carer) can understand the instructions supplied with the ORT sachets or effervescent tablets and can measure the necessary amounts of clean water.

Recommence normal feeds and diet after 24hr (or earlier if diarrhoea has settled or the patient is hungry). Give further ORT if the diarrhoea continues. A child with acute diarrhoea requires daily review (usually by the GP), but should be seen earlier if he becomes more ill (especially if drowsy or pyrexial), or if vomiting and/or diarrhoea worsens. Home-made salt and sugar mixtures may be dangerously inaccurate for ORT, but if nothing else is available, one could use salt 2.5mL (half a 5mL spoonful) and sugar 20mL (4 × 5mL spoonfuls) in 1 pint (500mL) of cooled boiled water.

Drugs other than ORT are rarely needed in gastroenteritis. In adults an anti-emetic (prochlorperazine 12.5mg IM or 3mg buccal) may be helpful, but in children prochlorperazine often causes troublesome side effects. However, oral ondansetron (0.1–0.15mg/kg, max 8mg) reduces vomiting and the need for IV fluids and admission. Prolonged vomiting requires investigation and hospital admission.

Anti-diarrhoeal drugs (eg kaolin, codeine phosphate, loperamide) are contraindicated in children and rarely needed in adults: they may aggravate nausea and vomiting and occasionally cause ileus.

Antibiotics are only needed in special circumstances. Most episodes of gastroenteritis are brief and many are caused by viruses and not helped by antibiotics. Patients with amoebiasis, giardiasis, *Campylobacter* or *Shigella* infections may need antibiotics: refer to an Infectious Diseases unit for treatment and follow-up. Antibiotics are occasionally useful in traveller's diarrhoea before a long journey or an important meeting: trimethoprim (200mg bd PO for 5 days) or ciprofloxacin (500mg bd PO for 2 days: see the *BNF* or data sheet about side effects and warnings).

Fish poisoning

Histamine fish poisoning

Also known as scombroid fish poisoning or scombrotoxin poisoning, this is caused by ingesting toxins in fish such as tuna, mackerel, and other dark-meat fish, which have been stored improperly. If the fish is not cooled rapidly after it is caught, an enzyme in bacteria converts histidine into histamine and other toxins, which are heat-stable and so are unaffected by cooking. The patient may notice that the fish tastes metallic, bitter, or peppery and the flesh looks honeycombed. Symptoms start within a few minutes to 2 hours, with flushing of the face and upper body, headache, nausea, vomiting, abdominal pain, diarrhoea, dizziness and palpitations. Urticaria and bronchospasm are less common. The symptoms usually settle within 6 hours without treatment, but resolve more quickly with antihistamines (eg chlorphenamine 10mg IV in adults, 250 micrograms/kg in children). In severe cases cimetidine and, rarely, adrenaline might be needed, with oxygen, IV fluids and bronchodilators.

The patient should be told that histamine fish poisoning is caused by improper fish handling and storage. It is not an allergic reaction and so the patient would not have to avoid eating fish in future.

Ciguatera fish poisoning

This is caused by a neurotoxin called ciguatoxin which is produced by a dinoflagellate (a unicellular plankton) associated with coral reefs. Fish imported from the tropics may cause ciguatera poisoning in the UK and elsewhere. Symptoms usually start 1–6 hours after ingestion with nausea, vomiting, watery diarrhoea and abdominal pain, followed by neurological symptoms, including paraesthesiae of the lips, tongue and feet, ataxia and muscle weakness. A classic feature is paradoxical temperature reversal (cold objects feel hot and hot objects feel cold). Alcohol makes these symptoms worse. Bradycardia and hypotension may occur. Treatment is symptomatic and supportive. Gastro-intestinal symptoms usually settle within 1 day, but paraesthesiae may persist for weeks or months.

Paralytic shellfish poisoning

This can be caused by eating molluscs such as mussels, clams, cockles and scallops which concentrate a neurotoxin called saxitoxin produced by dinoflagellate plankton. This plankton proliferates when sea temperatures rise in summer and may make the sea look red ('red tide'). Symptoms start 30 minutes to 10 hours after ingestion, with dizziness, ataxia, paraesthesiae and muscle weakness, which may progress to respiratory failure. Treatment is supportive, with assisted ventilation if necessary. Complete recovery is usual within 24 hours.

Infestations

Worms

The most common helminthic infection seen in the UK is the thread-worm *Enterobius vermicularis*. This causes anal itching, especially at night. Sometimes intact worms (length 5–13mm, diameter 0.1–0.5mm) are seen in the faeces. Unwashed fingers transmit ova from the perianal skin to the mouth. Personal hygiene is important in treatment and in prevention of reinfection (hand-washing and nail-scrubbing before each meal and after every visit to the toilet). A bath immediately after getting up removes ova laid overnight. All members of the family require treatment with mebendazole or piperazine (see *BNF*).

Other helminthic infections include roundworms, hookworms and tapeworms. Obtain advice from departments of Infectious Diseases or Tropical Medicine (see 📖 p.246).

Lice

Humans may be infected by the body louse (*Pediculosis humanis corporis*), head louse (*Pediculosis humanis capitis*), or the 'crab'/pubic louse (*Phthirus pubis*).

Head lice are common in school children. Infection is not related to lack of hygiene or the length of hair. Adult lice are 3–4mm long, vary in colour from white to grey-black and attach themselves firmly to the scalp at the base of hairs. The egg cases ('nits') are white and 1–2mm in diameter, glued firmly to the base of hairs and moving outwards as the hair grows. Head lice cause intense itching, which may suggest the diagnosis. Secondary infection may result in impetigo. Head lice are usually treated with malathion, phenothrin or simeticone, repeated after 7 days (see *BNF*). Drug-resistant lice occur in some areas. Wet combing to remove head lice takes time and is possibly less effective than drug treatment.

Infection by body lice is related to poor hygiene and infrequent washing of clothes. Body lice are found in the seams of clothing, and sometimes in body hair. Treatment is with malathion. Clothes can be disinfected by boiling or by machine laundering and ironing. Body lice may transmit rickettsial diseases (louse-borne typhus) and other infections.

Crab lice are usually transmitted sexually. They cause itching in pubic hair areas. Occasionally, children become infested on eyelashes or eyebrows. Treat with permethrin or malathion (see *BNF*). Sexual partners or other family members may also need treatment. There may be other co-existing sexually transmitted diseases.

Fleas

There are many different types of flea. They cause itchy bites with linear erythematous papules. Treat with calamine lotion and an oral antihista-mine (eg chlorphenamine) if itching is severe. A long-acting insecticide is needed in the house, especially in cracks in the floor and under furniture. All household cats and dogs must be treated for fleas. Fleas can transmit many infections, including plague, typhus and Q fever.

Scabies

Scabies is caused by infestation with a mite, *Sarcoptes scabiei*, which is about 0.2–0.4mm long and burrows into the skin. It is most often found in the finger webs and on the flexor aspect of the wrists. After 4–6 weeks, intense itching occurs, especially at night or after a hot shower. Burrows (3–15mm long) may be apparent, especially on palpation of affected skin. Genital lesions are reddish and nodular. Secondary bacterial infection may occur. Scabies can be confirmed by microscopy of scrapings from suspected lesions. Treat with permethrin or malathion (see *BNF*). Treat all members of the household at once. Calamine lotion and an oral antihistamine may help to relieve itching.

Ticks

Ticks may be acquired from domestic animals or while walking through undergrowth or exploring caves. Ticks may be removed with tweezers or curved forceps. They can carry several diseases, including Lyme disease (see below), tick-borne encephalitis, typhus, and Rocky Mountain spotted fever. Tick paralysis occurs in North America and Australia, with progressive paralysis which is often misdiagnosed as poliomyelitis. However, the risk of infection from tick bites is low in most areas, and so routine prophylaxis with antibiotics is not recommended.

Lyme disease (Lyme borreliosis) is caused by a tick-borne spirochaete, *Borrelia burgdorferi*, and occurs in the UK, most of Europe, the USA, and parts of Asia and Australia. Most cases occur in the summer and early autumn, and are transmitted by ticks from deer or sheep. The initial tick bite may go unnoticed. Clinical illness develops after about 7–14 days (range 2–30 days) with an expanding red area around the site of the bite (erythema migrans). The second clinical stage of the disease occurs some weeks or months later, with fever, muscle and joint pains, and sometimes facial palsy or other cranial nerve or peripheral nerve palsies. Meningitis, encephalitis and arthritis may develop. Myocarditis and heart block occur occasionally. Refer to an Infectious Diseases specialist for confirmation and treatment if Lyme disease is suspected.

Tuberculosis[ND]

The Mycobacterium genus is characterized by acid-fast staining (ie it is not decolourized by acid after staining with hot carbol fuchsin).

Infection with *Mycobacterium tuberculosis* is common throughout the world. There is growing concern about the re-emergence of TB in the UK and other countries. Many cases of TB occur in the lower socio-economic groups, ethnic minorities and the immunocompromised.

The *incidence* of TB ↑ with age.

Presentation

TB can involve almost any organ of the body.

Primary infection is usually pulmonary and often asymptomatic.

Post-primary infection may present with malaise, weight loss and night sweats, with localized symptoms depending on the organs involved.

Pulmonary TB may result in cough, haemoptysis, pneumonia and pleural effusion (□ p.103).

Miliary TB, with blood-borne infection of many organs, develops over 1–2 weeks with fever, weight loss, malaise and breathlessness: CXR may show multiple small opacities throughout the lung fields, and choroidal tubercles may be visible in the optic fundi.

TB meningitis causes headaches and vomiting, sometimes with neck stiffness, cranial nerve palsies and papilloedema (see □ p.224).

Tuberculous osteomyelitis usually affects the spine, with collapse of adjacent vertebrae and a paravertebral abscess.

Patients may present with swollen lymph nodes from *tuberculous lymphadenitis* or with sinuses or cold abscesses from bone or soft tissue infection: microscopy of the discharge will show acid-fast bacilli.

Treatment

Refer patients with suspected TB to an appropriate specialist for assessment and treatment. Isolation is required for patients with untreated pulmonary TB. Notify the local Health Protection department (□ p.221).

AnthraxND

Anthrax is caused by the bacterium *Bacillus anthracis* which affects cows and other herbivorous animals, especially in warm climates. The bacterium forms spores, which may remain infective for years. Most human cases of anthrax are *cutaneous anthrax* caused by direct skin contact with infected tissues and occur in people working with animal products such as imported hides. Less common, but more serious, are *inhalation anthrax* caused by inhalation of anthrax spores, and *intestinal anthrax* which is a rare form of food poisoning caused by under-cooked infected meat. Anthrax spores released deliberately in terrorist attacks could cause cutaneous anthrax or inhalation anthrax, which is often fatal.

Cutaneous anthrax starts 2–7 days after infection, with a red papule which develops into an ulcer with a black leathery eschar, surrounded by non-pitting oedema. The lesion is painless but may itch. Small satellite lesions may surround the original lesion. Malaise and fever may occur, with septicaemia in 10–20% of cases. Penicillin ↓ risk of complications from cutaneous anthrax. Clinical diagnosis is confirmed by microscopy and culture of the pustule.

Inhalation anthrax starts within 48 hours of exposure (rarely up to 6 weeks) with a flu-like illness, followed by breathlessness, cyanosis, stridor and sweating, often with subcutaneous oedema of the chest and neck. CXR and CT show mediastinal widening from lymphadenopathy and pleural effusions. Shock, septicaemia and meningitis are common and usually fatal, despite antibiotics and intensive treatment.

Airborne transmission of anthrax from one person to another does not occur, but cutaneous anthrax could result from direct contact with anthrax lesions. Obtain expert advice immediately if anthrax is suspected. It is a notifiable disease (📖 p.221). Post-exposure antibiotics can prevent anthrax if started early enough. Press enquiries must be anticipated after any case of anthrax, especially if anthrax has been released deliberately. Further information is available from: www.hpa.org.uk/infections.

Anthrax in drug users After a serious anthrax outbreak in heroin users in Scotland in 2010, Health Protection Scotland (www.hps.scot.nhs.uk) advised doctors to suspect anthrax in a drug user presenting with any of the following:
• Severe soft tissue infection and/or signs of severe sepsis/meningitis.
• Clinical features of inhalational anthrax.
• Respiratory symptoms + features of meningitis or intracranial bleeding.
• GI symptoms (eg pain, bleeding, nausea, vomiting, diarrhoea, ascites).

Approach Get expert help early to advise on management (microbiology, hospital infection control team, Public Health, ICU, surgeons). Start IV antibiotics according to advice (eg combination of ciprofloxacin, clindamycin + penicillin, or if there is soft tissue infection: ciprofloxacin, clindamycin, penicillin, flucloxacillin + metronidazole). Experts will advise on whether to use anthrax immune globulin.

Streptococcal infections

Streptococcus pyogenes and other streptococci may reside in the pharynx without symptoms, but can cause sore throats (📖 p.554), soft tissue infections (📖 pp.413 and 528), scarlet fever, and occasionally endocarditis and septicaemia. Later, non-suppurative sequelae of streptococcal infections include erythema nodosum, rheumatic fever (📖 p.496) and glomerulonephritis. Streptococci and Staphylococci may cause necrotizing fasciitis, impetigo, and toxic shock.

Scarlet fever[ND]

Some streptococcal infections are associated with scarlet fever. A diffuse blanching scarlet rash often involves the neck, chest, axillae and groin. Occlusion of sweat glands makes the skin feel rough, like sandpaper. During the first 1–2 days of illness there is a 'white strawberry tongue', with red papillae protruding through white furry material. After a few days the white fur separates, leaving a shiny 'raspberry tongue'. 10–14 days after onset of the rash, skin may peel from palms and soles. Treat with penicillin or erythromycin for 14 days. Complete recovery is usual.

Infective endocarditis

Endocarditis may develop on previously normal heart valves, as well as on diseased or prosthetic valves. The commonest organism is *Strep. viridans*, but many others have been implicated. Many acute cases present with heart failure and involve *Staphylococcus aureus*. Injecting drug users are liable to staphylococcal infection of the tricuspid valve, with fever and pneumonia from septic PE.
Clinical features Fever and changing murmurs suggest endocarditis. Emboli may cause strokes. Ask about weight loss, malaise, night sweats. Look for clubbing, splinter haemorrhages, splenomegaly, anaemia, microscopic haematuria.
Treatment On suspicion of endocarditis, admit immediately for investigation (blood cultures, echocardiography) and treatment.

Cellulitis and erysipelas

Treat these bacterial skin infections as described in 📖 p.528.

Necrotizing fasciitis

This is a rare and severe bacterial infection of soft tissues. It can occur with or without obvious trauma and may follow illicit IM heroin injection ('muscle popping'). *Strep. pyogenes* is often involved, sometimes with *Staph. aureus* or other bacteria. Often there are both aerobic and anaerobic organisms. Infection involves fascia and subcutaneous tissues, with gas formation and development of gangrene. Infection may spread to adjacent muscles, causing myonecrosis or pyogenic myositis. Similar infections may involve the abdomen and groin (Fournier's gangrene).
Initial symptoms and signs may be vague, with very severe pain, but little to find on examination: the affected area may be tender, sometimes with slight erythema and swelling. The patient is usually pyrexial. Infection can spread rapidly and cause marked soft tissue swelling with discolouration, bruising, haemorrhagic blisters, or overlying skin necrosis. Toxic shock may develop and the mortality rate is high. X-rays may show gas in the soft tissues but may be normal.
Treatment involves resuscitation with IV fluids and antibiotics (penicillin and clindamycin), urgent surgery to debride the affected area and excise necrotic tissues, and intensive care.

Staphylococcal infections

Staphylococcus aureus is involved in many infections of wounds, soft tissues (📖 p.413), joints and bones (📖 p.494 and 705). Staphylococci may also cause impetigo, scalded skin syndrome, food poisoning, toxic shock syndrome, endocarditis, pneumonia, septicaemia and meningitis.

Impetigo

A highly infectious superficial skin infection caused by staphylococci or streptococci. It may involve normal skin or complicate a pre-existing condition, such as eczema or scabies. Lesions often start around the mouth and nose, spreading rapidly on the face and to other parts of the body. Irregular golden-yellow crusted lesions occur, particularly in strep-tococcal infections. Staphylococci may cause bullous impetigo, with bullae containing pus which rupture and dry to form crusts. Treat with topical fusidic acid or mupirocin (usually for 7 days, max. 10 days) and give oral flucloxacillin or erythromycin if lesions are widespread or there is cellulitis or pyrexia.

Scalded skin syndrome

Staph. aureus may produce an exotoxin causing separation of the outer layers of the epidermis, large sections of which slide off with minimal pressure, leaving large raw areas resembling a severe scald. Drug allergies can cause similar lesions. Most cases of scalded skin syndrome (toxic epidermal necrolysis, Lyell's syndrome) occur in children. Admit for nursing and medical care.

Toxic shock syndrome

This is caused by exotoxins from *Staph. aureus* or (less commonly) *Strep. pyogenes*. Some cases during menstruation are related to tampons, other cases occur after surgical operations, burns, other trauma, or local infections. There is high fever, a generalized erythematous rash, confusion, diarrhoea, muscle pains, hypotension, and renal failure. Subsequently, scales of skin separate from hands and feet. Death may occur from multiple organ failure. Treat for septic shock with IV fluids and anti-staphylococcal antibiotics. Remove tampons and send for culture. Refer to ICU. Involve a surgeon if an associated abscess requires drainage.

Staphylococcal septicaemia

Occurs particularly in debilitated or immune-compromised patients and in injecting drug users. There may be endocarditis with metastatic infection of lungs, bone or soft tissues and gangrene due to emboli or arterial thrombosis. Signs of meningitis and DIC may suggest meningo-coccal septicaemia (📖 p.224) and the rash may be similar.

Meticillin resistant *Staphylococcus aureus* (MRSA)

MRSA causes particular concern because of antibiotic resistance and is carried by many asymptomatic people (patients and staff). Transmission is minimized by hand washing (📖 p.32) and other infection control measures. An information leaflet about MRSA for patients is available at www.hpa.org.uk/infections/topics_az/staphylo/mrsa_leaflet.htm

Tetanus[ND]

An acute and often fatal disease, common in much of Asia, Africa, and South America, especially in neonates. Now rare in developed countries: 30–40 cases/year in UK, many involving the elderly. Injecting drug users (eg those 'skin popping') are also at particular risk. Spores of the Gram +ve organism *Clostridium tetani* (common in soil and animal faeces) contaminate a wound, which may be trivial. The spores germinate in anaerobic conditions, producing tetanospasmin, an exotoxin which blocks inhibitory neurones in the CNS and causes muscle spasm and rigidity.

Incubation period is usually 4–14 days, but may be 1 day to 3 months. In 20% of cases there is no known wound. Tetanus occasionally occurs after surgery or IM injections.

Clinical features

Stiffness of masseter muscles causes difficulty in opening the mouth (trismus, lockjaw). Muscle stiffness may spread to all facial and skeletal muscles and muscles of swallowing. Characteristically, the eyes are partly closed, the lips pursed and stretched (risus sardonicus). Spasm of chest muscles may restrict breathing. There may be abdominal rigidity, stiffness of limbs and forced extension of the back (opisthotonus). In severe cases, prolonged muscle spasms affect breathing and swallowing. Pyrexia is common. Autonomic disturbances cause profuse sweating, tachycardia and hypertension, alternating with bradycardia and hypotension. Cardiac arrhythmias and arrest may occur.

Differential diagnoses

Dystonic reaction to metoclopramide or phenothiazines, strychnine poisoning, quinsy, dental abscess, meningitis, rabies. Procyclidine relieves muscle spasms from drug-induced dystonia, but will not affect tetanus; diazepam may relieve dystonia or tetanic spasms.

Management

Obtain senior medical and anaesthetic help. Monitor breathing, ECG and BP. Refer to ICU. Control spasms with diazepam. Paralyse and ventilate if breathing becomes inadequate. Clean and debride wounds. Give penicillin and metronidazole and human tetanus immune globulin.

Prognosis

Depends on severity of disease and quality of care. Short incubation (<4 days) and rapid progression suggest severe disease with a high mortality. With expert intensive care, the mortality in adults is <10%, but neonatal tetanus is often fatal.

Immunization

Tetanus is eminently preventable by immunization and by proper care of wounds (📖 p.406, 📖 p.410).

Gas gangrene

This is a rapidly spreading infection of muscle caused by toxin-producing Clostridial bacteria (anaerobic Gram +ve bacilli), usually *C. perfringens*. It is fatal if untreated. It may involve wounds of the buttocks, amputations for vascular disease or severe muscle injuries (eg gunshot wounds). Occasionally gas gangrene of the perineum occurs without trauma.

Incubation period is usually <4 days (sometimes a few hours). Sudden severe pain occurs at the wound site. Generalized toxicity develops, with tachycardia, sweating and fever. Swelling and skin discolouration occur around the wound, with a serous ooze, marked tenderness and sometimes haemorrhagic vesicles and crepitus. Shock and renal failure develop, with death often within 2 days of the first symptoms.

Diagnosis depends on clinical features. Severe pain necessitates wound inspection (remove or window any plaster of paris (POP)). Obtain immediate senior surgical advice if gas gangrene is suspected. The wound discharge may contain Gram +ve bacilli. X-rays may show soft tissue gas, but its absence does not exclude gas gangrene.

Treatment IV antibiotics (penicillin and clindamycin), immediate surgical removal of all infected tissue, and intensive care. Hyperbaric O_2 and gas gangrene antitoxin are rarely available and of no proven benefit.

BotulismND

The exotoxin of *Clostridium botulinum* paralyses autonomic and motor nerves by blocking acetylcholine release at neuromuscular junctions and nerve synapses. Infection occurs from eating tinned or preserved food contaminated with *C. botulinum* spores: cases have involved sausage, tinned salmon, hazelnut yoghurt and other foods. Rarely, *C. botulinum* infects wounds or colonizes the gut. Injecting drug users may develop botulism after IM or SC injections of contaminated drugs.

Incubation period is 12–72hr. Initial symptoms may be GI (nausea, vomiting, abdominal discomfort, dryness of the mouth) or neurological (dizziness, blurred vision, diplopia). Later problems include dysarthria, dysphagia, muscle weakness or paralysis, constipation and urinary retention, respiratory failure, and sudden death. Susceptibility varies: some people who eat contaminated food develop no symptoms or suffer only mild fatigue.

Clinical signs result from involvement of autonomic and motor nerves: dry mouth, cranial nerve palsies (ptosis, squint, fixed pupils, weakness of tongue), limb weakness with flacid muscles. Consciousness and sensation are preserved. Hypotension and ileus may occur. Fever is unusual.

Differential diagnoses are Guillain–Barré syndrome, myasthenia, brainstem stroke, diphtheria, poisoning (anticholinergics or organophosphates), paralytic rabies. Botulism may be misdiagnosed as staphylococcal food poisoning, paralytic shellfish poisoning, CO or mushroom poisoning.

Management Get senior help. Assess breathing, ventilate if necessary and admit to ICU. Botulinum antitoxin reduces mortality and morbidity: see *BNF* and TOXBASE (📖 p.181). Inform Public Health: others who have eaten contaminated food may need urgent treatment. Anticipate media enquiries and the arrival of worried people with tins of suspicious food.

Sexually transmitted diseases

The commonest sexually transmitted disease (STD) is non-specific genital infection. Other common diseases include chlamydia, gonorrhoea, genital herpes, trichomoniasis, genital warts, pediculosis pubis, HIV, and syphilis. Many patients have more than one disease. Suspicion of STD necessitates prompt referral to a genitourinary (GU) medicine clinic for proper diagnosis, treatment and follow-up of the patient and contacts. Some GU departments provide an on-call service. Only prescribe antibiotics for suspected STDs on the advice of a GU specialist.

Genital ulcers and sores

Most genital ulcers/erosions are either multiple and painful or single and painless. In the UK, multiple genital ulcers are most often due to herpes simplex; other causes are Behçet's disease and (rarely) chancroid or scabies. Multiple painful sores may occur with gonorrhoea, candida, or other conditions. Painless genital ulceration should suggest syphilis (primary chancre is a single ulcer, secondary syphilis often multiple: both are highly infectious and incidence has ↑ recently). Other causes of painless ulcers include carcinoma and trauma (possibly self-inflicted).

Urethritis

In men, dysuria and urethral discharge are the commonest presenting symptoms of an STD. However, 5–10% of men with gonococcal or non-gonococcal urethritis have no symptoms. Urethritis may result from physical trauma, foreign bodies or attempts at self-treatment with intra-urethral chemicals.

Gonorrhoea usually has a shorter incubation period (3–5 days) than non-gonococcal urethritis (eg chlamydia 7–14 days), but do not rely on a clinical diagnosis: refer to a GU clinic for diagnosis, management and follow-up. If no GU advice is available and treatment cannot wait for attendance at a GU clinic, give doxycycline 200mg PO stat and then 100mg PO daily (or tetracycline 500mg PO qds). If possible, make a glass slide of the discharge, dried in air, for the patient to take to the clinic. He should be told not to pass urine for 4 hours before the appointment, in order to allow serial urine samples to be taken.

Reiter's disease is a rare complication of non-gonococcal urethritis. There is arthritis (mainly of knees, ankles and feet) and sometimes conjunctivitis, rashes and cardiac and neurological problems.

Gonorrhoea

Gonorrhoea may infect the urethra, cervix, rectum, pharynx or conjunctiva. Men usually have dysuria and urethral discharge, with rectal discharge and tenesmus in homosexuals. Women are often asymptomatic, but may have dysuria and vaginal discharge.

Complications include prostatitis, epididymitis, salpingitis, Bartholin's abscess; rarely septicaemia with arthritis, fever, rash (maculopapular initially, then pustular) and endocarditis.

Hepatitis[ND]

Hepatitis A (infectious hepatitis)[ND]

Hepatitis A occurs throughout the world, but is particularly common in the tropics and subtropics. It is transmitted by contamination of food or water with infected faeces or urine. Many infections are asymptomatic. The incubation period is 2–6 weeks (usually ≈4 weeks). Fever, malaise, anorexia and nausea may last for 2–7 days before jaundice develops. Jaundice is more common in adults than in children and is associated with dark urine, pale stools and tender hepatomegaly.

Treatment is symptomatic, but alcohol should be avoided. Infectivity is greatest before jaundice develops, so isolation is of little value. Arrange follow-up by a specialist or GP. Complete recovery is usual. Hepatitis A vaccine should be considered for close contacts (see *BNF*).

Hepatitis B[ND]

Hepatitis B is transmitted by infected blood (eg shared needles in drug abusers, tattooing, needlestick injury) and by sexual intercourse. The incubation period is 6 weeks to 6 months. The symptoms are similar to hepatitis A, often with arthralgia and skin rashes. Most patients with hepatitis B recover completely. A few patients develop liver failure or chronic hepatitis, with a risk of primary liver cancer. Refer to a specialist for follow-up. Asymptomatic carriers of hepatitis B virus are common (≈0.1% of the population in the UK, but ≈20% in parts of Africa and Asia). Because of the high risk of infection, all health care workers should be immunized against hepatitis B and use 'standard precautions' (📖 p.32) when handling all blood samples and 'sharps'. The management of needlestick injury is described on 📖 p.418.

Hepatitis C, D, and E[ND]

Hepatitis C and D are spread in the same way as hepatitis B, and may cause hepatic failure or chronic liver disease. No immunization is available.

Hepatitis E is similar to hepatitis A, but has a high mortality in pregnancy. Refer to a specialist for follow-up.

Leptospirosis (Weil's disease)[ND]

Leptospirosis, caused by the spirochaete *Leptospira interrogans* and other Leptospira species, is spread by contact with infected rat's urine, often in rivers, canals or sewers. The leptospires enter the body through small breaks in the skin or via mucous membranes of the eyes or nose. About 10 days after exposure (range 2–26 days) the illness starts with fever, severe muscle pains, headache, sore throat, nausea and vomiting. Conjunctival reddening is common. A haemorrhagic rash, jaundice, renal failure and pulmonary haemorrhage may occur (Weil's disease).

Refer to an Infectious Diseases unit. Treatment is with penicillin or doxycycline with supportive care and haemodialysis if necessary. Prophylactic doxycycline is reasonable for people who fall into waterways likely to be contaminated with leptospires.

Herpes virus infections

Varicella zoster

Chickenpox results from primary infection with varicella zoster virus, which then remains dormant in the dorsal root ganglia. Reactivation of the virus causes *shingles*. Chickenpox is usually a mild disease of childhood. An itchy vesicular rash appears, most densely on the trunk and face, but decreasing peripherally. The lesions appear in crops and crust over in 3–4 days. Fever, malaise and muscle aches may occur in adults. Infectivity starts 3 days before the rash appears and lasts until the last lesion has crusted.

Treat symptomatically, eg calamine lotion for itching and paracetamol for fever. Occasionally, antibiotics are needed for secondary bacterial skin infection (usually *Staph.* or *Strep.*). Pneumonia is rare and in children is usually staphylococcal, but in adults may be caused by chickenpox virus. Chickenpox may be severe in neonates and in patients with cystic fibrosis or immune deficiency, who need specialist assessment and treatment with aciclovir and/or varicella-zoster immune globulin. Consider aciclovir also for adults and older adolescents (see *BNF*).

Shingles often occurs in the elderly and may affect any dermatome, most often thoracic. The pain of shingles may cause diagnostic difficulty until the rash appears, usually after 1–4 days. Erythema is followed by vesicles and then crusting of lesions in a unilateral distribution over 1 dermatome or 2 adjacent dermatomes. Ophthalmic shingles may affect the eye via the long ciliary nerves: skin lesions on the side of the tip of the nose imply a high risk of eye involvement. Oral lesions occur in maxillary and mandibular shingles. Infection of the geniculate ganglion causes a facial palsy with lesions in the pinna of the ear and on the side of the tongue and hard palate *(Ramsay–Hunt syndrome)*. In severe shingles there may be weakness of muscles supplied by nerves of the same spinal root.

Antiviral treatment (aciclovir, famciclovir, or valaciclovir) ↓ risk of post-herpetic pain if given early (within 72hr of start of rash). Dose: aciclovir 800mg 5 times daily for 7 days. In renal failure antiviral drugs may cause severe toxicity, so use much smaller or less frequent doses. Patients with immune deficiency or ophthalmic zoster need immediate specialist referral and antiviral treatment. Give analgesia. Antibiotics may be required for secondary infection.

Herpes simplex

Primary herpes simplex infection causes painful vesicles and ulceration of the mouth or genitalia (📖 p.238). The virus may be inoculated into skin by trauma (herpes gladiatorum, scrumpox) or by contamination of fingers causing herpetic paronychia (whitlow). Infection of the cornea may cause dendritic ulcers (📖 p.543). *Herpes simplex meningitis and encephalitis*[ND] are uncommon, but may be fatal, especially in immunodeficient patients.

The herpes simplex virus persists in sensory ganglia and may be reactivated by stimuli such as sun, cold, trauma, or viral infections. Recurrence of cold sores of the lips is often preceded by tingling: aciclovir cream or tablets may prevent the development of vesicles. Secondary bacterial infection may require antibiotics. Do not incise a suspected whitlow. Cover it with a dressing and advise care to avoid spreading infection to the lips or eyes.

Infectious mononucleosis (glandular fever)

Infection with the *Epstein–Barr virus* is common in children and young adults and is spread by saliva or droplets. Infection often occurs without clinical disease. In glandular fever there is malaise, fever, a sore throat, and cervical lymphadenopathy. The throat may be very red and in 25% of cases there is also infection with a β-haemolytic streptococcus. In severe cases there is marked oedema of the throat with tonsillar swelling and a membranous exudate ('anginose' infectious mononucleosis) with difficulty in swallowing and breathing. A rash is uncommon unless ampicillin or amoxicillin are given, causing a widespread erythematous maculopapular rash (which does not signify allergy to penicillins in general).

Complications of infectious mononucleosis include respiratory obstruction, ruptured spleen (spontaneously or after minor trauma), thrombocytopenia, jaundice, meningitis, encephalitis, facial palsy, and acute polyneuritis (occasionally causing respiratory failure).

Investigations FBC and blood film (for atypical lymphocytes), Monospot test or Paul–Bunnell test (which may be –ve initially).

Differential diagnosis includes cytomegalovirus and toxoplasmosis.

Treatment is unnecessary in most patients. Severe or complicated cases need specialist assessment and follow-up. In anginose infectious mono-nucleosis, a short course of high dose oral steroids gives rapid relief of symptoms (prednisolone 80mg on day 1; 15mg tds on days 2–3; 10mg tds on days 4–5; 5mg tds on days 6–7). Steroids are also helpful in patients with neurological complications. Concurrent β-haemolytic streptococcal infection requires erythromycin (500mg qds), which would also treat the rare unrecognized case of diphtheria.

Human immunodeficiency virus (HIV)

First reports of acquired immune deficiency syndrome (AIDS) involved homosexuals in the USA in 1981. HIV (previously called HTLV-III, LAV, or ARV) was identified as the causative agent in Paris in 1983.

Structure and pathogenesis

HIV is an RNA retrovirus. Retroviruses are characterized by having the enzyme reverse transcriptase. This allows viral RNA to be transcribed (copied) into DNA and incorporated into host cells, which then make a new virus. This mechanism has proved difficult to overcome: no 'cure' or 'vaccine' is yet available.

Glycoproteins on the surface of HIV bind to specific receptors on target cells. The cellular receptor for HIV is the CD4 molecule. CD4 receptors are found on a variety of cells, particularly helper/inducer T lymphocytes ('CD4 cells'), but also monocytes and macrophages. CD4 cells normally play a crucial role in co-ordinating the immune response: as HIV infection progresses and CD4 cell counts ↓, the patient develops profound cellular immunodeficiency. Although other complex mechanisms are also involved, CD4 cell counts provide a useful index of disease stage and progress.

Transmission

HIV has been found in many body fluids, but is mostly transmitted via blood, semen, cervical secretions and, perhaps, breast milk. It may be acquired by:
- Sexual intercourse (vaginal or anal), with ↑ risk of transmission where individuals already have a genital mucosal breach (eg co-existent STD).
- Risk of transmission from HIV +ve pregnant mother to baby is ≈15%.
- Transfusion of unscreened blood/blood products (screening started in 1985 in the UK).
- Contaminated needles shared amongst IV drug abusers. Needlestick injuries from an HIV positive source carry a risk of ≈0.3%.

Diagnosis and HIV testing

Antibodies to HIV provide evidence of infection and form the basis of current blood tests, but these antibodies may not appear until 3 months after exposure. HIV testing is not appropriate in the ED, but reserved for clinics where informed consent and counselling are available. Refer patients requesting HIV tests to local Infectious Diseases/GU clinics or advisory organizations, eg Terrence Higgins Trust (tel. 0808 802 1221), or the NHS Sexual Health Helpline (24hr freephone 0800 567 123).

Natural history of HIV infection

HIV infection progresses through phases, which form the basis of the two commonly used classification systems (World Health Organization (WHO) and CDC systems).

Acute infection is often sub-clinical, but 2–6 weeks after exposure there may be a non-specific febrile illness with lethargy, myalgia, sore throat, lymphadenopathy, and often a maculopapular rash on the face and trunk. This illness usually resolves after 1–2 weeks but sometimes persists for longer. A long asymptomatic period (≈10 years) follows the initial illness.

Some patients develop persistent generalized lymphadenopathy (PGL), with lymphadenopathy (>1cm) at two non-inguinal sites for 3 months. Patients become symptomatic as their immunity ↓, developing unusual infections and tumours. Many are 'AIDS-defining diseases' (see below). The label 'AIDS' has significant psychological connotations. Most patients with AIDS survive >2 years.

Anti-retroviral drugs (AZT and other drugs) delay the onset of AIDS in asymptomatic patients and ↑ length of survival. 'HAART' (highly active antiretroviral therapy) is a regime combining 3 or more anti-HIV drugs.

Initial presentation of HIV to the emergency department

Many HIV +ve patients attending the ED are aware of their HIV status. Some patients, however, present with HIV-related illness, without knowing (or admitting) that they are HIV +ve. Presentation of any of the diseases listed below should arouse particular suspicion.

Centers for Disease Control classification of HIV infection

Group I   Acute infection
Group II   Asymptomatic
Group III   Persistent generalized lymphadenopathy
Group IV Symptomatic infection with subgroups:
                A—constitutional disease (fever, diarrhoea, weight loss)
                B—neurological disease (dementia, peripheral neuropathy)
                C—secondary infectious diseases
                D—secondary cancers (lymphomas, Kaposi's sarcoma)
                E—other conditions

Some AIDS-defining diseases in HIV +ve patients

- *Pneumocystis jiroveci* pneumonia (previously called *P. carinii*).
- Kaposi's sarcoma.
- Tracheobronchial or oesophageal candidiasis.
- Cerebral toxoplasmosis.
- Pulmonary TB.
- Cytomegalovirus retinitis.
- Cerebral lymphoma.
- Recurrent *Salmonella* septicaemia.
- Disseminated histoplasmosis.
- Invasive cervical carcinoma.
- Disseminated coccidioidomycosis.
- Cryptococcosis.
- Cryptosporidiosis.
- Progressive multifocal leucoencephalopathy.
- Oesophageal or bronchial herpes simplex.

CD4 counts and AIDS

CD4 counts provide an indication of disease progression: many HIV +ve patients know what their last count was. In the USA, CD4 counts <200/mm^3 may also be used to define AIDS.

Presentation of HIV +ve patients

Many patients with symptomatic HIV infection bypass the ED and liaise directly with the specialist unit caring for them. Assessment of HIV +ve patients is difficult in the ED, where advanced infections may present with relatively few signs and little past history is available. Similarly, interpretation of investigations is difficult without knowledge of previous results. It is therefore reasonable to have a low threshold for specialist referral. HIV +ve patients may present with a variety of complications:

Respiratory problems

As CD4 counts ↓, pneumonia due to *Pneumocystis jiroveci* (previously *Pneumocystis carinii*) becomes more likely and it is a common indicator diagnosis of AIDS. A non-productive cough occurs with dyspnoea and fever. CXR may show bilateral interstitial mid-zone shadowing, but may be normal. Obtain blood and sputum cultures, rehydrate with IV fluids as necessary and refer urgently for IV co-trimoxazole or pentamidine ± steroids. Occasionally, *Pneumocystis* infection may present with fulminant respiratory failure needing emergency tracheal intubation and IPPV. Other common infections include *Aspergillus*, *Cryptococcus* and TB. Injecting drug users are at increased risk of bacterial infection, especially *Haemophilus influenzae* and *Strep. pneumoniae*.

Neurological problems

Cryptococcus neoformans meningitis may present with headache, fever and sometimes ↓ conscious level. Neck stiffness and photophobia are rare. Obtain a CT scan to exclude space-occupying lesions before LP and CSF examination. *Cerebral toxoplasmosis* may present similarly, often with focal signs or fits. Neurological problems may also be caused by cerebral lymphoma, progressive leucoencephalopathy (focal deficits secondary to papovaviruses), CMV encephalitis (retinopathy is usually present—see below) and HIV-associated delirium or dementia.

Eye problems

The most significant eye problem is *Cytomegalovirus (CMV) retinitis*, occurring in 15% of patients. This presents with blurred vision, blind spots, 'floaters' or flashing lights, and ↓ VA. Characteristic retinal changes are irregular yellow-white lesions and perivascular haemorrhages that have been called 'pizza pie'. Retinal detachment may occur. Refer urgently for ophthalmological assessment and treatment with ganciclovir or foscarnet.

Mucocutaneous problems

Oral candidiasis, seborrhoeic dermatitis, and oral hairy leukoplakia (white ridges on lateral border of tongue) are often seen before AIDS develops. As immunity ↓, patients may develop herpes simplex, herpes zoster and molluscum contagiosum. Gum bleeding and dental problems are common: the former may be due to thrombocytopenia. Kaposi's sarcoma is seen in skin and mucous membranes, particularly in homosexuals with AIDS. It is rarely life-threatening, but requires specialist evaluation and treatment.

Gastrointestinal problems

Nausea, vomiting, diarrhoea and weight loss are common complaints and can be due to drug therapy. Dysphagia may result from oesophageal candidiasis, herpes simplex, CMV, or Kaposi's sarcoma, all of which require specialist investigation and treatment.

CMV colitis can cause a serious illness, characterized by abdominal pain, diarrhoea and fever. Obtain plain X-rays if the recognized complication of toxic dilatation is suspected. Other frequently implicated infective causes of diarrhoea include cryptosporidium, *Giardia*, microsporidium and *Salmonella*. Send stool specimens (including for *Clostridium difficile*) and treat severe diarrhoea by IV rehydration and correction of electrolyte imbalance before referral.

Hepatitis viruses are likely to complicate the picture in injecting drug users, many of whom are infected with hepatitis B and C.

Drug reactions and side effects

Many patients will present with symptoms due to drug therapy. This may not be initially apparent: the safest approach is to exclude tumours and opportunistic infection first.

HIV and emergency department staff

ED staff are often concerned about the possibility of acquiring HIV from patients. The need to perform invasive emergency procedures on 'high risk' patients makes these concerns understandable. Additionally, apparently 'low risk' patients may also pose a threat. Therefore treat every patient as if he is 'high risk'. The risk to ED staff is largely in the form of needlestick injury (although the risk of acquiring HIV following needlestick from a HIV +ve source can be ↓ by post-exposure prophylaxis—see 📖 p.418). Safe practice is reflected in the recommended standard precautions (see 📖 p.32)—follow these in all patients. Pregnant staff should not treat patients with AIDS (because of concern about CMV and herpes simplex virus).

Handling HIV +ve patients

Despite vigorous attempts to educate the general public, HIV and AIDS remain taboo subjects amongst many in society. It is imperative to treat all patients, including those who are HIV +ve, with sensitivity and compassion. Touching and shaking hands with HIV +ve patients is perfectly safe, and may help to reassure them that the discrimination and irrational treatment they may have received outside hospital does not extend into the ED. In view of prevailing attitudes towards HIV, patient confidentiality is of the utmost importance. Remember that family and friends accompanying the patient may be unaware of his HIV status.

HIV +ve staff

The risk to patients from ED staff infected with HIV is minimal, but remains a theoretical possibility. Staff who believe that they may be HIV +ve must obtain and follow occupational health advice.

Needlestick injury: See 📖 p.418.

Imported infectious diseases

Patients may present to the ED with infectious diseases acquired abroad. It is essential to ask where a patient has been, especially in the 6 weeks before the onset of symptoms. The most common imported diseases are bowel infections causing diarrhoea (📖 p.226). Less common, but very important diseases include malaria (📖 p.247), typhoid (📖 p.248), Legionnaires' disease (📖 p.110) and hepatitis (📖 p.239). Rabies (📖 p.249) and viral haemorrhagic fevers, such as Lassa fever (📖 p.250) are very rare in the UK.

Occasionally, tropical diseases are acquired in Britain from bites by infected insects carried by plane (eg 'airport malaria').

Advice about tropical diseases is available from departments of Infectious Diseases or Tropical Medicine:

- *Birmingham* (Heartlands Hospital). www.heartofengland.nhs.uk Telephone 0121 424 2000.
- *Liverpool* (School of Tropical Medicine). www.liv.ac.uk/lstm Telephone 0151 705 3100.
- *London* (Hospital for Tropical Diseases) www.thehtd.org/Emergencies. aspx Telephone 0845 155 5000.
- *Oxford* (Churchill Hospital) Telephone 01865 741 841.
- *Glasgow* (Brownlee Centre for Infectious and Communicable Diseases, Gartnavel General Hospital) Telephone 0141 211 3000.
- A public access website provided by the NHS which gives information for people travelling abroad from the UK is www.fitfortravel.scot. nhs.uk

Pyrexia of unknown origin in travellers

Think of and check for malaria (📖 p.247) in any febrile patient who has been in a malarious area. Consider Lassa fever (📖 p.250) in someone who has been in West Africa in the previous 3 weeks. Typhoid (📖 p.248) often presents as a septicaemic illness with constipation, rather than diarrhoea. TB (📖 p.232) and brucellosis may cause fever and sweating at night.

Investigations (warn lab of possible risks)

FBC, thick and thin blood films for malaria, U&E, blood glucose, blood culture, urine stick testing, microscopy and culture, CXR.

Further investigations may include LFTs and viral titres.

Management Barrier nurse in a cubicle (use a negative pressure room if available). Wear gown, gloves, goggles and mask. Record vaccination and prophylaxis history, with countries and areas visited, and dates of travel and onset of symptoms. Look particularly for confusion, dehydration, jaundice, rashes, chest signs, liver and spleen enlargement and tenderness, lymphadenopathy, neck stiffness, photophobia. Seek expert advice at once if the patient is very ill or there is concern about typhoid or Lassa fever or other viral haemorrhagic fevers. Refer to an Infectious Diseases specialist.

Malaria[ND]

Malaria is very common in the tropics and subtropical regions, and is a parasitic infection transmitted by mosquitoes. The five species which cause malaria in humans are *Plasmodium falciparum*, *P. vivax*, *P. malariae*, *P. ovale*, and *P. knowlesi*. Falciparum ('malignant tertian') malaria is the most important, since it may be rapidly fatal and drug-resistant strains are common. Serious complications are unusual in the other types of malaria, but they may cause febrile convulsions in children.

In the UK malaria occurs in travellers from malarious areas, especially *P. vivax* from the Indian subcontinent and *P. falciparum* from Africa, South-East Asia, and Central and South America. Malaria often develops despite antimalarial tablets, because of drug resistance or incorrect dosage. Check for malaria in any febrile illness within 2 months of visiting a malarious area. Common misdiagnoses are influenza and viral hepatitis.

Clinical features

The incubation period is usually 7–14 days for *P. falciparum* and 12–40 days for other types of malaria, but occasionally it is much longer (>1 year), especially in *P. malariae* and *P. vivax* infections. There is malaise, fatigue, fever and headache followed by paroxysms lasting 8–12hr of rigors, vomiting and then severe sweating. The fever may be periodic (classically 48hr in *P. ovale* or *P. vivax*, and 72hr in *P. malariae*). Haemolytic anaemia, jaundice and splenomegaly may occur, but lymphadenopathy is not a feature. *P. falciparum* may cause cerebral malaria with coma, fits and focal neurological signs. Diarrhoea, cardiac failure, pulmonary oedema and shock may occur. Deterioration can be rapid.

Investigations

Consider Lassa fever (📖 p.250) in recent visitors to West Africa. In any ill patient who has been in a malarious area send blood for thin and thick film examination for malaria. Repeated blood films may be needed. Also arrange FBC (since malaria may cause anaemia, thrombocytopenia and neutropenia), blood glucose (hypoglycaemia may be severe), U&E (renal failure is possible), and test the urine for blood ('black water fever').

Treatment of falciparum malaria[1]

Careful monitoring is needed ± ICU. Obtain expert advice from a tropical disease specialist (📖 p.246), especially if the patient is severely ill or has come from south-east Asia, where there is widespread drug resistance.

Give quinine, orally or IV depending on the severity of illness: oral quinine sulphate 600mg (adult) or 10mg/kg (child) every 8hr for 7 days, followed by doxycycline 200mg od for 7 days, clindamycin 450mg tds for 5 days or Fansidar® 3 tablets. Alternative oral drugs are Malarone® (proguanil with atovaquone) or Riamet® (artemether with lumefantrine): for details see *BNF*. For algorithm[1] see www.britishinfectionsociety.org.

Treatment of benign malarias (*P. vivax, ovale, malariae*)[1]

The usual treatment is chloroquine (see *BNF*). A course of primaquine is also needed to prevent relapse in vivax and ovale infections, but glucose-6-phosphate dehydrogenase levels should be checked before primaquine is used, since it may cause haemolysis in G6PD deficient patients. In the UK refer to an Infectious Diseases unit for treatment and follow-up.

---

1 Lalloo DG *et al.* (2007) UK malaria treatment guidelines. *Journal of Infection* **54**: 111–121.

Typhoid[ND] and paratyphoid[ND] (enteric fever)

These fevers, caused by *Salmonella typhi* and *S. paratyphi A, B, or C,* occur throughout the world, especially where hygiene is inadequate. They are spread by contamination of food or water by urine or faeces from a patient or an asymptomatic carrier. Typhoid may occur despite immunization. Typhoid and malaria are the first diseases to consider if fever develops soon after a visit to the tropics. The *incubation period* is usually 7–14 days, but may range from 3–60 days.

Initial symptoms

Headache, fever, and a dry cough, with abdominal discomfort and anorexia. Constipation is common, but diarrhoea may occur, especially in children. Confusion and hallucinations may develop.

Physical examination

This may be normal except for fever. There may be a relative brady-cardia (ie less than the usual 15 beats/min ↑ in pulse rate per °C of fever). Splenomegaly and abdominal tenderness occur, but there is no lymphadenopathy. 'Rose spots' are pink macular spots on the lower chest or upper abdomen which blanch on pressure. There may be signs of pneumonia or dehydration. Intestinal perforation or haemorrhage occur occasionally.

Investigations

FBC (mild anaemia is common, WBC usually normal), blood films for malaria, U&E, LFTs, blood cultures, CXR (for signs of TB or pneumonia).

Treatment

Isolate and barrier nurse. Admit suspected cases to an Infectious Diseases unit and notify the local consultant in Communicable Disease Control. The usual drug treatment is with ciprofloxacin or cefotaxime but other antibiotics may be needed for drug-resistant infections.

Dengue

Dengue is a mosquito-borne viral infection which is common in southern Asia, the western Pacific, central Africa and central and south America. Most infections are asymptomatic. Symptoms start after an incubation period of 4–7 days with fever, malaise, nausea and vomiting, headache, severe muscle and bone pains ('break bone fever'). Some patients have a transient macular rash, petechiae, lymphadenopathy, hepatomegaly, ↓ WCC and platelets and ↑ liver enzymes.

Most patients recover after 3–7 days with symptomatic treatment. A few develop dengue shock syndrome (DSS) with hypotension, pleural effusions, ascites, ↓ plasma protein and bleeding problems. Abdominal pain may be severe. Treatment is supportive, with careful fluid balance management and IV fluids in DSS. With expert care most patients with severe dengue eventually make a full recovery.

PoliomyelitisND

Paralytic poliomyelitis is rare in developed countries where vaccination is routine. Fever is followed by signs of meningitis, pain and spasm in limb muscles. Respiratory failure may be fatal.

Resuscitate and ventilate if necessary and refer to ICU.

The differential diagnosis includes Guillain–Barré syndrome (📖 p.142) and organophosphate poisoning (📖 p.206).

RabiesND

Rabies is a viral infection of mammals that occurs in most parts of the world, including much of the Arctic, as well as tropical and temperate regions. At present it is not endemic in the UK, Norway, Sweden, Iceland, Australasia, or Japan. Human and animal rabies is most common in the Indian subcontinent, China, Thailand, the Philippines, and parts of South America. Most human infections result from dog bites, but rabies can be transmitted by many other domesticated or wild animals, such as cats and foxes. Rabies virus in an animal's saliva may cause infection by contamination of a bite or scratch or by absorption through mucous membranes of the eye, mouth or nose. Rarely, infection occurs from inhalation of the virus in bat-infested caves.

Prevention of rabies after a bite is described on 📖 p.415.

Advice about post-exposure treatment and suspected cases of rabies is available in the UK from the Health Protection Agency. For details see www.hpa.org.uk/Topics/InfectiousDiseases/InfectionsAZ/Rabies

Clinical features

The *incubation period* of rabies is usually 3–12 weeks, but can vary from a few days to >2 years.

The first symptoms are itching, tingling or pain at the site of the bite wound. Headache, fever, and malaise occur, with spreading paralysis and episodes of confusion, hallucination and agitation. Hydrophobia is characteristic: attempts at drinking cause spasm of muscles involved in breathing and swallowing and also profound terror. In ≈20% of cases there is 'dumb rabies' with increasing paralysis but no episodes of spasm or hyperactivity. Rabies is almost always fatal, even with ICU treatment.

Management

If rabies is suspected, barrier nurse the patient in a quiet room with the minimum of staff, who must wear gowns, gloves, eye protection and masks. Obtain advice immediately from a specialist in Infectious Diseases. Anticipate press enquiries. Record the names of all staff involved, so that they can be offered rabies immunization.

Viral haemorrhagic fevers[ND]

Lassa fever

Lassa fever occurs in many rural parts of West Africa. It is a viral infection acquired from infected blood or secretions, transmitted by inadvertent innoculation (eg needlestick injuries) or contamination of mucous membranes or broken skin. In Africa it is transmitted by multimammate rats. The incubation period is up to 3 weeks. There is a high mortality.

Early symptoms are non-specific with fever, malaise, headache, sore throat, retrosternal chest pain and backache. Periorbital oedema, swelling of the neck and conjunctival injection are common. Suspect Lassa fever in any pyrexial patient who has been in rural West Africa (south of the Sahara) in the previous 3 weeks. However, malaria and typhoid are much more common and need urgent diagnosis and treatment.

Management If Lassa fever is possible, barrier nurse the patient in a cubicle by staff wearing gloves, gowns, goggles and masks. Take special care to avoid needlestick injuries, which may cause fatal infection. Before taking any blood samples, discuss the case with a tropical diseases specialist and the local consultant in Communicable Disease Control. Start treatment immediately for falciparum malaria (📖 p.247). Warn the laboratory about Lassa fever and send blood for examination for malaria. The patient will be admitted to an isolation bed, possibly in a high security Infectious Diseases unit.

Ebola fever and Marburg fever

These are viral haemorrhagic fevers which occur in West and Central Africa (Zaire, Uganda, Kenya and Sudan), and have similar clinical features and a high mortality. Transmission is usually by infected blood, but the viruses may be acquired from monkeys or apes. The incubation period is usually 4–10 days. Illness starts suddenly with severe headache, high fever, and generalized pains, especially in the back, followed by severe diarrhoea, abdominal pain, dry throat, a maculopapular rash, conjunctivitis, and gastrointestinal bleeding. Isolate and treat as for suspected Lassa fever.

Other viral haemorrhagic fevers

Diseases with similar features (plus in some cases jaundice) include dengue (see 📖 p.248), Crimean-Congo fever (central Africa, parts of Eastern Europe, and Asia) and yellow fever (Africa and South America). The initial management is the same as for Lassa fever.

Severe acute respiratory syndrome

Background

Severe acute respiratory syndrome (SARS) is a viral respiratory illness caused by a coronavirus. SARS was first recognized in March 2003, but probably originated in November 2002 in the Guangdong province of China, where the virus has been found in wild animals. SARS spread to several countries, causing deaths in south-east Asia and Canada in March to May 2003. Few cases have occurred since then. No cases are known at the time of writing, but there is concern that SARS may re-emerge from China.

Spread

SARS is spread by respiratory droplets produced when an infected person coughs, sneezes, or uses a nebulizer. The virus can also spread when someone touches an object contaminated by infectious droplets and then touches his/her mouth, nose, or eyes.

Features

The incubation period of SARS is usually 2–7 days, but may be up to 10 days. The illness starts with fever (>38°C), usually associated with rigors, headache, muscle pains and malaise. Diarrhoea may occur. Some patients have mild respiratory symptoms initially. A dry cough develops after 2–7 days, with increasing breathlessness from hypoxia caused by pneumonia. Consider the possibility of SARS in a patient with these symptoms who, within 10 days of the onset of illness, has visited an area where SARS may occur (especially China) or worked in a laboratory holding SARS virus samples.

CXR may be normal or may show patchy infiltrates, and later areas of consolidation. WCC is usually normal or ↓ initially (lymphopenia).

Management

If SARS is suspected, get expert help (ED consultant, Infectious Diseases specialist, and infection control staff) and isolate the patient (if possible in a negative pressure room). Ensure that the minimum number of staff have contact with the patient. Staff who do have contact must wear masks or respirators (of FFP3 standard), goggles, gowns and gloves, with strict handwashing and careful disposal of all items. Provide the patient with an N95 mask or a surgical mask. Record SpO$_2$ and give O$_2$ if necessary, but avoid flow rates of >6L/min, to minimize virus aerolization. If bronchodilators are needed, use a spacer inhaler rather than a nebulizer. Maintain a list of all contacts. Expect press enquiries.

An expert will help to assess to decide about admission. Those admitted should ideally be placed in a negative pressure isolation room with full infection control measures. Treat as for community-acquired pneumonia (📖 p.110).

Further information about SARS is available from:
- www.hpa.org.uk/Topics/InfectiousDiseases/InfectionsAZ/ SevereAcuteRespiratorySyndrome/ (Health Protection Agency, UK).
- www.who.int/csr/sars/en/index.html (World Health Organization).

Influenza pandemics, avian flu, and swine flu

Background

Influenza is common in the UK and many other countries, particularly during winter. Most people are ill for only a few days with fever, muscle aches, coughing and nausea, but there are some deaths, especially in elderly people.

Pandemic influenza occurs when a new subtype of influenza A emerges, which can spread easily from person to person and which is different from previous strains (so there is no pre-existing immunity). Influenza pandemics occurred in 1918–1919 (with 40–50 million deaths worldwide, including many children and young adults), and also in 1957 and 1968. Another pandemic could develop at any time. There was concern about influenza A subtype H5N1, which infected poultry in Hong Kong in 1997 and 2003 and spread to birds across south-east Asia, with carriage by migrating birds across Asia and to Europe and Africa. This *avian flu* infected many millions of birds and some people in south-east Asia and Turkey who had been in close contact with infected chickens. The mortality in these cases was high. In 2009 influenza A subtype H1N1 caused a pandemic of *swine flu* which started in Mexico and spread to many other countries. Most patients with swine flu had only mild illness but a minority developed severe infection, and some died.

Human-to-human spread of H1N1 or H5N1 flu is rare, at the time of writing, but another pandemic could develop if the virus mutates again.

Spread

Like SARS (see ☐ p.251) flu is spread by droplets coughed or sneezed into the air, or by direct contact with hands contaminated with the virus.

Features

Consider the possibility of avian flu or swine flu in a patient with fever ≥38°C and cough or breathlessness, who in the last 7 days has been in an area affected by H1N1 or H5N1 influenza. Laboratory staff and health care workers in contact with cases of severe unexplained respiratory illness could also be at risk.

Management

Isolate the patient and treat with precautions against transmission of the virus, as for SARS (☐ p.251). Antiviral treatment with oseltamivir or zanimivir may be considered, depending on current guidelines.

Further information

Clinical guidelines about the assessment of suspected cases and the management of influenza patients will be updated as the situation changes and if another pandemic develops. Information is available from the UK Health Protection Agency: www.hpa.org.uk/infections/topics_az/influenza/pandemic

Environmental emergencies

Hypothermia: presentation

Definitions
Hypothermia exists when the core temperature (T°)<35°C.

Hypothermia may be classified as follows:

Mild hypothermia	= 32–35°C
Moderate hypothermia	= 30–32°C
Severe hypothermia	= <30°C

Background
Infants and the elderly are at particular risk. In young adults hypothermia is usually due to environmental exposure (eg hill-walking or cold water immersion), or to immobility and impaired conscious level from alcohol or drugs. In the elderly, it is more often a prolonged state of multifactorial origin: common precipitants include unsatisfactory housing, poverty, immobility, lack of cold awareness (autonomic neuropathy, dementia), drugs (sedatives, antidepressants), alcohol, acute confusion, hypothyroidism and infections.

Clinical features
Severe hypothermia may mimic death. Wide variations occur, but as core T° ↓, cerebral and cardiovascular function deteriorate. At 32–35°C, apathy, amnesia, ataxia and dysarthria are common. At <32°C, conscious-ness falls progressively, leading to coma, ↓ BP, arrhythmias (check pulse for at least 1min before diagnosing cardiac arrest), respiratory depression and muscular rigidity. Shivering is an unreliable sign. VF may occur sponta-neously when T° falls <28°C and may be provoked by limb movement or invasive procedures (especially in the presence of hypoxia).

Diagnosis
Check tympanic T° (or rectal T° with an electronic probe or low-reading thermometer). Tympanic and rectal T° may lag behind core (cardiac) T° during rewarming. Oesophageal T° reflects core levels more accurately, but requires special equipment.

Investigations
- U&E.
- FBC, toxicology and clotting screens. Note that hypothermia can cause or aggravate coagulation disturbances.
- Blood glucose (BMG reading may be falsely ↓).
- Amylase (↑ levels common, but do not necessarily imply pancreatitis).
- Blood cultures.
- ABG.
- ECG: look for prolongation of elements in the PQRST complex, J-waves, and arrhythmias (AF and bradycardias are the commonest) (Fig. 6.1).
- CXR: look for pneumonia, aspiration, left ventricular failure. Other X-rays may be required after rewarming (eg for suspected fractured neck of femur).
- CT scan may be indicated if head injury or stroke is suspected.

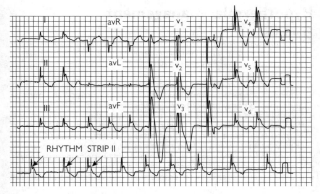

Fig. 6.1 ECG in hypothermia.

Notes on this ECG

- Rhythm disturbance: atrial fibrillation with slow ventricular response.
- Prolongation of QRS.
- Delayed repolarization 'J-waves' (arrowed).
- ST–T wave abnormalities.

Hypothermia: management

Principles
- Treat in a warm room (>21°C).
- Handle the patient gently (to ↓ risk of VF).
- Remove wet clothes and dry the skin.
- Monitor ECG.
- Give warmed, humidified O_2 by mask.
- Intubation, if needed, should be preceded by oxygenation and must be performed expertly to avoid precipitating arrhythmias.
- Secure IV access. IV fluid is rarely required unless there is loss of volume from another cause. If BP ↓ during rewarming, give 300–500mL of warmed 0.9% saline or colloid. In unstable patients, consider CVP and urinary catheter. Warm IV fluid administration is an inefficient rewarming method and runs the risks of fluid overload and precipitating arrhythmias.
- Correct hypoglycaemia if present with IV glucose.
- If CPR is required, give chest compressions and ventilations at standard rates.
- In hypothermic cardiac arrest, the heart may be unresponsive to defibrillation, pacing and drug therapy. Drug metabolism is ↓ and unpredictable: avoid drugs until core T°>30°C.
- Defibrillation is appropriate at normal energy levels if VF/VT occurs. If 3 shocks are unsuccessful, defer further shocks until core T°>30°C.

Rewarming methods
The choice depends upon the severity and duration of the condition, available facilities and the individual patient:

Passive rewarming
Easy, non-invasive, and suitable for mild cases (T°>32°C). ↓ evaporative and conductive losses by wrapping in warm blankets (remember to cover the back and sides of the head) ± polythene sheets. Avoid space blankets which are noisy and have no advantages over polythene sheets. Endogenous metabolism and shivering usually generate enough heat to allow spontaneous rewarming. Aim for a rate of 0.5–2°C/hr, but do not rewarm the elderly with prolonged hypothermia too rapidly (>0.6°C/hr), as hypotension or cerebral/pulmonary oedema may develop.

Active rewarming
A water bath at ≈41°C is rapid and useful for immersion hypothermia, but cannot be used in injured patients or if CPR is required. Airway care, ventilation and monitoring are difficult, and hazards include core T° after-drop and BP ↓ due to peripheral vasodilation. Hot water bottles and heat pads are less efficient and can cause burns. A hot air blanket is more convenient than a water bath, provides some heat and reduces heat loss.

Core rewarming
- Airway warming with heated (40–45°C) humidified O_2 provides some additional heat and reduces heat loss. It can be combined with other rewarming methods. It may reduce the risk of cardiac arrhythmias.
- Peritoneal lavage is simple, and quick to set up. Saline at 45°C is run in via a DPL catheter (🕮 p.347), left for 10–20mins and replaced with a fresh warm supply. The fluid directly heats the liver and retroperitoneal structures including blood in the IVC.

Extracorporeal rewarming with cardiopulmonary bypass maintains brain and organ perfusion and, if available, is the method of choice in patients with severe hypothermia or cardiac arrest. Cardiopulmonary bypass can result in rapid rewarming with core T° ↑ at 1–2°C/5min.

Frostbite and non-freezing cold injury

Frostbite[1, 2]

Frostbite occurs when tissues freeze at sub-zero temperatures. Predisposing factors include inadequate clothing/footwear, hypothermia, exhaustion, alcohol (which impairs judgement), drugs (eg beta-blockers), peripheral vascular disease, smoking, and previous cold injury. Frostbite usually involves extremities, especially fingers, toes, nose and ears.

Frostnip may precede frostbite. The skin of the nose, face or fingers goes white and numb, but recovers rapidly on protection from the cold, with transient paraesthesiae but no tissue loss and no permanent damage.

Superficial frostbite involves skin and subcutaneous tissues. The frozen area is numb, and looks white and waxy. Tissues feel firm or hard but are still pliable. Rewarming is painful. Oedematous hyperaemic skin becomes mottled or purple, with serum-filled blisters. A hard black eschar forms, and after ≈3 weeks this separates, revealing sensitive red shiny skin.

Deep frostbite involves muscles, nerves and sometimes bone, as well as skin and superficial tissues. The damaged area is hard and remains grey or white after rewarming. Blood-filled blisters develop. The dead tissue mummifies and then separates after several weeks or months.

Treatment of frostbite varies with the situation and facilities. Only frostnip should be treated in the field. Frostbitten tissues need rewarming as soon as possible but further damage must be avoided: it is better to walk out on frozen feet than on partially thawed feet. Treat hypothermia before frostbite. Rewarm frostbitten limbs in water at 37−39°C until skin circulation returns (usually ≈30min). Give analgesia and ibuprofen (which inhibits prostaglandins). After rewarming let the area dry in warm air (do not towel dry). Elevate the limb. Expose the area, with a bed cradle to avoid pressure of bedclothes. Clean the area daily in a whirlpool bath and encourage movement. If necessary split eschar to relieve stiffness, but avoid surgical debridement and amputations and allow the eschar to separate spontaneously: premature surgery causes avoidable tissue loss. Expert advice is helpful in severe frostbite: the British Mountaineerng Council (www.thebmc.co.uk) has a frostbite advice service. Bone scans or MRI/MRA may help to define deep tissue injury. In severe frostbite early thrombolysis with tPA may reduce the risk of eventual amputations.

Non-freezing cold injury[1, 2]

Trench foot (immersion foot) is caused by prolonged immersion in cold water or wet boots at temperatures just above freezing. Vasoconstriction causes tissue ischaemia and nerve damage. The feet are initially cold, numb and pale or mottled. On rewarming they become red, swollen and very painful. Blisters may develop.

Treatment: keep the feet clean, warm and dry, elevated to reduce oedema.

Outcome: most patients recover fully, but some have continued pain, paraesthesiae and sensitivity to cold.

1 State of Alaska Cold Injury Guidelines. www.chems.alaska.gov/EMS/documents/AKColdInj2005. pdf
2 Imray C et al. (2009) Cold damage to the extremities: frostbite and non-freezing cold injuries. *Postgraduate Medical Journal* **85**: 481–8.

Drowning and near drowning

Definitions

Drowning is death by suffocation from submersion in any liquid. Drowning is a common cause of death in young people. 40% of drownings occur in children aged <4 years.

Near drowning is survival (at least temporarily). In adults, the commonest predisposing factor is alcohol, sometimes with other drugs. A significant proportion reflect attempted suicide. In the UK, marine near drowning is usually associated with hypothermia (p.254).

Pathophysiology

Wet drowning Involves significant aspiration of fluid into the lungs. This causes pulmonary vasoconstriction and hypertension with ventilation/perfusion mismatch, aggravated by surfactant destruction and washout, ↓ lung compliance and atelectasis. Acute respiratory failure is common. ABG shows hypoxia, hypercarbia, and mixed respiratory/metabolic acidosis. The onset of symptoms can occur rapidly, but in lesser insults, symptoms may be delayed.

Contamination Water contaminated with chemical waste, detergents etc., may induce further lung injury.

Electrolytes Irrespective of whether aspirated water is salt, fresh, or swimming pool, changes in serum electrolytes and blood volume are similar, and are rarely immediately life-threatening.

Gastric fluid Swallowing of fluid into the stomach, with gastric dilatation, vomiting, and aspiration, is common.

Dry drowning In ≈10–20% of deaths from drowning, a small amount of water entering the larynx causes persistent laryngospasm, which results in asphyxia and an immediate outpouring of thick mucus, froth, and foam, but without significant aspiration—this is 'dry drowning'.

Secondary drowning A deterioration in a previously apparently well patient following successful resuscitation after submersion. It may occur in 5–10% of initial survivors.

The mammalian diving reflex

This is probably seen only in young children, but may explain why successful resuscitation without neurological deficit can occur after prolonged immersion. Cold water stimulates facial nerve afferents, while hypoxia stimulates the carotid body chemoreceptors. These effects reflexively ↓ heart rate and vasoconstrict skin, GI tract and skeletal muscle vessels, redistributing blood to the brain and heart. Associated hypothermia results in ↓ metabolic demands, delaying cerebral hypoxia.

Management

- Consider associated injury (eg to the cervical spine from diving into a shallow pool or surfing), and treat appropriately.
- Maintain the airway. Remove regurgitated fluid/debris by suction of the upper airway. Ensure adequate ventilation and correction of hypoxia. If the patient does not have a gag reflex or is apnoeic, ventilate with a bag and mask and proceed to early tracheal intubation and IPPV. In spontaneously breathing patients, give the highest FiO_2 possible. IPPV will be required if hypoxia and/or hypercapnia are present despite O_2 therapy, or if there are signs of pulmonary oedema. Ventilation with PEEP may significantly improve oxygenation by ↑ functional residual capacity, improving V/Q mismatch and enhancing fluid resorption from the pulmonary bed. However, PEEP may ↓ venous return to the heart.
- If the patient is in cardiac arrest, commence CPR (📖 p.46). Defibrillation may not be successful until core T°>30°C (📖 p.256). Appropriate rapid core rewarming techniques are required.
- Remove all wet/cold clothing.
- Monitor core T° and start rewarming (📖 p.256).
- NG tube to relieve gastric dilatation.
- Check U&E, blood glucose, ABG, FBC, CXR, ECG.
- Consider the possibility of alcohol, illegal drugs or drug overdose. Keep urine and blood samples and test if appropriate, eg paracetamol.
- Do not use 'prophylactic' steroids or barbiturates.
- Antibiotics may be warranted if contaminated water (eg sewage) is involved (see 📖 Leptospirosis, p.239).
- Inhalation of mud/sand etc may require bronchoscopy for clearance.

Outcome

Resuscitation without cerebral deficit is possible after prolonged submersion (even >60min), particularly if associated with hypothermia. 50% of children recovered apparently lifeless will survive, and even adults with $GCS^{3-4}/_{15}$ and fixed dilated pupils can survive unimpaired.

Respiratory effort is a sensitive prognostic sign, but in hypothermic patients its absence does not necessarily imply poor outcome. Note the time to the first spontaneous inspiratory gasp.

Poor prognostic factors include extremes of age, severe acidosis, immersion >5 min, and coma on admission.

Good prognostic factors include patients who are alert on admission, hypothermia, older children/adults, brief submersion time, and those who receive rapid on-scene basic life support and respond to initial resuscitation measures.

Asymptomatic patients who have no abnormality on repeated clinical examination, ABG and CXR require observation for at least 4–6 hours prior to considering discharge. Admit all others to ICU or general ward as appropriate.

Diving emergencies: 1

Consider any symptom developing within 48 hours of a dive as related to the dive until proven otherwise. On suspicion of a diving-related episode, seek specialist advice urgently (see Table 6.1).

Diving related emergencies fall into four main categories: drowning (📖 p.258), barotrauma, decompression illness, and marine bites or stings (📖 p.416).

Barotrauma

May occur in any gas-containing body cavity during descent or ascent.

Descent barotrauma ('squeeze') results from compression of gas in enclosed spaces as the ambient pressure ↑. Commonly, the ears, sinuses and skin are affected. Middle ear squeeze may be precipitated by Eustachian tube congestion and leads to erythema, haemorrhage, or tympanic membrane perforation with conductive hearing loss. Round or oval window rupture (inner ear squeeze) occurs with sudden pressure changes between the middle and inner ear and results in acute tinnitus, vertigo and deafness, and a perilymphatic fistula. ENT opinion is urgently required if a perilymphatic fistula is suspected and for cases of severe or continuing symptoms. If tympanic membrane rupture has not occurred, middle ear squeeze can usually be managed with decongestants/simple analgesics. If it has ruptured, give antibiotics (📖 p.551). Instruct the patient not to dive until the symptoms have resolved and the drum has completely healed.

Sinus barotrauma has a similar aetiology to middle ear injury and is often associated with URTI, mucosal polyps and sinusitis. Treat similarly to ear barotrauma.

Divers who fail to exhale periodically via the nose into their face mask during descent may develop 'face mask squeeze' (skin barotrauma). Erythema, bruising, and petechial and conjunctival haemorrhages develop in the enclosed area. Skin tightly enclosed by parts of the diving suit can have similar appearances. Usually no treatment is required.

Ascent barotrauma is the reverse of squeeze, and particularly affects the lungs. It may be caused by breath-holding during rapid uncontrolled ascent or by air trapping in patients with asthma or congenital lung bullae. Mediastinal emphysema is the commonest event and presents with ↑ hoarseness, neck swelling, and retrosternal chest discomfort. Symptoms usually resolve spontaneously with high concentrations of O_2. Pneumothorax is a potentially life-threatening complication if it develops during the dive, as the intrapleural gas cannot be vented and increasing ascent will precipitate tension. Conventional treatment by needle decompression, aspiration or chest drain insertion (📖 p.336) is required.

Dental pain may occur on ascent or descent in carious teeth or those which have had recent fillings. The affected tooth is tender on tapping. Treat symptomatically with analgesics and arrange dental referral.

Table 6.1 Sources of advice on diving emergencies and hyperbaric chambers

England, Wales, Northern Ireland

- Diving Incident Telephone Advice Line, Institute of Naval Medicine Gosport, Hampshire

  Telephone 07831 151523 (24 hrs)
  Ask for Duty Diving Medical Officer

- Diving Diseases Research Centre Plymouth
  www.ddrc.org

  Telephone 01752 209999 (24 hrs)
  Ask for the Duty Diving Doctor

Scotland

- Hyperbaric Medicine Unit Aberdeen Royal Infirmary
  www.hyperchamber.com

  Telephone 0845 408 6008
  State 'diving emergency'. Give your name and telephone number. Ask for the Duty Hyperbaric Doctor

In the event of any difficulties in contacting these agencies in the UK, telephone 999 and ask for COASTGUARD

Other countries

- Divers Alert Network
  www.diversalertnetwork.org

  DAN Diving Emergency Hotline (USA) +1 919 684 8111

This has links to diving emergency contact numbers throughout the world

Further information

Diving and Hyperbaric Medicine Division, Institute of Naval Medicine (Gosport, Hampshire, England). http://www.royalnavy.mod.uk/training-and-people/rn-life/medical-branch/institute-of-naval-medicine/diving-and-hyperbaric-medicine-division-dhmd/

Diving Diseases Research Centre (Hyperbaric Medical Centre, Plymouth, England). www.ddrc.org

British Hyperbaric Association. www.hyperbaric.org.uk/

Scottish Diving Medicine. www.sdm.scot.nhs.uk

Divers Alert Network. www.diversalertnetwork.org

Diving emergencies: 2

Decompression illness

There are two forms of decompression illness. The first occurs when dissolved nitrogen in blood and tissues is not expelled at a sufficient rate to prevent bubble formation. The second occurs when air bubbles are released into the circulation because of pulmonary barotrauma. This follows if air bubbles enter the pulmonary capillaries from ruptured alveoli. The bubbles travel via the left side of the heart to the systemic circulation. Cerebral air embolism usually causes symptoms as the diver surfaces, with loss of consciousness, fits, cardiovascular collapse and chest pain. Clinically, differentiation between the two forms is difficult and initial management is the same. In general, the sooner the onset of symptoms, the greater the likely severity. Symptoms may be attributed by the patient (and the unwary doctor) to musculoskeletal sprains/strains or other minor injury.

Decompression illness is more likely in divers who have not followed safe ascent recommendations, the obese, in cold water, and when excessive exercise has occurred during the dive. It may be precipitated by air travel if insufficient time is left between diving and flying for residual nitrogen to leave the body in a controlled fashion. Bubbles have direct mechanical and local inflammatory effects, commonly involving joints, skin, CNS, lungs and ears.

Joint pain, 'the bends', most often affects shoulders and elbows. A dull aching sensation, ↑ by movement but without localized tenderness is common. Pruritic rashes, local swelling and a *peau d'orange* effect may occur. Back pain, limb weakness, sensory abnormalities or urinary retention imply spinal cord involvement. Central effects include focal deficits, cerebellar disturbance and mood changes.

Treatment for decompression illness is recompression. If delayed, risks of permanent damage to brain and spinal cord greatly ↑. The diagnosis of decompression sickness may only follow the response to recompression. Pending this, give the highest possible concentration of O_2. Analgesics and sedatives can mask recompression responses and should only be used on specialist advice. Entonox® is absolutely contraindicated.

If intubation is required, inflate the ET tube cuff with sterile water, since during recompression an air-filled cuff will deflate. IV fluids (0.9% saline or a plasma expander) assist oxygenation of ischaemic tissues and facilitate discharge of excess tissue nitrogen load into the venous system by ensuring adequate circulating volume. Some centres may recommend aspirin and/or dextran solutions to ↓ capillary sludging which accompanies severe decompression sickness.

Despite dry or wet suits, hypothermia is common. Treat with appropriate passive or active rewarming (📖 p.256).

Air evacuation If, after consultation with the diving medical centre, air evacuation is necessary, unpressurized aircraft should not fly above 300m. The diver should breathe 100% O_2. On reaching the diving centre, recompression to a simulated depth of 18m with 100% O_2 occurs, interspersed with periods of air breathing to ↓ O_2 toxicity risk. Slow decompression then follows standard treatment protocols.

Divers usually dive in pairs. If a diver has symptoms of decompression sickness or pulmonary barotrauma, his 'buddy' will be at risk also. Although recompression may not be required in the buddy, transfer him/her along with the affected diver and their diving equipment to the recompression facility.

Obtain the following information before referral, if possible:
- The patient's current condition, progression since onset, and response to treatment.
- Time of onset of symptoms related to the dive.
- Dive profile and history (depth, duration, activity during the dive, speed of ascent including details of any stoppages, environmental conditions (water temperature, currents, etc.), pre-dive exercise, alcohol, drugs and food, type and condition of diving equipment used, clothing worn, other recent dives). Many divers store much of this information in a dive computer.
- Previous medical history, previous diving-related episodes, drug history.

Heat illness

Body T° is normally kept at 36–38°C by homeostatic mechanisms which are controlled by the hypothalamus. Hyperthermia occurs when these mechanisms are overwhelmed by factors acting individually, or (commonly) together. These conditions can occur even in temperate climates. At-risk groups include the young and the elderly in conditions of ↑ temperature and humidity, and patients with unaccustomed or prolonged muscular activity (eg at 'raves', associated with ecstasy or other drugs), grand mal fitting, athletes, marathon runners and armed forces recruits.

Predisposing medical factors include
- Alcohol use or withdrawal (including delirium tremens).
- Cardiac disease.
- Any condition which may cause or aggravate Na^+/H_2O loss (eg gastroenteritis, cystic fibrosis).
- Drugs, including: alcohol, diuretics, salicylates, anticholinergics (antihistamines, tricyclic antidepressants), sympathomimetics (amphetamines, ecstasy, LSD, cocaine, phencyclidine, appetite suppressants), phenothiazines, antipsychotics, MAOI, SSRI.

Heat illness has a spectrum of severity:

Heat cramps ⇔ Heat exhaustion ⇔ Heat stroke

In *heat cramps/exhaustion*, homeostatic mechanisms still function, but are overwhelmed.

In *heat stroke*, all thermoregulatory control is lost, body temperature ↑ rapidly to very high levels (>41°C) causing widespread severe tissue and organ damage. Mortality may exceed 10%.

Heat cramps

Core T° of 37–39°C. Mental function is normal. Sweating during exercise and replacement with hypotonic fluid leads to Na^+ deficiency. Brief cramps occur in muscles used in heavy work, usually after exertion.

Heat exhaustion

Core T°<40°C. Mental function is normal. Characterized by mixed Na^+/H_2O depletion. Sweating and tachycardia are usually present. Symptoms of weakness, fatigue, headache, vertigo, nausea and vomiting, postural dizziness, syncope. Patients will recover with rest and fluids.

In mild cases, remove from heat and use simple cooling techniques. Rehydrate with oral electrolyte solutions.

More severe cases require IV 0.9% saline or 0.45% saline/5% dextrose. Use clinical assessment, U&E and haematocrit to guide infusion rate. Up to 4L of fluid may be required over 6–12hr. Avoid over-rapid infusion which may cause pulmonary and/or cerebral oedema.

Measurement of core temperature

Tympanic or rectal T° measurement is appropriate in the ED, but may underestimate core T° and respond slowly as this changes. Oesophageal and intravascular probes give the most accurate readings of core T° but require special equipment.

Heat stroke

Suspect in collapse during or after exercise and in high risk groups. Core T° is >41°C (but significant cooling can occur before arrival in the ED). There is multi-system damage especially to the CNS. Outcome depends upon the height and duration of ↑ T°. Mortality is ≈10%.

- *CNS*: oedema + petechial haemorrhages cause focal/generalized damage.
- *Muscle injury* releases enzymes, myoglobin, urate, K^+, PO_4^{3-}.
- *Liver*: damaged cells release enzymes. Jaundice commonly develops after 24hr.
- *Kidneys*: ARF from hypovolaemia, muscle breakdown products, acidosis, DIC.
- *Blood*: DIC, thrombocytopenia, leucocytosis.
- *Metabolic*: ↑ or ↓ K^+, metabolic acidosis, respiratory alkalosis, hypoglycaemia.

Features

Sweating may be present. The skin surface may feel deceptively cool due to peripheral vasoconstriction.

- *CNS*: confusion, delirium, fitting, coma, oculogyric crisis, dilated pupils, tremor, muscle rigidity, decerebrate posturing, cerebellar dysfunction.
- *CVS*: tachycardia, hypotension, arrhythmias.
- *Coagulopathy*: purpura, conjunctival haemorrhages, melaena, haematuria.

Investigations

ABG, U&E, BMG, CK, clotting screen, LFTs, urate, Ca^{2+}, PO_4^{3-}, ECG, CXR.

Treatment

- Rapid therapy is vital. Do not wait for the results of investigations.
- Remove the patient from the hot environment and remove all clothing.
- Secure the airway (intubation and IPPV if needed). Give high FiO_2.
- Cooling techniques depend upon facilities available and the clinical state of the patient. Do not give 'antipyretics' such as aspirin/paracetamol. Evaporative cooling is the most efficient and applicable treatment. Spray the naked patient with tepid tap water and blow air over the body with fans. Ice-packs can be applied to the axillae, groins, neck, and scalp (but avoid prolonged contact). Consider cold gastric or peritoneal lavage, or cardiopulmonary bypass if these techniques fail. Aim for cooling rate of at least 0.1°C/min. When core T° <39°C stop active cooling as hypothermia may develop.
- *IV fluids*: give 50mL 50% dextrose IV if BMG <3mmol/litre. Severe hypovolaemia is uncommon. If hypotension persists despite ↓ T°, give IV 0.9% saline (1–1.5L over 1–2hr). Avoid overloading circulation with risk of pulmonary/cerebral oedema. CVP monitoring may be needed. CVP may be initially ↑ due to peripheral vasoconstriction.
- Insert a urinary catheter. If myoglobinuria is present, aim for ↑ urine output, and consider giving IV bicarbonate and/or mannitol.
- If fits occur, give IV lorazepam—but beware of respiratory depression.

Neuroleptic malignant syndrome is an idiosyncratic reaction in patients on antipsychotics (especially haloperidol, thioridazine, chlorpromazine). Features are muscle rigidity, extrapyramidal signs, autonomic dysfunction, severe dyskinesia. Stop the antipsychotic, cool the patient, and give dantrolene.

Malignant hyperpyrexia is a rare autosomal dominant condition related to use of suxamethonium and volatile anaesthetics. Dantrolene prevents Ca^{2+} release from skeletal muscle and is very effective: initial dose is 2–3mg/kg IV, then 1 mg/kg as needed, max total dose 10 mg/kg. See guidelines: www.aagbi.org/publications/guidelines/docs/malignanthyp07amended.pdf

Electrical injuries

An electric shock can cause cardiac and respiratory arrest. The heart often restarts spontaneously, but the respiratory arrest may be prolonged, causing fatal hypoxia. Thermal injury from the electric current produces burns and muscle damage. Muscle spasms from a shock may result in dislocations or fractures or precipitate a fall causing major trauma. Fatal electrocution can occur from domestic electricity (in the UK 230 volts, alternating current at 50cycles/sec), but severe injury is more common with high voltage shocks (>1000V).

Lightning causes a direct current (DC) shock at a very high voltage (up to 100,000,000V), but short duration (0.1–1msec).

Electrical flash and arc burns

An electrical short-circuit near to a person may cause sudden vaporization of metal and deposition of a thin layer of hot metal on the skin, without any electricity passing through the casualty. Electrical flash burns may look dramatic because of discolouration of the skin, but are often superficial and heal uneventfully. In contrast, electrical arcing produces high temperatures, and may cause deep dermal or full thickness burns, especially if clothing is set alight.

Contact burns

If electricity has passed through the patient there are usually two or more entry or exit wounds, which are full thickness burns with white or charred edges. Tissue damage is more extensive than the visible burns, especially with high voltage injuries. Deeper layers of skeletal muscle may be involved and muscle damage can cause myoglobinuria and renal failure. Myonecrosis and oedema of muscles may produce a compartment syndrome (📖 p.398).

If current passes through the torso, cardiac arrhythmias are more likely than if only a single limb is involved. Myocardial damage may occur, often in association with vascular injuries.

Neurological effects of electric shocks include coma, fits, headaches, transient paralysis, peripheral neuropathy, and mood disturbances.

Ophthalmic injuries are common after electrical burns of the head. Cataracts and glaucoma may develop later.

Electrocution in pregnancy has major risks for the foetus (spontaneous abortion has been reported). Obtain obstetric advice.

Lightning

The sudden vaporization of sweat and rain water caused by lightning may explode clothes and shoes off the victim and rupture ear drums. Lightning burns are superficial, often with a characteristic feathered or fern-like appearance. The limbs are often cold and mottled due to arterial spasm, which usually resolves over a few hours. Deep muscle damage and myoglobinuria are rare. Coma may result from direct brain injury, head injury due to a fall, or cardiac arrest. CPR, if indicated, may be successful even if required for prolonged periods. Survivors may be confused and amnesic for several days and may have fits and temporary paralysis. Cataracts are common.

Management

- At the scene, make sure that the current is turned off before anyone approaches or touches the casualty. Remember that high voltage electricity can arc through the air or pass through the ground.
- Check the airway, breathing and circulation. Electrical burns of the mouth and throat may cause oedema and airway obstruction.
- Perform CPR if necessary, but minimize movement of the spine in case of trauma.
- Examine thoroughly for head, chest, abdominal and skeletal injuries.
- Examine all over for skin entry/exit burns, and check pulses and sensation.
- Check the ECG: there may be arrhythmias (eg atrial fibrillation), conduction defects, ST elevation and T wave changes.
- Check FBC, U&E and creatine kinase (except in minor low-voltage burns).
- Test the urine for blood. If the stick test is +ve for blood, but there are no red blood cells on microscopy, treat for myoglobinuria to prevent renal failure: obtain specialist advice, maintain a high urine output, and consider using mannitol ± isotonic sodium bicarbonate.
- Fluid loss into muscles results in hypovolaemia: IV fluids are often required. After high voltage injuries, widespread fasciotomies may be needed, with excision or amputation of non-viable tissues and inspection and further debridement after 48 hours.

Admission

It is reasonable to allow home asymptomatic patients with domestic and minor low voltage burns, a normal ECG, no history suggestive of arrhythmia (eg palpitations) and no myoglobinuria, but advise review if any problem develops.

Admit children who bite electric flexes for observation, because of the risk of delayed bleeding from labial blood vessels.

Many patients with electrical injuries will need admission for observation and monitoring. Admit all patients with high voltage conduction injuries, cardiac arrhythmias, chest pain or ECG abnormalities, vascular injury or myoglobinuria.

Radiation incidents

In the UK, 24 hour advice and assistance is available via NAIR (National Arrangements for Incidents involving Radioactivity) on telephone 0800 834153 or via the police. Try to distinguish between external irradiation of a person and contamination with radioactive material. Someone exposed to X-rays or to gamma rays in a radiation sterilizing unit receives no further radiation after removal from the source, and there is no risk of contaminating anyone else. However, a person contaminated with radioactive material is still exposed to radiation and needs urgent, careful decontamination to minimize the risks to himself and to other people. Some hospitals are officially designated for the care of casualties contaminated with radioactive substances, but in an emergency a patient may be taken to any ED, where a plan for such events should exist.

Anticipation of a radiation accident

- Inform the ED consultant on duty immediately if a patient from a radiation incident arrives or is expected.
- Get advice and help from a radiation physicist (from Medical Physics or radiotherapy department).
- Implement the appropriate Radiation Incident Plan to deal with the patient.
- Expect media enquiries.

Treatment of contaminated casualties

Where possible, treatment should take place in a designated decontamination room. This room should have a separate entrance, ventilation arrangements, decontamination facilities with shower, and contaminated water collection facilities. Cover the floor of this room and entrance/exit corridors with disposable sheeting. All staff must themselves be decontaminated and checked before leaving this area.

- Turn off air conditioning.
- Pregnant and potentially pregnant staff should not be involved.
- Provide any necessary life-saving treatment, but avoid spreading contamination.
- 'Barrier nurse', as for an infectious disease.
- Assume patients are contaminated until they have been checked by the radiation physicist.
- Instruct patients and staff not to eat, drink, or smoke.
- Involve the minimum number of staff, who should wear facemasks, theatre clothing with impermeable gowns or plastic aprons, two pairs of gloves, and overshoes or rubber boots.
- Restrict and record movements of people in and out of the room.
- Ensure that the ambulance crew waits for monitoring of themselves and their vehicle.
- Keep everything that may be contaminated for radiation testing.
- Collect the patient's clothes, dressings, swabs, and any equipment used in plastic bags, and keep them in the decontamination room.
- All blood/urine samples must be specially labelled and the laboratories informed of the radiation risk.
- Life-threatening injuries may take precedence over all of the above, such that patients may need to be managed in the resuscitation room.

Decontamination of the patient

The radiation physicist should determine the sites of contamination and monitor the effectiveness of treatment. The object is to remove any contaminating substance and minimize absorption into the body, especially via the mouth, nose, and wounds.

- Cover any wounds prior to decontamination.
- Avoid splashing.
- Radioactive material can usually be removed from intact skin by washing with soap and water. Gentle scrubbing may be needed, but it is important to avoid damaging the skin. Carefully clean wounds and irrigate with water or saline.
- Clean the mouth using a mouthwash and a soft toothbrush, with care to avoid swallowing any fluid.
- Instruct the patient to blow their nose into paper handkerchiefs. If the nose is still contaminated irrigate it with small amounts of water.
- Irrigate each eye from the medial side outwards to avoid draining contaminated water into the nasolacrimal duct.
- Clean the hair by washing with shampoo and by clipping if contamination persists, but do not shave the scalp.
- If monitoring shows that all contamination has been removed, treat the patient as for an irradiated, but uncontaminated patient. However, if contamination persists, or if radioactive material has been ingested or inhaled, further treatment will be needed after discussion with a radiation specialist.
- Check all staff involved in treating the patient for radioactive contamination before they leave the treatment area.

The irradiated patient

A patient who has been irradiated or contaminated with radiation may be at risk of radiation sickness or other ill effects. Admit to a designated unit for assessment and follow-up by a radiotherapist or other specialist.

Initial symptoms of radiation sickness are malaise, nausea, vomiting, and diarrhoea, starting a few hours after exposure. There is then a latent period before the main effects of radiation sickness appear. Record any symptoms and the time of onset. The effects of anxiety and stress may be similar to the early features of radiation sickness.

Take blood for FBC, U&E, and blood group, recording the time on the blood tubes and in the notes. Measurement of the lymphocyte count and analysis of chromosomes at known times after exposure are helpful in assessing the amount of radiation received and determining the prognosis. A low (<1.0 × 10^9/L) or falling lymphocyte count indicates serious radiation exposure.

Further information

Radiation incidents

http://www.hpa.org.uk/Topics/Radiation/UnderstandingRadiation/UnderstandingRadiationTopics/RadiationIncidents/incid_Nair/
www.hpa.org.uk (Health Protection Agency).

Deliberate release and CBRN incidents (see also 📖 p.210)
www.hpa.org.uk/emergency/CBRN.htm

Analgesia and anaesthesia

Pain relief

Many patients who come to the ED are in pain. Knowledge of the site and characteristics of the pain is often important in diagnosing the problem. Relief of pain is an essential and urgent part of treatment. Pain and distress may prevent patients giving useful details of history and symptoms and may not allow them to co-operate with investigations or treatment.

Methods of pain relief

Relieving pain often requires analgesic drugs, but other types of treatment are sometimes more important. If an injury is more painful than expected consider the possibility of infection (eg necrotizing fasciitis, 📖 p.234) or vascular compromise. Severe pain despite immobilization of a fracture suggests a vascular injury, compartment syndrome (📖 p.398) or a tight plaster (📖 p.424). Reflex sympathetic dystrophy (Sudeck's atrophy) may also cause severe pain starting a few days after relatively minor trauma.

Splintage

Immobilization of a fracture helps to relieve pain and ↓ requirement for analgesic drugs. Inhalation analgesia with Entonox® (📖 p.278) is often helpful while the splint or cast is being applied.

Elevation

Many limb injuries produce considerable swelling, which causes pain and stiffness. Elevate the limb to ↓ swelling, relieve the pain, and allow mobilization as soon as possible.

Cold

Cool burns as soon as possible, usually in cold water, to relieve the pain and stop any continuing thermal injury. Chemical burns from hydrofluoric acid (📖 p.397) are often extremely painful and need prolonged cooling in iced water. Pain from recent sprains and muscle injuries may be ↓ by cooling with ice-packs (or a pack of frozen peas) applied for 10–15min at a time, with a piece of towelling between the ice-pack and the skin.

Heat

Pain following sprains and strains of the neck, back, and limbs is often caused by muscle spasm. It may be eased by heat from a hot bath, hot water bottle, or heat lamp.

Dressings

Pain from minor burns and fingertip injuries often resolves after a suitable dressing is applied.

Local anaesthesia (LA)

LA provides excellent pain relief for fractured shaft of femur (📖 p.304, 472) and for some finger and hand injuries (📖 p.292). Strongly consider giving analgesia with LA before obtaining X-rays. Check for any possible nerve injury before injecting LA.

Definitive treatment

Reducing a pulled elbow or trephining a subungual haematoma usually gives immediate relief of pain, so no analgesia is needed.

Psychological aspects of pain relief

Anxiety and distress accompany pain and worsen patients' suffering. Psychological support is needed, as well as physical relief from pain. Patients are helped by caring staff who explain what is happening and provide support and reassurance. The presence of family members or a close friend is often helpful.

Analgesics

Many different analgesic drugs are available, but it is best to use only a few and become familiar with their actions, dosages, side effects, and contraindications. Most hospitals have analgesic policies and limit the choice of drugs which may be used. Before prescribing any drug, check what treatment has been given. The patient may already be taking analgesia or have supplies at home. Many drugs interact with others: important drug interactions are listed in the *BNF*. Ask about drug allergies and record them. Before giving aspirin or NSAIDs ask and record about indigestion, peptic ulceration and asthma.

Analgesics: aspirin and paracetamol

Aspirin

Aspirin is a good analgesic for headaches, musculoskeletal pain and dysmenorrhea, and has antipyretic and mild anti-inflammatory actions. It interacts with warfarin, some anticonvulsants and other drugs, and may exacerbate asthma and cause gastric irritation.

- Do not use aspirin in children <16 years or during breast feeding.
- Adult dose PO is 300–900mg 4–6 hourly (max 4g daily).

Paracetamol ('acetaminophen' in USA)

Paracetamol has similar analgesic and antipyretic actions to aspirin, but has no anti-inflammatory effects and causes less gastric irritation.

- The therapeutic dose range of paracetamol in children and adults is 10–15 mg/kg. In severe symptoms maximum single dose is 20 mg/kg. Adults and children who are small for age should be weighed and the dose calculated. In most patients the dose can safely be based on age.
- The adult dose is 0.5–1g 4–6 hourly (maximum 4g in 24 hours).
- For children aged less than 6 years use paracetamol infant suspension (120 mg/5 mL).
  - 2–3 months (babies with weight > 4 kg, born after 37 weeks): 2.5 mL (60 mg). If necessary a second 2.5 mL dose may be given after 4–6 hours. Do not give more than two doses in 24 hours.
  - 3–6 months: 2.5 mL (60 mg)
  - 6–24 months: 5 mL (120 mg)
  - 2–4 years: 7.5 mL (180 mg)
  - 4–6 years: 10 mL (240 mg).
- For children aged 6 years and over use paracetamol six plus suspension (250 mg/5 mL):
  - 6–8 years: 5 mL (250 mg)
  - 8–10 years: 7.5 mL (375 mg)
  - 10–12 years: 10 mL (500 mg).
- Paracetamol may be repeated 4–6 hourly. Adults, and children older than 3 months, may have a maximum of four doses in 24 hours.
- Overdosage can cause liver and renal damage (📖 p.190).

Compound analgesics (paracetamol + opioid)

Compound analgesic tablets containing paracetamol and low doses of opioids are widely used, but have little benefit over paracetamol alone and cause more side effects, such as constipation and dizziness, particularly in elderly people. These compound preparations include:

- *Co-codamol 8/500* (codeine phosphate 8mg, paracetamol 500mg).
- *Co-dydramol* (dihydrocodeine tartrate 10mg, paracetamol 500mg).

Compound preparations of paracetamol and full doses of opioids, eg co-codamol 30/500 (codeine phosphate 30mg, paracetamol 500mg), are more potent than paracetamol alone, but may cause opioid side effects, including nausea, vomiting, constipation, dizziness, drowsiness and respiratory depression. Opioid dependency can occur with prolonged usage.

Analgesics: NSAIDs

Non-steroidal anti-inflammatory drugs

NSAIDs are often used to treat musculoskeletal pain, with or without inflammation, although in many cases non-drug treatment (heat or cold, elevation) and paracetamol should be tried first. NSAIDs can cause gastric irritation, diarrhoea, GI bleeding and perforation, with ↑ risk at higher drug dosage and in patients aged >60 years and those with a history of peptic ulcer. NSAIDs may exacerbate asthma and can precipitate renal failure in patients with heart failure, cirrhosis or renal insufficiency. Interactions occur with diuretics, warfarin, lithium and other drugs (see *BNF*). When possible, advise that NSAIDs be taken after food to ↓ risk of GI side effects. If NSAID treatment is essential in patients at high risk of GI problems consider prophylactic treatment with misoprostol (see *BNF*).

Many NSAIDs are available and all can cause serious adverse effects, but ibuprofen, diclofenac and naproxen are relatively safe and cover most requirements. Ibuprofen has the lowest incidence of side effects, is the cheapest of these drugs and may be bought without prescription. Ibuprofen is useful in children as an analgesic and antipyretic, especially when paracetamol is insufficient.

- *Ibuprofen dosage* 1.2–1.8g daily in 3–4 divided doses (max 2.4g daily). Child (>7kg): 20mg/kg daily in 3–4 divided doses.
- *Diclofenac* (oral or rectal) 75–150mg daily in 2–3 divided doses.
- *Naproxen* 500mg initially, then 250mg 6–8-hourly (max 1.25g daily). *Acute gout* 750mg initially, then 250mg 8-hourly until pain resolves.

Injectable NSAIDs

Some NSAIDs may be given by injection for musculoskeletal pain (eg acute low back pain), or for renal or biliary colic. The contraindications and side effects are the same as for oral treatment. Intramuscular (IM) injections are painful and can cause sterile abscesses, so oral or rectal treatment is preferable. NSAIDs provide effective analgesia for renal colic, but the onset is slower than with IV opioids, which some prefer. A NSAID is particularly useful in suspected drug addicts who claim to have renal colic.

- *Ketorolac* may be given IM or slowly IV (initial dose 10mg over at least 15sec: see *BNF*). It is useful as an adjunct for MUAs.
- *Diclofenac* must be given by deep IM injection (not IV, which causes venous thrombosis). Dose: 75mg, repeated if necessary after 30min (max 150mg in 24 hours).

Topical NSAIDs

NSAID gels or creams applied to painful areas provide some analgesia, but are less effective than oral treatment. Systemic absorption may occur and cause adverse effects as for oral NSAIDs.

Analgesics: opioids

Morphine

Morphine is the standard analgesic for severe pain. As well as providing analgesia, it is sometimes used for cardiogenic pulmonary oedema (📖 p.101) to relieve distress and to help increase venous capacitance.

Morphine often causes nausea and vomiting in adults, so consider giving an anti-emetic (cyclizine 50mg IV/IM or prochlorperazine 12.5mg IM). Anti-emetics are not usually necessary in children aged < 10years.

Other side-effects of opioids include drowsiness and constipation. Respiratory depression and hypotension may occur, especially with large doses. Pinpoint pupils can complicate neurological assessment. Naloxone (📖 p.188) reverses the effects of opioids.

In acute conditions, give morphine by slow IV injection, which provides rapid but controlled analgesia. The dose varies with the patient and the degree of pain. Titrate the dose depending on the response: 2mg may be adequate in a frail old lady, but sometimes >20mg is needed in a young fit person with severe injuries. Dilute morphine with 0.9% saline to 1mg/mL (label the syringe clearly) and give it slowly IV (1–2mg/min in adults) in 1mg increments until pain is relieved. Give further analgesia if pain recurs. IV morphine dose in children is 100–200micrograms/kg, given in increments, repeated as necessary. Patient-controlled analgesia using a computerized syringe pump is very good for post-operative analgesia, but rarely appropriate in the ED.

IM injections provide slower and less controlled effects than IV analgesia: avoid their use, especially in shocked patients. IM morphine could be used in children needing strong analgesia but not IV fluids (eg while dressing superficial burns), but oral or nasal analgesia is preferable.

• *Morphine* may be given orally as *Oramorph*® oral solution:
  • *child aged 1–5 years:* max dose 5mg (2.5mL);
  • *child aged 6–12 years:* max dose 5–10mg (2.5–5mL).
• *Codeine* is given orally for moderate pain (30–60mg 4hrly, max 240mg daily) and has side effects similar to morphine. Codeine may also be given IM (but not IV, because it may cause hypotension).
• *Dihydrocodeine* is very similar to codeine.
• *Diamorphine (heroin)* has similar effects to morphine, but is more soluble and so can be dissolved in a very small volume of diluent. Nasal diamorphine provides effective analgesia in children (📖 p.281).
• *Fentanyl* is a short-acting opioid which is often used in anaesthesia.
• *Pethidine* provides rapid but brief analgesia, but is less potent than morphine. It is sometimes used for renal or biliary colic in preference to morphine, which occasionally causes smooth muscle spasm (📖 p.277). Pethidine is given slowly IV, titrated as necessary (usual adult dose 50mg IV), or less effectively IM (50–100mg). Give an anti-emetic with it.

Smooth muscle spasm due to opioid analgesics

In a few patients opioids such as morphine can cause severe pain due to smooth muscle spasm, especially spasm of the sphincter of Oddi. About 5–20 minutes after morphine has been given, severe colicky abdominal pain develops. This may be typical of biliary colic but can mimic renal colic, intestinal perforation or myocardial infarction.

Pain from spasm of the sphincter of Oddi may be relieved by glucagon (1mg IV, repeated if necessary) although this is liable to cause vomiting. Naloxone (0.2mg IV, repeated if necessary) is also effective, but may reverse desired analgesia. GTN can also relieve smooth muscle spasm of the sphincter of Oddi. Glucagon is probably the treatment of choice for this rare complication of opioid analgesia.

Analgesics: Entonox® and ketamine

Entonox®

Entonox® is a mixture of 50% N_2O and 50% O_2. It is stored as a compressed gas in blue cylinders with a blue and white shoulder. It is unsuitable for use at <−6°C, since the gases separate and a hypoxic mixture could be given. Entonox® diffuses more rapidly than nitrogen and so is *contraindicated* with the following: undrained pneumothorax (since it may produce a tension pneumothorax), after diving (↑ risk of decompression sickness), facial injury, base of skull fracture, intestinal obstruction, ↓ conscious level.

Entonox® is controlled by a demand valve and inhaled through a mask or mouthpiece, often held by the patient. It gives rapid and effective analgesia and is widely used in prehospital care. In the ED, Entonox® is useful for initial analgesia, eg while splinting limb injuries, and for many minor procedures, such as reduction of a dislocated patella or finger. Tell the patient to breathe deeply through the mask or mouthpiece, and warn that he may feel drowsy or drunk, but that this will wear off within a few minutes.

Ketamine

Ketamine is a dissociative anaesthetic drug which may be given IM or IV by experts, and which provides strong analgesia in sub-anaesthetic dosage. It is rarely used in hospital practice for adults, because it may cause severe hallucinations, but these are less of a problem in children. It is very useful for sedation of children for procedures such as suturing of minor wounds. Ketamine is particularly useful in prehospital care and is the most appropriate drug in the rare cases when a GA is needed outside hospital for extrication or emergency amputation.

Airway-protective reflexes are maintained better with ketamine than with other induction agents, but airway obstruction and aspiration of gastric contents are still potential hazards. Respiratory depression is uncommon at normal dosage. Ketamine is a bronchodilator and may be used in asthmatics. It stimulates the cardiovascular system and often causes tachycardia and hypertension, so avoid it in severe hypertension. Hallucinations are less likely if a small dose of midazolam is given and the patient is not disturbed during recovery from anaesthesia.

Ketamine is available in *3 strengths*: 10, 50, and 100mg/mL, which are easily confused. The IV dose for GA is 1–2mg/kg over 1min, which is effective after 2–7min and provides surgical anaesthesia for 5–10min. The IM dose for GA is 10mg/kg, which is effective after 4–15min and gives surgical anaesthesia for 12–25min. Further doses (10–20mg IV or 20–50mg IM) can be given if major limb movements or ↑ muscle tone prevent extrication of the patient.

For sedation of children undergoing suturing or other minor procedures, ketamine may be given IM (2.5mg/kg) or IV (1mg/kg over at least 1min). With this dose of ketamine, LA is needed for cleaning and suturing of wounds, but little physical restraint should be needed to allow the procedure to take place. Occasionally, a second dose of ketamine (1mg/kg IM or 0.5mg/kg IV) is required to achieve adequate sedation. Larger initial doses provide deeper sedation, but are more likely to cause side effects (eg vomiting or agitation) during recovery. With low doses of ketamine, agitation is unlikely and there is no need to add midazolam.

Analgesia for trauma

Multiple injuries

Entonox® may be useful for analgesia during transport and initial resuscitation, but only allows administration of 50% O_2 and should not be used if there is an undrained pneumothorax. As soon as practicable use other forms of analgesia, usually IV morphine (📖 p.276) and/or nerve blocks (📖 p.292), and splint fractures to ↓ pain and ↓ blood loss.

Head injury

Relief of pain is particularly important in head-injured patients, since pain and restlessness ↑ ICP, which can exacerbate secondary brain injury. Headache following a head injury can usually be treated with paracetamol, diclofenac or codeine phosphate (which may cause less central depression than stronger opioids such as morphine). If the headache is severe or increasing, arrange a CT scan to look for an intracranial haematoma. Try to avoid strong opioids, because of concern about sedation and respiratory depression, but if pain is severe give morphine in small IV increments: the effects can be reversed if necessary with naloxone. Femoral nerve block is particularly useful in a patient with a head injury and a fractured femur, since it ↓ or avoids the need for opioids.

Small children with minor head injuries often deny having headaches, but look and feel much better if given paracetamol (📖 p.274). Give further doses if necessary over the following 12–24 hours.

Chest injury

Chest injuries are often extremely painful. Good analgesia is essential to relieve distress and ↓ risk of complications such as pneumonia and respiratory failure. Avoid Entonox® if a pneumothorax is a possibility, until this has been excluded or drained. Give high concentration O_2 as soon as possible and check SpO_2 and ABG. Give morphine in slow IV increments (📖 p.276) and monitor for respiratory problems. Intercostal nerve blocks (📖 p.303) provide good analgesia for fractured ribs, but may cause a pneumothorax and should only be used in patients being admitted. In severe chest injuries get anaesthetic or ICU help: thoracic epidural anaesthesia can sometimes avoid the need for IPPV. Before a thoracic epidural is performed, check X-rays of the thoracic spine for fractures.

Analgesia in specific situations

Children

Injured children are distressed by both fear and pain. Parental support can be very helpful. Sensitive treatment, explanation and reassurance are important, but give analgesia whenever necessary.

Oral analgesia is usually with paracetamol (📖 p.274), but if this is inadequate add ibuprofen (📖 p.275), dihydrocodeine elixir, or Oramorph®:

- *Ibuprofen dose:* 20mg/kg daily in divided doses as ibuprofen suspension (100mg in 5mL) 1–2 years: 2.5mL; 3–7 years: 5mL; 8–12 years: 10mL; all 3–4 times daily.
- *Dihydrocodeine elixir dose:* 0.5–1mg/kg PO 4–6-hourly.
- Children in severe pain may benefit from oral morphine (as Oramorph® oral solution—📖 p.276).

Entonox® (📖 p.278) gives rapid analgesia without the need for an injection.

IV morphine is appropriate in severe injuries, but take particular care if there is a head injury, since sedation may occur.

Femoral nerve block (📖 p.304) provides good analgesia for femoral fractures and is usually well tolerated.

Digital nerve block with bupivacaine (📖 p.294) is useful for painful finger injuries, especially crush injuries. Provide this before X-ray: when the child returns from X-ray the finger may then be cleaned and dressed painlessly.

IM morphine could be used to provide analgesia for small burns or fractured arms, but oral morphine or nasal diamorphine are preferable, since IM injections are painful and unpleasant.

Nasal diamorphine is not licensed, but is playing an increasing role in the provision of pain relief in children (see Table 7.1).

Acute abdominal pain

It is cruel and unnecessary to withhold analgesia from patients with acute abdominal pain. Adequate analgesia allows the patient to give a clearer history, and often facilitates examination and diagnosis: tenderness and rigidity become more localized, and masses more readily palpable. Good X-rays cannot be obtained if the patient is distressed and restless because of renal colic or a perforated ulcer.

Morphine by slow IV injection (📖 p.276) is appropriate in severe pain, unless this is due to renal or biliary colic, in which an NSAID (📖 p.275) may be preferred. Morphine occasionally causes severe abdominal pain due to smooth muscle spasm of the sphincter of Oddi (📖 p.277).

Toothache

Toothache or pain after dental extractions can often be eased by aspirin, a NSAID or paracetamol. Do not give opioids such as codeine or dihydrocodeine, which may make the pain worse. Drainage of a dental abscess may be required to relieve toothache.

Nasal diamorphine for analgesia in children[1,2]

In the UK, diamorphine is licensed for use IV, IM, SC and PO. Nasal diamorphine is unlicensed, but clinical studies and experience have shown that this is an effective and acceptable method of analgesia for children with limb fractures or small burns who do not need immediate venous access. It should be given as soon as possible, prior to X-rays.

Contraindications: age <1 year (or weight <10kg), nasal obstruction or injury, basal skull fracture, opioid sensitivity.

Verbal consent for nasal diamorphine should be obtained from the child's parents (and the child if appropriate), since this is an unlicensed route of administration of this drug. Follow local protocols.

The dose of nasal diamorphine is 0.1mg/kg, given in a syringe in a volume of 0.2mL. The child is weighed. The appropriate concentration of solution for the weight of child is achieved by adding a suitable volume of 0.9% saline to a 10mg ampoule of diamorphine.

Table 7.1 Dosage of nasal diamorphine in children

Weight (kg)	Volume of saline (mL)	Dose of diamorphine (mg) in 0.2mL
10	2.0	1.0
15	1.3	1.5
20	1.0	2.0
25	0.8	2.5
30	0.7	2.9
35	0.6	3.3
40	0.5	4.0
50	0.4	5.0
60	0.3	6.7

0.2mL of this solution is drawn up into a syringe and given in one or both nostrils, whilst the child's head is tilted backwards. Turn the head to each side, maintaining each position for several secs. A small syringe can be used to drip the solution into the nose, but if possible use an aerosol device (eg MAD®), allowing for the dead space of the device (0.1mL for MAD, so draw up 0.3mL). Record the time of administration. Monitor conscious level for 20min. Respiratory depression is unlikely, but resuscitation facilities and naloxone must be available. Nasal diamorphine provides rapid analgesia which lasts up to 4 hr.

Fentanyl may also be used nasally (initial dose 2micrograms/kg) as an alternative to nasal diamorphine.

1 College of Emergency Medicine Clinical Effectiveness Committee (2009). *Guideline for the management of pain in children*. College of Emergency Medicine, London.
2 http://intranasal.net/PainControl/default.htm

Local anaesthesia (LA)

Indications for LA in the emergency department

LA is indicated in any situation in which it will provide satisfactory analgesia or safe and adequate conditions for operations or procedures. These include the following:

- *Insertion of venous cannulae* (0.1mL of 1% lidocaine SC 30 secs prior to cannulation ↓ pain of cannulation without affecting the success rate).
- *Cleaning, exploration and suturing* of many wounds.
- *Analgesia for some fractures,* eg shaft of femur.
- *Minor operations/procedures,* eg manipulation of some fractures and dislocations, insertion of chest drain, drainage of paronychia, removal of corneal FB.

Contraindications to local anaesthetic

- *Refusal or poor co-operation by the patient.*
- *Allergy to local anaesthetic* Severe allergic reactions to LA are rare, but anaphylaxis can occur. If allergy to a LA is alleged, obtain full details of the circumstances and the drug involved and check with a senior before giving any LA. It may be possible to use a different drug. Some reactions are caused by the preservative in multi-dose vials, rather than the drug itself, so single dose ampoules may not cause a problem. Some alleged 'allergies' are actually toxic effects due to overdosage, or faints due to fear and pain.
- *Infection at the proposed injection site* Injection into an inflamed area is painful and could spread infection. High tissue acidity from inflammation ↓ effectiveness of LA drugs. Hyperaemia causes rapid removal of the drug and so a short duration of action and ↑ risk of toxicity. LA nerve block at a site away from the infected area can provide good anaesthesia, eg digital nerve block for paronychia or nerve blocks at the ankle for an abscess on the sole of the foot.
- *Bleeding disorder* Anticoagulant therapy and thrombocytopenia are contraindications for nerve blocks in which there is a risk of inadvertent arterial puncture.

Special cautions (↑ risk of toxicity)

- Small children.
- Elderly or debilitated.
- Heart block.
- Low cardiac output.
- Epilepsy.
- Myasthenia gravis.
- Hepatic impairment.
- Porphyria.
- Anti-arrhythmic or β-blocker therapy (risk of myocardial depression).
- Cimetidine therapy (inhibits metabolism of lidocaine).

Lidocaine (lignocaine)

Lidocaine is the LA used most often for local infiltration and for nerve blocks. It is available in 0.5%, 1% and 2% solutions, either 'plain' (without adrenaline) or with adrenaline 1:200,000. For routine use the most suitable choice is 1% plain lidocaine.

Duration of action Lidocaine acts rapidly and the effects last from 30–60min (for plain lidocaine) to 90min (lidocaine with adrenaline). The duration of action varies with the dosage and the local circulation.

For *plain lidocaine* the maximum dose is 200mg (20mL of 1% solution) in a healthy adult or 3mg/kg in a child.

For *lidocaine with adrenaline* the maximum dose is 500mg (50mL of 1% solution) in a healthy adult or 7mg/kg in a child.

These are the maximum total doses for one or more injections of LA given together for local infiltration or nerve block (with care to avoid intravascular injection). Reduce the dose in debilitated or elderly patients, or if there is a particular risk of toxicity (see opposite).

Lidocaine can also be used for anaesthesia of the skin (with prilocaine in EMLA® cream, 📖 p.288), urethra and cornea, and also as a spray for anaesthetizing mucous membranes in the mouth and throat.

Bupivacaine

Bupivacaine is particularly useful for nerve blocks since it has a long duration of action (3–8hr), although its onset of anaesthesia is slower than lidocaine. It may also be used for local infiltration, but *not* for Bier's block (📖 p.290). Bupivacaine is available in concentrations of 0.25 and 0.5% with or without adrenaline: the usual choice is 0.5% bupivacaine without adrenaline. The maximum dose of bupivacaine (with or without adrenaline) for a fit adult is 150mg (30mL of 0.5% or 60mL of 0.25%) and for a child 2mg/kg.

Prilocaine

Prilocaine has a similar duration of action to lidocaine. It can be used for local infiltration or nerve blocks, but is particularly useful for Bier's block (📖 p.290). High doses (usually >600mg) may cause methaemoglobinaemia. The maximum dose of prilocaine for a healthy adult is 400mg (40mL of 1% solution) and for a child 6mg/kg.

Tetracaine (amethocaine)

Tetracaine is used for topical local anaesthesia of the cornea (📖 p.535) and skin (📖 p.288).

Proxymetacaine

Proxymetacaine is also used for topical local anaesthesia of the cornea. It causes less initial stinging than tetracaine and is particularly useful in children.

Local anaesthetic toxicity

Toxic effects

These result from overdosage of LA or inadvertent intravascular injection. The first symptoms and signs are usually neurological, with numbness of the mouth and tongue, slurring of speech, lightheadedness, tinnitus, confusion and drowsiness. Muscle twitching, convulsions and coma can occur.

Cardiovascular toxicity may initially result in tachycardia and hypertension, but later there is hypotension with a bradycardia and heart block. Ventricular arrhythmias and cardiac arrest occur occasionally, especially with bupivacaine.

Early signs of toxicity

These may be detected if the doctor maintains a conversation with the patient while injecting LA. Toxic effects may start immediately if an intravascular injection is given. However, peak blood levels usually occur ≈10–25min after injection—so if a relatively large dose has been given, do not leave the patient alone while anaesthesia develops.

Occasionally, patients initially agree to LA, but become hysterical or faint (even while lying flat) when an injection is given. In such circumstances it may be difficult to distinguish immediately between the effects of anxiety and those of drug toxicity.

Treatment of LA toxicity

- Stop the procedure.
- Call for help.
- Clear and maintain the airway.
- Give 100% O_2 and ensure adequate lung ventilation.
- Obtain reliable IV access. If possible take blood for U&E.
- Monitor ECG. Record pulse, BP, respiratory rate and conscious level.
- If convulsions occur ensure adequate oxygenation and give lorazepam (adult dose 2–4mg slowly IV; child: 100micrograms/kg, max 4mg) or diazepam (adult 5–10mg slowly IV; child 100micrograms/kg).
- Treat hypotension by raising the foot of the trolley. If systolic BP remains <90mmHg in an adult, give IV fluids (eg colloid 500mL). In a child give 20mL/kg if systolic BP <70mmHg.
- Bradycardia usually resolves without treatment. If bradycardia and hypotension persist give atropine and consider IV lipid emulsion.
- In cardiac arrest due to LA toxicity, give lipid emulsion using Intralipid® 20% 1.5mL/kg over 1min (bolus of 100mL for 70kg patient) then 15mL/kg/hr (500mL over 30min for 70kg patient). Continue CPR. If circulation is still inadequate repeat IV bolus of Intralipid twice at 5min intervals then IVI 30mL/kg/hr (500mL over 15min). Maximum total dose of 20% lipid emulsion is 12mL/kg).
- See 📖 p.187 and http://www.aagbi.org/publications/guidelines/docs/la_toxicity_2010.pdf

Adrenaline (epinephrine) in local anaesthesia

Most local anaesthetics cause vasodilatation, so adrenaline is sometimes added as a vasoconstrictor. This ↓ blood loss, ↑ duration of anaesthesia and ↓ toxicity by delaying absorption of the LA. Lidocaine with adrenaline is often useful in scalp wounds, in which bleeding can be profuse but the bleeding point is not visible.

Bupivacaine with adrenaline is recommended for intercostal nerve block to ↓ risk of toxicity from rapid absorption in a relatively vascular area.

Lidocaine with adrenaline can be used in some situations (see below for contraindications) if a relatively large volume of LA is needed, since the max dose for a healthy adult is 500mg (50mL of 1% solution) compared to 200mg (20mL of 1%) for plain lidocaine. Other possibilities in such circumstances include 0.5% lidocaine, prilocaine (max dose: 40mL of 1% solution) or GA.

The maximum concentration of adrenaline in LA is 1 in 200,000, except for dental anaesthesia in which 1 in 80,000 may be used. The maximum total dose of adrenaline in a healthy adult is 500micrograms.

Contraindications and cautions

Never use adrenaline for injections in the nose, ears, or penis, nor in Bier's block (📖 p.290). Avoid adrenaline for injections in or near flap lacerations, since vasoconstriction could cause ischaemic necrosis. Adrenaline is traditionally regarded as dangerous in digital nerve blocks of fingers and toes, because of the risk of ischaemia, but some hand surgeons have used LA with adrenaline uneventfully to reduce bleeding and avoid the need for a finger tourniquet However, LA without adrenaline is advisable for routine use in fingers and toes, to avoid concerns about ischaemia.

Avoid adrenaline in:
• Ischaemic heart disease.
• Hypertension.
• Peripheral vascular disease.
• Thyrotoxicosis.
• Phaeochromocytoma.
• Patients on beta-blockers.

The *BNF* states that LA with adrenaline appears to be safe in patients on tricyclic antidepressants.

Storage Keep ampoules and vials of LA with adrenaline in a locked cupboard separate from those without adrenaline, so that they are only available by special request and are not used inadvertently or inappropriately.

General principles of local anaesthesia

Obtain a brief medical history and record drug treatment and allergies. Think about possible contraindications and cautions for LA (📖 p.282). Obtain expert advice if you have any query.

Consent for local anaesthetic

Explain to the patient what is planned. Verbal consent is adequate for most LA procedures in the ED.

Written consent is needed:
• If there is a significant risk of a toxic reaction or complication, including procedures needing large doses of LA.
• Bier's block (📖 p.290).
• Intercostal nerve block (risk of pneumothorax).

Safety

Ensure that resuscitation equipment and drugs for toxic reactions are readily available. Monitoring and IV access are not needed for routine simple LA, but are essential if there is a risk of complications or toxicity. Calculate the maximum dose of LA that could be used (📖 p.283) and think how much might be needed. Before drawing up any LA check the drug label carefully, especially if adrenaline is contraindicated.

Giving local anaesthetic

• Lie the patient down in a comfortable position with the site of injection accessible and supported. Some patients faint if LA is injected while they are sitting up.
• Warm the LA to body temperature prior to use.
• Wash your hands, use gloves, and clean the skin.
• Use a fine needle if possible. Before inserting the needle warn the patient and hold the relevant part firmly to prevent movement.
• Aspirate and check for blood in the syringe before injecting any LA. If the needle moves, aspirate again.
• Inject LA slowly to ↓ pain. Do not use force if there is resistance to injection.
• Maintain a conversation with the patient, to allay anxieties and also to detect any early signs of toxicity (📖 p.284).

Further details of techniques and precautions are listed on other pages:

Topical anaesthesia: 📖 p.288.

Local infiltration and field blocks: 📖 p.289.

Haematoma block for fractures: 📖 p.289.

Bier's block (IV regional anaesthesia): 📖 p.290.

Nerve blocks: 📖 pp.292–306.

Recording the local anaesthetic

Write clearly in the notes to record the time and site of injection and the type and quantity of LA given.

Local anaesthesia in children

The general principles are the same as for adults. LA is very useful in children, but requires experienced staff. Many children tolerate LA without any problem, but in some sedation with midazolam (📖 p.308) or ketamine (📖 p.278) can be helpful.

Weigh the child if possible and calculate the maximum dose of LA (📖 p.283). In an average size child a simple initial estimate of the maximum dose of 1% plain lidocaine is 1mL per year of age (ie 3mL for a 3-year-old child). If a larger volume may be needed, consider using 0.5% solution or lidocaine with adrenaline (📖 p.285), or possibly a GA instead.

Prepare everything before bringing the child into the room—rattling equipment and drawing up LA within sight of a patient causes unnecessary anxiety. Most parents prefer to stay with their child during the procedure and this is often helpful. Position the child and parent comfortably. Explain simply and honestly what is going to happen. Have adequate help to keep the child still. Use a small needle if possible and inject slowly to minimize pain from the injection.

Topical anaesthesia

LA applied directly to mucous membranes of the mouth, throat or urethra will diffuse through and block sensory nerve endings. Development of anaesthesia may take several minutes and the duration is relatively short because of the good blood supply. Over-dosage is dangerously easy because most topical preparations contain high concentrations of lidocaine (2% in lidocaine gel, 5% in ointment, and 4% or 10% in lidocaine spray).

Lidocaine gel has been used to allow cleaning of gravel burns, but this is not advisable: absorption of lidocaine can easily cause toxicity and the degree of anaesthesia is rarely satisfactory. Scrubbing is often necessary to remove embedded gravel, so proper anaesthesia is essential. Field block may be adequate for a small area, but GA is often necessary for cleaning large or multiple gravel burns, in order to avoid tattooing.

Topical anaesthesia

EMLA® cream

'Eutectic mixture of local anaesthetics' (EMLA®) cream contains lidocaine 2.5% and prilocaine 2.5%, and is used for topical anaesthesia of the skin. EMLA® is of limited value in the ED because it must only be applied to intact skin (not wounds) and the onset of anaesthesia is slow, usually ≈1 hour. EMLA® must not be used in children aged <1 year and caution is needed in patients with anaemia or methaemoglobinaemia.

EMLA® can usefully ↓ pain of an injection or cannulation. Apply a thick layer of EMLA® cream to the skin and cover it with an occlusive dressing, which must be left undisturbed for 1 hour.

Tetracaine (amethocaine) gel (Ametop®)

This is similar to EMLA®, but acts more quickly and causes vasodilatation, which aids venous cannulation. It must not be used in wounds because of the risk of rapid absorption and toxicity.

Other topical LA agents

Topical agents such as TAC (tetracaine, adrenaline, and cocaine) or LET (lidocaine, epinephrine and tetracaine) are sometimes used to provide anaesthesia for wound repair. These preparations can provide effective anaesthesia, but toxic effects may occur from excessive absorption (especially of cocaine) and they are not licensed in the UK.

Ethyl chloride

Ethyl chloride is a clear fluid which boils at 12.5°C. Spraying the liquid on the skin causes rapid cooling and freezing of the surface. In the past ethyl chloride was used for incision of paronychias and small abscesses, but it rarely provides adequate anaesthesia and it cannot be recommended. Ethyl chloride is highly inflammable and is a GA, so it must be handled with care if it is used at all.

Local anaesthetic administration

Local infiltration anaesthesia

Local infiltration is the technique used most often in the ED. The LA injected subcutaneously in the immediate area of the wound acts within 1–2min. Anaesthesia lasts 30–60min with plain lidocaine or ≈90min with lidocaine and adrenaline.

In clean wounds the pain of injection can often be ↓ by inserting the needle through the cut surface of the wound. Do not do this in dirty or old wounds, because of the risk of spreading infection. Less pain is produced by injecting slowly through a thin needle, injecting in a fan-shaped area from a single injection site, and by inserting the needle in an area already numbed by an earlier injection. Rapid injection of LA, especially in scalp wounds, can cause spraying of solution from the tip of the needle or from separation of the needle from the syringe. Slow injection and the use of goggles should ↓ risk of transmission of infection.

Field block

This involves infiltration of LA subcutaneously around the operative field. Sometimes it is only necessary to block one side of the area, depending on the direction of the nerve supply. Field block can be useful for ragged and dirty wounds, and for cleaning gravel abrasions. Check the max safe dose before starting a field block. If relatively large volumes of anaesthetic might be needed, consider 0.5% lidocaine or lidocaine with adrenaline (📖 p.285).

Haematoma block

A Colles' fracture (📖 p.444) can be manipulated after infiltration of LA into the fracture haematoma and around the ulnar styloid. This often provides less effective anaesthesia than Bier's block (📖 p.290) and a poorer reduction. It converts a closed fracture into an open one and so there is a theoretical risk of infection, but in practice this is rare.

Contraindications and warnings
- Fractures >24 hours old (since organization of the haematoma would prevent spread of the LA).
- Infection of the skin over the fracture.
- Methaemoglobinaemia (avoid prilocaine).

Drug and dosage 15mL of 1% plain prilocaine. Lidocaine can be used, but there is a lower margin of safety. Never use solutions containing adrenaline.

Technique Use a 20mL syringe and 0.6 × 25mm needle. Full asepsis is essential. Insert the needle into the fracture haematoma and aspirate blood to confirm this. Inject slowly to minimize pain and reduce the risk of high blood levels and toxicity. Anaesthesia develops in ≈5min and lasts for 30–60min. Sometimes anaesthesia is inadequate for proper manipulation and so an alternative anaesthetic is needed.

Bier's block

Bier's block (IV regional anaesthesia) is often used to provide anaesthesia for reduction of Colles' fractures or for minor surgery below the elbow. Bier's block uses a large dose of LA and so there is a risk of a toxic reaction, although this is minimized by correct technique. Ensure that the patient has fasted for 4 hours. Pre-operative assessment is necessary, including recording of BP and weight. Obtain written consent for the operation. Bier's block should only be performed by doctors who are competent to deal with severe toxic reactions. At least two trained staff must be present throughout the procedure.

Contraindications

- Severe hypertension or obesity.
- Severe peripheral vascular disease.
- Raynaud's syndrome.
- Sickle cell disease or trait.
- Methaemoglobinaemia.
- Children aged <7 years.
- Uncooperative or confused patient.
- Procedures needed in both arms.
- Surgery that may last >30min.
- Surgery that may need the tourniquet to be released.

Proceed with caution in epileptic patients because of the risk of a fit from LA toxicity.

Drug and dose

The only drug suitable for Bier's block is prilocaine, from a single dose vial without preservative. Never use solutions with adrenaline. Do not use lidocaine or bupivacaine, which are more likely than prilocaine to cause toxic effects. The ideal concentration of prilocaine is 0.5%. If only 1% prilocaine is available dilute it with an equal volume of 0.9% saline to make 0.5% prilocaine.

The dose of prilocaine is 3mg/kg, which is 42mL of 0.5% prilocaine for a 70kg adult, or 30mL of 0.5 % prilocaine for a 50kg patient.

Equipment

- Special tourniquet apparatus is essential, with a 15cm wide cuff for adults.
- Check the tourniquet apparatus and cuff regularly.
- Ordinary BP cuffs and sphygmomanometers are not reliable enough, and should not be used for Bier's blocks.
- Check that resuscitation equipment and drugs are available to hand.
- Ensure that the patient is on a tipping trolley.
- Monitor the ECG, BP and SpO_2 throughout.

Technique for Bier's block[1]

- Insert a small IV cannula in the dorsum of the hand on the side of operation (ready for injection of prilocaine) and another IV cannula in the opposite arm (for emergency use if needed).
- Check the radial pulse. Place the tourniquet high on the arm over padding, but do not inflate it yet.
- Elevate the arm for 3min while pressing over the brachial artery, to try to exsanguinate the limb. (Do not use an Esmarch bandage for this purpose, because of pain.)
- While the arm is elevated inflate the tourniquet to 300mmHg, or at least 100mmHg above the systolic BP. Lower the arm on to a pillow and check that the tourniquet is not leaking.
- Record the tourniquet time. A trained person must observe the tourniquet pressure constantly during the procedure.
- Slowly inject the correct volume of 0.5% plain prilocaine into the isolated limb, which will become mottled. If the operation is on the hand, squeeze the forearm during injection to direct LA peripherally. Test for anaesthesia after 5min. If anaesthesia is inadequate inject 10–15mL 0.9% saline to flush the prilocaine into the arm. Occasionally, no adequate anaesthesia is achieved and GA is needed instead.
- Complete the manipulation or operation. Before applying a POP back slab remove the cannula from the injured arm.
- The tourniquet cuff must remain inflated for at least 20min and a maximum of 45min.
- Obtain a check X-ray while the tourniquet cuff is still inflated (in case remanipulation is required).
- If the check X-ray is satisfactory deflate the tourniquet slowly and record the time. Maintain a conversation with the patient and watch carefully for any sign of toxicity. If any toxic effects occur re-inflate the tourniquet and give any necessary treatment (📖 p.284).
- After release of the tourniquet the arm becomes warm and flushed. Sensation returns after a few minutes.
- Observe the patient carefully for at least 30mins after a Bier's block in case of delayed toxicity. Check the circulation of the limb before the patient is discharged home. Reactive swelling can occur: elevate the limb in a sling and give POP instructions.

1 College of Emergency Medicine Clinical Effectiveness Committee (2010) *Intravenous regional anaesthesia for distal forearm fractures (Bier's block)*. College of Emergency Medicine, London.

Local anaesthetic nerve blocks

LA nerve blocks are very useful in the ED for many minor operations and to provide analgesia. Several nerve blocks are described in the following sections. Many other nerve blocks and regional blocks are possible, but are not normally appropriate in the ED. Some should only be performed by doctors with anaesthetic training, or in a few cases, dental training.

Equipment for nerve blocks

Ordinary injection needles can be used for most local blocks in the ED. Anaesthetists sometimes use special pencil-point or short bevel needles when blocking large nerve trunks and plexuses.

General procedure for nerve blocks

- Follow the general principles of LA (📖 p.282).
- Review the relevant anatomy for the block. Determine the site of injection by feeling for local structures such as arteries or tendons.
- When performing a nerve block hold the needle with the bevel in the line of the nerve (rather than across it), to reduce the risk of cutting nerve fibres.
- Ask the patient about tingling in the area supplied by the nerve. Do not try to elicit paraesthesiae. If paraesthesiae occur withdraw the needle 2–3mm before injecting.
- Wait for the nerve block to work, but do not leave the patient alone during this time. Tell the nurse when to call you back, in case you are busy with other patients. Estimate when a nerve block should be effective and do not test sensation before then. Small nerves may be blocked in 5min, but large nerves may take up to 40min.

Failed nerve block

If a nerve block does not work, consider waiting longer or giving another injection. Before giving any more LA, review relevant anatomy, consider using ultrasound guidance, and check that the maximum safe dose of the drug will not be exceeded. Entonox® can be helpful as a supplement to LA for some procedures, such as reduction of dislocations. Alternatively, sedation (📖 p.308) may be useful in some cases. Occasionally, one has to abandon LA and arrange GA instead.

Ultrasound guidance for nerve blocks[1]

Ultrasound guidance can help in identifying nerves and other structures and allows visualization of the needle position and the spread of LA. Precise injection of LA adjacent to a nerve gives a faster onset and longer duration of anaesthesia with a smaller volume of LA, less pain and a reduced risk of complications. Ultrasound is unnecessary for some nerve blocks, eg digital nerves and supraorbital nerve block. Ultrasound allows nerve blockade away from identifying structures, eg medial nerve block in the forearm.

Successful use of ultrasound for LA requires appropriate equipment, knowledge of relevant anatomy, and training in ultrasound techniques.

1 Marhofer P (2008) *Ultrasound Guidance for Nerve Blocks.* Oxford University Press, Oxford.

Digital nerve block

Digital nerve block

Digital nerve block is used frequently for simple operations on the fingers and toes. (The term 'ring block' is often used, but is incorrect since it implies that LA is injected in a ring around the finger, which is unnecessary and might cause ischaemia due to vascular compression).

A dorsal and a palmar digital nerve run along each side of the finger and thumb. Similarly, there are dorsal and plantar nerves in the toes.

1% plain lidocaine is often used, but bupivacaine (0.5% plain) is preferable because it is less painful on injection, and gives prolonged anaesthesia and analgesia. The traditional advice is never to use adrenaline or any other vasoconstrictor. In an adult use 1–2mL of LA on each side of the finger, thumb, or big toe. Use smaller volumes in the other toes or in children.

Technique

- Use a 0.6 × 25 mm (23G) needle (0.5 × 16 mm, 25G, in small children).
- Insert the needle from the dorsum on the lateral side of the base of the digit, angled slightly inwards towards the midline of the digit, until the needle can be felt under the skin on the flexor aspect.
- Aspirate to check the needle is not in a blood vessel.
- Slowly inject 0.5–1mL. Continue injecting as the needle is withdrawn.
- Repeat on the medial side of the digit.
- If anaesthesia is needed for the nail bed of the great toe give an additional injection of LA subcutaneously across the dorsum of the base of the proximal phalanx, to block the dorsal digital nerves and their branches. This is also required for anaesthesia of the dorsum of the digit proximal to the middle phalanx.

Anaesthesia develops after ≈5min. Autonomic nerve fibres are blocked, as well as sensory nerve fibres, so when the block works the skin feels dry and warm. Occasionally, anaesthesia remains inadequate and another injection is needed. The maximum volume that can be used in a finger, thumb, or big toe is 5mL. Use less in the other toes or in children.

Single injection digital nerve block

Anaesthesia of the distal phalanx and DIP joint can be achieved by a single subcutaneous injection in the volar aspect of the base of the finger. Pinch the soft tissues just distal to the proximal skin crease. Insert a 25G needle just beneath the skin at the midpoint of the skin crease and inject 2–3mL of 0.5% bupivacaine. Massage the LA into the soft tissues.

Digital nerve block at metacarpal level

Digital nerves can be blocked where they run in the interspaces between the metacarpals. Insert a thin needle in the palm through the distal palmar crease, between the flexor tendons of adjacent fingers. Injection of 3–4mL of 1% plain lidocaine will block the adjacent sides of these two fingers. Anaesthesia develops after 5–10min. Alternatively, a dorsal approach can be used: this is often preferred because it is less painful, but there is an ↑ risk of inadvertent venepuncture and the digital nerves are further from the dorsal surface, so a deep injection is needed.

Digital nerve block

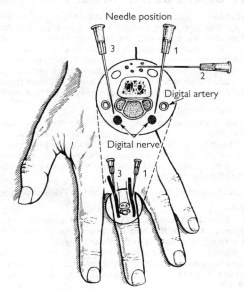

Needle position

Digital artery

Digital nerve

Digital nerve block at the base of the finger

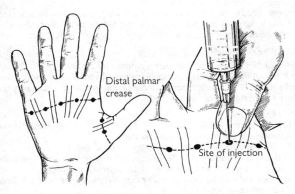

Distal palmar crease

Site of injection

Digital nerve block at metacarpal level

Fig. 7.1 Digital nerve block.

Nerve blocks at the wrist: 1

The median nerve supplies sensation to the radial half of the palm, the thumb, index and middle finger, and the radial side of the ring finger. The ulnar nerve supplies the ulnar side of the hand, the little finger, and the ulnar side of the ring finger. The radial nerve supplies the dorsum of the radial side of the hand. The different nerve distributions overlap. In some people, the radial side of the ring finger and the ulnar side of the middle finger are supplied by the ulnar, rather than median nerve. LA block of one or more nerves at the wrist provides good anaesthesia for minor surgery on the hand and fingers.

Median nerve block

At the wrist the median nerve lies under the flexor retinaculum on the anterior aspect of the wrist, under or immediately radial to the tendon of palmaris longus and 5–10mm medial to the tendon of flexor carpi radialis. Just proximal to the flexor retinaculum, the median nerve gives off the palmar cutaneous branch, which travels superficially to supply the skin of the thenar eminence and the central palm.

Carpal tunnel syndrome is a contraindication to median nerve block.

Technique
- Use a 0. 6mm (23G) needle and ≈5–10mL of 1% lidocaine.
- Ask the patient to flex the wrist slightly and bend the thumb to touch the little finger, in order to identify palmaris longus.
- Insert the needle vertically at the proximal wrist skin crease, between palmaris longus and flexor carpi radialis, angled slightly towards palmaris longus, to a depth of 1 cm. If paraesthesiae occur withdraw the needle by 2–3 mm.
- Inject ≈5mL of LA slowly.
- Block the palmar cutaneous branch by injecting another 1–2mL SC while withdrawing the needle.
- Some people do not have a palmaris longus tendon—in this case, identify flexor carpi radialis and insert the needle on its ulnar side.
- Ultrasound allows blockade of the median nerve in the forearm.

Ulnar nerve block

In the distal forearm the ulnar nerve divides into a palmar branch (which travels with the ulnar artery to supply the hypothenar eminence and palm) and a dorsal branch (which passes under flexor carpi ulnaris to supply the ulnar side of the dorsum of the hand).

Technique
- Use a 0.6mm (23G) needle and 5–10mL of 1% lidocaine. Avoid adrenaline in peripheral vascular disease.
- Check the radial pulse before blocking the ulnar nerve.
- Feel the ulnar artery and flexor carpi ulnaris tendon and insert the needle between them at the level of the ulnar styloid process.
- Aspirate and look for blood in the syringe. Withdraw the needle 2–3mm if paraesthesiae occur.
- Inject 5mL of LA.
- Block the dorsal branch of the ulnar nerve by SC infiltration of 3–5mL of LA from flexor carpi ulnaris around the ulnar border of the wrist.

Nerve blocks at the wrist

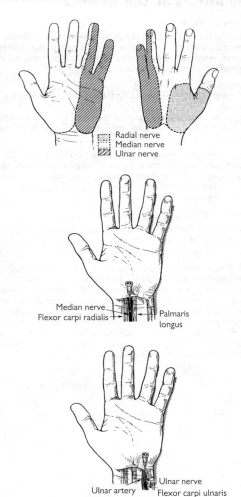

Fig. 7.2 Nerve blocks at the wrist.

Nerve blocks at the wrist: 2

Radial nerve block

In the distal part of the forearm the radial nerve passes under the tendon of brachioradialis and lies subcutaneously on the dorsum of the radial side of the wrist, where it separates into several branches and supplies the radial side of the dorsum of the hand.

Technique

- Use a 0.6mm (23G) needle and 5mL of 1% lidocaine, with or without adrenaline.
- Infiltrate LA subcutaneously around the radial side and dorsum of the wrist from the tendon of flexor carpi radialis to the radio-ulnar joint. Beware of inadvertent IV injection.

Radial nerve block involves an infiltration technique and often has a more rapid onset and shorter duration of action than median nerve and ulnar nerve blocks. In combined blocks, experts may use lidocaine with adrenaline in order to prolong the anaesthetic and ↓ the risk of lidocaine toxicity.

Other nerve blocks in the arm

Nerve blocks at the elbow The median, ulnar, and radial nerves can be blocked at the level of the elbow, but this is rarely necessary. The onset of anaesthesia is slower than with blocks at the wrist.

Brachial plexus blocks These should only be used by doctors with anaesthetic training. Brachial plexus blocks can provide good anaesthesia for operations on the arm but the onset of anaesthesia is often slow (30–45min) and there is a risk of LA toxicity because of the large dose required. The axillary approach can be used in outpatients. If the supraclavicular approach is used, admission to hospital is necessary, because of the risk of a pneumothorax. Ultrasound guidance helps to allow accurate positioning of the injection, which improves the effectiveness of the block and reduces the risk of complications.

Radial nerve block at the wrist

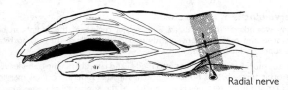

Radial nerve

Fig. 7.3 Radial nerve block at the wrist.

Nerve blocks of forehead and ear

Nerve blocks of the forehead

Many wounds of the forehead and frontal region of the scalp can be explored and repaired conveniently under LA block of the supraorbital and supratrochlear nerves.

The supraorbital nerve divides into medial and lateral branches, and leaves the orbit through two holes or notches in the superior orbital margin, ≈2.5 cm from the midline. The branches of the supraorbital nerve supply sensation to most of the forehead and the frontal region of the scalp.

The supratrochlear nerve emerges from the upper medial corner of the orbit and supplies sensation to the medial part of the forehead.

Technique
- Use 5–10mL of 1% lidocaine, with or without adrenaline.
- Insert the needle in the midline between the eyebrows and direct it laterally.
- Inject LA subcutaneously from the point of insertion along the upper margin of the eyebrow.
- If the wound extends into the lateral part of the forehead SC infiltration of LA may be needed lateral to the eyebrow to block the zygomatico-temporal and auriculotemporal nerves.

Possible complications
- Injury to the eye can occur if the patient moves during the injection.
- It is possible to block the supraorbital nerve at the supraorbital foramen, but this is not advisable since inadvertent injection into the orbit may cause temporary blindness if the LA reaches the optic nerve.

Nerve blocks of the ear

The auricle (pinna) of the ear is supplied by branches of the greater auricular nerve (from inferiorly), lesser occipital nerve (posteriorly), and the auriculotemporal nerve (anteriorly/superiorly). These nerves can be blocked by SC infiltration of up to 10mL of 1% plain lidocaine in the appropriate area, or in a ring around the ear.

To block the *greater auricular nerve* infiltrate 1cm below the ear lobe from the posterior border of the sternomastoid muscle to the angle of the mandible.

Block the *lesser occipital nerve* by infiltration just behind the ear.

When blocking the *auriculotemporal nerve* by infiltration just anterior to the external auditory meatus, aspirate carefully to avoid inadvertent injection into the superficial temporal artery.

Nerve blocks: forehead and ear

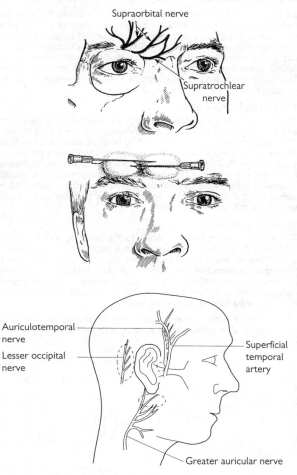

Fig. 7.4 Nerve blocks of the forehead and ear.

Dental anaesthesia

Intraoral injections of local anaesthetic are used frequently for dental procedures, but can also be useful for cleaning and repair of wounds of the lips, cheeks, and chin. Instruction by a dentist or oral surgeon is required. Give dental anaesthetics with dental syringes and cartridges of LA. An appropriate drug for most purposes is lidocaine 2% with adrenaline 1 in 80,000. Some dental syringes do not allow aspiration prior to injection. Disposable dental syringes are preferable to reusable syringes, to ↓ risk of needlestick injury from resheathing of needles.

Infra-orbital nerve block

The infra-orbital nerve supplies the skin and mucous membrane of the cheek and upper lip, and also the lower eyelid and the side of the nose. The nerve emerges from the infra-orbital foramen, which is 0.5cm below the infra-orbital margin and vertically below the pupil when the eyes are looking forwards. The nerve can be blocked at the infra-orbital foramen by injection through the skin, but the intraoral approach is preferable, because it is less unpleasant for the patient. Insert the needle into the buccogingival fold between the first and second premolars, and direct it up towards the infra-orbital foramen.

Mental nerve block

The mental nerve supplies sensation to the lower lip and the chin. It emerges from the mental foramen, which is palpable on the mandible on a line between the first and second premolar teeth. The nerve can be blocked at the mental foramen with 1–2mL of LA, using either an intra- or extra-oral approach. Avoid injecting into the mental canal, since this may damage the nerve. If the wound to be repaired extends across the midline bilateral mental nerve blocks will be needed.

The nerves to a single lower incisor may be blocked by submucous infiltration of LA in the buccal sulcus adjacent to the tooth.

Intercostal nerve block

Intercostal nerve blocks can give useful analgesia for patients with rib fractures who are admitted to hospital, but it is not a routine procedure and requires training and experience. These blocks must not be used in outpatients and should not be performed bilaterally because of the risk of pneumothorax. Patients with obesity or severe obstructive airways disease have ↑ risk of complications. Alternative procedures used in ICU are interpleural analgesia and thoracic epidurals, but these are not appropriate in the ED.

Femoral nerve block

Femoral nerve block is a simple technique and provides good analgesia within a few minutes for pain from a fractured shaft of femur. It may be used in children, as well as in adults. Perform femoral block on the clinical diagnosis of a fractured shaft of femur, before X-ray or the application of a traction splint.

Femoral nerve block can be used with a block of the lateral cutaneous nerve of the thigh for anaesthetizing a skin donor site.

Anatomy

The femoral nerve passes under the inguinal ligament, where it lies lateral to the femoral artery. The femoral nerve supplies the hip and knee joints, the skin of the medial and anterior aspects of the thigh, and the quadriceps, sartorius and pectineus muscles in the anterior compartment of the thigh.

Technique

- Use a mixture of lidocaine and bupivacaine to give both rapid onset and prolonged anaesthesia. In an adult give 5mL of 1% lidocaine and 5mL of 0.5% bupivacaine. In a child use 0.1mL/kg of 1% lidocaine and 0.1mL/kg of 0.5% bupivacaine. Check the maximum dose carefully, especially in children or if bilateral femoral nerve blocks are needed.
- Use a 0.8 × 40 mm (21G) needle in adults and a 0.6 × 25 mm (23G) needle in children.
- Blocking the right femoral nerve is best performed from the patient's left side (and vice versa).
- Using your non-dominant hand palpate the femoral artery just below the inguinal ligament.
- Clean the skin.
- Insert the needle perpendicular to the skin and 1cm lateral to the artery to a depth of ≈3cm. If paraesthesiae occurs, withdraw the needle 2–3mm.
- Aspirate and check for blood.
- Inject LA while moving the needle up and down and fanning out laterally to ≈3cm from the artery. (The distances quoted refer to adults.)
- If the femoral artery is punctured compress it for 5–10min. If no bleeding is apparent, continue with the femoral nerve block.
- This 'blind' technique for femoral nerve block has a high success rate and usually provides rapid and effective analgesia. However, ultrasound (📖 p.292) can be helpful to delineate the anatomy of the femoral nerve (which can vary between patients) and to allow precise positioning of the injection adjacent to the nerve.

Femoral nerve block

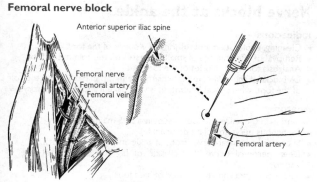

Anterior superior iliac spine

Femoral nerve
Femoral artery
Femoral vein

Femoral artery

Fig. 7.5 Femoral nerve block.

Nerve blocks at the ankle

Indications
- Cleaning, exploration and suturing of wounds of the foot.
- Removal of FB. Drainage of small abscesses on the sole of the foot.
- Analgesia for crush injuries of the forefoot.
- LA blocks at the ankle are particularly useful for anaesthetizing the sole of the foot, where local infiltration is very painful and unsatisfactory.

Anatomy
Sensation in the ankle and foot is supplied by 5 main nerves:
- Saphenous nerve (medial side of ankle).
- Superficial peroneal nerve (front of ankle and dorsum of foot).
- Deep peroneal nerve (lateral side of big toe and medial side of 2nd toe).
- Sural nerve (heel and lateral side of hind foot).
- Tibial nerve (which forms the medial and lateral plantar nerves, supplying the anterior half of the sole).

There are individual variations and significant overlap between the areas supplied by different nerves, especially on the sole of the foot. It is often necessary to block more than one nerve.

For each of these blocks use a 0.6mm (23G) needle and 5mL of 1% lidocaine (with or without adrenaline) or 0.5% bupivacaine. Check the maximum dose (📖 p.283), especially for multiple blocks. Ultrasound can help to allow accurate injection of LA, so smaller amounts are needed.

Do not use adrenaline in patients with peripheral vascular disease.

Saphenous nerve
Infiltrate LA subcutaneously around the great saphenous vein, anterior to and just above the medial malleolus. Aspirate carefully because of the risk of IV injection.

Superficial peroneal nerve
Infiltrate LA subcutaneously above the ankle joint from the anterior border of the tibia to the lateral malleolus.

Deep peroneal nerve
Insert the needle above the ankle joint between the tendons of tibialis anterior and extensor hallucis longus. Inject 5mL of LA.

Sural nerve
Lie the patient prone. Insert the needle lateral to the Achilles tendon and infiltrate subcutaneously to the lateral malleolus.

Tibial nerve
Lie the patient prone. Palpate the posterior tibial artery. Insert the needle medial to the Achilles tendon and level with the upper border of the medial malleolus, so the needle tip is just lateral to the artery. Withdraw slightly if paraesthesiae occur. Aspirate. Inject 5–10mL.

Nerve blocks at the ankle

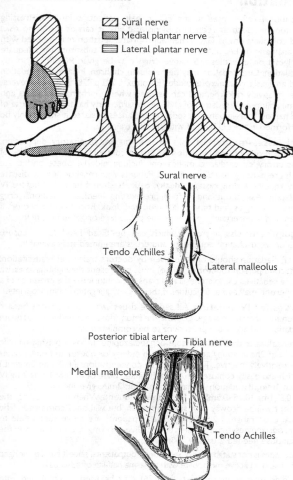

Sural nerve
Medial plantar nerve
Lateral plantar nerve

Sural nerve

Tendo Achilles

Lateral malleolus

Posterior tibial artery   Tibial nerve

Medial malleolus

Tendo Achilles

Fig. 7.6 Nerve blocks at the ankle.

Sedation

Sedation is often used in the ED to help patients tolerate distressing procedures, such as reduction of dislocations. It carries the same risks and complications as GA. When appropriate, sedation may be used with an analgesic or LA, but do not use sedation as a substitute for adequate analgesia or anaesthesia. Sedative drugs may be given PO, IM, IV, or by inhalation. Oral sedation may be helpful in children. Inhalational sedation and analgesia with nitrous oxide (Entonox®, 🕮 p.278) is rapidly reversible, relatively risk-free, and can be used when appropriate in adults and some children. IV sedation of children is particularly hazardous because of the narrow margin between sedation and anaesthesia, so it should only be performed in the ED by staff with specific training.

Risk assessment Main risks of sedation are respiratory depression, ↓ cardiac output and inhalation of gastric contents. Patients at ↑ risk of respiratory or cardiac complications include elderly, obese and those with pre-existing heart/lung disease. Patients with renal or hepatic disease may require ↓ drug dosage. Ideally, patients should be fasted before IV sedation. Ask about and record pre-existing medical conditions, drug therapy, allergies, and time of last food and drink. Record pulse and BP. If there is any uncertainty, postpone the procedure or get expert help.

Equipment Use a trolley which can be tilted head-down. Ensure suction, resuscitation equipment and drugs are immediately available.

Staff Sedation should only be given by doctors trained in resuscitation. A second person (doctor or nurse) must be present throughout to assist. Some sedatives cause amnesia and transient confusion—the presence of a chaperone may avoid difficulties if there is any allegation of impropriety.

Drugs for IV sedation All sedative drugs will produce anaesthesia if given in excessive dosage. Use the minimum dose that will give adequate sedation and allow the procedure to be completed satisfactorily.

Midazolam is the most suitable benzodiazepine. It has a plasma half-life of about 2hr in young adults (longer in elderly or obese) and metabolites are relatively inactive. There are three concentrations (1, 2, and 5mg/mL) which are easily confused. In fit adults initial dose of midazolam is 2mg IV over 1min. If sedation is inadequate after 2min, give incremental doses of 0.5–1mg (0.25–0.5mL of 10mg/5mL solution). When fully sedated, the patient will be drowsy with slurred speech, but will obey commands. The usual dose range is 2.5–7.5mg. Elderly patients are more susceptible to benzodiazepines—give smaller doses. Give 0.5–1mg as an initial dose: the total dose needed is usually 1–3mg.

Diazepam is not suitable for IV sedation of outpatients, since it has a prolonged action and an active metabolite with a plasma half-life of ≈3–5 days.

Opioids such as morphine (🕮 p.276) may be used IV combined with midazolam, but there may be a synergistic effect with ↑ risk of respiratory depression. Give the opioid first in ↓ dosage, followed by careful titration of midazolam.

Other drugs Propofol (🕮 p.316) can give excellent sedation for short procedures, with rapid recovery, but its use requires anaesthetic training. Ketamine (🕮 p.278) may be given IV or IM, but requires special training.

Monitoring during IV sedation

Ensure patients given IV sedation receive O_2, pulse oximetry monitoring and have a venous cannula. Monitor ECG.

Antagonists

The specific antagonists flumazenil (for benzodiazepines) and naloxone (for opioids) must be available immediately, but should be needed very rarely. If respiratory depression occurs, standard techniques to maintain the airway and breathing are more important than giving antagonists. Flumazenil and naloxone have shorter durations of action than the drugs they antagonize, so careful observation is essential if either drug is used.

Recovery and discharge after sedation

If IV sedation is used, monitor the patient carefully until recovery is complete.

Monitoring and resuscitation equipment and drugs must be available.

Minimum criteria for discharging a patient are:
• Stable vital signs.
• Ability to walk without support.
• Toleration of oral fluids and minimal nausea.
• Adequate analgesia.
• Adequate supervision at home by a responsible adult.

Instruct the patient (both verbally and in writing) not to drive, operate machinery, make any important decisions or drink alcohol for 24 hours. Arrange appropriate follow-up. Ensure the adult accompanying the patient knows who to contact if there is any problem.

Sedation in children

Many children (and their parents and staff) are distressed by procedures such as suturing of minor wounds under LA. Sedation is helpful to prevent distress and allows procedures to take place with minimal physical restraint. Sedation may be given by oral or nasal routes, IM or IV. Paediatric IV sedation requires anaesthetic experience because of the narrow therapeutic margin between sedation and anaesthesia.

Ketamine given IM in a dose of 2–2.5mg/kg is currently the method of choice for paediatric sedation in the ED by doctors with appropriate training (📖 p.278). This dose of ketamine does not provide full anaesthesia and so local anaesthesia is required for cleaning and suturing of wounds.

Oral midazolam is advocated by some specialists. Oral sedation with *promethazine* is not advisable, since it is often ineffective.

General anaesthesia in the emergency department

GA may be needed in the ED for many different conditions:
- Minor surgery (eg drainage of abscesses, manipulation of fractures).
- Cardioversion.
- Airway problems (eg facial trauma, burns, epiglottitis).
- Respiratory failure (eg asthma, chronic obstructive airways disease, pulmonary oedema, chest injuries).
- To protect the airway and control ventilation after head injuries and to keep the patient immobile for a CT scan.
- To protect the airway and maintain ventilation in status epilepticus unresponsive to standard drug therapy.
- Immediate major surgery (eg thoracotomy or laparotomy for trauma, ruptured ectopic pregnancy or aortic aneurysm). If at all possible take the patient to the operating theatre before anaesthesia, as the loss of sympathetic tone after the onset of anaesthesia can cause catastrophic hypotension in a hypovolaemic patient. In extreme emergencies, it may be necessary to operate in the ED.

GA in the ED tends to be stressful for the anaesthetist and potentially hazardous for the patient, who is usually unprepared for anaesthesia, with a full stomach and increased risk of aspiration. GA should only be given by doctors with anaesthetic training, but other staff should know what is required so they can help when necessary.

Pre-operative assessment

This is essential for safe anaesthesia. If time allows, assess the patient before contacting the anaesthetist to arrange the anaesthetic. However, if emergency anaesthesia is needed, call the anaesthetist immediately so that he/she can come and assess the patient, and get senior help if necessary. A checklist of questions to ask before GA is shown opposite.

Fitness for GA The American Society of Anaesthesiologists (ASA) classification of pre-operative fitness is widely used by anaesthetists:
1 Healthy patient with no systemic disease.
2 Patient with a mild to moderate disease which does not limit their activity in any way (eg treated hypertension, mild diabetes, smoker).
3 Patient with a severe systemic disturbance from any cause which limits activity (eg IHD with ↓ exercise tolerance, severe COPD).
4 Patient with a severe systemic disease which is a constant threat to life (eg severe chronic bronchitis, advanced liver disease).
5 Moribund patient who is unlikely to survive 24 hours with or without treatment.

The risk of complications from GA correlates well with ASA group. Only patients in ASA groups 1 and 2 should be given an elective anaesthetic by a junior anaesthetist in the ED. Children aged <7 years should not usually have a GA in the ED, except in an emergency.

Pre-operative investigations

No investigation except 'dipstick' urinalysis is needed, unless pre-operative assessment reveals a problem. Measure Hb in any patient who appears anaemic. Check for sickle cell disease in any patient of Afro-Caribbean, Cypriot or Indian origin. Measure U&E in patients on diuretics, and blood glucose in diabetics. ECG and CXR are not needed, unless clinically indicated. Perform a pregnancy test if pregnancy is possible.

Checklist for pre-operative assessment in the ED

- Age.
- Weight.
- Time of last drink.
- Time of last food.
- Drugs.
- Drugs given in the ED.
- Time of last analgesia.
- Allergies.
- Sickle cell risk?
- Infection risk?
- Family history of GA problems?
- Airway problem?
- Dentures/crowns/loose teeth?
- Chest disease?
- Smoker?
- Cardiac disease?
- Blood pressure.
- GI problem?
- Other illness?
- Possibility of pregnancy?
- Previous GA? (problems?)
- Consent form signed?
- Is the patient expected to go home after recovery from anaesthetic?
- Is there a responsible adult who can look after the patient at home?

Preparation for GA

Ideally, the patient should have nothing to drink for 4 hours and no food for 6 hours before anaesthesia. Explain why this is necessary. Fasting does not guarantee an empty stomach. Trauma, pregnancy and opioids delay gastric emptying.

If the patient is in pain, give analgesia and an antiemetic. Discuss with the anaesthetist any other drug treatment that is required. Patients with a hiatus hernia or gastro-oesophageal reflux need antacid prophylaxis (eg ranitidine 50mg IV and an antacid).

Explain the proposed operation and anaesthetic to the patient (and relatives if appropriate) and ensure valid consent is obtained. The patient must be clearly labelled with a wrist-band. Remove contact lenses, false teeth and dental plates.

Recovery and discharge after anaesthesia

When the operation has finished, place the patient in the recovery position and ensure continuous observation by trained staff until recovery is complete. The anaesthetist should stay with the patient until consciousness is regained and the airway is controlled. Monitoring and resuscitation equipment and drugs must be available. The minimum criteria for discharging a patient are the same as following sedation (📖 p.309).

Importantly, tell the patient (both verbally and in writing) not to drive, operate machinery, make any important decisions or drink alcohol for 24 hours. Arrange appropriate follow-up and make sure that the adult accompanying the patient knows who to contact if there is a problem.

Emergency anaesthesia and rapid sequence induction

Emergency anaesthesia and intubation are often needed to protect the airway and provide adequate ventilation in a patient with a head injury or multiple trauma. There is a high risk of aspiration of gastric contents into the lungs, so use a cuffed ET tube (uncuffed in small children). In a patient with a gag reflex any attempt to intubate without anaesthesia may cause vomiting and aspiration. Anaesthesia before intubation is essential in head-injured patients to minimize the ↑ in ICP.

Rapid sequence induction (RSI)

RSI involves administration of a sedative or induction agent virtually simultaneously with a neuromuscular blocking agent to allow rapid tracheal intubation. *RSI should only be performed by staff who have had specific training and experience in the techniques and the drugs used, and the recognition and management of possible problems.* However, it is useful if ED staff who have not had such training understand the principles of RSI, so that they can assist as needed.

- Call for senior ED/anaesthetic/ICU help.
- Check all drugs and equipment, including suction, bag and masks, laryngoscope (and spare with large blade), tracheal tubes and introducers, syringe and valve or clamp for ET tube cuff, connectors.
- Check that the trolley can be tilted head-down easily.
- Check monitoring equipment (ECG, BP, pulse oximeter, end-tidal CO_2 monitor).
- Explain the procedure to the patient if possible.
- Assess the risks and any conditions which might cause problems with intubation (eg trauma to the face or neck, ↓ mouth opening, receding chin). Identify a back-up plan (📖 p.314) and communicate this to the team.
- Establish monitoring (ECG and pulse oximetry) and secure IV access.
- Protect the cervical spine in all trauma patients: an assistant should provide in-line immobilization during intubation. In other patients, use a pillow and position the head and neck to aid intubation.
- If possible, pre-oxygenate for 3min with 100% O_2 via a tight-fitting mask, with the patient breathing spontaneously. If breathing is inadequate, ventilate for 2min on 100% O_2 with a bag and mask, with an assistant applying cricoid pressure by pressing firmly downwards with a thumb and index finger on the cricoid cartilage, while supporting the patient's neck with the other hand.
- Give an induction agent (eg thiopental or etomidate) quickly to provide rapid anaesthesia. Cricoid pressure must be maintained continuously until the airway is secure.
- Follow the induction agent immediately with a muscle relaxant (usually suxamethonium).
- Keep the face mask tightly applied until the anaesthetic and relaxant are effective. Then intubate and inflate the cuff quickly.

- Try to confirm tracheal placement of the tube: ideally it will have been seen passing through the cords, but this may not be possible in an emergency intubation. Check air entry in both sides of the chest. Check end-tidal CO_2 (but this may be misleading if oesophageal intubation occurs in a patient who has recently consumed antacids or fizzy drinks). If CO_2 is not detected, oesophageal intubation has occurred.
- Cricoid pressure can be released when the ET tube is correctly positioned, the cuff has been inflated and ventilation is satisfactory.
- Secure the tracheal tube.
- Continue observation and monitoring.

Difficult intubation

Difficulties with intubation may result from problems with the equipment, the patient, the circumstances of intubation, and from lack of experience or skill.

Equipment

Proper working equipment must be available where intubation may be needed—pillow, suction, laryngoscope (and spare) with interchangeable blades, ET tubes of different diameters (cut to suitable lengths, but with uncut tubes available), syringe and clamp for cuff, connectors, flexible stylet, gum-elastic bougie, lubricating jelly, Magill's forceps, tape for securing ET tube. A face mask and ventilating bag, and oral/nasal airways must be immediately available. Laryngeal masks and cricothyroidotomy equipment must be accessible. Fibre-optic laryngoscopes are useful in skilled hands, but are not routinely kept in EDs.

The patient

Patients may be difficult to intubate because of facial deformity or swelling, protruding teeth, ↓ mouth opening from trismus or trauma, ↓ neck movement or instability of the cervical spine, epiglottitis or laryngeal problems, tracheal narrowing or deviation, blood, vomit or FB in the airway.

Circumstances and skills

Intubation is much easier in the controlled environment of an operating theatre than in an emergency in the ED or in pre-hospital care. Skilled help is vital—in-line immobilization of the neck, cricoid pressure, and assistance with equipment and cuff inflation are needed. Practice intubating manikins regularly.

Practical points

Before attempting intubation, oxygenate by bag and mask ventilation. Take a deep breath as you start intubation—if the patient is not intubated successfully when you have to breathe again, remove the ET tube and laryngoscope, and ventilate with O_2 for 1–2min using a bag and mask before making another attempt. Consider adjusting the patient's position, using a different size of laryngoscope blade or ET tube or a stylet or bougie. Cricoid pressure can help by pushing the larynx backwards into view. The BURP manoeuvre (Backwards Upwards Rightwards Pressure on the thyroid cartilage) may be useful in a difficult intubation.

Oesophageal intubation

Fatal if unrecognized. The best way of confirming tracheal intubation is to see the ET tube pass between the vocal cords. Inadvertent oesophageal intubation can produce misleadingly normal chest movements and breath sounds. End-tidal CO_2 measurement helps to confirm tracheal intubation, but end-tidal CO_2 can be misleadingly ↑ in patients who have taken antacids or fizzy drinks. If in doubt, remove the ET tube and ventilate with bag and mask.

Failed intubation drill

Persistent unsuccessful attempts at intubation cause hypoxia and ↑ risk of aspiration and damage to teeth and other structures. If three attempts at intubation are unsuccessful, follow a failed intubation drill:

- Inform all staff that intubation attempts have ceased and get senior help.
- Ventilate the patient on 100% O_2 using bag and mask, and an oral or nasal airway, while an assistant maintains cricoid pressure.
- If ventilation is impossible, turn the patient onto the left side and tilt the trolley head down, while maintaining cricoid pressure. If ventilation is still impossible release cricoid pressure slowly and attempt to ventilate again.
- A laryngeal mask airway (LMA) can be very useful in this situation but requires training. Practice the technique of LMA insertion on manikins and on patients in the operating theatre whenever possible.
- Cricothyroidotomy (📖 p.326) is rarely needed, but must be performed promptly if necessary.
- In non-emergency cases, the patient can be allowed to wake up, but this is not an option in a life-threatening emergency. Discuss the problem with a senior anaesthetist.
- Warn the patient and GP if the difficulty with intubation is liable to recur.

Laryngospasm

Laryngospasm occurs when the laryngeal muscles contract and occlude the airway, preventing ventilation and causing hypoxia.

Causes
- Stimulation of the patient during light anaesthesia.
- Irritation of the airway by secretions, vomit, blood or an oropharyngeal airway.
- Irritant anaesthetic vapours.
- Extubation of a lightly anaesthetized patient.

Treatment
- Give 100% O_2.
- Clear the airway of secretions, using gentle suction.
- Gently ventilate the patient using a bag and mask. Over-inflation is liable to fill the stomach and cause regurgitation.
- Monitor the ECG for bradycardia or arrhythmias.

In severe laryngospasm, an experienced anaesthetist may consider deepening anaesthesia or giving suxamethonium to allow intubation, or ventilation with a bag and mask. In a hypoxic patient, suxamethonium may cause bradycardia requiring treatment with atropine.

General anaesthetic drugs

GA should only be given after anaesthetic training.

IV anaesthetic induction agents are used for induction of anaesthesia, as the sole drug for short procedures (eg cardioversion), for treatment of status epilepticus unresponsive to other anticonvulsants (🕮 p.149), for total IV anaesthesia and for sedation of a ventilated patient. They are particularly hazardous in patients with upper airway obstruction or severe hypovolaemia. Thiopental, etomidate and many other drugs are unsafe in acute porphyria (see 🕮 p.165 and *BNF*).

Propofol is particularly useful in day-case surgery, and for manipulation of fractures and dislocations, because recovery is rapid. The injection may be painful. Hypotension is common and severe bradycardia may occur. Induction dose is 1.5–2.5mg/kg.

Etomidate causes less hypotension than propofol or thiopental (and so may be useful in patients who are already hypotensive), and recovery is rapid. However, the injection is painful, and uncontrolled muscle movements and adrenocortical suppression may occur. Induction dose is up to 0.3mg/kg.

Ketamine (🕮 p.278) is used mainly in prehospital care, but may be useful for rapid sequence intubation in hypotensive patients and in acute asthma. Induction dose is 1–2mg/kg IV.

Thiopental (thiopentone) is a barbiturate drug. Thiopentone solution is unstable and has to be prepared from powder to form a 2.5% solution (25mg/mL). Care is needed with injections because extravasation causes irritation, and arterial injection is particularly dangerous. Hypotension may occur, especially with overdosage. The induction dose in a fit adult is up to 4mg/kg (child: 2–7mg/kg).

Muscle relaxants

Suxamethonium is a short-acting depolarizing muscle relaxant, which is often used to allow intubation, especially in rapid sequence induction of anaesthesia (🕮 p.312). In a dose of 1mg/kg it causes muscle fasciculation followed rapidly by flaccid paralysis. Suxamethonium is contra-indicated in hyperkalaemia and also in burns, paraplegia or crush injuries, where dangerous hyperkalaemia may develop if suxamethonium is used 5–120 days after injury. Suxamethonium causes ↑ ICP and ↑ intraocular pressure. Usual duration of action is ≈5min, but prolonged paralysis occurs in patients with abnormal pseudo-cholinesterase enzymes.

Rocuronium is a muscle relaxant that may be used for intubation if suxamethonium is contraindicated.

Atracurium and vecuronium are non-depolarizing muscle relaxants, which act for ≈20–30min. They cause fewer adverse effects than older relaxants (eg pancuronium). Paralysis from these drugs can be reversed with neostigmine, which is given with atropine or glycopyrronium to prevent bradycardia.

Inhalational anaesthetics

These can be used for analgesia (especially Entonox®), induction of anaesthesia (particularly in upper airway obstruction, when IV induction of anaesthesia is hazardous), and for maintenance of anaesthesia.

Nitrous oxide (N_2O) is widely used for analgesia as Entonox®, a 50:50 mixture with O_2 (📖 p.278). It is also used frequently in GA in a concentration of 50–70% in O_2, in combination with other inhaled or IV anaesthetics. N_2O is contraindicated in certain circumstances (eg undrained pneumothorax)—see 📖 p.278.

Halothane, enflurane, isoflurane, and sevoflurane are inhalational anaesthetic agents that are given using specially calibrated vaporizers in O_2, or a mixture of N_2O and O_2. Sevoflurane is particularly useful for gas induction of anaesthesia in upper airway obstruction. Halothane is also effective for gas induction, but now rarely used because of the risk of hepatotoxicity, especially after repeated use. Halothane sensitizes the heart to catecholamines, so adrenaline must not be used with halothane. These inhalational anaesthetic drugs can cause malignant hyperpyrexia (📖 p.265) in susceptible patients.

Major trauma

Major trauma: treatment principles

Patients who present with serious (or apparently serious) injuries require immediate assessment and resuscitation. The finer points of history taking may have to wait until later. However, suspect major trauma in:
• High speed road collisions, vehicle ejection, rollover, prolonged extrication.
• Death of another individual in the same collision.
• Pedestrians thrown up or run over by a vehicle.
• Falls of more than 2m.

Management of specific injuries is outlined in subsequent pages. Although treatment should be tailored to the needs of each individual patient, many therapeutic interventions are common to all patients:

Airway control

Use basic manoeuvres (suction, chin lift, oropharyngeal airway) to open the airway and apply O_2 by face mask (p.324). Avoid tilting the head or moving the neck if there is a chance of neck injury. If the airway remains obstructed despite these measures, get ED and ICU and/or anaesthesia help and consider advanced manoeuvres (p.326).

O_2

Provide high flow O_2 to all. Patients who are apnoeic or hypoventilating require assistance by bag and mask ventilation prior to tracheal intubation and IPPV.

Cervical spine control

This is the first priority in any patient who presents with possible spine injury (eg neck pain, loss of consciousness). Provide immediate in-line manual cervical immobilization by placing one hand on each side of the patient's head and holding it steady (without traction) and in line with the remainder of the spine. Whilst maintaining manual immobilization, ask an assistant to apply an appropriately sized hard cervical collar. Adhesive tape and sandbags may be applied, but may cause problems in certain patients (eg patients who are vomiting or uncooperative patients who have consumed alcohol).

IV fluids

Insert 2 large cannulae into forearm or antecubital fossae veins. If initial attempts fail, consider a femoral venous line or an intra-osseous line. If these fail or are inappropriate, consider a central line or a cut-down onto the long saphenous vein. However, bear in mind the difficulties and potential hazards of attempting central venous access in hypovolaemic patients.

Commence IV fluids for patients with hypovolaemic shock with 1L of 0.9% saline (or Hartmann's solution) in adults (20mL/kg in children). Consider urgent blood transfusion if >2L (in an adult) have been given (p.174) and look for sources of bleeding—chest, abdomen, and pelvis.

Analgesia

Adequate pain relief is often forgotten or deferred. Give morphine IV (diluted in saline to 1mg/mL) titrated in small increments according to response. Provide an antiemetic (eg cyclizine 50mg IV) at the same time. Consider other forms of analgesia (eg regional nerve blocks, immobilization, and splintage of fractures).

Antibiotics

Give prophylactic IV antibiotics for compound fractures and penetrating wounds of the head, chest or abdomen. Antibiotic choice follows local policy—a broad spectrum antibiotic (eg cefuroxime) is useful.

Tetanus

Ensure tetanus prophylaxis in all patients (□ p.410).

Advanced trauma life support (ATLS®)

The ATLS concept was introduced by the American College of Surgeons in an attempt to improve the immediate treatment of patients with serious injury. The ATLS® approach has enabled some standardization of trauma resuscitation. According to ATLS®, treatment of all patients with major trauma passes through the same phases:

- Primary survey.
- Resuscitation phase.
- Secondary survey.
- Definitive care phase.

A key feature of ATLS® is frequent re-evaluation of the patient's problems and the response to treatment. Any deterioration necessitates a return to evaluate the 'ABC' (airway, breathing, and circulation).

Primary survey

On initial reception of a seriously injured patient, life-threatening problems should be identified and addressed as rapidly as possible. An 'ABC' approach is adopted, with each of the following aspects being quickly evaluated and treated:

A—airway maintenance with cervical spine control.

B—breathing and ventilation.

C—circulation and haemorrhage control.

D—disability (rapid assessment of neurological status).

E—exposure (the patient is completely undressed to allow full examination).

With optimum staffing and direction, instead of considering each of these aspects sequentially (from 'A' to 'E'), aim to address them simultaneously.

Resuscitation phase

During this period, treatment continues for the problems identified during the primary survey. Further practical procedures (eg insertion of oro/nasogastric tube, chest drain and urinary catheter) are performed. Occasionally, immediate surgery (damage control surgery) is required for haemorrhage control before the secondary survey.

Secondary survey

This is a head to toe examination to identify other injuries. This should be accompanied by relevant imaging and other investigations. Monitor the patient closely—any deterioration requires a repeat ABC assessment. A high index of suspicion is essential to avoid missing occult injuries—particularly in the severely injured and those with ↓ conscious level.

Definitive care phase

The early management of all injuries is addressed, including fracture stabilization and emergency operative intervention.

Investigations in major trauma

Select specific investigations according to the presentation, but bear in mind that all patients with major trauma require: group and save/X-match, BMG, X-rays, ABG. Consider measuring lactate levels.

BMG

This is mandatory for all patients with major trauma and particularly important on any patient with GCS<15/15.

SpO₂

Attach a pulse oximeter on ED arrival, then monitor continuously.

Blood tests

Check U&E, FBC, and glucose in all patients. If there is any possibility of significant haemorrhage, request a group and save, or cross-match. Request a baseline clotting screen in patients with major haemorrhage or those at special risk (eg alcoholics or those on anticoagulants). Request fresh frozen plasma and platelets early for patients with major haemorrhage.

X-rays

Multiply injured patients often require multiple X-rays. Obtain CXR and pelvic X-rays as a minimum. Cervical spine X-rays do not change the initial management in the resuscitation room and can be deferred to the secondary survey. Don lead aprons and gloves, and remain with the patient whilst X-rays are taken—in particular, ensure satisfactory immobilization of the cervical spine throughout. Accompany the patient if he needs to be taken to the radiology department for further imaging.

Urinalysis

Test the urine for blood if there is suspicion of abdominal injury. Microscopic haematuria is a useful marker of intra-abdominal injury.

Arterial blood gas

Provides useful information about the degree of hypoxia, hypoventilation and acidosis. In critically ill patients (especially those requiring ventilatory support or those destined for neurosurgery/ICU) repeat as necessary and consider inserting an intra-arterial line to continuously monitor BP.

Electrocardiogram

Monitor all patients; record an ECG if >50 years or significant chest trauma.

Computed tomography scan

CT is increasingly used to evaluate head, neck and truncal injuries. An appropriately trained doctor should accompany the patient to the CT scanner and monitoring must continue. Local protocols will dictate which patients have a total body 'pan scan' rather than selective imaging. Patients with haemodynamic instability should not go to the CT scanner.

USS (FAST) and DPL

Focused assessment with sonography for trauma (FAST; 📖 p.346) is a USS technique to identify free fluid in the peritoneal or pericardial cavities. It can be performed by a trained ED doctor, surgeon, or radiologist. Local policy and expertise will determine individual ED practice. DPL (📖 p.347) is rarely used now in developed countries given the availability of FAST and CT. DPL still plays an important role if FAST and CT are not available.

Other investigations

Angiography is indicated in certain specific circumstances (major pelvic fracture, aortic injury). Occasionally, other tests requiring specialist expertise (eg echocardiography) may prove to be useful.

Trauma scoring

Trauma scoring is often used in research on the epidemiology and management of trauma. A basic understanding of the accepted system of trauma scoring may be of benefit to those treating injured patients.

Injury Severity Score (ISS)

The ISS is widely used to retrospectively score the anatomical injuries of an individual patient. The score is obtained by first scoring each individual injury using the Abbreviated Injury Scale (AIS), which attributes a score between 1 and 6 to each individual injury, as follows:

AIS 1 = minor injury   AIS 4 = severe injury

AIS 2 = moderate injury   AIS 5 = critical injury

AIS 3 = serious injury   AIS 6 = inevitably fatal injury

To calculate the ISS from an array of AIS scores for a patient, the 3 highest AIS scores in different body *regions* are squared then added together. ISS considers the body to comprise 6 regions: head/neck; face; chest; abdomen; extremities; external (skin). Possible ISS scores range from 1 to 75. Any patient with an AIS = 6 is automatically given an ISS of 75. See www.aast.org/Library/TraumaTools/InjuryScoringScales.aspx

For example, see Table 8.1.

Table 8.1

Injuries	AIS (body region)
Closed linear temporal skull fracture	AIS = 2 (head/neck)
Major aortic arch rupture at its root	AIS = 5 (chest)
Bilateral pulmonary contusions	AIS = 4 (chest)
Massive splenic rupture with hilar disruption	AIS = 5 (abdomen)
Multiple widespread superficial abrasions	AIS = 1 (external)

$ISS = (5)^2 + (5)^2 + (2)^2 = 54$. The ISS is non-linear and some scores (eg 15) are impossible. One accepted definition of 'major trauma' is an ISS >15.

The Revised Trauma Score

The Revised Trauma Score (RTS) is used to assess the physiological disturbance of a trauma patient. The score is calculated from the respiratory rate, systolic BP and GCS. Each of these parameters are assigned a code (value) to which a weighting factor is applied. The 3 resultant scores are then added together to give the RTS. The RTS ranges from 0 (worst possible) to 7.84 (best).

TRISS methodology

Combining the ISS with the RTS and adding a weighting factor according to the age of the patient, it is possible to calculate a 'Probability of Survival' (Ps) for each patient, based upon the national norm. Patients who survive with Ps<0.5 are regarded as 'unexpected survivors'; patients who die with Ps>0.5 as 'unexpected deaths'. By analysing the results of treating a large number of patients, TRISS methodology may be used to compare 'performances' (eg of one hospital against the national norm).

Airway obstruction: basic measures

Severely injured patients die rapidly unless oxygenated blood reaches the brain and other vital organs. Clear, maintain, and protect the airway, ensure that ventilation is adequate and give O_2 in as high a concentration as possible. The most urgent priority is to clear an obstructed airway, but avoid causing or exacerbating any neck injury: instruct someone to hold the head and neck in a neutral position until the neck is satisfactorily immobilized. Ensure you always wear personal protective equipment.

When treating any seriously injured patient, always ensure that O_2, suction and airway equipment are readily available. Get senior ED ICU/anaesthetic help early if a patient with a serious airway problem arrives or is expected.

Causes of airway obstruction

- Coma from any cause can result in airway obstruction and loss of protective airway reflexes.
- Blood or vomit may block the airway.
- The airway may be disrupted by trauma of the face or larynx, or may be occluded by a haematoma or by oedema following burns.

Assessment of airway obstruction

Talk to the patient and see if he responds. A lucid reply shows that the airway is patent, that he is breathing and that some blood is reaching the brain, at least for the moment. Ensure that the neck does not move until it has been checked and cleared of injury (📖 p.320).

Look and listen to check how the patient is breathing. Complete airway obstruction in someone who is still trying to breathe results in paradoxical movements of the chest and abdomen, but no breath sounds. Gurgling, snoring and stridor are signs of partial obstruction.

Management of airway obstruction

- Look in the mouth and pharynx for FBs, blood, and vomit. The tip of a laryngoscope may be useful as an illuminated tongue depressor.
- Remove any FB with Magill's forceps and suck out any liquid with a large rigid suction catheter. See if the patient responds and has a gag reflex, but beware of precipitating coughing or vomiting.
- If vomiting occurs, tilt the trolley head down and suck out any vomit.
- Lift the chin and use the jaw thrust manoeuvre (see opposite) to open the airway, but do not flex or extend the neck.
- After any airway intervention, look, listen, and feel to reassess airway patency and efficacy of breathing.
- If the gag reflex is absent or poor, insert an *oropharyngeal airway* (see opposite). This helps to hold the tongue forwards, but can cause vomiting or coughing if there is a gag reflex. If the gag reflex is present or the patient's jaws are clenched, consider a *nasopharyngeal airway*. Although a nasopharyngeal airway is useful in some situations, avoid its use if there is evidence of severe facial or head injury.
- If the airway is now patent and the patient is breathing, give high concentration O_2 (15L/min via a non-rebreathing reservoir mask).
- If the airway is patent, but breathing inadequate, ventilate the patient with O_2 bag and mask device and prepare for tracheal intubation. If possible, one person should hold the mask on the face with both hands to ensure a good seal, whilst a second person squeezes the ventilation bag.

Insertion of oropharyngeal airway

- Select the appropriate size of airway.
- Hold an airway against the patient's face. A correctly sized airway reaches from the corner of the mouth to the external auditory canal. A large adult usually needs a size 4 airway, most men require size 3, some women need a size 2. An incorrectly sized airway may make the obstruction worse, rather than better.
- Open the patient's mouth and use a rigid suction catheter with high power suction to suck out any fluid or blood from the oropharynx.
- Insert the oropharyngeal airway 'upside down' for 4–5cm (half way), then rotate it 180° and insert it until the flange is at the teeth.
- In children, use a laryngoscope as a tongue depressor and insert the airway the 'correct way up' to avoid trauma to the palate.
- Re-check the airway and breathing and give high flow O_2.
- Ventilate the patient if breathing is inadequate.

Insertion of nasopharyngeal airway

- Select an appropriate airway, usually a 7.0mm for adult males and a 6.0mm for adult females. A safety pin through the flange end will prevent displacement into the nose or nasopharynx.
- Lubricate the airway with water or a water-soluble lubricant.
- Insert the tip of the airway into one nostril and direct the airway posteriorly, aiming the tip at the tragus of the ear.
- The airway should slide easily into the nose until the flange abuts the nostril and the tip is just visible in the pharynx. Never force a nasopharyngeal airway into the nostril—any bleeding produced will markedly aggravate the airway problem.
- Re-check the airway and breathing and give high flow O_2.

Jaw thrust manoeuvre

The aim of this is to open the upper airway with minimum movement of the cervical spine. Place the forefingers of both hands immediately behind the angles of the mandible and push the mandible anteriorly. This will lift the tongue anteriorly and thus away from the posterior pharyngeal wall.

Tracheal intubation in trauma

An injured patient who has no gag reflex needs tracheal intubation to maintain the airway and protect it against blood and vomit. Intubation may also be needed because of: apnoea (after initial ventilation with a bag-valve-mask), respiratory inadequacy, to prevent potential obstruction from facial burns or to allow manipulation of ventilation in patients with ↑ ICP). Intubation in such circumstances requires emergency anaesthesia: suitable expertise, appropriate equipment and assistance are essential (📖 p.312). An assistant must hold the head to prevent movement of the neck during intubation, while another assistant provides cricoid pressure.

Confirm correct tracheal tube placement by:
- Seeing the tube pass through the cords.
- Observing symmetrical chest movement.
- Listening over both axillae for symmetrical breath sounds.
- Confirming placement with end-tidal carbon dioxide (CO_2) monitoring.

If airway obstruction is complete, the obstruction cannot be relieved and intubation is impossible, an urgent surgical airway is needed (📖 p.326).

Airway obstruction: surgical airway

Surgical cricothyroidotomy or jet insufflation of the airway via a *needle cricothyroidotomy* is needed if the airway is obstructed by trauma, oedema or infection, and the trachea cannot be intubated. Emergency tracheostomy is not indicated in this situation because it is too time-consuming to perform and the necessary expertise may not be available.

Needle cricothyroidotomy

This is a rapid temporizing measure whilst preparation is made for a definitive airway (eg surgical cricothyroidotomy). Jet insufflation via a cannula placed through the cricothyroid membrane can provide up to 45min of oxygenation of a patient with partial airway obstruction (Fig. 8.1).

• Use a large IV cannula-over-needle (adults: 12 or 14G; children: 16 or 18G), attached to a syringe. If right-handed, stand on the patient's left.
• Palpate the cricothyroid membrane between the thyroid and cricoid cartilages. Hold the cricoid cartilage firmly with the left hand.
• Pass the needle and cannula at a 45° angle to the skin in the midline through the lower half of the cricothyroid membrane into the trachea.
• Aspirate whilst advancing the needle. Aspiration of air confirms entry into the trachea. Withdraw the needle whilst advancing the cannula down into position in the trachea.
• Connect the cannula via a Y connector or O_2 tubing with a side hole to wall O_2 at 15L/min (in a child the rate should initially be set in L/min at the child's age in years, increasing if necessary until capable of causing chest movement). Hold the cannula firmly in position. Occlude the side hole or the end of the Y connector with a thumb for 1 in 5sec to give intermittent insufflation of O_2.

Spontaneous breathing through the small airway of a cannula is very difficult, but the patient should be able to exhale partially in the 4sec between jets of O_2. However, CO_2 retention occurs and limits the time that jet insufflation can be tolerated. Proceed immediately to a definitive airway (call a senior ENT or maxillofacial surgeon).

Surgical cricothyroidotomy

This technique is not appropriate in children aged <12 years.
• Stand on the patient's right. Feel the thyroid and cricoid cartilages and the cricothyroid membrane between them.
• Clean the area and give LA (if the patient is conscious and time allows).
• Hold the thyroid cartilage with the left hand and make a transverse incision through the skin and the cricothyroid membrane.
• Use a tracheal dilator or curved artery forceps to open the hole into the trachea. Do not worry about any bleeding at this time.
• Insert a lubricated tracheostomy tube (5–7mm diameter) through the cricothyroid membrane into the trachea.
• Remove the introducer from the tracheostomy tube, inflate the cuff and connect the tube to a catheter mount and ventilation bag.
• Confirm correct placement with end-tidal CO_2 monitoring.
• Ventilate the patient with O_2 and secure the tracheal tube.
• Examine the chest and check for adequacy of ventilation.

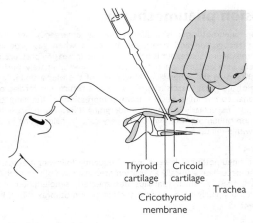

Thyroid cartilage | Cricoid cartilage | Trachea
Cricothyroid membrane

Fig. 8.1 Needle cricothyroidotomy.

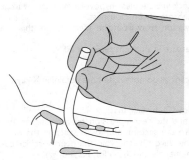

Fig. 8.2 Surgical cricothyroidotomy.

Tension pneumothorax

Tension pneumothorax is a life-threatening emergency and requires prompt recognition and treatment. It occurs when gas progressively enters the pleural space, but is unable to leave. Increasing pressure causes complete lung collapse on the affected side and ultimately pushes the mediastinum to the other side. Movement of the mediastinum leads to kinking of the great vessels, thereby ↓ venous return and cardiac output. Additional compromise results from compression of the lung on the other side, particularly in patients undergoing IPPV. The process leading to tension pneumothorax may occur very rapidly, culminating in cardiac arrest within minutes.

Causes

Tension pneumothorax is seen most frequently following trauma, but it may also occur iatrogenically after attempted insertion of a central venous line (🕮 p.56). A small (perhaps unsuspected) simple pneumothorax is particularly likely to become a tension pneumothorax when IPPV is commenced.

Features

- Dyspnoea, tachypnoea, and acute respiratory distress.
- Absent breath sounds on the affected side.
- Hyper-resonance over the affected lung (difficult to demonstrate in a noisy environment).
- Distended neck veins (unless hypovolaemic), tachycardia, hypotension, and ultimately, loss of consciousness.
- Tracheal deviation away from the affected side (this is rarely clinically apparent).
- ↑ Airway pressure in a patient receiving IPPV.

Diagnosis

This is *entirely clinical*: do not waste time obtaining X-rays.

Treatment

- Apply high flow O$_2$ by face mask.
- Perform immediate decompression by inserting an IV cannula (16G or larger) into the second intercostal space in the mid-clavicular line, just above the third rib (to avoid the neurovascular bundle; Fig. 8.3). Withdraw the needle and listen for a hiss of gas.
- Tape the cannula to the chest wall.
- Insert an axillary chest drain on the affected side immediately (🕮 p.336).
- Remove the cannula and apply an adhesive film dressing.
- Check the patient and obtain a CXR.

Note: the risk of causing a pneumothorax by needle decompression in a patient who did not have one is approximately 10%. If the patient is very muscular or obese, consider using a longer cannula than normal (e.g. central venous line) to ensure that the pleural cavity is reached.

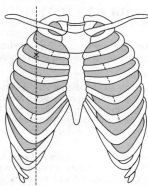

Fig. 8.3 Site for needle decompression of right tension pneumothorax.

Chest wall injury 1

Background

Blunt chest wall trauma is extremely common—both as an isolated injury and as part of multiple injuries. It can cause great morbidity in the elderly.

Isolated rib fracture

A history of trauma with subsequent musculoskeletal pain suggests rib fracture. The diagnosis is confirmed by localized chest wall tenderness—the diagnosis of a single rib fracture is a clinical one. Check for features which are suggestive of pneumothorax (dyspnoea, ↓ air entry, see 📖 p.334), secondary pneumonia or multiple rib fractures, and if any are present, obtain a CXR.

Treat uncomplicated isolated rib fracture with oral analgesia (eg co-codamol ± NSAID). Warn the patient that the rib may remain painful for ≥3 weeks and to seek medical advice if additional symptoms develop.

Multiple rib fractures

Observe the chest wall carefully for possible flail segment, and look for clinical evidence of pneumothorax or, in late presentations, secondary pneumonia.

Check SpO$_2$, ABG, and obtain a CXR. Note that up to 50% of rib fractures may not be apparent on CXR.

Treat Flail segment and pneumothorax (📖 p.332). Treat patients with uncomplicated multiple rib fractures according to the presence of other injuries and pre-existing medical problems as follows:

In patients with other injuries requiring IPPV, discuss the potential need for chest drains with the ICU team (↑ risk of pneumothorax).

Patients with pre-existing pulmonary disease and limited respiratory reserve require admission for analgesia and physiotherapy.

Patients with chest infection often require admission for analgesia, antibiotics and physiotherapy, depending upon past medical history, clinical, and radiological findings.

Sternal fracture

Sternal fracture frequently occurs during road traffic collisions, either due to impact against the steering wheel or seat belt. The injury may be associated with myocardial contusion, great vessel injury and spinal injury (see below).

Features Anterior chest pain with localized tenderness over the sternum.

Investigations
- Place on a cardiac monitor.
- Record an ECG to exclude arrhythmias, MI (📖 p.70) or myocardial contusion (look for ST changes, particularly elevation). Consider further investigation with echocardiography.
- Check cardiac specific enzymes (troponins) if there are ECG changes.
- Request CXR and lateral sternal X-ray: the latter will demonstrate the fracture (which is usually transverse), the former, associated injuries.

Treatment Provide O_2 and analgesia. Admit patients who have evidence of myocardial contusion or injuries elsewhere. Only consider discharging those patients who have an isolated sternal fracture, with a normal ECG, no associated injuries and normal pre-existing cardiopulmonary function. Patients who are discharged require oral analgesia (eg co-codamol ± NSAID) and GP follow-up.

Note Rarely, forced flexion of the chest causes a displaced sternal fracture with wedge fractures of upper thoracic vertebrae. Check the spine carefully, ask about pain, and look for kyphosis and tenderness (which may not be apparent). Lateral thoracic X-rays often fail to show the upper thoracic vertebrae, so if injury is suspected there, consider requesting a CT scan.

Chest wall injury 2

Flail segment

Fractures of ≥3 ribs in 2 places allows part of the chest wall to move independently. This flail segment usually indicates significant injury to the underlying lung (typically pulmonary contusions). Large flail segments occur laterally when several ribs on one side fracture anteriorly and posteriorly. Similarly, an anterior flail segment is produced by bilateral fractures of all ribs anteriorly—in this case, the free portion comprises the sternum, costal cartilages, and the medial parts of the fractured ribs (see Fig. 8.4).

Presentation The flail segment causes pain and moves paradoxically compared with the rest of the chest wall, limiting the effectiveness of respiration. The diagnosis is a clinical one, but it can be difficult to make. Look tangentially at the chest for areas which move paradoxically (ie inwards during inspiration and outwards during expiration). There may be associated features of respiratory distress (cyanosis, tachypnoea). Check for pneumothorax or haemothorax (📖 p.334).

Investigations Assessment of the extent of respiratory compromise is largely clinical, aided by a few simple investigations:
- SpO_2 on pulse oximetry.
- ABG—the combination of hypoxia and respiratory acidosis (↑ pCO_2, ↑ H^+) indicates severe respiratory compromise.
- CXR will demonstrate fractures and associated injuries (eg pulmonary contusions, pneumothorax, haemothorax).

Treatment
- Provide high flow O_2 and treat associated life-threatening problems.
- Contact the ICU/anaesthesia team and carefully consider the need for immediate or urgent tracheal intubation with IPPV.
- Careful observation and monitoring in an high dependency unit (HDU) or ICU is required.
- Consider inserting an intra-arterial line for frequent ABG analyses.
- Selected patients may benefit from epidural analgesia in ICU.

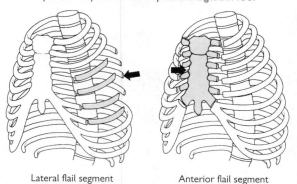

Lateral flail segment   Anterior flail segment

Fig. 8.4 Lateral (left) and anterior (right) flail segments.

Ruptured diaphragm

Left-sided ruptures predominate (75%).

Major rupture of the diaphragm, with associated herniation of abdominal contents into the chest, is a severe injury resulting from a significant traumatic insult (often massive abdominal crushing). Depending upon the extent of the injuries, the patient may present with hypovolaemic shock and respiratory compromise. Note that a ruptured diaphragm may have some clinical features similar to a tension pneumothorax. Call a surgeon and anaesthetist : the patient will require urgent intubation and IPPV.

Minor rupture, with less dramatic herniation, may present in more subtle fashion and result from penetrating injury. The diagnosis is difficult to identify on CT scanning and is frequently missed initially—it is important because:
- It is often associated with injury to both abdominal and thoracic contents.
- There are possible late complications (eg bowel herniation/obstruction).
- It does not heal spontaneously.

Suspect a ruptured diaphragm from the mechanism of injury, and an abnormal or high hemi-diaphragm contour on erect CXR. Look for stomach or bowel loops in the chest: the gastric tube may be seen coiled in the intra-thoracic stomach. If a ruptured diaphragm is suspected, resuscitate the patient and refer to a surgeon.

Oesophageal rupture

Traumatic (non-iatrogenic) rupture of the oesophagus is uncommon, but may follow blunt or penetrating injury. Suspect it if the patient complains of chest and back/neck pain in the presence of a normal ECG. Look for surgical emphysema in the neck. CXR may demonstrate pneumomediastinum (a layer of gas around the heart/mediastinum), a left sided pleural effusion or pneumothorax. Provide O_2, IV analgesia, and start IV antibiotics (eg cefuroxime 1.5g). Resuscitate, treat other injuries, and refer to a cardiothoracic surgeon.

Boerhaave's syndrome is 'spontaneous' rupture of the oesophagus associated with overindulgence and vomiting. Patients are classically middle-aged and present with severe chest pain, signs of shock, and subcutaneous emphysema. If this condition is suspected, treat as outlined above for traumatic oesophageal rupture.

Traumatic pneumothorax

Background

Pneumothorax frequently results from blunt injury with associated rib fractures or from penetrating injury (knife stabbing or gunshot wound). It may also be iatrogenic, secondary to attempted insertion of a central venous line.

Clinical features

Patients are likely to complain of symptoms relating to the associated injuries (eg rib fractures, 📖 p.330). The degree of breathlessness resulting from a pneumothorax depends largely upon its size. Other features may be present, including surgical emphysema, cyanosis, ↓ air entry over the affected lung. Severe dyspnoea and distended neck veins/hypotension suggest tension pneumothorax (📖 p.328).

CXR demonstrates the pneumothorax. Both inspiratory and expiratory X-rays are not required. Wherever possible, obtain an erect CXR. X-rays taken with the patient lying supine may not show a free lung edge, despite a considerable pneumothorax, because in this position air tends to lie anteriorly in the pleural space. If there is no definite pneumothorax visible on a supine CXR, features which are suggestive of a pneumothorax are:

- Hyperinflation of the affected hemithorax with depressed hemidiaphragm.
- Double contour of a hemidiaphragm.
- Basal hyperlucency of the affected lung.
- Visualization of apical pericardial fat tags.

CT scan obtained to assess other injuries will easily demonstrate a pneumothorax. SpO_2 and ABG may reveal hypoxia.

Treatment

Tension pneumothorax is an emergency requiring immediate needle decompression (📖 p.328). Provide O_2 and drain other traumatic pneumothoraces using a chest drain and open technique, as described on 📖 p.336.

Note: although not currently considered to be 'standard practice', there is increasing experience with initially managing some patients who have isolated chest injury and small traumatic pneumothoraces in a conservative fashion, using close observation and no chest drain. Further experience will be needed before this approach can be widely recommended. Patients who have multiple injuries and/or other injuries (particularly those requiring GA and IPPV) certainly require chest drain insertion in the ED.

Haemothorax

Blood may collect in the pleural cavity in association with a pneumothorax (haemopneumothorax) or without (haemothorax). A large amount of bleeding into the pleural space sufficient to produce hypovolaemic shock is termed *massive haemothorax*.

Clinical features

The clinical presentation is similar to that seen in traumatic pneumo-thorax, except that there may be dullness to percussion over the affected lung and, with massive haemothorax, evidence of hypovolaemia.

CXR Blood from a haemothorax collects under the affected lung, showing up as ↑ shadowing on a supine X-ray, with no visible fluid level. It may be very difficult to distinguish haemothorax from pulmonary contusions on supine X-ray, but haemothorax may produce blurring of a hemidiaphragm contour or of the costophrenic angles.

Treatment

Give O_2 and insert 2 large venous cannulae (sending blood for X-matching). If hypovolaemic, start IV fluids before inserting a large (≥32FG) chest drain. Although it is common practice to try to direct the chest drain towards the diaphragm, this seldom makes a difference in practice—it is more important to use a chest tube of sufficient calibre in order to minimize blockages due to blood clots.

Chest drain insertion

Use the 'open' technique, as described below. Explain the procedure, obtain consent and confirm that the patient has venous access, is breathing O_2, and is fully monitored. Ensure that all equipment is ready and a good light and assistance are available. Give adequate IV opioid analgesia to conscious patients as this procedure can be painful.

- Abduct the ipsilateral arm fully.
- Don a sterile gown and gloves, and use a face shield to protect against blood splashes.
- Clean the skin with antiseptic and cover with sterile drapes.
- Identify the 5th intercostal space just anterior to the mid-axillary line (count down and across from the angle of Louis at the level of the 2nd rib) (Fig. 8.5, top).
- Generously infiltrate LA (1% lidocaine ± adrenaline) under the skin and down to the periosteum at the upper edge of the 6th rib.
- Prepare the chest drain; remove and discard the trocar (in adults, use a size 28–32FG; in children, use the largest size that will comfortably pass between the ribs).
- Make a 2–3cm skin incision in the line of the ribs (Fig. 8.5).
- Use blunt dissection with artery forceps to open the tissues down to the pleural space, just above the 6th rib.
- Puncture the pleura with the artery forceps.
- Insert a gloved index finger into the pleural cavity to ensure there are no adhesions and that you are within the thoracic cavity (Fig. 8.5).
- Insert the chest drain ensuring that all drainage holes are inside the chest (typically ≈15–20cm in adults).
- Connect the drain to an underwater seal and look for 'swinging'.
- Suture the drain securely in place (eg with heavy silk) and cover with an adhesive film dressing and adhesive tape (Fig. 8.5). Whilst securing it, get an assistant to hold the drain so that it does not inadvertently fall out. It is useful to insert two untied sutures at the site of exit of the chest drain, so that these can be later tied to close the exit site when the drain is removed.
- Check the underwater seal is 'swinging' in the tube with respiration.
- Listen for air entry and check the patient.
- Obtain a CXR to confirm placement: if the tube has been inserted too far (eg so that it is touching the mediastinum), pull it back slightly and re-suture in place.
- Afterwards, keep the water seal drainage bottle below the level of the patient. Avoid clamping the tube.

Referral to a thoracic surgeon If the chest drain initially yields >1500mL of blood, or subsequently drains >200mL/hr for 2hr, refer urgently to a thoracic surgeon for possible urgent thoracotomy.

Ruptured bronchus Persistent, continuing bubbling of gas through the underwater drain may reflect a major rupture of the tracheobronchial tree, especially if the lung fails to re-expand. Bronchial rupture may also present with haemoptysis or tension pneumothorax. Involve a thoracic surgeon at an early stage.

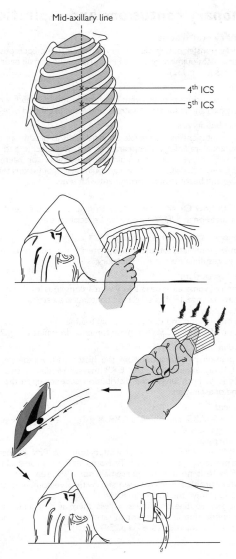

Fig. 8.5 Chest drain insertion.

Pulmonary contusions and aspiration

Pulmonary contusions

High energy transfer during blunt injury (eg road traffic collisions or high falls) often causes pulmonary contusions. Suspect these in all patients with flail segments (📖 p.332).

Clinical features

Pulmonary contusions produce ventilation-perfusion mismatch which may lead to hypoxia and respiratory distress, and ↑ the likelihood of ARDS.

Radiological appearances

Pulmonary contusions may be visible on initial CXR as patchy opacification. However, initial radiological appearances are non-specific and may be confused with those seen after pulmonary aspiration or haemothorax (📖 p.335). X-ray changes resulting from pulmonary contusions tend to be progressive and become more prominent with time.

Management

Provide high flow O_2 and check ABG to help assess the need for GA, tracheal intubation and IPPV. Involve ICU specialists early.

Pulmonary aspiration (📖 see p.112)

Inhalation of vomit and other foreign material may add considerably to the damage resulting from the initial injury.

Common associations

- Inhalation of vomit after head injury with ↓ conscious level and impaired protective laryngeal reflexes: gastric contents are particularly irritant to the respiratory tract.
- Inhalation of blood and teeth after facial trauma.
- Inhalation of water and foreign matter in near drowning (📖 p.258).

Presentation

Suspect pulmonary aspiration from the history, associated respiratory signs and X-ray appearance. The CXR may show diffuse opacification affecting one or both lungs—the distribution depends upon the position at the time of aspiration.

Management

- Check SpO_2, ABG, and obtain a CXR.
- Provide high flow O_2.
- Treat other injuries.
- Consider the need for GA, tracheal intubation, and IPPV. Bronchoscopy may be needed to remove large FBs from within the bronchial tree.
- Even if there is no urgent requirement for IPPV, remember that the respiratory problem is likely to worsen (with development of infection/ARDS), so involve the ICU team early.
- Do not give routine antibiotics, unless there is a specific indication, such as immersion in sewage or in rat-infested water with the risk of developing leptospirosis (see 📖 p.239).

Penetrating chest injury 1

In the UK, unlike the USA, chest 'stabbing' is far more frequent than 'shooting'. Both types of injury can pose a serious threat to life.

Initial assessment and resuscitation

Do not be misled by seemingly innocuous wounds. The size of the external wound has no correlation with the potential for internal injury. All patients need O_2, venous access (send blood for cross-matching, or group and save) and resuscitation according to an evaluation of the airway/cervical spine, breathing, and circulation. Remove all of the patient's clothes and log roll to check for wounds to the back of the trunk and perineum. Particularly in gunshot injuries, make a quick early check for evidence of spinal cord injury. Remember also that penetrating chest injury often involves the abdomen (and vice-versa). During initial assessment aim to exclude or identify and treat the following:

- Tension pneumothorax (📖 p.328).
- Sucking chest wound (📖 p.342).
- Cardiac tamponade (📖 p.342).
- Massive haemothorax (📖 p.334 and 335).

Further management depends partially upon haemodynamic status.

The stable patient

Many patients present without overt evidence of significant injury:

- Provide O_2, secure venous access, and send blood for group and save.
- Monitor SpO_2, pulse, BP, and respiratory rate.
- Administer minimal or no intravenous fluids.
- Perform a FAST scan if possible to look for cardiac tamponade (📖 p.346).
- Obtain a CXR (ideally postero-anterior (PA) erect).
- Record an ECG.
- Provide IV analgesia as required (see 📖 p.320).
- Consider tetanus status and the need for prophylactic antibiotics (eg 1.5g IV cefuroxime—according to local policy).
- Cover the chest wound with a sterile dressing (for sucking chest wound—see 📖 p.342).
- Drain any pneumothorax with a chest drain (having decompressed any tension pneumothorax—📖 p.328). *Do not* insert the drain through the wound (this ↑ the risk of infection).
- Refer all patients for admission, observation, formal wound cleaning, exploration, and closure. If the patient remains stable overnight, with no clinical or radiological abnormalities (on repeat CXR ≥6hr after the first), they may be safely discharged with arrangements for review.
- Carefully document the size, position and other features of the chest wound, remembering the potential medicolegal significance (📖 p.402).

The unstable patient

Haemodynamic instability may be due to tension pneumothorax, massive haemothorax, sucking chest wound, or cardiac tamponade. Treat each of these as outlined on 📖 p.342 involving a senior surgeon at an early stage.

Indications for thoracotomy

Thoracotomy in theatre will be required for significant haemorrhage, which typically means:

• >1.5 L of free blood obtained by initial chest drainage, or.
• >200mL of blood draining per hr, via the chest drain.

Penetrating chest injury 2

Open chest injury

An open wound between the pleural cavity and the outside may cause respiratory insufficiency. When the chest expands on inspiration there is less resistance to air movement through the open chest wound than down the tracheobronchial tree. Air flow into the lungs is reduced and the lung collapses as air enters the pleural space and produces a pneumothorax. Hypoxia develops rapidly.

Features
Look for respiratory distress, tachypnea, and cyanosis.

Management
- Provide high flow O_2.
- Cover the chest wound with a square of polythene or sterile dressing.
- Secure 3 sides of the dressing to the chest wall with adhesive tape, leaving one side free. This will allow air to exit through the chest wall during expiration, but prevent air entry into the chest cavity.
- Insert a chest drain (not through the wound) to drain the pneumothorax.
- Provide further resuscitation as necessary.
- Call a thoracic surgeon to arrange formal wound closure.

Cardiac tamponade

Haemorrhage into the pericardial sac may compromise cardiac output. Continuing bleeding leads to cardiac tamponade, culminating in cardiac arrest. Cardiac tamponade usually results from penetrating trauma but may occur after blunt trauma.

Features
Clinical diagnosis requires a high index of suspicion. The oft-quoted Beck's triad comprises distended neck veins, hypotension, and muffled heart sounds. Identifying muffled heart sounds is rarely easy in a noisy ED and neck veins may not be distended in a hypovolaemic patient. Kussmaul's sign and pulsus paradoxus are classical, but rarely helpful.

Investigation
The investigation of choice is a FAST scan (📕 p.346) in the ED resuscitation room to identify the presence of pericardial fluid. USS signs of cardiac tamponade include right ventricular collapse. Formal echocardiography is rarely available immediately. CXR and ECG are rarely helpful, but may exclude co-existent conditions (eg pneumothorax).

Treatment
- Provide O_2, insert 2 IV lines, commence IV fluid infusion if severely shocked and monitor ECG.
- Request that the thoracotomy tray be made ready.
- Contact the most senior available cardiothoracic/general/trauma surgeon and anaesthetist and alert the operating theatre.
- If the patient's condition permits, arrange immediate transfer for thoracotomy in theatre. Theatre thoracotomies have better outcomes than those done in the ED.

- If the patient deteriorates to a peri-arrest state, consider pericardiocentesis using a long 18G needle connected to a 20mL syringe and 3-way tap. Puncture the skin 1–2cm below the xiphisternum at 45° to the skin. Aspirate while advancing the needle cephalad, aiming towards the tip of the left scapula. ST and T wave changes, widened QRS or arrhythmias imply that the needle has been advanced too far.
- Aspiration of a small amount of blood (eg 20–40mL) may improve cardiac output temporarily and 'buy time' to organize thoracotomy.
- Pericardiocentesis is often unsuccessful due to clots which have formed in the pericardial sac and which cannot be aspirated.
- Perform immediate thoracotomy in the ED for cardiac arrest from penetrating trauma. Do not waste time on pericardiocentesis.

Thoracotomy for cardiac tamponade

Thoracotomy in the ED may be required in certain life-threatening emergencies, including cardiac arrest due to penetrating chest injury: the principal aim is to decompress the pericardium and relieve tamponade. First exclude and treat other reversible causes of cardiac arrest (upper airway obstruction, 📖 p.324; tension pneumothorax, 📖 p.328). Thoracotomy is not indicated for cardiac arrest following blunt injury.

Procedure

- Summon expert help (ED consultant; cardiothoracic, general or trauma surgeon; anaesthetist) and proceed immediately. Do not wait.
- Whilst the thoracotomy tray is being opened, don gloves, a face shield and an apron, ensure that the patient is being ventilated with O_2 via a tracheal tube, and start external chest compressions (📖 p.49). Continue rapid IV infusion via multiple lines and obtain blood for transfusion.
- Standing on the patient's left side, abduct the left arm, stop chest compressions and open the left chest wall. Start the incision at the medial end of the 5th intercostal space and cut laterally just above the 6th rib into the axilla. Use a rib retractor to access the thoracic cavity. If necessary, improve access further by continuing the incision medially using strong scissors to cut through the sternum and into the right 5th intercostal space (clamshell thoracotomy). Speed is of the essence.
- Identify the heart: carefully incise vertically through the bulging pericardium over its anterior surface, avoiding the left phrenic nerve.
- Evacuate blood from the pericardial sac and identify the damage.
- Place a finger over the cardiac defect and perform internal cardiac massage by compressing the heart between 2 flat hands, with fingers placed over defects. Close myocardial wounds using interrupted 4/0 prolene sutures, using teflon or pericardial buttresses if necessary. Once sutures are in place, stop internal cardiac massage and check cardiac rhythm and output. If the heart is fibrillating, defibrillate using internal defibrillation paddles, by placing a paddle over each side of the heart. Start with 5J energy initially, ↑ as necessary to max of 50J. Use an external defibrillator if no internal paddles are available.
- Once a pulse has been restored, ensure that hypovolaemia is corrected. Give cefuroxime 1.5g IV, insert an arterial line and urinary catheter, recheck U&E, glucose, FBC, and clotting.
- The cardiothoracic surgeon will direct further surgical management.

Aortic injury

The vast majority of aortic injuries (≈90%) are sustained during high energy blunt trauma (eg road traffic collisions, high falls). Only a small proportion of these patients reach hospital with signs of life. The usual site of rupture is just distal to the origin of the left subclavian artery, possibly caused by differential shearing forces between the mobile arch and the fixed descending thoracic aorta. An alternative proposed mechanism is that during rapid deceleration the first rib and clavicle swing down and directly 'nip' the aorta ('osseous pinch' theory). The injury is relatively unusual in children, who are perhaps protected by having more elastic tissues.

Features

Patients who reach hospital alive are most likely to have a partial or contained rupture, with a haematoma confined by aortic adventitia. They may complain of chest and back pain and there may be a harsh systolic murmur, absent or ↓ pulses (with differential BP between arms and legs), and evidence of hypovolaemic shock: features of other significant non-aortic injuries may predominate.

Diagnosis

The diagnosis of aortic injury can be difficult: adopt a high index of suspicion. An erect CXR is invaluable provided that the patient's condition permits it.

CXR features suggesting aortic injury include:
• Widened mediastinum (>8cm on PA film).
• Abnormal aortic arch contour.
• Deviation of the trachea to the right side.
• Deviation of an orogastric/NG tube to the right side (such that it lies to the right of the T4 spinous process).
• Depression of the left main bronchus >40° below the horizontal.
• Left pleural cap or fractured first/second ribs are often quoted, but are of little diagnostic value.
• The CXR may be normal!

Management

Resuscitate and treat other injuries. Aortic injuries are associated with other severe chest injuries, eg flail segments, pulmonary contusions. As a minimum, provide O_2, insert two IV cannulae, start IV fluids, provide analgesia, monitor vital signs and SpO_2. Check U&E, glucose, FBC, clotting, ABG, and cross-match. Insert urinary catheter and arterial line.

Involve a cardiothoracic surgeon or a vascular surgeon with expertise in aortic injury. Refer urgently for specialist investigation (CT scan and/or aortography). Involve anaesthetist/ICU. Control BP (avoid over-infusion of IV fluids; use glyceryl trinitrate (GTN) infusion IV to maintain systolic BP ≈90mmHg) prior to treatment. This usually involves open surgical repair, but some centres have reported good short-term results using endovascular stents.

Focused assessment with sonography for trauma (FAST) scan

Increasingly used in the ED resuscitation room to assess the chest and abdomen of acutely injured patients, especially those with shock.

Can be performed by a trained ED doctor, surgeon, or radiologist.

Advantages
- Can be done in ED.
- Quick: takes 2–3min.
- Non-invasive.
- Repeatable if concerns persist or the patient's condition changes.

Disadvantages
- Operator dependent.
- Does not define injured organ, only presence of blood or fluid in abdomen or pericardium.

Ideally performed with a portable or hand-held USS scanner.

Looks at four areas for the presence of free fluid only:
- Hepatorenal recess (Morrison's pouch).
- Splenorenal recess.
- Pelvis (Pouch of Douglas).
- Pericardium.

The scan is usually done in that order, as the hepatorenal recess is the first to fill with fluid in the supine position, and is most easily identified.

If the indication for FAST scanning is to identify cardiac tamponade, the first view should be the pericardial view.

Free fluid appears as a black echo-free area:
- Between the liver and the right kidney.
- Between the spleen and the left kidney.
- Behind the bladder in the pelvis.
- Around the heart in the pericardium.

A positive FAST scan is one which identifies any free fluid in the abdomen or in the pericardium.

Visible free fluid in the abdomen implies a minimum volume of ≈500mL.

The finding of blood in the pericardium after trauma is an indication for emergency thoracotomy, ideally in the operating theatre; however, thoracotomy should be performed in the ED if the patient arrests.

FAST scanning requires training prior to use on trauma patients; there is a significant false-negative rate in inexperienced hands.[1]

---

1 See http://www.trauma.org/index.php/main/article/214/

Diagnostic peritoneal lavage (DPL)

DPL is helpful in situations where clinical evidence of intra-abdominal injury is equivocal and neither CT nor USS is available. DPL may also be useful to search for intra-abdominal bleeding in shocked head-injured patients, or those whose massive pelvic fracture is being externally fixed (see 📖 p.466). DPL is used less often now that FAST scanning and CT have become more readily available. Also, some injuries are treated conservatively (eg 'minor' splenic injury in children) and so a +ve DPL is of less value than a specific diagnosis made by CT. The open technique of DPL is shown below. Ideally, DPL is done by the surgeon who will perform the laparotomy if the DPL is +ve.

How to perform diagnostic peritoneal lavage

- Explain the procedure and obtain consent if conscious.
- Ensure that the bladder has been decompressed by a urinary catheter.
- Ensure that an orogastric/NG tube has been passed.
- Enlist an assistant and bright light.
- Clean the skin with antiseptic and drape with sterile towels.
- Infiltrate LA (1% lidocaine with adrenaline) around the proposed site of incision.
- Make a vertical midline skin incision ≈3cm long at a point one-third of the distance from the umbilicus to the symphysis pubis. However, use a supra-umbilical site if the patient has lower abdominal scars, is pregnant, or has a pelvic fracture. Request that the assistant exerts gentle pressure on the wound edges, in order to minimize bleeding.
- Divide the linea alba, identify the peritoneum and grasp it between 2 surgical clips.
- Gently bring the peritoneum into the wound and feel its edge between finger and thumb to ensure that no bowel has been caught in the clips.
- Make a tiny peritoneal incision, insert a peritoneal dialysis catheter (without the needle) and direct it downwards into the pelvis.
- Gently twist the peritoneal clip to obtain a good seal around the catheter. Attempt to aspirate any free fluid.
- If obvious enteric contents or >5mL blood is aspirated—stop, the *DPL is* +ve and the patient requires a laparotomy.
- Infuse 1L of warmed 0.9% saline. Keep the catheter and seal in place and allow 5min for the fluid to mix. Agitate the abdomen gently.
- Place the empty bag on the floor and allow the fluid to siphon out.
- Send fluid for laboratory analysis. Since a +ve DPL commits the surgeon to a laparotomy, an objective measurement is helpful.
- Close the abdomen in layers.

Criteria for +ve DPL

- Aspiration of >5mL free blood or obvious enteric contents.
- RBC count >100,000/mm^3.
- WBC count >500/mm^3.
- Food debris or other enteric contents (eg vegetable fibres).

Note: air enters the peritoneal cavity during DPL and may be visible on subsequent CXR or abdominal X-rays.

Blunt abdominal trauma

Blunt injury to the abdomen may be isolated or associated with injuries elsewhere. Evaluation of the abdomen may be particularly difficult in the latter situation. The mechanisms of injury responsible are diverse and include road traffic collisions, crushing injuries, high falls, and direct blows (eg kicks and punches). Remember that lower chest injury may be associated with splenic or liver injuries.

Examination

- *Assess* for hypovolaemia. Check pulse, BP, and capillary refill.
- *Look* for bruising (eg 'lap belt' imprint). (Measurements of abdominal girth are unhelpful and unreliable as a means of assessing intra-abdominal haemorrhage).
- *Feel* for tenderness and evidence of peritonism. Listening for bowel sounds is not helpful: their presence or absence is not a discriminating feature.
- *Check* for femoral pulses.
- *Log roll* to check for loin tenderness and back injury.
- *Examine the perineum* and perform a *rectal examination*, checking perineal sensation, anal tone, rectal integrity/blood and in the male, the position of the prostate. A high-riding, 'boggy' or impalpable prostate may indicate urethral injury (see 📖 p.352).

Investigations

The need for and choice of investigation depend upon individual circumstances, local policy, facilities, and expertise. Patients who are haemodynamically unstable or who have peritonism require immediate referral for laparotomy.

Perform urinalysis in all patients. A positive urinalysis is a marker for intra-abdominal solid organ injury, not just renal tract injury. Insert a urinary catheter in patients who present with haemodynamic disturbance or who are critically ill (unless there is evidence of urethral injury, see 📖 p.352). Perform a pregnancy test in all women of child bearing age.

Serum amylase does not discriminate between those with significant intra-abdominal injury and those without; it is unhelpful in the early stages of trauma resuscitation.

Plain abdominal X-ray is rarely useful, unless associated bony injury or bowel perforation is suspected: free intraperitoneal gas may be demonstrated on an erect CXR.

FAST (USS) provides a rapid, repeatable, non-invasive bedside test. It is operator-dependent. Haemoperitoneum is identified by scanning the hepatorenal and splenorenal recesses, and the pelvis. The pericardium can also be scanned to look for tamponade. See 📖 p.346.

CT scans are extensively used to evaluate abdominal injuries as well as identifying injuries in other regions (eg retroperitoneum, brain, chest). The major advantage of CT is the ability to diagnose the injured organ(s) within the abdomen and to quantify injuries (minor laceration of liver or spleen vs. multiple deep lacerations with significant haemoperitoneum).

Initial stabilization (see 📖 p.320)

- Provide O_2.
- Treat airway and breathing problems.
- Insert 2 wide bore (>16G) IV lines.
- Send blood for U&E, glucose, FBC, clotting screen, and cross-matching.
- Give IV fluids according to initial evidence of hypovolaemia and response to treatment. Give blood ± blood products early if unstable.
- Provide IV analgesia as necessary (contrary to popular opinion, this does not compromise clinical abdominal evaluation).
- Consider the need for orogastric/NG tube and urinary catheter.
- Involve a surgeon at an early stage.
- Inform the senior surgeon, duty anaesthetist and theatre staff if an urgent laparotomy is needed.

Further evaluation and treatment

Once resuscitation is under way, further evaluation and treatment will depend largely upon the clinical situation:

Haemodynamically unstable Refer urgently to a senior surgeon for laparotomy. Inform the operating theatre and the duty anaesthetist immediately. There is no need (or time) to attempt to define the intra-abdominal injury. Damage control surgery should be considered in unstable, acidotic or cold patients.

Clinical peritonism Resuscitate as above, provide IV antibiotics (eg cefuroxime 1.5g) and refer urgently to a surgeon for laparotomy.

Haemodynamically stable, no peritonism Refer to a surgeon for further investigation and observation. FAST (USS) and abdominal CT scans are very useful in further assessment of these patients. Depending on local policy, others may be appropriately managed with regular observations and clinical re-examination.

Possible abdominal injury in the multiply injured These patients provide a diagnostic challenge: tailor investigations and management to individual circumstances. FAST (USS) and DPL are rapid, simple, and useful tools to help to identify significant intra-abdominal haemorrhage in the multiply injured patient. CT has superior diagnostic accuracy, but it is time-consuming and requires transfer and IV contrast. If the patient is haemodynamically stable, abdominal CT is conveniently performed simultaneously with head CT. A patient who is haemodynamically unstable should be transferred to theatre, never to the CT scanner.

Abdominal trauma in pregnancy

Involve a senior obstetrician and gynaecologist at an early stage. USS can demonstrate fetal viability and look for signs of abruption and uterine rupture. Remember to check Rhesus/antibody status—📖 p.594.

Penetrating abdominal trauma

Most penetrating abdominal injuries are caused by knives or guns. The size of the external wound bears no relationship to the severity of intra-abdominal injuries. These injuries have medicolegal implications (📖 p.403).

Initial approach
On receiving the patient, provide O_2, secure venous access and resuscitate according to an initial assessment of:
- *Airway and cervical spine.*
- *Breathing.*
- *Circulation.*

Obtain complete exposure at an early stage in order to check for additional wounds to the chest, back, loins, buttocks, and perineum.

Evaluation of abdominal injury
Unless the patient presents with hypovolaemic shock, it may be difficult to decide the extent and severity of the abdominal injury on clinical grounds. In addition to standard monitoring and palpation of the abdomen, perform a digital rectal examination and (especially in gunshot injuries) check carefully for spinal cord/cauda equina injury (📖 p.380).

Investigations
Urinalysis Check the urine for blood.

Blood Check BMG, U&E, glucose, FBC, clotting, group and save/cross-match.

X-rays Obtain an erect CXR if possible to check for free gas under the diaphragm and a supine abdominal X-ray to identify bullet fragments, etc.

FAST (USS) FAST scanning will rapidly identify the presence of free intra-abdominal fluid which would mandate a laparotomy (📖 p.346).

DPL This is rarely helpful in penetrating injuries.

Management
- Give O_2; insert two IV cannulas and send blood as outlined above.
- In the unstable patient, give IV fluid as necessary, but do not give excessive IV fluids—aggressive infusion worsens outcome. A systolic BP ≈90mmHg in a conscious patient is enough until the start of surgery.
- Provide IV analgesia (eg titrated increments of morphine) as required.
- Give IV antibiotics (eg cefuroxime 1.5g + metronidazole 500mg).
- Consider the need for tetanus prophylaxis (📖 p.410).
- Cover the wound with a sterile dressing. Never probe or explore the wound in the ED to try and define depth and possible peritoneal penetration. Involve the surgeon early to decide further management.
- Patients who are haemodynamically unstable, have gunshot wounds, or have obvious protruding bowel contents require urgent resuscitation and immediate laparotomy. Cover protruding omentum or bowel with saline soaked sterile swabs and do not push it back into the abdomen.
- Investigation and treatment of other patients varies according to local policy. Some patients may be managed conservatively with monitoring and close observation.

Renal trauma

Most renal injuries result from direct blunt abdominal trauma, the kidney being crushed against the paravertebral muscles or between the 12th rib and the spine. Indirect trauma (eg a fall from a height) can tear the major blood vessels at the renal pedicle or rupture the ureter at the pelvi-ureteric junction. Penetrating injuries are relatively rare. Many patients with renal trauma also have other important injuries, which may obscure the diagnosis of the renal injury.

Children are particularly prone to renal injuries. Trauma may uncover congenital abnormalities, hydronephrosis, or occasionally incidental tumours.

Clinical features

Most patients give a history of a blow to the loin or flank and have loin pain followed by haematuria (which may be delayed). The loin is tender and there may be visible bruising or abrasions. Worsening renal pain may indicate progressive renal ischaemia. Perinephric bleeding can cause loin swelling and a palpable mass. Haematuria *may be absent* in severe injuries in which there are renal vascular tears, thrombosis or complete ureteric avulsion.

Investigations

Look for and record visible haematuria and test for microscopic haematuria. Get venous access, send blood for FBC, U&E, glucose, clotting screen, and group and save.

IVU was the standard investigation for suspected renal injuries, but this has been largely replaced by abdominal CT. If CT is not available, IVU can be used to elucidate the form and function of an injured kidney and confirm a functioning contra-lateral kidney. An unstable patient requiring immediate laparotomy may need an intra-operative IVU to diagnose a renal injury and to check that the other kidney is functioning.

CT Urgent abdominal CT is needed if there is frank haematuria or if the patient was shocked (but is now stable) and has frank or microscopic haematuria. The surgical team should be involved before CT is arranged. Patients should be haemodynamically stable for transfer to CT. IVU is unnecessary if contrast enhanced CT is planned or has been done.

FAST (USS) shows renal morphology and confirms the presence of two kidneys, but does not demonstrate function.

Selective angiography is occasionally helpful.

Stable patients with isolated microscopic haematuria do not need urgent IVU or CT, but require review and appropriate follow-up.

Management

Most *blunt renal injuries* settle with bed rest and analgesia. Give prophylactic antibiotics after consulting the surgical team and according to local policy. Repeat and record pulse, BP, and T°.

Patients with *penetrating renal injuries* and *severe blunt renal trauma* need urgent expert urological assessment ± emergency surgery: the warm ischaemic time of a kidney is only ≈2hr. Resuscitate with IV fluids and give IV analgesia and antibiotics.

Bladder, urethral, and testicular trauma

Bladder injury

Most bladder ruptures are into the peritoneal cavity, caused by direct blows to the lower abdomen. These injuries often occur in people with distended bladders. Bone fragments from a fractured pelvis may also penetrate the bladder (□ p.466).

Clinical features

Lower abdominal pain ± peritonism may be associated with haematuria or an inability to pass urine. Look for perineal bruising and blood at the external urethral meatus. Perform a rectal examination to check for the position of the prostate and the integrity of the rectum.

Investigations and management

X-ray the pelvis to check for fractures. If there is no sign of urethral injury, pass a catheter to check for haematuria. Refer to the urology team. A cystogram will show extravasation from a bladder injury. Intra-peritoneal ruptures need laparotomy and repair. Extraperitoneal ruptures may heal with catheter drainage and antibiotics.

Urethral injuries

Posterior urethral tears are often associated with pelvic fractures. Urethral injury may also result from blows to the perineum (especially falling astride).

Look for perineal bruising and blood at the external urethral meatus and perform a rectal examination (an abnormally high-riding prostate or inability to palpate the prostate imply urethral injury).

If urethral injury is suspected, do not attempt urethral catheterization, but refer urgently to the urology team. Some urologists perform a retrograde urethrogram to assess urethral injury, but many prefer suprapubic catheterization and subsequent imaging.

Penile injuries

See □ p.523.

Testicular trauma

Injury to the scrotum/testis may result in a scrotal haematoma or testicular rupture. Both conditions require good analgesia. Further treatment depends upon the exact diagnosis. USS may help to distinguish between scrotal haematoma and testicular rupture. Scrotal haematoma may respond to conservative measures. Testicular rupture requires urgent surgical exploration and repair.

Scrotal injuries

Wounds involving the scrotal skin may need to be sutured (preferably with absorbable sutures)—most heal rapidly. Refer for investigation if there is complete scrotal penetration with the attendant risk of damage to the testis, epididymis or vas deferens. If the testis is visible through the wound, refer for surgical exploration and repair in theatre.

Head injury: introduction

The size of the problem

Many patients with serious or fatal trauma have suffered a head injury. Additionally, minor head injuries are a frequent reason for attendance at an ED. Blunt injury is far more common than penetrating injury.

Common causes of head injury
- Road traffic collisions of all types.
- Falls.
- Assaults.
- Sporting and leisure injuries.
- Workplace injuries.
- Other mishaps.

Pathophysiology

Brain injury may be primary or secondary.

Primary injury occurs at the time of the head injury. This takes the form of axonal shearing and disruption, with associated areas of haemorrhage. This primary damage may be widespread ('diffuse axonal injury' in a fall hitting the occiput) or localized (eg 'contre-coup' frontal contusions in a fall hitting the occiput).

Secondary injury occurs later, due to various problems that commonly co-exist. Many of these are preventable or treatable, and should thus be the focus during resuscitation:
- Hypoxia.
- Hypovolaemia and cerebral hypoperfusion.
- Intracranial haematoma with localized pressure effects and ↑ ICP.
- Other causes of ↑ ICP, including cerebral oedema and hypercapnia.
- Epileptic fits.
- Infection.

The role of intracranial pressure

Once the skull sutures have fused, the cranium is a closed box. Thus, a small ↑ in volume (eg from swelling or haematoma) results in a large ↑ in ICP (see Fig. 8.6). As ICP ↑, cerebral perfusion pressure ↓, since:

Cerebral perfusion pressure = Mean arterial pressure − ICP

Once cerebral perfusion pressure falls <70mmHg, significant secondary brain injury may occur. Control of ICP and BP (including avoiding wild swings in BP) is an important treatment goal, especially as the normal cerebrovascular auto-regulatory mechanisms are impaired after head injury. Cerebral arterioles remain sensitive to pCO_2, however, with an ↑ pCO_2 resulting in marked arterial vasodilatation and unwanted ↑ ICP. Controlling pCO_2 to within normal levels is therefore important.

↑ ICP produces a diminishing conscious level and causes herniation of the temporal lobe through the tentorial hiatus, compressing the oculomotor nerve, resulting in ipsilateral pupillary dilatation. This may progress to contralateral hemiparesis and brainstem compression with cardiorespiratory arrest. ↑ ICP leads to a reflex ↑ in systemic arterial BP together with bradycardia: this combination is the *Cushing response*.

Indications for referral to hospital

Any one of the following criteria indicates the need for hospital assessment:
• Impaired conscious level at any time.
• Amnesia for the incident or subsequent events.
• Neurological symptoms (vomiting, severe and persistent headache, seizures).
• Clinical evidence of a skull fracture (cerebrospinal fluid leak, peri-orbital haematoma).
• Significant extracranial injuries.
• Worrying mechanism (high energy, possible non-accidental injury, possible penetrating injury).
• Continuing uncertainty about the diagnosis after first assessment.
• Medical co-morbidity (anticoagulant use, alcohol abuse).
• Adverse social factors (eg alone at home).

The following are highly recommended:
• The SIGN (Scottish Intercollegiate Guidelines Network) guideline on head injury is accessible at www.sign.ac.uk
• The NICE (National Institute for Health and Clinical Excellence) clinical guidelines on head injury published in 2007 and accessible at www.nice.org.uk

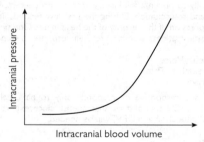

Fig. 8.6 ICP according to intracranial blood volume.

Head injury: triage and monitoring

Triage

Every ED requires a system for the rapid initial assessment of head-injured patients. The exact system will depend upon local policy, expertise and facilities. It must enable patients with significant injuries to receive immediate resuscitation and ensure urgent treatment of those patients liable to complications. Experienced nursing staff can quickly identify those patients in need of urgent attention, based upon:

- The mechanism of injury.
- History from the ambulance crew.
- An assessment of vital signs.
- Conscious level according to the Glasgow Coma Scale (📖 p.361).
- Limb power.
- Pupil responses.
- BMG.

For patients who are *haemodynamically stable, alert and orientated*, with no neurological deficit and an apparently minor head injury, it is appropriate to proceed to obtaining a full history, as outlined on 📖 p.358.

For patients with *multiple injuries and/or a serious head injury*, there will be no time initially to obtain a full history. Instead, proceed rapidly to initial assessment and resuscitation. During the first few seconds, it is useful to obtain an impression of the severity of the head injury. One simple method (AVPU) classifies patients according to their response to stimulation:

- **A**lert.
- Responsive to **V**oice.
- Responsive only to **P**ain.
- **U**nresponsive.

If a patient is unresponsive or responds only to pain, call for senior ED help and an ICU specialist or anaesthetist, since expert airway care (RSI, tracheal intubation and IPPV) will be needed.

Monitoring

Every head-injured patient requires regular neurological observations. These should include measurements of GCS, pupil response, limb power, pulse, BP and respiratory rate on a standard chart, such as the one shown in Fig. 8.7. This monitoring is critical if complications such as intracranial haematomas, fits and hypovolaemia from other injuries are to be detected and treated at an early stage. Any deterioration in GCS is an emergency: re-examine the patient and correct identifiable problems promptly whilst obtaining urgent senior help.

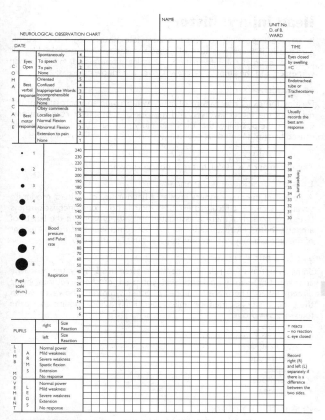

Fig. 8.7 An example of a neurological observation chart.

Head injury: history

It may be impossible to obtain a complete history from the patient, particularly if there was loss of consciousness and/or amnesia. Use all available sources of information, including friends and family, other witnesses, and the ambulance crew. Cover the following areas:

Mechanism of injury

Eliciting the exact mechanism of injury will provide an impression of the nature of the forces involved and the risk of subsequent complications. Consider the possibility that the head injury may have been preceded and caused by another medical problem (eg arrhythmia, epilepsy, diabetes).

Time of injury

This information is useful, but may not be known.

Loss of consciousness/amnesia

A period of unconsciousness implies a head injury of at least moderate severity. It can be difficult to establish exactly how long unconsciousness lasted, particularly if there is associated amnesia. Document the length of amnesia (both before and after injury), but remember that the full extent of the amnesia may not become apparent until much later.

Subsequent symptoms

Some symptoms are relatively common after head injury (eg headache and vomiting)—many patients will complain of these without being directly asked. There are a number of other symptoms, however, which the patient may not mention unless specifically asked. Enquire about the following symptoms:
• Headache.
• Nausea and vomiting.
• Limb weakness.
• Paraesthesiae.
• Diplopia.
• Rhinorrhoea.
• Otorrhoea.

Past medical history

Document pre-existing illnesses and symptoms, particularly those that may have caused the head injury (eg cardiac arrhythmias, epilepsy, diabetes), or might make the consequences more severe (eg bleeding tendency). Enquire about previous head injury (an old skull fracture visible on new X-rays may otherwise be confusing).

Drug history

Ask particularly about recent alcohol and other drug ingestion and whether or not the patient is taking anticoagulant drugs (eg warfarin). This is very important, since patients with bleeding disorders and/or on anticoagulants have a much higher risk of intracranial problems after head injury, often require CT and must be admitted to hospital (📖 p.366).

Social history
Before contemplating discharge of any head-injured patient, find out if there is a responsible adult at home, or if there is someone else with whom the patient could go and stay.

Tetanus status
If there are any wounds, consider the need for tetanus prophylaxis.

Head injury: examination

Resuscitation proceeds with examination, according to problems identified in the primary survey. Follow initial brief neurological examination (GCS, pupil reactions, limb weakness) by definitive complete examination:

Cervical spine injury

Consider this possibility in all cases (see 📖 p.320).

Glasgow Coma Scale

Determining the conscious level is a crucial part of the neurological examination. The adult score ranges from a minimum of 3 to a maximum of 15 and is calculated as shown in Table 8.2. Repeated GCS recordings are a crucial part of monitoring the head injured patient. A fall in GCS indicates a potentially serious deterioration and mandates a search for correctable conditions.

Vital signs

Record pulse, BP, and respiratory rate.

BMG

This is essential in all patients with altered conscious level.

Alcohol

Record if the patient smells of alcoholic drinks but *never* assume ↓ GCS is due to alcohol.

Eye signs

Document pupil size (in mm) and reaction to light. Unilateral pupillary dilatation may reflect orbital injury or oculomotor nerve compression due to ↑ ICP (📖 p.354). Check for a full range of eye movements and the presence of diplopia or nystagmus. Look in the fundi, although papilloedema is a late sign of ↑ ICP. If there is any suspicion of eye injury, measure VA (📖 p.534). In infants, check for retinal haemorrhages (📖 p.731).

Scalp, face, and head

Examine the cranial nerves and search for abnormal cerebellar signs (nystagmus, hypotonia, intention tremor, dysdiadochokinesia). Carefully record scalp, ear or facial injury. Examination of facial injuries is on 📖 p.370.

The limbs

Check limb tone, power, sensation and reflexes. Abnormalities (eg hemiparesis) may result from the primary brain insult or be a consequence of a developing intracranial haematoma requiring urgent intervention. A stroke can cause a fall resulting in a head injury.

Other injuries

The presence of a head injury can render identification of non-cranial injuries difficult. Intra-abdominal injuries often co-exist with serious head injuries and are difficult to detect; have a low threshold for FAST ± CT. In particular, relatively minor non-life-threatening orthopaedic injuries (eg finger dislocations, wrist fractures) are easily missed. Ensure full examination, including palpation of all limbs for possible injury.

Signs of base of skull fracture

This is often a clinical diagnosis. One or more of the following may be seen:
- Bilateral orbital bruising confined to the orbital margin ('panda eyes').
- Subconjunctival haemorrhage (no posterior margin of bleeding seen).
- Haemotympanum or bleeding from the auditory meatus.
- CSF otorrhoea or rhinorrhoea (± anosmia). Fluid mixtures containing relatively similar quantities of blood and CSF will separate into a 'double ring' when dropped onto blotting paper.
- Battle's sign: bruising over the mastoid process without local direct trauma follows petrous temporal bone fracture, but takes several days to appear.

Glasgow Coma Scale (adults)

The GCS assesses the level of consciousness by scoring three aspects of the patient's response and adding up the scores to reach a final score.

Table 8.2 Glasgow Coma Scale

Eye response	open spontaneously	4
	open to verbal command	3
	open to pain	2
	no response	1
Verbal response	talking and orientated	5
	confused/disorientated	4
	inappropriate words	3
	incomprehensible sounds	2
	no response	1
Motor response	obeys commands	6
	localizes pain	5
	flexion/withdrawal	4
	abnormal flexion	3
	extension	2
	no response	1
Total (GCS)		Range 3–15

Notes
- Record GCS in shorthand showing its component parts (for example, GCS 10/15 (E3, V2, M5) means that the patient opens eyes to verbal commands, speaks incomprehensible sounds, localizes a painful stimulus). Similarly, when communicating with other health professionals describe the total score (GCS) and list its components.
- Unconsciousness is generally taken to mean no eye response and GCS ≤8.
- 'Abnormal flexion' implies decorticate rigidity; and 'abnormal extension' implies decerebrate rigidity.
- The GCS is difficult to apply to small children, but may be modified as outlined on 📖 p.717.

Head injury: imaging

Traditional use of X-rays has largely been replaced by CT scanning; EDs in some countries have abandoned skull X-rays altogether, so be aware of local policies and protocols. In the UK, Scottish Intercollegiate Guidelines Network (SIGN) guidelines on the early management of patients with a head injury (www.sign.ac.uk) were updated in 2009. In England and Wales, National Institute for Health and Clinical Excellence (NICE) guidance, published in 2007, is available at www.nice.org.uk

The role of CT scanning

CT scanning is used to identify and define the brain injury, especially intracranial haematomas amenable to surgical treatment. Ensure adequate resuscitation before transferring for CT scan. In many cases, this will include RSI, tracheal intubation, and IPPV. Always arrange for appropriately trained staff to accompany the patient to the CT scanner. When clinical features point strongly to an intracranial haematoma (eg the emergence of focal signs or a deteriorating GCS), discuss promptly with a neurosurgeon the benefits of transferring the patient to a centre that has both CT scanning facilities and an emergency neurosurgical service.

Indications for CT scan

Request CT scan for any of the following (see www.nice.org.uk):
- GCS $<^{13}/_{15}$ at any point since injury.
- GCS $^{13-14}/_{15}$ at 2hr post-injury.
- Suspected open or depressed skull fracture.
- Any sign of basal skull fracture.
- Post-traumatic seizure.
- Focal neurological deficit.
- >1 episode of vomiting (except in children <12 years, where clinical judgement is required).
- Amnesia for >30min of events before impact[*].
- Loss of consciousness and/or amnesia combined with one of: age >65 years, coagulopathy (including clotting disorder, anticoagulant drug treatment) or dangerous mechanism[*] (eg pedestrian hit by car, fall >1m or 5 steps).

Most requests will be urgent (scan performed and interpreted within an hour), except for the two indications marked with an asterisk[*], which if isolated, may allow CT scan to be obtained less urgently (within 8hr), depending upon locally agreed policy.

Interpretation of CT scan

CT scans must be assessed by someone with appropriate expertise.
- Skull fractures are obvious, as is the degree of depression of fragments.
- Intracranial haematomas may cause midline shift and take several forms: extradural haematomas (🔲 p.365) appears as a high density (white) lens-shaped lesions. Subdurals conform more to the surface of the brain (🔲 p.365). Extradural and subdural haematomas can co-exist.
- Cerebral contusions appear as patches of low or mixed attenuation.
- Cerebral swelling may take some time to develop, causing the ventricles to appear smaller than normal.

Skull X-rays: rationale

Skull X-rays are quick, cheap, and easy to obtain but they should only be used when CT scanning is not available in adult patients with minor head injury who do not need an immediate CT scan. Standard views are: antero-posterior (AP), lateral and Towne's. They are useful to detect skull vault fractures, but do not define any intracranial lesion. Identification of skull fractures has been traditionally held to be important because of the ↑ risk of intracranial haematoma, particularly if the conscious level is impaired (see Table 8.3). If CT is planned, do not waste time doing skull X-rays.

Table 8.3 Risks of operable intracranial haematoma after head injury

GCS $^{15}/_{15}$	Overall	1 in 6000
GCS $^{15}/_{15}$	With no other features	1 in 31,300
GCS $^{15}/_{15}$	With post traumatic amnesia	1 in 6,700
GCS $^{15}/_{15}$	With skull fracture	1 in 81
GCS $^{15}/_{15}$	With skull fracture and amnesia	1 in 29
GCS $^{9-14}/_{15}$	Overall	1 in 51
GCS $^{9-14}/_{15}$	With no skull fracture	1 in 180
GCS $^{9-14}/_{15}$	With skull fracture	1 in 5
GCS $^{3-8}/_{15}$	Overall	1 in 7
GCS $^{3-8}/_{15}$	With no skull fracture	1 in 27
GCS $^{3-8}/_{15}$	With skull fracture	1 in 4

Adapted from Teasdale et al.

Indications for skull X-rays

Skull X-rays should no longer be used when CT scanning is immediately available. If CT is not available, it can be used to identify adult patients with skull vault fractures, who will then require transfer for CT scanning. They have virtually no role now in the assessment of head injuries.

Interpretation of skull X-rays

It can be difficult to distinguish fractures from vascular markings and suture lines. If in doubt, examine the relevant part of the head for sign of injury and seek a senior opinion. Linear fractures appear as sharp-edged lucent lines, which have a different appearance from vascular markings. Depressed fractures take various forms, but tangential views may demonstrate the depressed bone. Base of skull fractures are often not visible, but there may be indirect evidence in the form of an intracranial aerocoele or fluid (air/blood) level in a sinus. Check each of the main sinuses (frontal, sphenoidal, maxillary) in turn, remembering that the lateral skull X-ray is usually obtained with the patient lying supine ('horizontal beam', ie occiput downwards). This will affect the orientation of the fluid level.

Management of serious head injury

Tailor management according to the needs of each individual patient.

Initial management

- Clear, establish and maintain the airway, provide O_2 and protect the cervical spine (📖 p.320).
- Check breathing—provide support with bag/valve/mask device as necessary. Examine for and treat any serious chest injury.
- Check BMG and treat hypoglycaemia if present (📖 p.322).
- Insert two large IV cannulae and send blood for X-matching, FBC, clotting screen, U&E, and glucose.
- Correct hypovolaemia, resuscitate, and treat other injuries.
- If GCS ≤ $^8/_{15}$, the patient will require urgent airway protection with RSI, tracheal intubation and IPPV (see 📖 p.312). Call for senior ED help and request help from ICU and/or anaesthesia. Check ABG and ventilate to pCO_2 of ≈4.5kPa.
- Liaise early with an anaesthetist, ICU and a neurosurgeon (see below).
- Contact a radiologist early to arrange a CT scan with minimum delay.
- In the multiply or seriously injured patient who will require a CT scan, concerns of opioid drugs masking pupillary signs are less important than ensuring adequate analgesia. Give titrated IV opioid analgesia (📖 p.320), after recording GCS, pupil reactions, and basic neurological examination.
- Give IV antibiotics for patients with compound skull fractures. Cefuroxime 1.5g IV is a suitable choice, but be guided by local policy. Regional neurosurgical centres vary as to whether or not they advise prophylactic antibiotics for clinical base of skull fracture (there is no compelling evidence that they prevent meningitis): follow local policy.
- Clean and close scalp wounds to control scalp bleeding (use simple interrupted silk sutures for rapid closure), but do not allow this to unduly delay CT scan or neurosurgical transfer.
- Insert a urinary catheter.
- Consider the need for an orogastric tube. Avoid using NG tubes in facial injury or any possibility of base of skull fracture.
- Consider the need for tetanus immunization.

Indications for neurosurgical referral

- CT shows a recent intracranial lesion.
- Patient fulfils the criteria for CT scan, but this cannot be done within an appropriate period of time.
- Persisting coma (GCS < $^9/_{15}$) after initial resuscitation.
- Confusion which persists >4hrs.
- Deterioration in conscious level after admission (a sustained drop of one point on the motor or verbal subscales, or two points on the eye opening subscale of the GCS).
- Progressive focal neurological signs.
- Seizure without full recovery.
- Depressed skull fracture.
- Definite or suspected penetrating injury.
- CSF leak or other sign of a basal fracture.

Treating complications

Early recognition and treatment of complications is essential to prevent secondary brain damage. It is crucially important to prevent hypoxia and hypovolaemia adding to the primary cerebral insult.

Seizures

Check BMG, glucose, and ABG. Treat with IV lorazepam 4mg. Repeat this once if not initially effective. Start an IV phenytoin infusion (loading dose 10–15mg/kg IV over 30min with ECG monitoring) to prevent further fits. Fits which continue for ≥10–15min or recur despite this treatment require senior ED and ICU help, RSI, tracheal intubation, and IPPV.

Deteriorating conscious level

Having corrected hypoxia, hypercapnia and hypovolaemia, a diminishing conscious level is likely to reflect intracranial pathology, leading to ↑ ICP, requiring urgent investigation and treatment. Bradycardia, hypertension, and a dilating pupil are very late signs of ↑ ICP. Speed is of the essence. Liaise with a neurosurgeon who will advise on use of agents to ↓ ICP (eg a bolus of 0.5g/kg IV mannitol—typically 200mL of 20% for an adult). Mannitol is an osmotic diuretic which may temporarily ↓ ICP and 'buy time' to get the patient to theatre for drainage of an intracranial haematoma.

Other examples of deterioration requiring urgent reassessment

- The development of agitation or abnormal behaviour.
- The development of severe or increasing headache or persistent vomiting.
- New or evolving neurological symptoms/signs (eg limb weakness).

Intracranial haematoma

Causes of neurological deterioration after head injury include hypoxia, hypovolaemia, seizures, cerebral swelling, and intracranial haematomas. Intracranial haematomas are important, as prompt surgery may save lives. Patients with bleeding disorders or on anticoagulants have a greatly ↑ risk of developing an intracranial haematoma after head injury.

Extradural haematoma

Classically, extradural haematoma follows bleeding from the middle meningeal artery's anterior branch after temporal bone fracture. Texts describe head injury with initial loss of consciousness, then return to full consciousness, before neurological deterioration as intracranial bleeding continues and ICP ↑. However, many patients deviate from classical 'talk and die' descriptions: extradural haemorrhage may occur in non-temporal areas, with no skull fracture and no initial loss of consciousness.

Subdural haematoma

Bridging vein bleeding between brain and dura causes subdural haematoma. Unlike extradural haematoma (which is separated from brain surface by the dura), subdural haematoma conforms to the brain surface. This helps distinguish extradural from subdural haematoma on CT. Subdural haematoma may be acute or chronic. *Acute subdural haematoma* is associated with a severe brain insult. *Chronic subdural haematoma* often occurs in elderly and alcoholics (↑ risk perhaps due to cerebral atrophy). Chronic subdural haematoma develops over several days, often presenting with fluctuating conscious level, sometimes with an obscure (or even no) history of head injury.

Minor head injury

Introduction

Assessment and management of patients who have sustained relatively minor primary brain insults can be difficult. This is especially true when assessment is rendered awkward by virtue of age, epilepsy, drug, or alcohol ingestion. In these circumstances, adopt a cautious approach and admit the patient for observation until the picture becomes clearer.

Golden rules for managing head injury are:
- Never attribute a ↓ GCS to alcohol alone.
- Never discharge a head-injured patient to go home alone.
- Admit patients with head injury and coexisting bleeding tendency (including those taking anticoagulant drugs).

Differential diagnosis

Consider whether another condition could be principally responsible for the patient's symptoms. For example, small children who vomit after head injury may be suffering from otitis media or a throat infection. Otitis media may be responsible for both the vomiting (with fever) and for the head injury (by causing unsteadiness of gait, resulting in a fall).

Indications for admission

- ↓ GCS (ie <$^{15}/_{15}$), neurological deficit or post-traumatic seizure.
- Significant neurological symptoms (severe headache, vomiting, irritability or abnormal behaviour, continuing amnesia >5min after injury).
- Significant medical problems, particularly bleeding tendency (including inherited diseases and anticoagulant drugs).
- Inability to assess due to epilepsy, consumption of alcohol or drugs.
- Clinical or radiological evidence of skull fracture.
- No one available at home or no safe home to go to (including suspected NAI and domestic violence).

Observation of those admitted

All patients require regular neurological observations (see 🕮 p.356). Act promptly if conscious level ↓ or neurological deficit develops. Remember that one of the principal reasons for admitting patients with apparently minor head injuries is to monitor for the development of intracranial problems. In these cases, resuscitate, liaise with a neurosurgeon and obtain an urgent CT scan.

If after 12–24hr of observation, the patient is symptom-free, haemodynamically stable and is GCS $^{15}/_{15}$ with no neurological deficit, it is reasonable to consider discharge. Patients who do not fall into this category (ie symptomatic, ↓ GCS or neurological deficit) require a CT scan.

Discharging patients

Most of the patients who present with minor head injury can be safely discharged directly from the ED. Ensure that there is a responsible adult available to accompany them home and someone to stay with them for 24hr once they get home. Warn the patient and the accompanying adult of the potential problems following a head injury (Box 8.1)—and what to do if any of these problems are experienced. Give advice regarding analgesia. Most EDs have standard written instructions which are given to the patient and accompanying adult. Examples of head injury warning instructions are shown below.

Box 8.1 An example of head injury warning instructions

Adults

- Ensure a responsible person is available to keep an eye on you for the next 24hr and show them this card.
- Rest for the next 24hr.
- Do take painkillers such as paracetamol to relieve pain and headache.
- DO NOT drink alcohol for the next 24hr.
- DO take your normal medication, but DO NOT take sleeping tablets or tranquilizers without consulting your doctor first.
- If any of the following symptoms occur then you should return or be brought back to the hospital or telephone the hospital immediately. Tel (01***)****** (24hr):
  - headache not relieved by painkillers such as paracetamol;
  - vomiting;
  - disturbance of vision;
  - problems with balance;
  - fits;
  - patient becomes unrousable.

Children

- Your child has sustained a head injury and following a thorough examination we are satisfied that the injury is not serious.
- Your child may be more tired than normal.
- Allow him/her to sleep if he/she wants to.
- Give Calpol® or Disprol® (paediatric paracetamol) for any pain or headache.
- Try to keep your child resting for 24hr.
- If your child should develop any of the following:
  - headache not relieved by paediatric paracetamol;
  - vomiting;
  - altered vision;
  - irritability;
  - fits;
  - becomes unrousable.
- Bring him/her back to the hospital or telephone for advice immediately: Tel (01***)****** (24hr).

Alternative suggested written advice is available from the National Institute for Clinical Excellence (www.nice.org.uk).

Post-concussion symptoms

Presentation

Post-concussion symptoms are common after head injury and cause much anxiety in patients and their relatives. The most frequent complaints are:

- Headache.
- Dizziness.
- Lethargy.
- Depression.
- Inability to concentrate.

Headaches occur in most patients admitted to hospital after head injuries: in ≈30% the headaches persist for >2 months. The headaches are usually intermittent and become worse during the day or on exertion. Some appear to be 'tension headaches' and are often not significantly helped by analgesics. Migraine attacks may become more frequent or severe after a head injury. Headaches that do not fit these patterns may reflect serious intracranial pathology.

Non-specific dizziness is common after concussion. Detailed questioning may distinguish dizziness from vertigo due to disturbance of the vestibular mechanisms. Dizziness may be caused by postural hypotension or by drugs (eg co-codamol and other analgesics) or alcohol (to which patients are often more sensitive after a head injury).

Diagnosis

Post-concussion symptoms are diagnosed by exclusion of other problems or complications following head injury. Take a careful history, including questions about drowsiness, intellectual function, neck pain, photophobia, vomiting, and rhinorrhoea.

Examine the patient for any specific cause of the symptoms and for any neurological deficit. Look particularly for evidence of meningitis or an intracranial haematoma. Check for papilloedema.

Elderly or alcoholic patients or those with a bleeding tendency are prone to develop chronic subdural haematomas, which may cause confusion or intellectual deterioration, often without localizing signs. Obtain a CT.

Treatment

After a careful history and examination, with appropriate investigations to exclude other problems, reassure the patient and explain that the symptoms are likely to resolve gradually. Reduced short-term memory and impaired concentration may make it difficult for a patient to return to work and cause additional stress and anxiety: give suitable explanations and discuss the provision of a sick note with the GP.

Follow-up

Since symptoms may last for some time, arrange appropriate follow-up. This usually involves the GP, who needs to be kept fully informed of the clinical findings and diagnosis.

Maxillofacial injuries: introduction

These injuries often look dramatic and can be life-threatening as well as causing significant long-term morbidity.

Common causes are road traffic collisions, assaults, and sport.

Emergency resuscitative measures

- Perform a rapid initial assessment to look for and treat airway obstruction or major bleeding (💭 p.320). Remember the possibility of an associated neck injury. Blood may rapidly accumulate in the pharynx requiring anterior ± posterior nasal packing for control (💭 p.552).
- Management of airway obstruction is complex, intubation often difficult and occasionally a surgical airway is required: obtain experienced ED and anaesthetic assistance early. Use jaw thrust, chin lift, and suction to establish a patent airway.
- With bilateral mandibular fractures, the tongue may fall backwards. Restore airway patency by pulling the fractured segment anteriorly or by inserting a large (0 silk) suture in the tongue and pulling anteriorly.
- Maxillary fractures may be displaced far enough backwards to compromise the airway by contact of the soft palate against the posterior pharyngeal wall. This can be relieved by hooking two fingers behind the hard palate, and pulling forwards and upwards, *but* this can produce considerable bleeding.

History

Important clues may be obtained from knowing the causative events both in relation to the facial injury itself and also of injury to the head, spine etc. Drug history (eg anticoagulants or bleeding tendency) may be important.

Examination

Inspect the face from the front, side and above (by standing above and behind the patient). Look for:
- Asymmetry.
- Flattening of the cheek (depressed zygomatic fracture).
- 'Dish face' deformity (flattened elongated face due to posterior and downward displacement of the maxilla).
- Nasal deviation or saddle deformity. Measure the intercanthal distance: if >3.5cm suspect naso-ethmoidal fracture—see below.
- Uneven pupillary levels (due to orbital floor fracture).
- CSF rhinorrhoea (causes 'tramline' effect with central CSF and blood either side).
- Subconjunctival haemorrhage without a posterior border (suggests an orbital wall or anterior cranial fossa fracture).

Palpate the facial bones systematically. Start over the superior orbital margins. Work down feeling both sides at the same time checking for pain, deformity, crepitus and movement. Feel specifically for steps in the inferior orbital margin and zygoma. Subcutaneous emphysema implies a compound fracture—often of the maxillary sinus.

Check for hypo/anaesthesia of the cheek, side of the nose and upper lip (infra-orbital nerve injury), and for numbness of the upper teeth (anterior superior alveolar nerve in the infra-orbital canal), and lower teeth and lip (inferior dental nerve damage due to mandibular fracture).

Examine inside the mouth, checking for dental malocclusion (ie the teeth do not meet together properly when the mouth is closed), loose, or lost teeth (this may need CXR), bruising and bleeding.

Examine the eyes carefully (📖 p.536): assume any laceration below the medial canthus involves the lacrimal duct until proven otherwise.

Investigations

In patients with multiple injuries, imaging of the chest, pelvis and cervical spine will take precedence. Even with 'isolated' facial injuries, perform imaging of the cervical spine and head, where indicated, before facial X-rays or CT scanning.

Facial X-rays are often both difficult to perform (because of poor patient cooperation) and difficult to interpret. Get maxillofacial specialist advice regarding the views required and their interpretation. CT scanning is often required prior to definitive maxillofacial surgery.

The commonly required views include:
• Occipitomental 10°, 30°, and 45°.
• Lateral.
• Orthopantomogram (for mandible).

Treatment

Treatment of specific facial fractures is considered in 📖 p.372, 📖 p.374, 📖 p.376. Remember that even in the absence of a visible fracture on X-ray, patients in whom there is clinical suspicion of facial fracture (swelling, tenderness, asymmetry, numbness, etc.) require expert attention and/or follow-up.

Middle third facial fractures

Dento-alveolar fractures

These injuries involve only the teeth and their bony support. Look for deranged occlusion and stepped malalignment of teeth, bruising of gums, and palpable fracture in the buccal sulcus.

Le Fort facial fractures (Fig. 8.8)

These lie between the frontal bone, the skull base and mandible. They involve the upper jaw, teeth, nose, maxillary, and ethmoid air sinuses

- *Le Fort I* involves the tooth-bearing portion of the maxilla. Look for lengthening of the face due to the dropped maxillary segment. There may be movement or a split of the hard palate, a haematoma of the soft palate/buccal sulcus, and malocclusion.
- *Le Fort II* involves the maxilla, nasal bones and the medial aspects of the orbits. Look for a 'dished-in' face, a step in the infra-orbital margin, infra-orbital nerve damage, malocclusion and surgical emphysema. The maxilla may be floating—if the upper teeth are pulled (gently!) the maxilla may move forward. Check for epistaxis, CSF rhinorrhoea, diplopia, and subconjunctival haematoma. Facial swelling occurs rapidly and is often severe. Later, bilateral peri-orbital bruising may be evident.
- *Le Fort III* involves the maxilla, zygoma, nasal bones, ethmoid and the small bones of the base of the skull. The entire midface is fractured from the base of the skull. Features include those of type II plus: flattened zygomatic bones (which may be mobile and tender), steps over the fronto-zygomatic sutures, movement and deformity of the zygomatic arch, and different pupillary levels. There is usually severe facial swelling and bruising. Pharyngeal bleeding may severely compromise the airway and cause hypovolaemic shock.

Le Fort fractures may be asymmetric (eg Le Fort II on the right and III on the left).

Naso-ethmoidal fractures

These produce a flattened nasal bridge with splaying of the nasal complex, saddle-shaped deformity of the nose, traumatic telecanthus, periorbital bruising, subconjunctival haematoma, epistaxis, CSF rhinorrhea, and supraorbital or supratrochlear nerve paraesthesia.

Management of middle third facial fractures

- Resuscitate and establish a clear airway as described on 🕮 p.324.
- Refer dentoalveolar fractures for repositioning and immobilization with acrylic/metal splints ± wiring.
- Refer all patients with middle third or naso-ethmoidal fractures to the maxillofacial surgeons for admission. Any continuing haemorrhage requires packing—leave this to the specialist. Tell the patient not to blow the nose (↑ subcutaneous emphysema and may drive bacteria into fracture sites and intracranially). Prophylactic antibiotics are often advised by maxillofacial surgeons. Ensure tetanus prophylaxis (🕮 p.410).
- Discuss patients with CSF leaks with the neurosurgeons.
- Clean and dress compound facial lacerations, but do not close them (unless actively bleeding); they may need formal debridement and they provide access to fractures for open reduction and internal fixation.

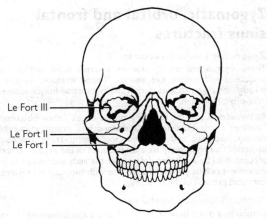

Le Fort III

Le Fort II
Le Fort I

Fig. 8.8 *Le Fort* classification of facial fractures.

Zygomatic, orbital and frontal sinus fractures

Zygomatic (malar) fractures

These injuries are usually due to a direct blow and are frequently associated with severe eye injuries. 'Tripod fractures' involve fractures through the zygomatico-temporal and zygomatico-frontal sutures, and the infra-orbital foramen.

Examination Look for flattening of the cheek (often obscured later by swelling), a palpable defect in the infra-orbital margin, infra-orbital nerve damage, diplopia, and subconjunctival haemorrhage (especially if no posterior margin is seen). Isolated fractures of the zygomatic arch may be accompanied by a palpable defect over the arch and limited or painful jaw movement resulting from interference with the normal movement of the coronoid process of the mandible.

Orbital 'blow-out' fractures

Caused by a direct blow to the globe of the eye (commonly from a squash ball or shuttlecock) resulting in a fracture of the orbital floor and prolapse of contents into the maxillary sinus.

Examination Check for diplopia due to inferior rectus entrapment (the patient cannot look up and medially), enophthalmos, and surgical emphysema. Carefully check the eye itself for injury (hyphaema, retinal detachment, glaucoma, blindness). Record the visual acuity. Test infra-orbital nerve function. Fractures of the floor of the orbit may not be easily visible on X-ray, but can often be inferred by the soft tissue mass in the roof of the maxillary sinus ('tear drop' sign), clouding of the sinus and surgical emphysema.

Management of zygomatic and orbital fractures
- Tell the patient not to blow his/her nose.
- Refer all patients (including those in whom a fracture is clinically suspected but not evident on X-ray) to maxillofacial specialists who will advise regarding prophylactic antibiotics and will arrange further investigation (usually CT scanning) and treatment.
- Involve the ophthalmologists if the eye is also injured.

Note: Patients with orbital emphysema who complain of sudden ↓ in vision may be suffering from a build-up of air under pressure which is compromising retinal blood flow. These patients need emergency decompression.

Frontal sinus fractures

Presenting features include supraorbital swelling, tenderness and crepitus, occasionally with supraorbital nerve anaesthesia. CT scanning will determine whether or not there are fractures of simply the anterior wall or of both anterior and posterior sinus walls (± depressed fragments). Give IV antibiotics and refer for admission and observation, which in the case of depressed fragments, should be to the neurosurgical team.

Mandibular injuries

Considerable force is required to fracture the mandible, so look for concurrent head or other injuries. The mandible may be fractured at a site distant from the point of impact (eg a fall on the chin may cause condylar fractures). There are often fractures at two or more sites (Fig. 8.9). The temporomandibular joint may be dislocated or the condyle driven through the temporal bone causing a skull base fracture.

Symptoms and signs

The patient usually presents with pain (aggravated by jaw movement or biting). Check for swelling, tenderness, or steps on palpation of the mandible. Look for malocclusion, loose or missing teeth, and intra-oral bruising. Numbness of the lower lip indicates injury to the inferior dental nerve where it passes through the ramus of the mandible.

X-rays

Request an orthopantomogram (OPG). Temporomandibular joint dislocation and condylar fractures are best shown by condylar views.

Management

Simple undisplaced single fractures not involving the teeth can be treated with analgesia, soft diet, prophylactic antibiotics (eg penicillin or co-amoxiclav), tetanus cover, and referral to the maxillofacial outpatient department. Refer displaced or multiple fractures to the on-call specialist.

Refer to the on-call specialist patients with bilateral condyle fractures or single fractures with malocclusion or deviation of the jaw on opening. Advise patients with unilateral asymptomatic fractures to take a soft diet and arrange outpatient follow-up.

Temporomandibular joint dislocation

This is almost invariably anterior, but can be uni- or bilateral. It may be caused by a direct blow to the (often open) jaw, or in patients with lax joint capsule/ligaments by yawning, eating, dystonic reactions or intubation. The patient cannot close the mouth, the jaw protrudes anteriorly and difficulty in swallowing leads to drooling of saliva. The pain is often over the temporal fossa, rather than the temporomandibular joint itself. Obtain X-rays only if there is a history of direct trauma.

Treatment If seen shortly after dislocation, reduction can usually be achieved simply and without anaesthesia or sedation (Fig. 8.10). Explain the process to the patient. Sit in front of him/her and with your gloved thumb(s) protected by a gauze swab press down and backwards on the lower molar teeth, while gently cupping and lifting the chin with the fingers. After reduction advise the patient to take a soft diet, and not to yawn (difficult!) or open the mouth widely for 24hr. Delayed presentations can be associated with muscle spasm requiring anaesthesia and muscle relaxants.

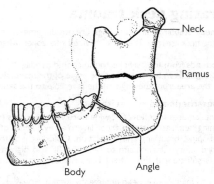

Fig. 8.9 Common fracture sites of the mandible.

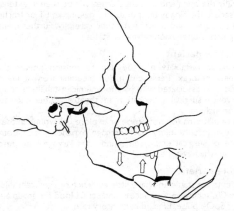

Fig. 8.10 Reduction of dislocated temporomandibular joint.

Penetrating neck trauma

In the UK, neck 'stabbings' and 'slashings' are not uncommon, but gunshot wounds to the neck are rare. The neck is divided into 'zones' when classifying wounds.

- *Zone 1* extends from the clavicles to the cricoid cartilage.
- *Zone 2* extends from the cricoid to the angle of the mandible.
- *Zone 3* is the area from the angle of the mandible to the skull base.

Initial assessment and resuscitation

Every patient requires high flow O_2, wide bore venous access (send blood for X-matching) and resuscitation according to an evaluation of the airway and cervical spine, breathing and circulation. Quickly check for evidence of spinal cord injury. Do not aim to raise the BP too high; a systolic of ≈90mmHg is sufficient if the patient is conscious. Look for and rapidly treat the following:

- Direct airway injury—may need emergency surgical airway (📖 p.326).
- Tension pneumothorax (📖 p.328).
- Major external haemorrhage—apply pressure to the wound.
- Massive haemothorax (📖 p.335).

Occasionally the open end of a cut trachea will be seen in extensive neck wounds; secure the airway temporarily by passing an ET or tracheostomy tube into the lumen and securing the tube carefully. Further management depends partially upon haemodynamic status:

The unstable patient

Haemodynamic instability may be due to tension pneumothorax or massive haemothorax. Persistent major bleeding from a neck wound (usually Zone 2) associated with haemodynamic instability is an indication for emergency surgical exploration in theatre. Other indications for exploration include:

- Breach of platysma (do not probe or explore the wound in the ED).
- Evidence of vascular injury (haemorrhage, expanding haematoma).
- Evidence of surgical emphysema (indicates laryngeal or oesophageal disruption which requires repair).

The stable patient

Many patients are stable and have little evidence of significant injury.

- Provide O_2, secure venous access, and send blood for group and save.
- Monitor SpO_2, pulse, BP, and respiratory rate.
- Obtain a CXR (to exclude pneumothorax/haemothorax).
- Provide IV analgesia as required (see 📖 p.320).
- Consider tetanus status and the need for prophylactic antibiotics (eg 1.5g IV cefuroxime—according to local policy).
- Investigations may include cervical spine X-rays and/or CT neck.
- Occasionally 4-vessel angiography or duplex ultrasound scanning (to exclude vascular injury) and a contrast swallow/oesophagoscopy (to exclude oesophageal injury) are required (usually Zone 1 or 3 injuries).
- Refer all patients to ENT or maxillofacial surgeons for admission, observation, formal wound cleaning, exploration and closure.
- Carefully document the size, position and other features of the neck wound, in view of the high medicolegal significance (📖 p.403).

Spine and spinal cord injury: 1

Consider the possibility of spinal injury when managing every injured patient. Careless manipulation or movement can cause additional spinal injury. Maintain a particularly high index of suspicion and provide spinal immobilization in patients with:

- Major trauma.
- 'Minor' trauma with spinal pain and/or neurological symptoms/signs.
- Altered consciousness after injury.
- A mechanism of injury with a possibility of spinal injury (eg road traffic collision, high fall, diving, and rugby injuries).
- Pre-existing spinal disease (eg rheumatoid arthritis, ankylosing spondylitis, severe osteoarthritis, osteoporosis, steroid therapy), as serious fractures or dislocations may follow apparently minor trauma.

The commonest sites of spinal injury are the cervical spine and the thoracolumbar junction.

Airway management and spinal immobilization

These two aspects demand immediate attention in any patient with possible spinal injury—manage them together. The neck is the commonest site of cord injury. If immobilization is not achieved with unstable injuries, it is the site at which most additional cord or nerve root damage can be produced.

- Perform manual immobilization rapidly (without traction), keeping the head and neck in the neutral position, by placing both hands around the neck and interlocking them behind, with the forearms preventing head movement (see Fig. 8.11).
- Apply a hard collar with continued manual stabilization or support with sand bags placed on either side of the head and tape applied to the forehead to prevent rotation. The collar should fit securely, but not occlude the airway or impair venous return from the head. Take care in patients with pre-existing neck deformity (eg ankylosing spondylitis— p.497) not to manipulate the neck or to force the collar into place.
- Ensure airway patency and adequate ventilation—hypoxia compromises an injured cord. Initially in an unconscious patient, jaw thrust and suction to the upper airway can be used. Remember that oropharyngeal stimulation can provoke severe bradyarrhythmias. Simple airway adjuncts such as oro- and nasopharyngeal airways often maintain upper airway patency, but sometimes tracheal intubation is required. This must be performed by an individual experienced in advanced anaesthetic techniques (usually RSI, rarely fibre-optic) with an assistant controlling the head/neck to limit cervical spine movement.
- Ventilation can deteriorate due to cord oedema/ischaemia, so look regularly for diaphragmatic breathing (diaphragm is supplied by C3/4/5) and the use of accessory muscles of respiration. Use pulse oximetry and regular ABG analysis to confirm adequate oxygenation and ventilation. Tracheal intubation and controlled ventilation may be required.
- Usually, patients will have been transported on a spinal board, which should be removed as soon as the primary survey is completed and resuscitation commenced (Fig. 8.12). Remove the board before imaging if possible.

Suspect spinal injury in patients with ↓ consciousness if there is:
- Flaccid arreflexia.
- ↓ Anal tone on PR examination.
- Diaphragmatic breathing.
- An ability to flex (C5/6), but not to extend (C6/7) the elbow.
- Response to painful stimulus above, but not below the clavicle.
- Hypotension with associated bradycardia.
- Priapism.

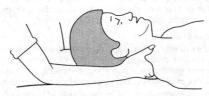

Fig. 8.11 Manual immobilization of the neck.

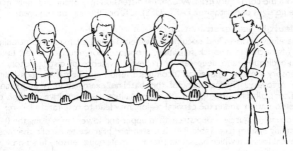

Fig. 8.12 Co-ordinated 4 person lift.

Spine and spinal cord injury: 2

Managing the circulation

Monitor ECG and BP. Interruption of the sympathetic system in the cord causes loss of vasomotor tone, with vasodilatation, ↑ venous pooling, and ↓ BP. Flaccidity and arreflexia, together with the absence of a reflex tachycardia or an associated (inappropriate) bradycardia are pointers to this, but before diagnosing 'neurogenic shock' exclude and treat other causes of hypotension (eg blood loss, tension pneumothorax). IV fluids (📖 p.320) usually correct any relative hypovolaemia, but inotropes may be needed if ↓ cardiac output persists despite adequate volume replacement and correction of bradyarrhythmias by atropine. Use CVP monitoring of patients in neurogenic shock to prevent fluid overload.

Other considerations

Insert a urinary catheter (strict aseptic technique) to monitor urine output and prevent bladder distension. If there is no craniofacial injury, an NG tube will prevent gastric distension (ileus commonly develops after cord injury), and ↓ risk of aspiration and respiratory embarrassment.

With blunt injury mechanisms, up to two-thirds of individuals with spinal cord injury have major injuries at other sites. Conscious patients can usually describe a sensory level and paralysis, with pain at the level of the vertebral injury. Have a high index of suspicion for thoracic/abdominal injury—clinical features may be obscured by sensory or motor deficits from the cord injury itself. Abdominal distension may occur and there may be no signs of peritonism. FAST (USS), CT, or DPL may be required.

Neurological examination

Carefully perform and document the neurological examination, including light touch and pinprick sensation, proprioception, muscle power, tone, co-ordination, and deep tendon reflexes. Evidence of distal, motor, or sensory function implies an incomplete lesion and hence the possibility of recovery. The accuracy of this baseline examination is important, since cephalad progression of abnormalities is a sensitive marker of deterioration, and in the cervical region, may lead to respiratory failure.

Document muscle group strength in upper and lower limbs using the 0–5 grading system (see Table 8.4). It is standard practice to record the most caudal location which has intact (normal) motor and sensory function.

Examine the perineum and perform a PR examination; look for voluntary contraction and anal tone. An intact bulbocavernosus reflex (squeezing glans penis → contraction of bulbocavernosus muscle—S2,3,4) and anal cutaneous reflex (scratching peri-anal skin → anal contraction—S4,5) imply sacral sparing.

Spinal examination

Log-roll the patient. The person controlling the head and neck directs movement. Carefully examine for tenderness, step-deformity, gibbus, widening of interspinous gaps and prominence of spinous processes. There may not be overlying tenderness with vertebral body fractures. Remove any debris from under the patient. Keep the patient covered and warm, as ↓ sympathetic vasomotor tone → ↑ risk of hypothermia. To ↓ risk of pressure sores, remove the patient rapidly from the spinal board.

Table 8.4 Grading muscle strength

Grading of muscle power	
0	Total paralysis
1	Palpable or visible contraction
2	Movement with gravity eliminated
3	Movement against gravity
4	Weaker than usual
5	Normal strength
Muscles supplied by various nerve roots	
C5	Shoulder abductor (deltoid)
C6	Wrist extensors (extensor carpi radialis)
C7	Elbow extensor (triceps)
C8	Middle finger flexor (flexor digitorum profundus)
T1	Little finger abductor (abductor digiti minimi)
L2	Hip flexors (iliopsoas)
L3	Knee extensors (quadriceps)
L4	Ankle dorsiflexors (tibialis anterior)
L5	Big toe extensor (extensor hallucis longus)
S1	Ankle plantar flexors (soleus, gastrocnemius)

Incomplete cord injury patterns

There are several recognized patterns of incomplete spinal cord injury. Although the resultant physical signs can be predicted from a detailed knowledge of neuroanatomy, bear in mind that some patients present with an atypical injury and therefore an atypical pattern of injury.

Anterior cord syndrome Loss of power and pain sensation below the injury, with preservation of touch and proprioception.

Posterior cord syndrome Loss of sensation, but power preserved.

Brown-Séquard syndrome Hemisection of the cord producing ipsilateral paralysis and sensory loss below the injury, with contralateral loss of pain and temperature. This syndrome occurs more frequently after penetrating injury than after closed injury.

Central cervical cord syndrome Typically seen in elderly patients following extension injuries to the neck, with degenerative changes being the only X-ray abnormality. It is characterized by incomplete tetraparesis, which affects the upper limbs more than the lower limbs (as nerves supplying the upper limbs lie more centrally within the cord). Sensory deficits are variable.

Spinal cord injury without radiographic abnormality

A significant proportion of children with spinal cord injury have no radiographic abnormality. The extent of both the neurological deficit and recovery is variable. Adults may similarly have spinal cord injury due to traumatic herniation of an intervertebral disc, epidural haematoma or ligamentous instability, yet plain radiographs may appear normal.

Spine and spinal cord injury: 3

Imaging (for indications for cervical spine X-rays see 📖 p.462) X-rays are readily available, but interpretation can be difficult. Whenever possible get senior expert help. Cord injury can occur without X-ray abnormality. This may be due to ↑ soft tissue elasticity allowing excessive movement (children), or cord compression from disc prolapse (younger patients), or vascular involvement, or spondylosis (older patients).

Cervical spine Request *AP, lateral* (must show C7/T1 junction) and *open-mouth odontoid peg views* if CT of the cervical spine is not indicated. Displacement (subluxation/dislocation) and fractures of vertebral bodies, spinous processes, and peg are best seen on lateral view. Unifacet dislocation causes anterior displacement ≤50% of AP diameter of vertebral body. Displacement >50% suggests bilateral facet dislocation. Look for swelling of prevertebral soft tissues.

AP views show injuries to the pedicles, facets, and lateral masses.

Open-mouth odontoid view usually demonstrates peg fractures.

Flexion/extension views to assess neck stability are rarely indicated soon after injury, as muscle spasm may inhibit movement and there is potential to aggravate cord damage. Obtain senior advice before requesting these views. CT is usually a more appropriate investigation.

Thoracolumbar spine Standard views are AP and lateral. In the thoracic region overlapping structures may make interpretation difficult and necessitate other imaging. If X-rays are of diagnostic quality, visualization of compression or burst fractures, and displacement is not difficult, but these have little relation to the degree of cord injury.

CT and MRI CT delineates bony abnormalities and the extent of spinal canal encroachment. CT of the cervical spine (base of skull to T4 level) is indicated for patients requiring CT brain for significant head injury or as part of a 'pan-scan' for multiple trauma (see SIGN and NICE guidelines). CT or magnetic resonance imaging (MRI) are useful for patients in whom there is clinical suspicion of injury (persistent pain, positive neurology) despite normal X-rays.

Further treatment

Immobilize cervical injuries using a firm, well-fitting cervical collar (eg Philadelphia), pending a decision to undertake skeletal traction. Skeletal traction using Gardner–Wells calipers, or halo devices and pulley/weight systems may be undertaken by orthopaedic/neurosurgical staff to reduce fracture-dislocations, improve spinal alignment and decompress the cord.

Thoracolumbar fracture-dislocations are normally treated by bed rest with lumbar support. In specialist units, unstable injuries may be surgically fixed. High dose steroid therapy is no longer widely recommended as part of the treatment for blunt spinal cord injury—follow local protocols.

With penetrating injuries, if the object is still in place, arrange removal in theatre where the spinal cord/canal injury can be directly seen.

Assessment of spinal X-rays

Interpreting spinal X-rays can be difficult. If in any doubt, get senior expert help. A systematic approach helps to prevent injuries from being missed:

- Check alignment of the vertebrae. The spine should be straight or follow gentle curves and should not exhibit any 'steps'. On the lateral X-ray assess the alignment by checking in turn: anterior vertebral border, posterior vertebral border, posterior facets, anterior border of spinous processes, and posterior border of spinous processes. Look also at interspinal distances.
- Check alignment on the AP film by following the spinous processes and the tips of the transverse processes (Fig. 8.13). Look for rotational deformity and asymmetry.
- Assess the integrity of each spinal vertebra, including the vertebral bodies, laminae, and pedicles.
- Be vigilant in assessing the odontoid peg view (Fig. 8.13), looking for asymmetry/displacement of the lateral masses of C1. Distinguish fractures (limited to bone area) from overlying soft tissue shadows (extend beyond area of bone). Note that the atlanto-odontoid distance should be ≤3mm in adults and ≤5mm in children.
- Look for indirect evidence of significant spinal injury (↑ prevertebral space). The normal soft tissue prevertebral thickness at the antero-inferior border of C3 (ie distance between pharynx and vertebral body) is <0.5cm.

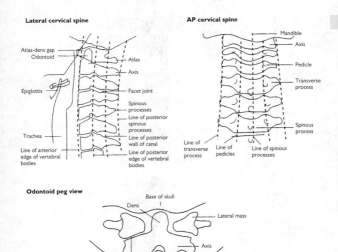

Fig. 8.13 Interpretation of spinal X-rays.

Dermatomes

Dermatomes front (Fig. 8.14)

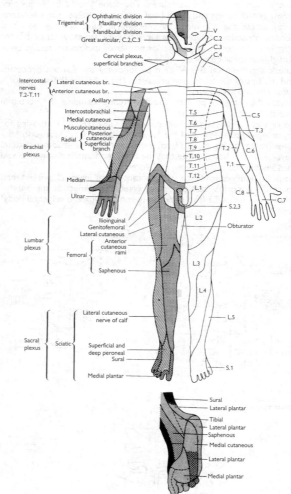

Fig. 8.14

Dermatomes back (Fig. 8.15)

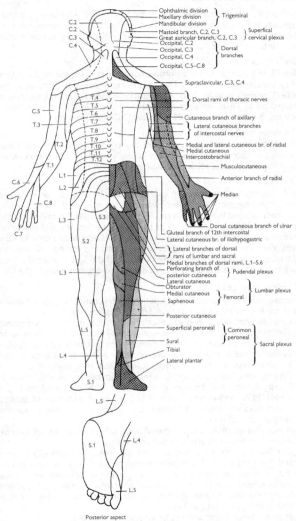

Fig. 8.15

Gunshot injuries

In the UK, inform the police as soon as possible whenever a patient presents with a gunshot wound. Wounds produced by bullets/missiles are determined by kinetic energy (KE) transfer, missile flight characteristics, and the tissue injured.

Kinetic energy transfer
The KE of a missile is directly proportional to its mass and to the square of its velocity (KE = $\frac{1}{2}mv^2$). Thus, tissue injury depends more upon the bullet's velocity than its mass. At velocities > speed of sound, the rate of dissipation of KE becomes proportional to the velocity[3] or even higher powers. Bullets travelling at >1,000ft/sec (300m/sec) are 'high velocity'.

The tissue itself
Tissue density affects a missile, and the energy dissipation and tissue destruction. Bone involvement may cause additional retardation, while bony fragments cause secondary injuries.

Cavitation
High velocity bullets transmit energy to the tissues, compressing and accelerating them at right angles away from the track. This leads to cavity formation around the track. Over a few micro-seconds the cavity enlarges and then collapses. Tissue elasticity perpetuates a process of cavity reformation and collapse, with rapidly ↓ amplitude of oscillations until all KE is expended. This causes highly destructive stretching, tearing and shearing of tissues, causing injury many times the size of the bullet. Since the pressure in the cavity is sub-atmospheric, debris and organisms are sucked in.

Clinical aspects
The principles of resuscitation of a patient with gunshot injury are identical to those for any major trauma case. Specific aspects are:
- Consider staff safety: involve police and check the patient for weapons.
- The magnitude of the external wounds may bear little relationship to the severity of internal injury. Remove the patient's clothes (police evidence) and examine the entire body for entrance/exit wounds that are often missed in hairy areas (eg scalp, axillae, and perineum).
- Patients are often young and fit: signs of hypovolaemia may be delayed.
- Chest injuries are commonly associated with pneumothorax (◻ p.334). PEA cardiac arrest should prompt rapid exclusion of tension pneumothorax then immediate thoracotomy to relieve cardiac tamponade (◻ p.343).
- Abdominal wounds are associated with a high incidence of internal injury and require laparotomy and antibiotic cover.
- Gunshot wounds are prone to anaerobic infection (especially tetanus and gas gangrene): clothing/fragments spread widely through tissues distant from the wound track. Extensive surgical debridement (wide excision/fasciotomy) is often required to remove devitalized tissue and foreign material. All high velocity injuries need delayed primary closure with grafting or suture at 3–5 days.
- Ensure tetanus cover and give prophylactic antibiotics.
- X-ray (AP + lateral) one body region above and one body region below any wound, as well as the region involved, to look for metallic FBs.

Blast injuries

Blast injuries may be due to explosions involving domestic gas, industrial sites (eg mines/mills), or bombs. Often several mechanisms co-exist to cause injury.

Blast wave (primary blast injury) This is an extremely short-lived pressure wave (lasting a few milliseconds only) which expands outwards from the explosive focus. It is produced by intense compression of air at the interface of the rapidly expanding hot gases. The effects can be dramatically aggravated and reinforced by reflection from solid surfaces, such as buildings. Blast wave injuries are caused by 3 mechanisms:

- Disruption at air/tissue interfaces (especially lungs and ears, producing blast lung and tympanic membrane rupture, respectively).
- Shearing injuries at tissue/tissue interfaces causing subserous and submucosal haemorrhage.
- Implosion of gas-filled organs leading to perforation of the GI tract and cerebral or coronary air embolism.

Blast winds These are fast moving columns of air that follow the initial blast wave. Their destructive force can be immense, leading to traumatic amputation or even complete dismemberment. Blast winds also carry debris (masonry, glass, etc.), which act as secondary missiles causing fragmentation injuries.

Fragmentation injuries Objects from a bomb (eg nails, casing, nuts, and bolts) or flying debris (masonry, wood, glass) cause lacerations or penetrating injuries. This is classified as *secondary blast injury.*

Flash burns These are usually superficial, affecting exposed skin in those close to the explosion. Smoke inhalation may also occur.

Tertiary blast injuries result from individuals being thrown by the blast wind, often causing severe multiple injuries.

Quaternary blast injuries include all explosion related injuries or illnesses not due to primary, secondary, or tertiary mechanisms listed above.

Psychological The psychological effects of blast injury are often severe, comprising acute fear, anxiety, and the potential for chronic sequelae.

General aspects of treatment

The principles of blast injury treatment are identical to those for patients with other causes of major trauma (📖 p.320).

Clinical features in blast injuries may be delayed, both in terms of onset and development of clinical signs. This particularly relates to lung and intra-abdominal complications; therefore, observe all patients for at least 48hr.

Search for pneumothorax (may be tension), respiratory failure/ARDS, peritonitis, abnormal neurological signs (suggesting air embolism), eardrum perforation, anosmia (direct olfactory nerve damage). Note that ventilation of patients with blast injuries is a highly specialized area, with potential risks of producing tension pneumothoraces and air embolism.

Other aspects For forensic reasons, ensure that all the patient's clothes, belongings, and any missile fragments are carefully retained, bagged, labelled, and kept secure until given to police officers.

Burns: assessment

Types of burns
- Thermal.
- Chemical.
- Electrical (📖 p.266).
- Radiation (📖 p.268).

History
Determination of the circumstances resulting in the patient being burned is essential to appreciate the nature of the insult and potential associated risks. Do not, however, delay resuscitation in an attempt to obtain a full history. Consider the following questions:
- Was there an explosion? (risk of blast injuries).
- Was the fire in an enclosed space? (CO poisoning, smoke inhalation).
- What was the burning material? (burning plastics release cyanide).
- When was the patient removed from the fire?
- How long was the patient exposed to fire and smoke?
- Was there a history of loss of consciousness?
- Did the patient fall or jump to escape the fire? (look for other injuries).
- What is the patient's past medical history and tetanus status?

Initial assessment
This proceeds with resuscitation. *Check*: Airway, Breathing and Circulation. Particular problems associated with burns are:
- *Airway burns*: suggested by hoarseness, stridor, dysphagia, facial and mouth burns, singeing of nasal hair, soot in nostrils, or on palate
- *Spinal injury*: particularly seen with blast injuries and in those who have jumped from buildings to escape fire
- *Breathing problems*: contracting full thickness circumferential burns ('eschar') of the chest wall may restrict chest movement
- *Circulatory problems*: hypovolaemic shock is a feature of severe burns and may also result from other associated injuries

Assessing extent
Estimation of the percentage of body surface area burnt is difficult for non-experts. Use Lund and Browder charts appropriate for the age of the patient (see Table 8.5, Fig. 8.16). The palmar surface of the patient's palm (not including the fingers) represents ≈0.75% body surface area.

Assessing depth
Burn depth varies with the temperature and duration of heat applied.

Superficial (first and second degree) burns range from minor erythema (first degree) through painful erythema with blistering, to deep partial thickness (second degree) burns, which do not blanch on pressure.

Full thickness (third degree) burns may be white, brown, or black and look 'leathery'. They do not blister and have no sensation.

On the day of injury it may be difficult to distinguish deep superficial (second degree) burns from full thickness (third degree) burns, but correctly making this distinction does not alter the initial management.

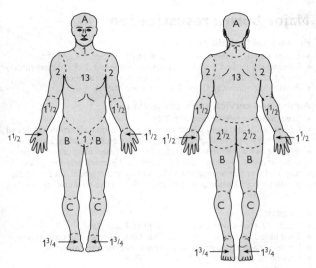

Fig. 8.16 Assessing extent of burns—Lund and Browder charts.

Table 8.5 Relative percentage of area affected by growth (age in years)

	0	1	5	10	15	Adult
A: half of head	$9^{1}/_{2}$	$8^{1}/_{2}$	$6^{1}/_{2}$	$5^{1}/_{2}$	$4^{1}/_{2}$	$3^{1}/_{2}$
B: half of thigh	$2^{3}/_{4}$	$3^{1}/_{4}$	4	$4^{1}/_{2}$	$4^{1}/_{2}$	$4^{3}/_{4}$
C: half of leg	$2^{1}/_{2}$	$2^{1}/_{2}$	$2^{3}/_{4}$	3	$3^{1}/_{4}$	$3^{1}/_{2}$

Adults rule of 9's:	head	= 9%
	each arm	= 9%
	each leg	= 18%
	front of trunk	= 18%
	back of trunk	= 18%
	perineum	= 1%
Infants rule of 5's:	head	= 20%
	each arm	= 10%
	each leg	= 20%
	front of trunk	= 10%
	back of trunk	= 10%

Major burns: resuscitation

Prehospital first aid measures

- Ensure rescuer safety first—be guided by the fire crew.
- Remove the patient from the burning environment. If clothes are smouldering, apply cold water and remove them, unless adherent.
- Provide high flow O_2. Cover burns in clean sheets.

Airway and cervical spine protection

- Treat airway obstruction (🕮 p.320).
- Continue O_2 and apply a hard cervical collar if there is any possibility of spinal injury—cervical spine imaging will be required subsequently.
- If there is any evidence of impending airway obstruction (stridor, oropharyngeal swelling—see 🕮 p.394), call immediately for senior ED help and a senior anaesthetist. Urgent GA and tracheal intubation may be life-saving. Use uncut endotracheal (ET) tubes to allow for swelling of lips and face.

Analgesia

- Obtain IV access with two large peripheral cannulae.
- Send blood: X-matching, FBC, COHb, U&E, glucose, and coagulation.
- Provide analgesia (IV morphine titrated according to response).
- Provide an antiemetic (eg IV cyclizine 50mg).

Fluid resuscitation

- Give IV fluids. Start with isotonic crystalloid (eg 0.9% saline) at 2–4mL of crystalloid per kg body weight per % body surface area burned, over the first 24hr following injury. Give half of this volume in the first 8hr.
- Check pulse, BP, and respiratory rate every 10–15min initially.
- Insert a urinary catheter and test the urine. Patients with myoglobinuria are at particularly high risk of acute renal failure—reduce this risk by adequate fluid resuscitation. Use urine output to guide fluid therapy.
- Review the rate of IV volume replacement frequently and adjust it according to haemodynamic parameters, in order to maintain a satisfactory urine output (>50mL/hr in adults; 1–2mL/kg/hr in children).
- Some burns units prefer a colloid (eg Gelofusine® or albumin) to form a component of the initial volume replacement: follow local policy.
- Patients with full thickness burns of body surface area >10% may require red cell transfusion in addition to the above measures.

Breathing

- Check COHb and ABG.
- Circumferential full thickness chest burns restricting chest movement require escharotomy. Cut the burnt areas down to viable tissue to release the constriction. Cutting diathermy can be helpful to reduce the significant blood loss involved in extensive escharotomy.
- Obtain a CXR.

The burn

- Measure the area of the burn as a % of body surface area.
- Irrigate chemical burns with warmed water (see 📖 p.396).
- Cover the burn with cling film or dry sterile sheets. Do not apply extensive burns dressings before assessment by a burns specialist.
- Involve a burn specialist at an early stage—in the UK, the National Burn Bed Bureau will help to locate a suitable bed (tel. 01384 215576).
- Ensure tetanus prophylaxis, but avoid 'routine' prophylactic antibiotics.

The burnt patient in cardiac arrest

- Follow standard guidelines.
- Give a large bolus of IV fluid.
- If there is a strong possibility of cyanide poisoning (eg burnt plastic furniture in a house fire), give appropriate antidote, eg dicobalt edetate (see 📖 p.207).

Vascular impairment to limbs and digits

Consider the need for longitudinal escharotomies. These are occasionally needed if ischaemia causes severe pain: get advice from a burns specialist.

Inhalation injury

The commonest inhalation injury is smoke inhalation accompanying burns in house fires. Inhalation injury alone may be fatal and it ↑ mortality for a given body surface area of burn. Smoke is a complex and unpredictably variable mixture of solid, liquid and gas constituents.

Common components of inhalation injury include:

- Direct thermal injury.
- Soot particles cause local injury to the cilia of the respiratory tract and obstruct small airways.
- ≈85% of fire deaths are caused by CO (📖 p.208).
- *Gas products of combustion*: oxides of sulphur, nitrogen, ammonia, chlorine, hydrogen cyanide, phosgene, isocyanates, ketones, and aldehydes are highly irritative and cause laryngospasm. Some react with water in the respiratory tract producing strong acids which cause bronchospasm, mucosal injury and oedema.

The nature of the inhaled insult determines the site, severity, and systemic features. The upper respiratory tract can dissipate heat efficiently, so that direct thermal injury to the lower respiratory tract is rare unless steam or other hot vapours are inhaled. In the lower airway, toxic components such as CO, oxides of sulphur, nitrogen, hydrogen cyanide, hydrogen chloride cause direct injury, and may act as systemic poisons.

Clinical features

Suspect smoke inhalation if any of the following features are present: exposure to smoke or fire in an enclosed space, confusion or altered/loss of consciousness, oropharyngeal burns, hoarseness/loss of voice, singed nasal hairs, soot in nostrils or sputum, wheeze, dysphagia, drooling or dribbling, stridor.

Investigations

Peak flow rate Determine this in all patients.

ABG Detection of hypoxia, hypercapnia, and acidosis may be helpful, but does not correlate well with the severity of inhalation injury. Note that pulse oximetry has limited value because of the difficulty in distinguishing between oxyhaemoglobin and COHb.

CXR Usually normal initially, later features of ARDS may develop.

Carboxyhaemoglobin (COHb) CO poisoning cannot be detected by physical examination, SpO_2, or pO_2. Either arterial or venous COHB can be measured. Clinical features correlate poorly with COHb levels. Use the nomogram opposite to estimate COHb levels at the time of exposure. The management of CO poisoning is covered on 📖 p.208.

ECG CO binds to myoglobin 3× more avidly than to Hb and by affecting the myocardium may produce arrhythmias, ischaemia, or even MI.

Fibre optic bronchoscopy, xenon lung scanning, ventilation-perfusion scans, or lung function testing may subsequently be required to assess lung problems due to inhalational injury.

Management

Signs of upper airway problems (facial burns, stridor, dysphagia, drooling, ↓ consciousness) indicate the need for *early tracheal intubation* by an experienced doctor (ED/ICU/anaesthesia) with appropriate training. Mucosal swelling in the oropharynx and epiglottis can progress rapidly and necessitate a surgical airway (📖 p.326). A surgical airway in these circumstances can be difficult due to burned skin and loss of landmarks. Meticulous preparation and planning for the airway are essential. Flexible bronchoscopy may help to assess thermal injury to the upper airway and help intubation. *Assisted ventilation with PEEP* may be indicated.

Give the highest possible concentration of *humidified* O_2. Hyperbaric O_2 may be indicated for CO poisoning, but remains controversial (📖 p.208).

If bronchospasm occurs, give *nebulized β_2 agonist* (salbutamol 5mg) via an O_2 powered nebulizer. ↑ in microvascular permeability leads to pulmonary oedema 2–3 days after injury and pneumonia after 7–14 days. Pulmonary fibrosis is common among survivors.

Inadequate IV fluid resuscitation is associated with greater pulmonary oedema. Burned patients who have smoke inhalation need larger amounts of IV fluids to maintain cardiac and urine output.

Inhalation of HCN from smouldering plastics (eg polyurethane) results in rapid systemic absorption. Measurement of blood CN concentration is difficult and takes several hours. *Cyanide poisoning* may be suggested by a severe metabolic acidosis, a high lactate and ↑ anion gap. Consider cyanide antidotes (📖 p.207), but they are potentially toxic so do not use blindly. There is no proven benefit from steroid therapy.

Nomogram of decay of COHb with time

This nomogram (Fig. 8.17) allows back-calculation estimation of the likely peak COHb level. It will considerably under-read for children and patients who received a high prehospital FiO_2.

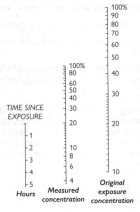

Fig. 8.17 Adapted from Clark *et al.* (1981).

Management of smaller burns

Assessment (📖 p.390)

First aid measures

Separate the patient and burning agent. Cool affected area with copious quantities of cold water, but beware of hypothermia in infants and young children.

Need for admission

Admit patients with large burns or significant smoke inhalation for IV fluids, resuscitation and analgesia. In the UK, the National Burn Bed Bureau will search for an appropriate bed (Tel: 01384 215576) after discussion with the local burns unit. Also refer for admission burns of suspected NAI origin and patients who would be unable to cope at home (eg an elderly person or if living in difficult social circumstances).

Referral to a burns specialist

Refer patients with the following:
- Airway burns.
- Significant full thickness burns, especially over joints.
- Burns >10%.
- Significant burns of special areas (hands, face, perineum, feet).

The burn wound

- Leave *full thickness burns* uncovered and refer to a specialist.
- Do not de-roof *partial thickness burns* with blistering—consider simple aspiration. Most can be cleaned and covered with an appropriate dressing (see below).

Hand burns Consider covering with soft paraffin inside a polythene bag or glove sealed at the wrist, changed after 24hr. Simple paraffin/tulle dressings are an alternative—follow local policy. Elevate to minimize swelling. Avoid silver sulphadiazine cream except on specialist advice.

Facial burns Leave uncovered, or consider application of soft paraffin.

Eye burns Check VA and refer to a specialist with prior irrigation if chemical burns (📖 p.538).

Perineal and foot burns Burns in these areas should be referred for burns unit admission as they require specialist nursing and wound care.

Burns dressings

The ideal burns dressing is sterile, non-adherent, and encourages wound healing in a moist environment. The diversity of dressings available reflects the fact that this ideal dressing remains elusive. Senior ED nursing staff will advise on local preference and policy. Accumulation of fluid means that many dressings need to be changed at ≈48hr—often this is appropriately done at a GP surgery.

Analgesia and tetanus

Unless there is a contraindication and/or if the patient is elderly, NSAID is appropriate and effective analgesia for many burns, which do not require admission. Ensure prophylaxis against tetanus.

Burns in children and non-accidental injury

Unintentional burns are common in children—use the opportunity to offer advice regarding injury prevention. A minority of burns may result from NAI. Suspect NAI (☐ p.730) and seek senior help in the following situations:

- When the explanation does not fit the burn.
- Late presentation.
- Other suspicious injuries.
- Stocking and glove distribution scalds (± sparing of the buttocks)—this implies forced immersion in hot water.
- Circular full thickness burns ≈0.75cm diameter may represent cigarette burns.

Chemical burns

Initial assessment is notoriously difficult. Alkalis tend to produce more severe burns and can continue to penetrate even after initial irrigation.

Treat chemical burns with copious irrigation with water, continued for at least 20min in alkali burns.

Hydrofluoric acid burns

Hydrofluoric acid is used industrially in a number of processes. Contact with the skin causes particularly severe burns, often with significant tissue damage and severe pain. This is because hydrofluoric acid rapidly crosses lipid membranes and penetrates the tissues deeply, where it releases the highly toxic fluoride ion. Fluoride ions may gain access to the circulation and produce a variety of systemic problems by a variety of mechanisms, including interfering with enzyme systems and producing hypocalcaemia by binding to calcium.

Manage hydrofluoric acid burns as follows:

- Provide copious lavage to the affected skin then apply iced water (this provides better pain relief than calcium gluconate gel).
- Call a plastic surgeon at an early stage.
- Check serum Ca^{2+} and Mg^{2+}, and U&E.
- Record an ECG and place on a cardiac monitor.
- Treat hypocalcaemia.

Cement burns

Wet cement or concrete can cause chemical burns due to the alkali contact. These are usually partial thickness, but may be full thickness. They often occur when wet cement falls into a work boot, but the burn is not initially noticed. Involve a specialist at an early stage.

Phenol burns

Phenol may be absorbed through the skin, resulting in systemic toxicity and renal failure. Get advice from Poisons Information Service (☐ p.181).

Crush syndrome

A spectrum of conditions characterized by skeletal muscle injury (rhabdomyolysis). Causes include :
- Direct injuries and severe burns causing muscle damage.
- Compartment syndromes: 'true' crush injuries produced by entrapment, or 'self-crushing' (eg an unconscious individual from drug overdose or alcohol excess lying on a hard surface). A vicious cycle is established where ↑ muscle compartment pressure obstructs blood flow, the muscles become ischaemic and oedematous, further ↑ compartment pressure and ↓ blood flow leading to more ischaemia and muscle cell death.
- Non-traumatic causes: metabolic disorders (diabetic states, ↓ K$^+$, ↓ PO$_4^{3-}$), myxoedema, neuroleptic malignant syndrome, myositis due to infection, or immunological disease.
- Exertional: from undue exertion, grand mal fitting, rave dancing (particularly associated with ecstasy or cocaine use), often complicated by hyperthermia.

Clinical features

Adopt a high index of suspicion. Symptoms depend on the underlying cause, but muscle pain, tenderness and swelling may not be present at the time of admission. In the lower limbs, the condition is commonly confused with DVT. The classic compartment syndrome with pain on passive muscle stretching and sensory deficits may take several days to develop and can pass unnoticed. The presence of distal pulses does *not* rule out a compartment syndrome.

Investigations

↑CPK levels reflect muscle damage. Check U&E, PO$_4^{3-}$, Ca^{2+} and urate. 70% have myoglobinuria and pigmented granular casts (urinary stix tests do not differentiate between Hb and myoglobin). However, absence of myoglobinuria does not exclude rhabdomyolysis, as myoglobin clears rapidly from plasma and its presence in urine depends upon the release rate, the degree of protein binding, GFR, and urine flow. If DIC is suspected, check a coagulation screen.

Treatment

Local problems Urgent orthopaedic referral is needed for compartment syndromes. If the difference between intra-compartmental and diastolic pressures is <30mmHg, fasciotomy, excision of dead muscle and even distal amputation may be required. These procedures may induce life-threatening electrolyte shifts, bleeding, local infection, and later generalized sepsis.

Systemic complications Severe metabolic complications start after revascularization. Hyperkalaemia may be life-threatening (p.162). Hypocalcaemia is common initially, but rarely symptomatic.

Acute renal failure can be produced by pre-renal, renal, and obstructive elements. Following restoration of circulation or release from entrapment, fluid leaks into damaged areas ↓ circulating plasma volume. Intracellular muscle contents enter the circulation and myoglobin and urate crystals can block the renal tubules. This process is aggravated by the ↓ intravascular volume and associated metabolic acidosis. DIC and drugs which inhibit intra-renal homeostatic mechanisms (eg NSAIDs and β-blockers) may also contribute.

Prompt correction of fluid deficits and acidosis (often with CVP monitoring) and establishing a good urinary flow is essential. Alkalinization of the urine may be required: early use of mannitol has been advocated, but can cause pulmonary oedema if renal impairment is already present. If renal failure occurs, dialysis may be needed, but prospects for renal recovery are good.

Wounds, fractures, orthopaedics

The approach to wounds

Wounds often have medicolegal implications—therefore record notes thoroughly, legibly, and accurately (📖 Note keeping, p.4). Resuscitation is the initial priority for the seriously wounded patient. Stop bleeding by applying direct pressure.

History

Key questions are:
- *What caused the wound?* (knives/glass may injure deep structures).
- *Was there a crush component?* (considerable swelling may ensue).
- *Where did it occur?* (contaminated or clean environment).
- *Was broken glass (or china) involved?* (if so, obtain an X-ray).
- *When did it occur?* (old wounds may need delayed closure + antibiotics).
- *Who caused it?* (has the patient a safe home to go to?).
- *Is tetanus cover required?* (see 📖 p.410).

Examination

Consider and record the following:
- *Length*: preferably measure. If not, use the term 'approximately' in the notes.
- *Site*: use diagrams whenever possible (rubber stamps are recommended). Consider taking digital photographs, particularly for compound fractures, in order to minimize the risk of infection by disturbing the wound as little as possible prior to surgery.
- *Orientation*: vertical, horizontal or oblique.
- *Contamination*: by dirt or other FBs may be obvious.
- *Infection*: either localized or spreading, is a feature of delayed presentations and is associated in particular with certain specific injuries (eg 'reverse fight bites'—see Bite wounds).
- *Neurological injury*: test and record motor and sensory components of relevant nerves. Be aware that complete nerve transection does not automatically result in complete loss of sensation—some feeling is likely to be preserved (particularly in the hand). Assume that any altered sensation reflects nerve injury.
- *Tendons*: complete division is usually apparent on testing. Partial tendon division is easily missed unless the wound is carefully examined—the tendon may still be capable of performing its usual function. Look in the wound whilst moving the relevant joint, and attempt to re-create the position of the injured part at the time of injury (eg clenched fist) to bring the injured structures into view.
- *Vascular injury*: check for distal pulses.
- *Depth*: wounds not fully penetrating the skin are 'superficial'. Do not try to judge depth of other wounds before exploration. In some circumstances (eg neck wounds), exploration is not appropriate in the ED.
- *Type of wound*: inspection often allows wounds to be described, helping to determine the mechanism of trauma (blunt or sharp injury) and hence the risk of associated injuries. The crucial distinction is whether a wound was caused by a sharp or blunt instrument. If in doubt, avoid any descriptive term and simply call it a 'wound'. This avoids inaccuracy and courtroom embarrassment! Use the terms as described opposite.

Forensic classification of wounds and injury

The expert forensic evaluation of injury is outside the remit of the ED specialist, but a simple understanding helps to avoid incorrect use of terminology with associated confusion (and sometimes embarrassment).

Incised wounds May also be referred to as 'cuts'. Caused by sharp injury (eg knives or broken glass) and characterized by clean-cut edges. These typically include *'stab'* wounds (which are deeper than they are wide) and *'slash'* wounds (which are longer than they are deep).

Lacerations Caused by blunt injury (eg impact of scalp against pavement or intact glass bottle), the skin is torn, resulting in irregular wound edges. Unlike most incised wounds, tissues adjacent to laceration wound edges are also injured by crushing and will exhibit evidence of bruising.

Puncture wounds Most result from injury with sharp objects, although a blunt object with sufficient force will also penetrate the skin.

Abrasions Commonly known as 'grazes', these result from blunt injury applied tangentially. Abrasions are often ingrained with dirt, with the risk of infection and in the longer term, unwanted, and unsightly skin 'tattooing'. Skin tags visible at one end of the abrasion indicate the edge of skin last in contact with the abrading surface and imply the direction in which the skin was abraded.

Burns See 📖 p.390.

Bruises Bruising reflects blunt force (crush) injury to the blood vessels within the tissues, resulting in tender swelling with discoloration: sometimes localized bleeding collects to form a *haematoma*. The term *'contusion'* is sometimes used as an alternative for bruise—it has no particular special meaning (or value). Record the site, size, colour, and characteristic features of any bruising. It is impossible to determine the exact age of a bruise from its colour. However, yellow colour within a bruise implies (except in the neonate) that it is >18hr old.

Scratches These may comprise either a 'very superficial incision' or a 'long, thin abrasion'—leave the distinction to an expert.

Interpersonal violence—medicolegal implications

Victims of violence frequently attend ED for treatment of their injuries. Some patients (particularly those who have suffered domestic violence) may not provide an accurate account of how the injuries occurred and may not seek involvement of the police. Classical defence wounds include:

- Isolated ulna shaft fracture as the arm is raised to protect against blunt injury.
- Incised wounds on the palmar aspects of the palms and fingers sustained in attempts to protect against knife attack.

In cases where the police are involved and where injuries are serious or extensive, the police may arrange to obtain photographs and a forensic physician (police surgeon) may be involved in the role of documenting injuries. Most ED patients who have suffered violence do not see a forensic physician (police surgeon). Therefore, ED staff have a dual role of treating injuries and recording them accurately for medicolegal purposes.

Further assessment of skin wounds

Investigation

X-ray if there is suspicion of fracture, involvement of joint, penetration of body cavity or FB. Specify on request forms that a FB is being sought, to allow appropriate views and exposure. Most metal (except aluminium) and glass objects >1mm in diameter will show up on X-ray. Some objects (eg wood) may not: USS may demonstrate these. CT or MRI are also occasionally helpful.

Note: X-ray all wounds from glass that fully penetrate the skin

During X-ray, use radio-opaque markers (eg paper clip) taped to the skin to identify the area of concern.

Wound swabs for bacteriology are unhelpful in fresh wounds, but obtain them from older wounds showing signs of infection.

By far the most important investigation is:

Wound exploration under appropriate anaesthesia

Allows full assessment and thorough cleaning of wounds that extend fully through the skin. Do not explore the following wounds in the ED:

- Stab wounds to the neck, chest, abdomen, or perineum.
- Compound fracture wounds requiring surgery in theatre.
- Wounds over suspected septic joints or infected tendon sheaths.
- Most wounds with obvious neurovascular/tendon injury needing repair.
- Other wounds requiring special expertise (eg eyelids).

Obtain relevant X-rays beforehand. Adequate anaesthesia is essential—in adults LA (eg 1% plain lidocaine) is often suitable (📖 p.282), but document any sensory loss first (if there is altered sensation, presume nerve injury and refer for formal exploration in theatre. Do not inject LA into the edges of an infected wound: it will not work in that acidic environment and it may spread the infection. GA may be the preferred option for treating some wounds in young children.

Inspect wounds for FBs and damage to underlying structures. Most problems with wound exploration relate to bleeding. If it proves difficult to obtain a good view:

- Obtain a good light and an assistant. The assistant retracting on a stitch placed on either side of the middle of the wound allows full exposure.
- Press on any bleeding point for ≥1min, then look again. Lidocaine with adrenaline (📖 p.283) is useful in scalp wounds which are bleeding profusely.
- If bleeding continues, consider a tourniquet for up to 15min. Consider a sphygmomanometer BP cuff inflated above systolic pressure (after limb elevation for 1min) on the limbs, or a 'finger' of a sterile rubber glove may be used on fingers or toes. Never leave a patient alone with a tourniquet on, lest it is forgotten. Ensure removal of the tourniquet afterwards. Record the time of application and removal.

If these measures fail, refer for specialist exploration in theatre. Do not blindly 'clip' bleeding points with artery forceps, for fear of causing iatrogenic neurovascular injury. Sometimes, small blood vessels in the subcutaneous tissues can be safely ligated using an appropriate absorbable suture (eg 4/0 or 6/0 Vicryl (braided polyglactin) or Dexon).

The approach to foreign bodies

FBs within soft tissues can cause pain, act as a focus for infection, or migrate and cause problems elsewhere. Therefore, remove FBs from recent wounds where possible, particularly if lying near a joint (but if FB is within a joint, refer to the orthopaedic team for formal exploration and removal). FBs which can be seen or felt or are causing infection are usually best removed. Finding FBs is frequently difficult without a bloodless field and good light. It may be appropriate to leave some FBs, such as gunshot deeply embedded in buttock soft tissues (antibiotic cover advised). However, most FBs of any size not removed in the ED warrant specialist consideration.

Patients not infrequently present with symptoms relating to (suspected) FBs under old healed wounds. In these circumstances, refer to an expert for exploration under appropriate conditions.

Fishhooks

The barbs on some fishhooks can make removal difficult. In some cases, it may be necessary to push a fishhook onwards (under LA) and thus out through the skin—wire cutters can then cut through the hook below the barb and allow release. Wear eye protection when doing this.

There are alternative methods for removing fishhooks. Smaller fishhooks that are relatively superficially embedded can sometimes be pulled back and removed through the entry wound once a hollow needle has been advanced alongside the hook to cover the barb.

Wound management

Wound cleaning

Thoroughly clean all wounds irrespective of whether closure is contemplated, to ↓risk of infection. The standard agent used for wound cleaning is 0.9% (normal) saline, possibly preceded by washing using tap water. Aqueous chlorhexidine or 1% cetrimide solutions are sometimes used. Do not use hydrogen peroxide or strong povidone iodine solutions. Wounds ingrained with dirt may respond to pressure saline irrigation (19G needle attached to 20mL syringe), or may require to be scrubbed with a toothbrush (use goggles to ↓chance of conjunctival 'splashback'). Devitalized or grossly contaminated wound edges usually need to be trimmed back (debrided), except on the hand or face. If dirt or other foreign material is visible despite these measures, refer to a specialist, who may choose to leave the wound open.

Wound closure

There are three recognized types of wound closure:

Primary closure Surgical closure (by whatever physical means) soon after injury.

Secondary closure No intervention: heals by granulation (secondary intention).

Delayed primary closure Surgical closure 3–5 days after injury.

If there is no underlying injury or FB, treat fresh wounds by primary closure as soon as possible. Accurate opposition of wound edges and obliteration of dead space provides the best cosmetic outcome with least infection risk.

Wounds not usually suitable for primary closure in the ED include:
• Stab wounds to the trunk and neck.
• Wounds with associated tendon, joint or neurovascular involvement.
• Wounds with associated crush injury or significant devitalized tissue/skin loss.
• Other heavily contaminated or infected wounds.
• Most wounds >12hr old (except clean facial wounds).

Methods of closure

If in doubt, sutures are usually the best option (see opposite).

Steri-Strips™ Adhesive skin closure strips allow skin edges to be opposed with even distribution of forces. They are inappropriate over joints, but useful for pretibial lacerations, where skin is notoriously thin and sutures are likely to 'cut out'. Before application, make Steri-Strips™ stickier by applying tincture of benzoin to dry skin around the wound. Leave 3–5mm gaps between Steri-Strips™. See also 🕮 Pretibial lacerations, p.481.

Skin tissue glue Particularly useful in children with superficial wounds and scalp wounds. After securing haemostasis, oppose the dried skin edges before applying glue to the wound. Hold the skin edges together for 30–60sec to allow the glue to set. Ensure that glue does not enter the wound. Do not use tissue glue near the eyes or to close wounds over joints.

Staples Quick and easy to apply, particularly suited to scalp wounds. Staple-removers are required for removal.

Sutures ('stitches' or 'ties') Traditional and most commonly used method to achieve primary closure. Oppose the skin aiming for slight eversion of wound edges, using strong non-absorbable inert monofilament suture material attached to curved cutting needles (eg prolene, polypropylene or nylon) with knots tied on the outside. Interrupted simple surgical knots tied using instruments are relatively easy, economical of thread and have a low risk of needlestick injuries. Specialized continuous sutures (eg subcuticular) are not appropriate for wounds in the ED. The size of thread used and time to removal vary according to the site. Use absorbable sutures (eg Vicryl) on the lips and inside the mouth. Absorbable sutures may also be used to close subcutaneous tissues to ↓chance of haematoma and infection. Suture choice and time to removal are given in Table 9.1.

Table 9.1 Suture choice and time to removal

Part of body	Suture and size	Time to removal
Scalp	2/0 or 3/0 non-absorbable† glue or staples	7 days
Trunk	3/0 non-absorbable†	10 days
Limbs	4/0 non-absorbable†	10 days
Hands	5/0 non-absorbable	10 days
Face	5/0 or 6/0 non-absorbable	3–5 days*
Lips, tongue, mouth	Absorbable eg 6/0 Vicryl/Dexon	–

†One size smaller may be appropriate for children.

*Sutures may be replaced with Steristrips at 3 days.

Key points when suturing

The technique of a basic instrument tie is shown in Figs 9.1–9.6.
- Tie sutures just tight enough for the edges to meet.
- Do not close a wound under tension.
- Handle the skin edges with toothed forceps only.
- Avoid too many deep absorbable sutures.
- Mattress sutures are useful on some deep wounds, but avoid on hands and face.
- Dispose of sharps as you use them—do not make a collection.
- Use strategic initial sutures to match up obvious points in irregular wounds.
- If a suture does not look right—take it out and try again.
- If it still does not look right—get help!

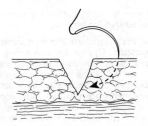

Fig. 9.1

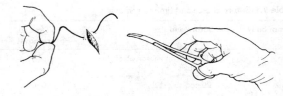

Fig. 9.2

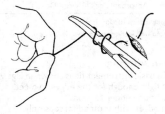

Fig. 9.3

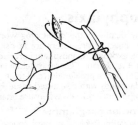

Fig. 9.4

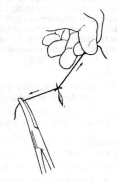

Fig. 9.5

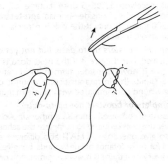

Fig. 9.6

Tetanus prophylaxis

Tetanus causes many deaths in the developing world. Occasional cases still occur in the UK. Injecting drug users are at risk (particularly if using SC or IM routes). The exotoxin tetanospasmin produced by the anaerobic, spore-forming Gram +ve bacillus *Clostridium tetani* interferes with neurotransmission (🕮 p.236). Spore proliferation and toxin production is likely in heavily contaminated wounds with devitalized tissue. However, any wound (including a burn) is a potential risk: always ensure tetanus prevention.

Tetanus immunization programme

Standard active immunization involves an initial course of 3 IM or deep SC doses of 0.5mL tetanus toxoid (formalin inactivated toxin) given at monthly intervals starting at 2months of age, followed by booster doses at 4 and 14years. A full course of 5 doses is considered to result in lifelong immunity. From 2006 in the UK, combined tetanus/diphtheria/inactivated polio vaccine replaced previous tetanus/diphtheria vaccine for adults and adolescents. Immunization required after injury depends upon immunization status of the patient and the injury. Inadequate immunity against tetanus is particularly likely in immigrants, the elderly, patients with ↓immunity and those who have refused vaccination.

Anti-tetanus prophylaxis

The need for tetanus immunization after injury depends upon a patient's tetanus immunity status and whether the wound is 'clean' or 'tetanus prone.'

The following are regarded as 'tetanus prone':
• Heavy contamination (especially with soil or faeces).
• Devitalized tissue.
• Infection or wounds >6hr old.
• Puncture wounds and animal bites.

Follow Department of Health guidelines. See www.dh.gov.uk

Do not give tetanus vaccine if there is a past history of a severe reaction: give HATI. Pregnancy is not a contraindication to giving tetanus prophylaxis.

Patient is already fully immunized
If the patient has received a full 5-dose course of tetanus vaccines, do not give further vaccines. Consider human anti-tetanus immunoglobulin ('HATI' 250–500units IM) only if the risk is especially high (eg wound contaminated with stable manure).

Initial course complete, boosters up-to-date, but not yet complete
Vaccine is not required, but do give it if the next dose is due soon and it is convenient to give it now. Consider human anti-tetanus immunoglobulin ('HATI' 250–500units IM) in tetanus prone wounds only if the risk is especially high (eg wound contaminated with stable manure).

Initial course incomplete or boosters not up-to-date
Give a reinforcing dose of combined tetanus/diphtheria/polio vaccine and refer to the GP for further doses as required to complete the schedule. For tetanus-prone wounds, also give one dose of HATI at a different site. The dose of HATI is 250units IM for most tetanus prone wounds, but give 500units if >24hr have elapsed since injury or if there is heavy contamination or following burns.

Not immunized or immunization status unknown or uncertain
Give a dose of combined tetanus/diphtheria/polio vaccine and refer to the GP for further doses as required. For tetanus-prone wounds, also give one dose of HATI (250–500units IM) at a different site.

Antibiotic prophylaxis

Antibiotics are not required for most wounds. Thorough cleaning is the best way of preventing infection. After cleaning and closure, consider oral antibiotic prophylaxis (eg penicillin + flucloxacillin) for certain wounds: compound fingertip fractures and wounds in those at extra risk (eg valvular heart disease, post-splenectomy). Co-amoxiclav has activity against anaerobes, and is appropriate for bites and heavily contaminated or infected wounds: leave these wounds open. Antibiotics are indicated for penetrating injuries which cannot be properly cleaned (📖 Puncture wounds, p.419). Although a scientific basis is lacking, antibiotics are frequently used for wounds >6hr old, complex intra-oral wounds and in workers at high risk (gardeners, farmers, fishermen).

Wound aftercare

Dressings

A large variety of dressings are available, with little scientific evidence to help choose between them: choice depends upon personal preference/prejudice and local departmental policy. A dry non-adherent dressing will protect most wounds from inadvertent contamination in the first few days. Dressings are not usually necessary for facial and scalp wounds. Beware circulatory problems resulting from encircling dressings/bandages applied too tightly to digits or other parts of limbs. Burns dressings are considered in 🕮 p.396.

General advice

Advise to keep wounds clean and dry for the first few days. Limb wounds require rest and elevation for the first 24hr. After this, restrict movements to avoid undue stress causing the suture line to open up (especially where the wound is over a joint). Warn all patients to return if features of infection develop (redness, ↑pain, swelling, fever, red streaks up the limb). Approximate times to suture removal are shown on Table 9.1—these need to be adjusted to meet the occasion. For example, sutures over joints are sensibly left 14 days to avoid dehiscence. Similarly, sutures may need to be left in for longer where wound healing may be delayed (eg DM, the elderly, malnourished, and those on steroids). Local policy will dictate where suture removal occurs (GP surgery or ED). If available, discharge with illustrated instructions about wound care and suture removal. This may particularly help patients with memory impairment or under the influence of alcohol.

Specific advice

Patients often ask when to return to work. If a question of personal safety or safety of the public or work colleagues is involved, advise to return to usual duties only once the wound has healed and sutures are out. This particularly applies to food handlers and some workers with machinery. Provide a sickness certificate for the patient's employer as appropriate.

Review and delayed primary closure

Arrange review of heavily contaminated wounds, infected wounds not requiring admission, and other wounds at particular risk of infection at ≈36hr. Check T° and look for wound discharge and erythema, ascending lymphangitis, and regional lymphadenopathy. Systemic symptoms or evidence of spreading infection despite oral antibiotics are indications for admission for wound toilet, rest, elevation, and IV antibiotics.

Treat other wounds deemed initially to be at less risk of infection, but not suitable for primary closure, with cleaning, light packing/dressing, and review at 3–5 days. Ideal dressings keep wounds moist, so consider the need for dressing changes prior to closure. If the wound is clean, employ delayed primary closure after wound cleaning and debridement under appropriate anaesthesia. If despite further cleaning and debridement, foreign material remains ingrained, consider if the patient requires admission. If there is much exudate and evidence of local infection, take wound swabs for culture, consider removing the sutures, clean and redress the wound, give oral antibiotics, and arrange further review.

Do not use 'loose closure' in contaminated wounds. The technique has all the risks of infection combined with a poor cosmetic result.

Infected wounds and cellulitis

Wound infection after injury

Although prompt treatment with cleaning and primary closure will ↓ risk, any wound may become infected. The risk of infection is ↑ by:

- Contamination (eg bites) and foreign material (including excess sutures).
- Haematoma.
- Devitalized tissue.
- Poor nutrition and ↓immunity (eg steroid therapy).

Pain is usually the first clue to wound infection. Note that many soft tissue infections (cellulitis, erysipelas) occur in the absence of an obvious wound (see 🕮 Cellulitis and erysipelas, p.528).

Examination Indicates the extent of the infection. Erythema and tenderness limited to the area around the wound suggest localized infection. Swelling and fluctuation are evidence of a collection of pus. Remove all sutures, together with pus and devitalized tissue, under appropriate anaesthetic. Send wound swabs for culture. Consider the possibility of a retained FB— X-ray/explore as appropriate. After thorough cleaning, leave the wound open, cover with a dressing and arrange review with a dressing change in 36hr. Consider the need for antibiotics (eg co-amoxiclav) particularly for cellulitis, for the immunocompromised and for patients at particular risk (eg those with prostheses and valvular heart disease).

Consider admission (for rest, elevation, analgesia, wound/blood cultures, and IV antibiotics) in patients with one or more of the following:

- A red line spreading proximally (ascending lymphangitis).
- Regional (sometimes tender) lymphadenopathy.
- Pyrexia >38°C.
- Systemic upset.

Soft tissue crepitus is ominous, suggesting gas-forming organisms (🕮 p.237).

Infected hand wounds

A particularly common problem is an infected wound on the dorsum of the hand over a MCPJ after a punch injury. These are often bite wounds, presenting late with infection in the region of the joint. Refer for exploration/washout in theatre and antibiotics (🕮 p.416).

Infected facial wounds

Take infected wounds of the cheek very seriously. They pose a significant threat of sepsis spreading intracranially, resulting in papilloedema and ophthalmoplegia due to cavernous sinus thrombosis. Adopt a low threshold for referring for admission and IV antibiotics.

Infected surgical wounds

Infection of a recent surgical wound after a planned procedure is a relatively common complication. In addition to the possible threat to life, wound infection can have disastrous implications as far as the success of the preceding operation is concerned (eg hernias may recur). Contact the team which performed the surgery as soon as possible, to allow the surgeon to treat the complication.

Bite wounds

Bites and infection

Bites cause contaminated puncture wounds, contaminated crush injuries, or both. All carry a high risk of bacterial infection, some also a risk of viral or other infections (eg rabies).

Bacterial infection is particularly likely in:
• Puncture wounds (cat/human bites).
• Hand wounds, wounds >24hr old.
• Wounds in alcoholics, diabetics, or the immunocompromised.

Bacteria responsible include: streptococci, *Staphylococcus aureus*, *Clostridium tetani*, *Pasteurella multocida* (cat bites/scratches), *Bacteroides*, *Eikenella corrodens* (human bites).

Approach

Establish what the biting animal was, how long ago and where the bite occurred. Obtain X-rays if fracture, joint involvement (look for air) or radio-opaque foreign body (FB) (tooth) is suspected.

Management of bite wounds

Cleaning

Explore fresh bite wounds under appropriate anaesthetic, debride and clean thoroughly with 'normal' saline (or by washing using tap water). Refer significant facial wounds and wounds involving tendons or joints to a specialist.

Closure

Cosmetic considerations usually outweigh risks of infection for most facial wounds, so aim for primary closure. Elsewhere, choose between primary or delayed primary closure—the latter is usually preferred in bite wounds affecting limbs, due to the increased risk of infection. Do not close puncture bite wounds that cannot be satisfactorily irrigated.

Antibiotic prophylaxis

Deciding whether or not to employ prophylactic antibiotics for bite wounds can be difficult and is controversial. Many departments advocate prophylactic antibiotics for all bite wounds. One approach is to give antibiotics for patients with any of the following:
• Puncture bites.
• Crush injuries with devitalized tissues.
• Bites to the hand, wrist, or genitals.
• Bites that are primarily closed.
• Bites from humans, cats, and rats.
• Bitten individuals who are immunocompromised (eg immunosuppressed, diabetes, post-splenectomy, rheumatoid arthritis, those with prosthetic joints).

Co-amoxiclav is an appropriate broad spectrum agent, effective against *Strep*, *Staph*, *Pasteurella*, and *Eikenella*. Alternatives for patients allergic to penicillin/amoxicillin include doxycycline + metronidazole or (especially if pregnant) ceftriaxone alone.

Do not use erythromycin or flucloxacillin alone as prophylaxis.

Tetanus
Bite wounds are tetanus-prone. Give prophylaxis accordingly (📖 p.410).

Rabies (covered fully in 📖 p.249)
Rabies results after the 'bullet-shaped' RNA rhabdovirus present in saliva of infected animals is transmitted to humans via a mucous membrane or skin break. After thorough cleaning, refer all patients who might have been in contact with a rabid animal to an Infectious Diseases specialist. Obtain further help from the Virus Reference Laboratory, London (020 8200 4400). The long incubation period of the rabies virus (14–90 days) allows successful post-exposure prophylaxis at even a relatively late stage, according to agreed guidelines.

Hepatitis, HIV
Consider possible risks of hepatitis B, C, and HIV in anyone who presents following a human bite and treat accordingly (see under 📖 Needlestick injury, p.418). Quantifying risks can be difficult, particularly for example, in 'reverse fight bites' (📖 p.416) where the other person involved may be unknown. If in doubt, take a baseline blood sample for storage (to allow later testing if necessary) and provide cover against hepatitis B.

Treatment of infected bites

Most bacterial infections occur >24hr after injury and are due to staphylococci or anaerobes. Pain, inflammation, swelling ±regional lymphadenopathy within 24hr suggests *P. multocida* infection. Take wound swabs of all infected wounds, then treat with cleaning, elevation, analgesia, and antibiotics. Oral co-amoxiclav and outpatient review at ≈36hr is appropriate for localized wound infection with no systemic symptoms and no suspected underlying joint involvement. Refer patients with spreading infection for IV antibiotics and admission.

Septicaemia is uncommon after bite injury, but has been reported with the Gram −ve bacillus *Capnocytophaga canimorsus*, previously known as *Dysgonic Fermenter 2 (DF-2)*. Infection produces a severe illness with septicaemia and DIC, often in immunocompromised (splenectomized individuals, diabetics, or alcoholics). Take wound swabs and blood cultures, then give IV antibiotics and refer.

Prevention of dog bites

Injury prevention measures aimed at preventing children from being bitten includes legislation relating to 'dangerous dogs' and education. Children may be taught the following:
• To treat dogs with respect.
• To avoid disturbing a dog that is sleeping, eating, or feeding puppies.
• To avoid shouting or running in the presence of a dog.
• Not to approach or play with unfamiliar dogs.

Specific bites and stings

Human bites and 'fight bites'

Many human bites occur 'in reverse', when an individual punches another in the mouth, causing wounds on the dorsum of the hand over the MCPJs. Underlying joint involvement is common and may progress to septic arthritis unless treated aggressively with exploration, irrigation and antibiotics. Refer all patients for this. Consider hepatitis B, C, and HIV, give appropriate prophylaxis (📖 Needlestick injuries, p.418) and arrange counselling.

Tick bites

Ticks are recognized vectors of a number of exotic diseases worldwide. In the UK, patients often present with embedded sheep ticks. Remove ticks by gentle traction with blunt forceps applied as close to the skin as possible. Avoid traditional folklore methods of removal, which may cause the tick to regurgitate, promoting infection. In areas where Lyme disease is endemic (see 📖 p.231), some physicians provide antibiotic prophylaxis with amoxicillin.

Insect bites

Minor local reactions are common. Treat with ice packs, rest, elevation, analgesia and antihistamines (eg chlorphenamine PO 4mg tds or a non-sedating alternative such as loratadine PO 10mg od). Occasionally, insect bites may be complicated by cellulitis and ascending lymphangitis requiring antibiotics (📖 Infected wounds and cellulitis, p.413).

Wasps and honey bee stings

May cause local reactions or anaphylaxis—treat promptly (📖 p.42). Flick out bee stings left in the skin. Treat local reactions as for insect bites.

Jellyfish stings and fish spines

Most jellyfish in UK coastal waters are harmless. Wash the bitten part in sea water then pour vinegar (5% acetic acid) over it to neutralize the toxin.

Fish spines (typically Weever fish) produce a heat labile toxin, which may be neutralized by immersion in hot water for 30min. Occasionally, tiny parts of the fish spines become embedded and cause long-term irritation. Localizing and removing these tiny FBs is difficult, so refer to an appropriate expert.

Contact with other wild animals

Contact with rats' urine may cause leptospirosis (Weil's disease)—see 📖 p.239. Provide prophylactic doxycycline to anyone who presents following an episode of significant exposure (eg immersion in river water or sewage). Unusual bites may pose specific threats, which infectious disease specialists will advise about (eg monkey bites may cause herpes simplex infection: give prophylactic oral aciclovir). Bats may carry rabies (📖 p.249).

Snake bites

The European adder is the only native venomous snake in the UK. It is grey/brown, with a V-shaped marking behind the head and dark zig-zag markings on the back. Most bites occur in summer. Venom is injected by a pair of fangs. The venom contains enzymes, polypeptides, and other low molecular weight substances. Only 50% of bites cause envenomation.

Features

Envenomation causes pain and swelling: look for 2 puncture marks 1cm apart. Vomiting, abdominal pain, diarrhoea, and hypotension may follow.

Investigation

Check urine, perform an ECG, and take blood for: FBC, U&E, LFTs, coagulation screen, and D-dimer.

Treatment

- *Prehospital*: rest (and avoid interference with) the bitten part.
- Clean and expose wound, give analgesia and IV fluids for hypotension.
- Treat anaphylaxis urgently according to standard guidelines
  (🕮 Anaphylaxis, p.42).
- Give prophylactic antibiotics (eg co-amoxiclav) and ensure tetanus cover.
- Antivenom has its own risk of anaphylaxis, but may be given for signs of systemic envenoming, hypotension, WCC>20 × 10⁹/L, ECG changes, elevated cardiac enzymes, metabolic acidosis or significant limb swelling (eg past the wrist for bites on the hand, or past the ankle for bites on the foot, within 4 hr).
- Obtain specific advice from a Poisons Information Centre (🕮 p.181).
- Observe for least 24hr, all patients who have any symptoms after snake bite.

Needlestick injury

A needlestick injury is a specialized puncture wound. In a clinical setting, it may represent failure to follow universal precautions (📖 p.32) and should provoke a review of policy and procedure.

Many infective agents have been transferred by needlestick: Blastomycosis, Brucellosis, Cryptococcosis, Diphtheria, Ebola fever, Gonorrhoea, Hepatitis B, Hepatitis C, Herpes zoster, HIV, Leptospirosis, Malaria, Mycobacteriosis, Mycoplasmosis, Rocky Mountain spotted fever, Scrub typhus, Sporotrichosis, *Staph aureus*, *Strep pyogenes*, Syphilis, Toxoplasmosis, TB.

In practice, the principal risks are hepatitis B and C and HIV. The risk of acquiring hepatitis B following a needlestick from a carrier has been estimated at 2–40%. All hospital workers should be immunized against hepatitis B and have regular checks of their antibody status. The risk of hepatitis C is believed to be 3–10%. In contrast, the risk of acquiring HIV after needlestick with HIV +ve source is much less (estimated at 0.2–0.5%, but may be higher if significant volumes are injected). There is a small (≈0.03%) risk of HIV transmission after mucocutaneous exposure (ie exposure of cuts, abrasions, mucous membranes including the eye). The (small) risk of acquiring HIV following needlestick injury from a person with known HIV may be reduced further by post-exposure prophylaxis, but time is of the essence (see below). No proven post-exposure prophylaxis currently exists for hepatitis C. Preventing needlestick injuries and exposure to these viruses is therefore crucial.

Management
- Wash the wound with soap and water.
- Ensure tetanus cover.
- Ensure hepatitis B cover: if not previously immunized, give hepatitis B immunoglobulin and start an active immunization course (give first vaccine in the ED and arrange subsequent doses). If previously immunized, check antibody titres. If satisfactory, take no further action. If low, give booster vaccine. If very low give both immunoglobulin and start vaccine course. Many local needlestick policies advise obtaining informed consent from the source patient, prior to taking blood to check hepatitis and HIV status. In practice, the identity of the source patient is not always clear: do not withhold hepatitis B prophylaxis if there is any doubt.
- If the source patient is known to be (or suspected of being) HIV +ve, follow local guidelines and/or refer immediately to an infectious diseases specialist to discuss post-exposure prophylaxis and follow-up. Follow Department of Health guidance on www.dh.gov.uk Combined prophylaxis therapy (eg 1 Truvada® tablet od and 2 Kaletra® tablets bd – ie 245mg tenofovir od + 200mg emtricitabine od + 400mg lopinavir bd + 100mg ritonavir bd) is most effective if started within an hour of exposure, but may be worth considering up to 72hr. However, prophylaxis has side effects, especially diarrhoea. Involve both healthcare worker and a local expert in deciding whether or not to start prophylaxis. Either way, advise the patient to use barrier contraception and not to give blood as a donor until subsequent HIV seroconversion has been ruled out.
- Take baseline blood for storing (serology for possible future testing), and in the case of a possible HIV source patient, also take FBC, U&E, LFTs, and amylase.
- If the incident occurred in hospital, report it to Occupational Health.

Puncture wounds

Puncture wounds are small skin wounds with possible deep penetration.

Stab wounds to the trunk and neck are considered elsewhere (☐ Penetrating chest injury, p.340).

Puncture wounds often involve the sole of the foot, patients having trodden on a nail. Examine to exclude neurovascular injury, then obtain an X-ray looking for FB. If significant foreign material is present radiologically, or the patient has associated fracture, tendon injury, or neurovascular deficit, refer for formal exploration and cleaning in theatre under a bloodless field. Otherwise:

- Irrigate and clean other wounds under local anaesthetic (LA) where possible (consider nerve blocks). For wounds to the sole of the foot this may be impractical. As a compromise, immerse foot in warm anti-septic (eg povidone iodine solution) for 15min.
- Apply a dressing and advise review/follow-up with GP as appropriate.
- Ensure adequate tetanus cover (☐ Tetanus prophylaxis, p.410).
- Prescribe simple analgesia.
- Strongly consider prophylactic oral antibiotic cover (eg co-amoxiclav).

Some puncture wounds may become infected despite treatment. This may be due to retained foreign material in the wound. *Pseudomonas osteitis* is an uncommon, but recognized complication of puncture wounds to the foot, particularly where a nail has gone through training shoes to cause the wound. Refer infected wounds for formal exploration and irrigation.

How to describe a fracture

Clear, precise, complete descriptions of fractures aid accuracy and save time when referring patients.

System for describing fractures

- State the age of the patient and how the injury occurred.
- If the fracture is compound, state this first (and Gustilo type— 📖 p.422).
- Name the bone (specify right or left, and for the hand, whether dominant).
- Describe the position of the fracture (eg proximal, supracondylar).
- Name the type of fracture (eg simple, spiral, comminuted, crush).
- Mention any intra-articular involvement.
- Describe deformity (eg displacement, angulation) from anatomical position.
- State grade or classification of fracture (eg Garden IV).
- State presence of any complications (eg pulse absent, paraesthesia, tissue loss).
- Other injuries and medical problems.

Example using this system

'29 year old male motorcyclist with a compound fracture of the left humerus. It is a transverse fracture of the humeral shaft and is Gustilo type I compound and minimally displaced with no neurovascular compromise ...'

Type of fracture

Simple Single transverse fracture of bone with only 2 main fragments.

Oblique Single oblique fracture with only 2 main fragments.

Spiral Seen in long bones as a result of twisting injuries, only 2 main fragments.

Comminuted Complex fracture resulting in >2 fragments.

Crush Loss of bone volume due to compression.

Wedge Compression to one area of bone resulting in wedge shape (eg vertebra).

Burst Comminuted compression fracture with scattering of fragments.

Impacted Bone ends driven into each other.

Avulsion Bony attachment of ligament or muscle is pulled off.

Hairline Barely visible lucency with no discernible displacement.

Greenstick Incomplete fracture of immature bone follows angulatory force, with one side of the bone failing in compression, the other side in tension.

Torus/buckle Kinking of the metaphyseal cortex follows axial compression.

Plastic deformation Deformation beyond the elastic limit but below the fracture point results in bending of bone ±microfractures (not apparent on X-ray).

Pathological Fracture due to underlying disease (eg osteoporosis, metastasis, Paget's disease).

Stress Certain bones are prone to fracture after repetitive minor injury.

Fracture-dislocation Fracture adjacent to or in combination with a dislocated joint.

Deformity Describe deformity using the terms displacement, angulation and rotation.

Displacement ('translation') Describe the relative position of two bone ends to each other. Further describe the direction that the distal fragment is displaced from the anatomical position (eg volar, lateral). Also estimate the degree of apposition of the bone ends (eg 50%).

Angulation This is usually described in terms of the position of the point of the angle (eg posterior angulation means that the distal fragment is pointing anteriorly). This can sometimes be confusing. Although a little long-winded, one way to avoid confusion is to describe the direction in which the distal part points, relative to the anatomical position (eg a Colles' fracture may be described as a 'fracture of the distal radius in which the distal fragment points dorsally'). Try to measure the angle on X-ray.

Rotation Describe the degree of rotation from the anatomical position, in terms of the direction (eg external or internal rotation) in which the distal part has moved.

Fractures—the role of osteoporosis

Osteoporosis is an important factor in a significant proportion of fractures seen in the ED. The following fractures are frequently (but by no means exclusively) associated with osteoporosis:

- Colles' fracture (📖 p.444).
- Fracture of surgical neck of humerus (📖 p.459).
- Lumbar spine vertebral fracture.
- Fracture of neck of femur (📖 p.470).
- Pubic rami fracture (📖 p.466).

Patients with post-menopausal osteoporosis may be treated with a biphosphonate in an attempt to ↓risk of future fractures, but do not commence this treatment in the ED.

Long bone anatomy

Each long bone has a shaft or diaphysis with an epiphysis at each end. While the bone is growing these are separated by an epiphyseal growth plate and this narrows down into the bone shaft. The transitional area of bone is the metaphysis. In addition to these landmarks, the femur and humerus have a ball-shaped head, a narrower neck, and at the lower ends a widened area consisting of the medial and lateral condyles of the femur, and the medial and lateral epicondyles of the humerus. Fractures proximal to these areas of the femur and humerus are termed supracondylar. Intercondylar fractures involve the central, distal, and juxta-articular portion. Fractures of the proximal femur between the greater and lesser trochanters are termed intertrochanteric.

Compound fractures

Compound (or open) fractures occur when a fracture is open to the air through a skin wound. They incur a risk of infection and can be associated with gross soft tissue damage, severe haemorrhage, or vascular injury. Treat as orthopaedic emergencies requiring rapid assessment and treatment.

Classification of compound injuries

Gustilo classification of compound injuries:

Type I Compound fracture where wound is <1cm long and appears clean.

Type II Compound fracture where wound >1cm, but is not associated with extensive soft tissue damage, tissue loss, or flap lacerations.

Type IIIA Either: compound fracture with adequate soft tissue coverage of bone despite extensive soft tissue damage or flap laceration or any fracture involving high energy trauma or bone shattering regardless of wound size.

Type IIIB Compound fracture with extensive soft tissue loss, periosteal stripping, and exposure of bone.

Type IIIC Compound fracture associated with vascular injury needing repair.

Management

Provide adequate fluid replacement, analgesia, splintage, antibiotics, and tetanus prophylaxis prior to surgical treatment. Rapidly complete the following steps while contacting orthopaedic service:

- Treat life-threatening injuries before limb threatening injuries. Do not be distracted from initial priorities by dramatic distal limb injuries.
- Control obvious haemorrhage by direct manual pressure whilst commencing IV fluids and/or blood replacement.
- Give analgesia in the form of incremental IV opioids (📖 p.276).
- Once analgesia is adequate, correct obvious severe deformities with gentle traction and splint. Certain dislocations may require immediate correction. Remove obvious contaminants if possible (eg large lumps of debris or plant matter).
- 'Routine' wound swabs for bacteriological culture are no longer recommended. They do not alter management and are poor predictors of deep infection.
- If available, take digital photographs of the wound (this helps to avoid the need for repeated inspection by different clinicians).
- Irrigate with saline, then cover the wound with a sterile moist dressing (eg saline soaked pads). Immobilize the limb in a POP backslab. Do not repeatedly inspect the wound as this greatly ↑ risk of infection. Once dressed and in POP, leave injuries covered until surgery.
- Give IV antibiotics (eg co-amoxiclav (1.2g) or cefuroxime (1.5g) according to local policy). Consider adding gentamicin or metronidazole if the wound is grossly contaminated.
- Give tetanus toxoid if indicated, and give HATI if gross wound contamination present (📖 p.410).

Record presence/absence of distal pulses/sensation and recheck frequently.

Limb salvage or amputation

Orthopaedic surgeons often face a difficult decision as to whether or not a limb can be salvaged. Gustilo type IIIC injuries are associated with a high rate of amputation. The Gustilo classification alone is not always an accurate predictor of outcome: other tools have been developed to assist. For example, the Mangled Extremity Severity Score takes into account the extent of skeletal and soft tissue damage, the extent and severity of limb ischaemia, associated shock, and age.

Dislocations

A dislocation involves complete loss of congruity between articular surfaces, whereas a subluxation implies movement of the bones of the joint, but with some parts of the articular surface still in contact. Describe dislocations in terms of the displacement of the distal bone. For example, the most common shoulder dislocation is described as 'anterior', with the humeral head lying in front of the glenoid. Aim to reduce dislocations as soon as possible in order to prevent neurovascular complications, ↓risk of recurrence and ↓pain. However, in general, aim to X-ray (to identify the exact dislocation ±associated fracture) before attempting a reduction. Exceptions to this principle are:

- Dislocations associated with considerable neurovascular compromise requiring urgent intervention (this includes some ankle fracture-dislocations).
- Uncomplicated patellar dislocations (see 📖 Knee fractures and dislocations, p.476).
- Uncomplicated mandibular dislocations (see 📖 Mandibular injuries, p.376).
- Some patients with (very) recurrent shoulder dislocations, where there may be longer-term concerns regarding radiation exposure.
- Some patients with collagen disorders resulting in hypermobility (eg Ehlers–Danlos syndrome) and unusual/recurrent dislocations without significant trauma.
- 'Pulled elbow' in young children (see 📖 Paediatric upper limb injuries, p.724).

Use analgesia/sedation/anaesthesia appropriate to the dislocation and the individual circumstances. For example, patellar dislocations often reduce under Entonox®, finger proximal interphalangeal joint (PIPJ) dislocations with LA digital nerve blocks, shoulder dislocations with IV analgesia ± sedation, whereas posterior hip dislocations typically require manipulation under GA. Except in very exceptional circumstances, X-ray after manipulation to confirm adequate reduction and also to check for fractures which may not have been apparent on initial X-rays.

Casts and their problems

Plaster of Paris (POP)

POP is cheap, easy to use and can be moulded. Usually applied in the form of a bandage or multiply folded as a supporting slab (see Figs 9.7 and 9.8). Disadvantages are susceptibility to damage (POP rapidly disintegrates if wet) and that it takes up to 48hr for larger casts to dry fully after application. Cut slabs to shape prior to use and apply over wool roll and stockinette. Mould with palms (not fingertips) to avoid point indentation of plaster.

Resin casts

More costly, but lighter and stronger than POP and more resistant to water or other damage. Made of cotton or fibreglass impregnated with resin that hardens after contact with water. Sets in 5–10min, maximally strong after 30min. Resin casts are more difficult to apply and remove. Being more rigid and harder to mould, there is ↑risk of problems from swelling or pressure necrosis. Remove/cover any sharp edges on the cast.

Complications of casts

Give all patients discharged with casts clear written instructions (including a contact phone number) to return if they develop pain or other symptoms in the immobilized limb. Formal cast checks within 24hr are only required if there is particular concern about swelling. Simple swelling or discolouration of fingers or toes usually responds to elevation and simple exercises.

Is the cast too tight?

Act immediately upon suspicion of circulatory compromise from a cast. Look for the 'five p's: pain, pallor, paraesthesia, paralysis, and 'perishing cold'. If any of these are present:
- Elevate limb.
- Cut wool and bandages of backslab until skin is visible along the whole length of limb.
- Split full casts and cut through all layers until skin is visible along the whole length of limb.

Any undivided layers will continue to obstruct the circulation until released. If this action fails to completely relieve the symptoms, contact orthopaedic and vascular surgery staff immediately, as angiography and urgent surgical intervention may be required. Note that compartment syndrome may occur in the presence of normal pulses.

Is the cast too loose?

Test by trying to move the plaster longitudinally along the limb. Replace excessively loose or damaged casts, unless there is an outweighing risk of fracture slippage.

Local discomfort

If there is local pressure discomfort (eg over a malleolus), cut a window in the cast to allow direct inspection of the skin. Trim or replace plasters, which restrict movement unduly.

Cast removal

Standard POP and selected resin casts may be removed with plaster shears. Use a plaster saw only after instruction in its proper use. In both cases, be careful to avoid skin damage.

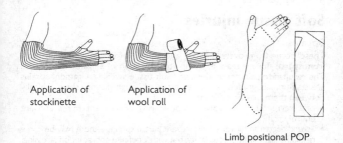

Application of
stockinette

Application of
wool roll

Limb positional POP
shape

Fig. 9.7 Application of a Colles' backslab POP.

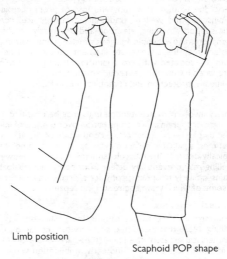

Limb position

Scaphoid POP shape

Fig. 9.8 Application of a scaphoid POP.

Soft tissue injuries

Sprains

These occur from overstretching and tearing of ligaments. Sprains vary from sparse fibrous tears to complete disruption of a ligament complex. The results are pain, tenderness, and soft tissue swelling. Ligament sprains are traditionally graded into three types, although distinguishing clinically between them may be difficult:

- *First degree sprains* involve minor tearing of ligament fibres and are entirely stable.
- *Second degree sprains* are more severe partial sprains—there may be some resultant slight ligamentous laxity, but with a definite end-point on stressing.
- *Third degree sprains* reflect completely torn ligaments causing significant laxity: patients sometimes report hearing a 'snap' at the time of injury.

Ligament sprains are very common, but there is a lack of reliable evidence about treatment. Prolonged immobilization seems to be detrimental to recovery, due to muscle wasting and loss of proprioception. Painful minor sprains respond well to traditional measures: ice, compression with elastic support/strapping, elevation and progressive mobilization as soon as symptoms allow. Simple analgesics such as paracetamol or NSAID (eg ibuprofen) may help. Complete ligament rupture can be relatively painless, but if associated with gross joint instability may require surgical repair. Associated haemarthroses require orthopaedic appraisal, aspiration, and often initially, protection and immobilization in POP.

Strains

Indirect injury involving muscle-tendon units may be classified in a similar fashion to ligament sprains. Pain on palpation over the site of injury is also reproduced by passive stress or active contraction of the affected muscle unit. Sometimes, a palpable defect may be apparent in complete ruptures (which typically occur at the musculotendinous junction). However, associated swelling may prevent any defect from being easily palpable. Treat minor strains similarly to sprains; consider specialist review for complete ruptures, some of which may require surgical repair.

Direct muscle injuries

These result from direct impact causing local pain, bruising, and soft tissue swelling. Note that associated bone contusions can occur, such as in the perimeniscal areas of the knee (these are visible on MRI). Treat minor injuries with ice, analgesia, and early mobilization within the limits of symptoms. For more significant injuries, consider and treat according to possible risks of compartment and crush syndromes (with rhabdomyolysis) and large haematomas (see next section).

Haematomas

Blood can accumulate as a result of traumatic disruption of the vascular structures in bone, muscle, or soft tissues. Deceptively large volumes of blood can be accommodated within the soft tissue planes of the chest wall or thigh. In the presence of massive visible bruising of the torso or a limb, check for shock and measure Hb and Hct. Perform a coagulation screen. Blood transfusion may be necessary. Treat minor haematomas with compression dressings, ice and consider ultrasound therapy. Large haematomas or supervening infection requires selective surgical drainage, haemostasis and antibiotics.

Other soft tissue problems

Myositis ossificans

After some muscle or joint injuries, calcification can occur within a hae-matoma leading to restriction of movement and loss of function. Frequent sites include calcification within a quadriceps haematoma (eg following a rugby injury) where inability to flex the knee >90° at 48hr after injury indicates an ↑risk of myositis ossificans. Other sites include the elbow and femur. Passive stretching movements of joints may be implicated in the development of myositis ossificans. This particularly applies at the shoulder, hip, and knee, where passive exercises are performed for spasticity following paraplegia or head injury.

Treatment involves immobilizing the limb or joint for a period of weeks, under specialist supervision. Early excision is contraindicated, as it is invariably followed by massive recurrence, but delayed excision (after 6–12 months) can improve function.

Tendonitis/tenosynovitis

This includes a wide range of conditions, some of which may have medico-legal implications ('overuse' or 'repetitive strain' injury). Examples include:
- *Classic tenosynovitis*: swelling along a tendon sheath, with pain on passive stretching or upon attempted active movement against resistance.
- *Chronic paratendonitis* (eg affecting Achilles tendon): swelling around the tendon with localized pain and tenderness.
- *Tendon insertion* inflammation causes epicondylitis in adults (see 🕮 p.452) and traction apophysitis in children (🕮 Osteochondritis, p.708).

Appropriate initial treatment usually includes rest, immobilization, and NSAID. Later, consider involving an appropriate specialist (eg physiotherapist or hand therapist).

Bursitis

Inflammation of bursae most frequently affects the subacromial, olecranon, and prepatellar bursae. There is localized swelling and tenderness: generalized joint effusion and/or tenderness along the whole joint line suggests an alternative diagnosis. In many instances, bursitis is non-infective, and responds to rest and NSAID. Significant warmth and erythema raise the possibility of an infective origin. In this case, consider aspiration for bacteriological culture and provide antibiotics (eg co-amoxiclav or penicillin + flucloxacillin).

Other problems

Other causes of joint or limb pain with no specific history of trauma in the adult patient include stress fractures, cellulitis, and other infections, osteoarthritis and other forms of acute arthritis, and nerve compression (eg carpal tunnel syndrome). Apparently atraumatic limb pain in children may present with limping—likely underlying causes vary according to the age (🕮 The limping child, p.704).

Physiotherapy in the ED

At its simplest, the term 'physiotherapy' in the ED includes the advice given to each patient following minor injury. At the other extreme, it encompasses the assessment and treatment of selected patients by skilled, experienced physiotherapists. It is valuable for a department to have close links with a physiotherapy unit, preferably with designated physiotherapy staff responsible for ED referrals. Find out local arrangements for access to and use of physiotherapy services.

'Everyday' physiotherapy

Minor soft tissue injuries are amongst the most commonly seen problems in EDs. Once bony injury has been excluded (clinically and/or radiologically) ensure that patients are discharged with clear, consistent advice on how to manage their own injuries in every case:

- Be clear and specific about what the patient is to do.
- Set a realistic time limit after which the patient should seek further attention if their symptoms are not improving.
- Give additional written instructions for reinforcement (eg ankle sprains, minor knee injuries) as patients forget much verbal advice.

Protection/rest/ice/compression/elevation (PRICE)

This forms the traditional basic framework for treatment of most acute soft tissue injuries.

Protection

Protect the injured part (eg using crutches or a walking stick).

Rest

With most acute injuries, advise a period of 24–48hr rest after an injury.

Ice

Ice is often advocated both in immediate first aid of soft tissue injuries, and in subsequent treatment. Crushed ice cubes wrapped in a damp cloth (to avoid direct contact with the skin) placed against an injured joint may ↓ swelling and pain. Do not apply for more than 10–15min at a time. Repeat every few hours initially. A cold pack or bag of frozen vegetables can be used (do not refreeze if for consumption!).

Compression

Despite a distinct lack of evidence, injured joints (particularly the ankle) are often treated in some support. The easiest to use is an elasticated tubular bandage (eg Tubigrip®), either single or doubled over. If provided, advise not to wear it in bed and to discard as soon as convenient. If not provided, explain why, or the patient may feel inadequately treated. Avoid providing support bandages to patients with elbow and knee injuries—the bandage tends to be uncomfortable and 'dig in' and in the case of the knee, may affect venous return and ↑ chance of DVT.

Elevation

Initially, advise elevation of injured limbs above horizontal to ↓ swelling and discomfort. This is particularly important in hand or foot injuries.

Exercise

Start gentle, controlled exercises for any injured joint as soon as symptoms allow. Demonstrate what is expected and confirm that the patient understands what to do.

Formal physiotherapy

Physiotherapists are trained in the rehabilitation and treatment of injury, based on a detailed knowledge of relevant limb and joint anatomy, bio-mechanics, and physiology. In the ED, physiotherapy staff are valuable in assessment and treatment of acute soft tissue injuries, patient education and advice, and in the provision of appropriate mobility aids after injury (particularly in the elderly). In order to make the best use of physiotherapy services, follow these guidelines:

- Refer early if required for acute injury. Aim for the patient to be seen for initial assessment the same day, so treatment needs can be properly assessed.
- Discuss the problem and treatment options with the physiotherapy staff prior to referral.
- Use the physiotherapy service for selected cases, not as a general rule.
- Never use the physiotherapy department to simply offload difficult or problematic patients.

Physiotherapists have a range of different treatments at their disposal, which typically focus upon regaining range of movement and mobility, improving strength and proprioception.

Approach to hand injuries

The history

Determine and record whether the patient is right- or left-handed, their occupation, and social situation. These points may have treatment implications (eg an elderly person living alone with little social support may not cope at home after a dominant hand injury).

Suspect patients presenting with wounds on the dorsum of the hand over the index, middle, ring, or little finger MC heads of having sustained a human bite ('fight bite') whatever history is given (📖 p.416).

Terminology

To avoid confusion always refer to fingers by name not number (index, middle, ring, little).

Use: palmar (or volar), dorsal, radial, ulnar (not anterior, posterior, lateral, medial).

Bones of the hand and wrist

There are 14 phalanges and 5 metacarpals (MCs). Name the metacarpals according to the corresponding fingers (ie thumb, index, middle, ring, and little). There are 8 carpal bones arranged in 2 rows. The proximal row (radial to ulnar) is comprised of scaphoid, lunate, triquetral, and pisiform (Fig. 9.9). The distal row (radial to ulnar) are trapezium, trapezoid, capitate, and hamate.

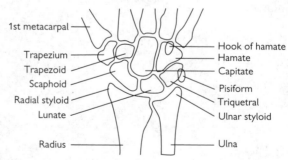

Fig. 9.9 AP view of normal wrist.

Anatomy of finger extensor tendon (Fig. 9.10)

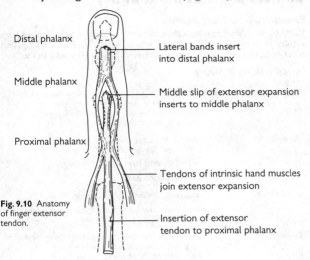

Distal phalanx

Middle phalanx

Proximal phalanx

Lateral bands insert into distal phalanx

Middle slip of extensor expansion inserts to middle phalanx

Tendons of intrinsic hand muscles join extensor expansion

Insertion of extensor tendon to proximal phalanx

Fig. 9.10 Anatomy of finger extensor tendon.

Anatomy of finger flexor tendon (Fig. 9.11)

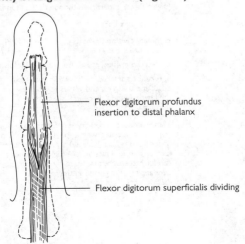

Flexor digitorum profundus insertion to distal phalanx

Flexor digitorum superficialis dividing

Fig. 9.11 Anatomy of finger flexor tendon.

Clinical signs of hand injury

Examination of hand injuries

Injury to the hand's rich collection of nerves, blood vessels, and tendons results in considerable functional deficit. Assess carefully, taking into account hand anatomy and clinical patterns of injury (Figs 9.12 and 9.13).

Specific signs of injury

Table 9.2 Specific signs of injury

Median nerve	↓sensation in the palm over radial 3½ digits
	unable to abduct thumb against resistance
Ulnar nerve	↓sensation palmar and dorsal 1½ fingers, little finger flexed (non-functioning lumbrical)
	unable to cross index and middle fingers
	↓abduction/adduction
Radial nerve	↓sensation dorsum first web space
	(no motor branches in hand, but proximal injury results in inability to extend wrist)
Digital nerve	↓sensation along radial or ulnar half of digit distally: note that some sensation is usually preserved, even with significant nerve injuries
Superficial flexor	hold other fingers straight (immobilizing all deep flexors), then unable to flex PIPJ (unreliable for index finger). Also, ≈10% of individuals do not have a flexor superficialis tendon to the little finger
Deep flexor	unable to flex DIPJ
Extensors	complete division prevents extension (at DIPJ causes mallet deformity)
	central slip division causes Boutonnière deformity
	in recent trauma, hold PIPJ at 90° over table edge, and try to extend versus resistance—DIPJ hyperextends in central slip division (Elson's test)
Deformity	a small amount of rotational deformity of a digit (typically associated with a spiral/oblique MC or finger fracture) can have a dramatic effect upon long-term hand function (see Fig. 9.14): check carefully to ensure that there is no abnormal overlapping of fingertips in the palm on making a fist

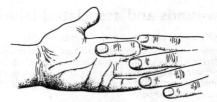

Fig. 9.12 Testing superficial flexor finger tendon.

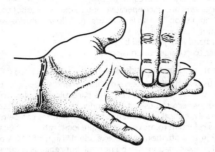

Fig. 9.13 Testing deep flexor finger tendon.

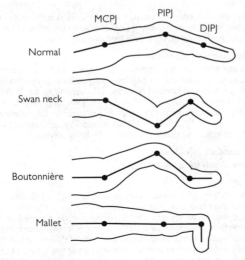

Fig. 9.14 Finger deformities.

Hand wounds and associated injuries

General principles of treating hand wounds

- Remove rings as soon as possible after any hand or arm injury as swelling can develop relatively rapidly. Try soap or water-based lubricant before using ring-cutters. Alternatively, pass string or 0/0 silk under the ring and wrap it firmly around the finger distally, allowing the ring to come off over the compressed tissues.
- Elevate to diminish swelling and pain.
- Avoid subcutaneous sutures.
- For patients who are uncooperative due to excess alcohol consumption, consider admission for a few hours to allow suturing with better co-operation later.
- X-ray any hand injury caused by glass.
- Remember to consider tetanus cover.

Exploration under anaesthesia

If it is obvious that surgical intervention by a hand surgeon is required, do not explore the wound in the ED. This particularly applies to suspected nerve injuries, where the use of LA renders subsequent assessment difficult. Conversely, clinical assessment of tendon injuries can be misleading if the patient is reluctant to move due to pain. Exploration under anaesthesia is necessary in this situation and to exclude division of >50% of a tendon (where clinical examination may be normal, but repair is required). Use an appropriate LA nerve block (as outlined on 🕮 Nerve blocks at the wrist, pp.296–299).

During exploration, consider the position of the hand at the time of injury: reproducing this may reveal injuries otherwise hidden. Therefore, put all mobile structures through their full range of movement.

Extensor tendon injuries

>50% or complete division needs repair (eg 4/0 or 5/0 non-absorbable monofilament using Bunnell or Kessler stitch) by an experienced surgeon. This may be achieved under LA in the ED, depending on facilities and expertise. Follow extensor tendon repair with appropriate immobilization (eg volar slab type POP with finger joints in full extension and slight flexion at the MCPJs). Treat <50% division by splintage in extension (eg POP slab as above) under the care of the hand surgeon.

Flexor tendon injuries

Refer immediately for specialist repair.

Nerve injuries

Complete division of a nerve may cause surprisingly little sensory loss, so take complaints of any altered sensation very seriously. Refer patients with suspected nerve injuries. Digital nerves can be repaired up to the level of the distal phalangeal joint (DIPJ), although it may be decided not to attempt to repair injuries which are distal to the PIPJ. Remember that it is functionally important to have intact sensation over the 'edges' of the hand (the thumb, the radial aspect of the index finger or ulnar aspect of the little finger). Patients sometimes present late after digital nerve injuries—repair can still be quite successful up to 2 weeks after injury.

Reverse fight bites
Treat and refer as outlined in 📖 Specific bites and stings, p.416. Consider transfer of blood-borne infection as discussed in 📖 Needlestick injury, p.418.

Amputations
Refer patients with partial or complete digital amputation with bony loss. Recent proximal amputations without crush injury in fit young patients may be suitable for re-implantation: others may be treated with 'terminalization' or advancement flap. Let the hand surgeon decide. Meanwhile, dress, bandage and elevate, give IV analgesia, tetanus cover, broad spectrum antibiotics (eg cephalosporin), and keep fasted. Wrap the amputated part in moist saline swabs and place in a sealed plastic bag, surrounded by ice/water mix at 4°C.

Note: Do not freeze or place the amputated part directly in solution.

Finger pad amputations
Skin loss less than $1cm^2$ without bony exposure may be allowed to heal with non-adherent dressings. Larger areas of tissue loss (particularly in adults) may require skin grafting or advancement flap, but some do heal satisfactorily with simple dressings.

Ring avulsions
Refer all circumferential and significant degloving injuries.

Compound injuries
Wounds over dislocations or fractures usually require specialist attention. Distal compound phalangeal fractures may be treated in the ED with wound cleaning, closure, review, and prophylactic antibiotics.

Crush injuries
Frequently cause 'burst' injury fingertip wounds. Clean the wounds and take into account the likely swelling when considering closure. Elevate, dress, give analgesia, and arrange review.

Nail bed lacerations
Accurate repair (eg 6/0 Vicryl) may prevent nail deformity. Nailfold-lacerations extending towards the nail bed require removal of the nail to allow suture. Consider replacing the nail after to act as a temporary dressing.

Foreign bodies under nail
Splinters and other FBs under fingernails are relatively common. Apply a digital block and remove with fine forceps. If the FB cannot be reached easily, cut away an appropriate piece of nail.

Subungual haematomas
Blood frequently collects under the nail after a crush injury, causing pain by pressure. If >50% of the nail is affected, trephine the nail distal to the lunula, using a red hot paper clip or battery operated drill.

High pressure injection injuries
Industrial grease or paint guns may cause small skin wounds, which initially appear trivial, disguising a devastating injury with risk of permanent stiffness and significant tissue loss. X-rays may help to identify the extent of foreign material. Refer all such patients to a hand surgeon for immediate exploration and debridement.

Hand fractures and dislocations

Distal phalangeal fractures

Treat closed fractures of the distal portion (tuft) of the distal phalanx with analgesia and elevation. Treat compound burst injuries (from crushing injuries or hammer blows) with meticulous exploration, wound toilet/ repair under LA and arrange follow-up. Give antibiotics (not a substitute for primary surgical treatment).

Mallet finger with fracture

'Mallet finger' injury may be associated with a small fracture at the base of the distal phalanx at the point of attachment of the extensor tendon. Treat as for (the more usual) mallet finger injury without fracture by plastic mallet splint for ≈6weeks, advice and follow-up (see details on 🕮 Soft tissue hand injuries, p.440). Refer larger bony fragments (>$^1/_3$ articular surface) with mallet deformity or those with subluxation for possible K-wire internal fixation.

Fig. 9.15 Mallet finger deformity.

Fig. 9.16 Mallet finger with avulsion fracture.

Proximal and middle phalangeal fractures

Treat undisplaced fractures with elevation, neighbour strapping (Fig. 9.17), and analgesia. Manipulate angulated proximal and middle phalangeal fractures under digital or wrist blocks. A useful tip for proximal phalangeal fractures is to use a needle-holder or pencil placed adjacent to the web space as a fulcrum. Maintain reduction using neighbour strapping and a volar slab POP or flexible padded aluminium (Zimmer) splint, although the latter can be difficult to secure. If reduction is unsatisfactory or cannot be maintained, refer for surgical fixation.

Index, middle, and ring metacarpal fractures

Check for displacement or rotational deformity and refer if present. Treat with analgesia, elevation, and protect in a volar slab POP. Internal fixation may be considered for midshaft MC fractures with marked angulation, but can be complicated by marked post-operative stiffness.

Phalangeal dislocations

X-ray all dislocations prior to reduction for presence of associated fractures. Reduce under digital or metacarpal nerve block (🕮 p.294) or Entonox® by traction and gentle manipulation, then check integrity of the collateral ligaments. Confirm reduction on X-ray and immobilize the finger by neighbour strapping. Elevate the hand, provide oral analgesia and arrange follow-up.

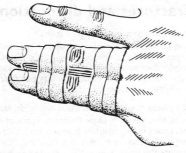

Fig. 9.17 Neighbour (buddy) strapping.

Little (5th) metacarpal fractures

Common result of punching. Check for rotational deformity by gently flexing fingers into the palm (they should point roughly to the thenar eminence and touch, but not overlap adjacent fingers on flexion). Angulation is common with neck fractures and rarely requires correction, with even up to 40° being accepted. Apply neighbour strapping, elevate and give analgesia. A volar slab POP for 2weeks is sometimes advocated—follow local protocols. Warn the patient that the 5th knuckle will be shorter than before. Arrange follow-up and advise hand exercises as soon as possible.

Refer to orthopaedic team if there is rotational deformity or significant angulation, particularly with base and shaft fractures, which may need surgery. Also refer patients with associated wounds, remembering that these may be compound human bites ('reverse fight-bites'—📖 Specific bites and stings, p.416).

Little (5th) metacarpal dislocations

Dislocations at the base of the 5th MC may be associated with a fracture. Refer for reduction and internal fixation.

Thumb fractures and dislocations

Dislocation at metacarpophalangeal joint

After X-rays and LA block, attempt reduction. If successful, assess and document the integrity of the collateral ligaments (see 📖 Soft tissue hand injuries, p.440), then immobilize in slight (≈15°) flexion in a POP and arrange follow-up in fracture clinic. Reduction may be unsuccessful due to 'button-holing'—in this case, refer for open reduction.

Gamekeeper's thumb with associated avulsion fracture

Most abduction injuries result in ulnar collateral ligament injury without fracture, but occasionally an avulsion fracture occurs at the point of ligament attachment instead. Treat this in a scaphoid POP and refer to fracture clinic, unless the bony fragment is displaced by more than 2mm, in which case internal fixation will probably be required.

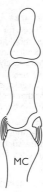

Fig. 9.18

If undisplaced, treat in scaphoid POP, and refer to fracture clinic, but if displaced, refer for internal fixation.

Thumb dislocations

Dislocations usually follow falls onto the thumb or hyperextension injuries. They can occur at any level, including at the interpahalangeal joint (IPJ), MCPJ, and at the carpometacarpal joint. Reduce dislocations by traction and local pressure under combined median and radial nerve blocks (📖 Nerve blocks at the wrist, p.296). Confirm reduction by X-ray, immobilize in a scaphoid POP, and arrange follow-up.

Bennett's fracture-dislocation (□ p.498)

This is a fracture through the base of the thumb (1st) MC with radial subluxation of the MC, leaving a small proximal fragment still joined to the trapezium (Fig. 9.19). The injury results from a fall onto the thumb or from a fall/blow onto a fist closed around the thumb. Deformity and swelling occur over the base of the thumb and may be mistaken clinically for a scaphoid injury. This is an unstable injury requiring expert attention. If undisplaced, apply a Bennett's type POP (similar to a scaphoid POP, but with the thumb abducted). If there is any displacement, refer for manipulation under anaesthetic (MUA)/fixation. Maintaining reduction often requires the use of screw or Kirschner wire fixation.

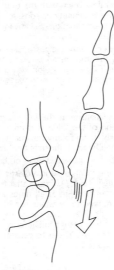

Fig. 9.19 Bennett's fracture-dislocation.

Soft tissue hand injuries

Gamekeeper's thumb

The thumb's ulnar collateral ligament is crucial for stability and function. It is typically injured in hyperabduction injuries (eg falls while skiing). Complete rupture usually results in the two parts of the ligament being separated by the adductor aponeurosis (the 'Stener lesion'), so satisfactory healing cannot occur. If tender over the ulnar collateral ligament of the thumb MCPJ, obtain X-rays: if these demonstrate a fracture, do not stress the joint, but treat appropriately instead (📖 Thumb fractures and dislocations, p.438). If no fracture, assess stability of the ulnar collateral ligament by gentle abduction of the MCPJ (compare with the other hand). Examine the ulnar collateral ligament with the thumb slightly (15°) flexed. If pain precludes adequate examination, consider Entonox® (and/or LA injection) and repeat the examination. Significant (>30°) laxity implies complete rupture and need for operative repair.

Treat uncomplicated sprains with analgesia, elevation, and either criss-cross adhesive strapping ('thumb spica') or a scaphoid POP if symptoms are severe, and arrange follow-up. Refer suspected or demonstrable ulnar collateral ligament rupture to the orthopaedic surgeon, to consider primary surgical repair.

Mallet finger

Injury to the extensor mechanism at the DIPJ is relatively common and results from forced flexion of the DIPJ or from a blow/fall directly onto the fingertip. In the elderly it can follow minimal trauma. There is loss of full active extension at the DIP joint. Normal flexion is preserved.

X-ray to exclude associated fracture—treated as outlined on 📖 p.436.

In the absence of a large fragment, treat in a plastic (mallet) splint secured with tape for ≈6weeks (see 📖 p.436). Ensure that the patient understands the importance of wearing the splint at all times and to keep the finger straight if the splint is removed for washing (eg hold finger against a flat surface until splint replaced). Warn that there may be a small degree of permanent flexion deformity. Arrange initial follow-up at ≈7–10 days, to ensure compliance with treatment and to reassess in case swelling has ↓ and a smaller splint is required.

Volar plate injury

These are significant injuries, often with prolonged morbidity. Hyperextension at the PIPJ injures the *volar plate* at the base of the middle phalanx with or without evidence of bony involvement. Examination shows fusiform swelling of the PIPJ with tenderness over the volar aspect. Treat with 'buddy strapping' to adjacent fingers (or 'Bedford splint'), elevate, provide analgesia, and begin mobilization immediately. Arrange review to ensure full mobility is regained.

A2 pulley injury

The finger flexor tendon sheath at the PIPJ is thickened and known as the A2 pulley. Occasionally (especially in rock climbers), the tendon cuts through the A2 pulley, causing characteristic bowstringing on flexion. There may be associated tendon injury. Treat conservatively with buddy strapping (or Bedford splint) and elevation. Arrange hand specialist follow-up.

Boutonnière deformity (📖 Eponymous fractures, p.498)

Characteristic deformity from untreated rupture/division of central slip finger extensor tendon may follow blunt or penetrating trauma.

Other soft tissue hand problems

Pulp infections

Infection of the pulp space at the fingertip may reflect underlying FB or osteomyelitis, so X-ray to search for these and treat accordingly. If X-rays are normal, incise the pointing area under LA digital block. Send pus for bacteriology, apply a dressing, commence oral antibiotics (eg flucloxacillin 250–500mg PO qds), and arrange follow-up.

Paronychia

Infection of the nailfold adjacent to the nail is common. In the early stages, oral antibiotics (eg co-amoxiclav or flucloxacillin) may cure.

Once pus has developed, drain this under LA digital block by an incision over the fluctuance (usually a small longitudinally-orientated incision adjacent to the proximal nailfold suffices, but pus under the nail may require removal of a segment of nail). Antibiotics are then unnecessary, unless there is spreading infection (in which case, consider co-amoxiclav).

Pyogenic flexor tenosynovitis

Infection of a finger flexor tendon sheath may follow penetrating injury. Classical signs (Kanavel's signs) are:

- Tenderness over the flexor tendon.
- Symmetrical swelling of the finger.
- Finger held in flexion.
- Extreme pain on passive extension.

Ensure tetanus prophylaxis, then refer urgently for exploration, irrigation, and IV antibiotics.

Other infections

These include palmar space infections and septic arthritis—refer immediately for specialist treatment.

Locked finger

Elderly patients with underlying osteoarthritis (OA) sometimes present with locking at a finger MCPJ. A fixed flexion deformity is present, such that the patient can flex, but not fully extend at the MCPJ. There is usually no particular history of trauma—the underlying cause is entrapment of the palmar plate on an osteophyte. Refer for an early hand surgeon opinion: surgery may be required.

Trigger finger/thumb

This is relatively common, but not particularly related to trauma. Most cases are satisfactorily treated by steroid injection into the flexor tendon sheath, but leave this to a specialist.

Carpal bone fractures and dislocations

Scaphoid fractures

Assess and document whether there is tenderness over the scaphoid in all wrist injuries. Scaphoid fractures occur from falling onto an outstretched hand or from 'kick-back' injuries (eg from a steering wheel in a car crash or football goalkeeper making a save). Pain and swelling over the wrist's radial aspect may be accompanied by difficulty gripping.

Look for
- Tenderness in anatomical snuffbox: compare both sides.
- Tenderness over palmar aspect of scaphoid (scaphoid tubercle).
- Scaphoid pain on compressing the thumb longitudinally.
- Scaphoid pain on gentle flexion and ulnar deviation of the wrist.
- Tenderness over dorsum of scaphoid.

X-rays Request specialized scaphoid (not wrist) views. Four views are usually taken (AP, lateral, right, and left obliques). Remember that scaphoid fractures may not be visible on initial X-rays. The scaphoid mostly fractures through the waist, but sometimes through the tubercle (the latter does not give rise to significant complications).

Treatment If there is clinical or radiological evidence of fracture, apply a scaphoid POP or splint, and arrange review in 10–14 days. Treat minimal snuffbox tenderness without radiologically visible fracture with analgesia, and a wrist splint and arrange review as above.

Complications Include non-union, avascular necrosis, and OA.

Follow-up of clinically suspected scaphoid fractures (but normal X-rays) is often undertaken in ED clinic. Review at 10–14 days after injury, when if there is no clinical evidence of fracture, patients may be discharged. If, however, there is continuing pain and/or scaphoid tenderness, repeat the X-rays: treat visible fractures in POP; but if X-rays are still normal, treat in splint or POP, and arrange MRI (or bone scan for those with claustrophobia or other contraindication to MRI) to definitively answer whether there is a fracture or significant carpal ligament injury.

Lunate dislocations

These injuries are rare, but often missed (Fig. 9.22). They follow falls onto the outstretched wrist, and result in pain and swelling anteriorly over the wrist. Median nerve paraesthesia may be a clue to the diagnosis. X-ray shows dislocation and rotation of the lunate so that it is shifted in front of the carpus and its concave surface faces towards the palm instead of distally. The AP view may look relatively normal, so carefully scrutinize lateral views. Refer for immediate MUA.

Complications Median nerve injury, avascular necrosis, Sudeck's atrophy.

Other carpal dislocations

Isolated dislocations of other carpal bones occur, but often injuries are more complicated and involve dislocations (and fractures) of one row of carpal bones (eg trans-scaphoid perilunate dislocation; Fig. 9.21). Surprisingly, perhaps, given almost inevitable significant swelling, these injuries can be missed. Give analgesia and refer for reduction by the orthopaedic team.

Flake avulsion carpal fractures

Small avulsions from the dorsum of the carpus are often from the triquetrum. Treat with immobilization in a POP backslab or wrist support splint, analgesia, and refer to fracture clinic.

Fractured hook of hamate

Local palmar tenderness may give rise to suspicion of a fracture of the hook of the hamate. Diagnosis can be difficult: specialized X-rays or CT may be required to demonstrate the fracture. Immobilize in POP and refer to fracture clinic.

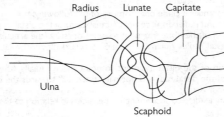

Fig. 9.20 Wrist: normal lateral.

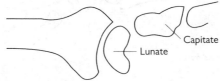

Fig. 9.21 Perilunate dislocation.

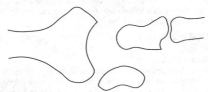

Fig. 9.22 Lunate dislocation.

Colles' fracture

Presentation

This fracture affects the radius within 2.5cm of the wrist, such that the distal fragment is angulated to point dorsally. It usually results from a fall onto an outstretched hand. Osteoporosis contributes to ↑frequency in post-menopausal women. Colles' fractures produce characteristic clinical deformity (sometimes likened to a 'dinnerfork'). Check for scaphoid tenderness, distal sensation, and pulses in all cases.

Radiological features

X-ray appearances include one or more of the following:
- Posterior and radial displacement (translation) of the distal fragment.
- Angulation of the distal fragment to point dorsally (the articular surface of the distal radius normally has a 5° forward tilt on the lateral wrist X-ray).
- Angulation of the distal fragment to point more radially (the articular surface of the distal radius is normally tilted 22° towards the ulnar side on AP wrist X-ray).
- Impaction, leading to shortening of the radius in relation to the ulna.

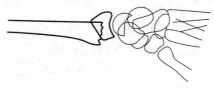

Fig. 9.23 Colles' fracture

Treatment

Provide analgesia, immobilize in a backslab POP, and elevate with a sling. Discharge those with undisplaced fractures (if they will manage at home) and arrange fracture clinic follow-up. Advise the patient to keep moving fingers, thumb, elbow, and shoulder.

Deciding if MUA is indicated

MUA is required for:
- Grossly displaced fractures.
- Loss of normal forward radial articular surface tilt on lateral wrist X-ray. Neutral or minimal tilt may be acceptable in the very young or very old (particularly in the non-dominant limb). Seek senior advice if unsure.

Timing of MUA

Patients with compound fractures and/or symptoms of nerve compression require urgent MUA. For many other patients, the timing of the procedure is less important. Many EDs undertake closed manipulation of Colles' fractures in adult patients at the time of initial presentation, whilst others arrange for the patient to return for the procedure within 1–2days to a specific theatre list as a day case.

MUA procedure for Colles' fractures

Consent

Discuss the risks and benefits of the procedure. In particular, explain that, if left untreated, an angulated Colles' fracture may result in long-term stiffness and a significantly weaker grip. The principal risks of manipulation are:

- Tears to the skin on the dorsum of the wrist (especially in those with thin skin (eg on steroids) and/or significant swelling (eg on warfarin).
- Late slippage of the bones requiring a further procedure.
- Risks of the anaesthetic employed.

Choice of anaesthetic

The anaesthetic options available include: haematoma block (📖 p.289), intravenous regional anaesthesia (📖 Bier's block, p.290), IV sedation (📖 p.308), GA (📖 p.310). The choice of anaesthetic will depend upon local protocols, as well as patient related factors, such as the type of fracture and extent of fasting. For example, a minimally angulated fracture in an elderly individual may be satisfactorily managed using a haematoma block, whereas a more dramatically angulated and displaced fracture may not. Evidence suggests that Bier's block is superior to haematoma block (see www.bestbets.org).

Technique

Different individuals may employ different techniques, but the aim is to attempt to return the anatomy to its previous position. In particular, it is important to correct the dorsal angulation ('restore the volar cortex'). Many descriptions of reduction techniques involve initial traction and 'dis-impaction' of the fragments, followed by wrist flexion and pronation with pressure over the distal radial fragment(s). Some operators focus more upon gentle direct manipulation of the distal fragment, rather than indirect measures (traction, wrist flexion, etc.).

Following manipulation, apply a backslab POP, whilst maintaining the reduction, with the wrist slightly flexed and pronated (avoid excessive flexion as this can cause additional long-term problems). Satisfactory reduction can be confirmed by image intensifier/X-ray. If the reduction is not satisfactory, repeat the manipulation procedure.

Medium and long-term complications of Colles' fracture

Patients may present to the ED with later complications following Colles' fracture (and the treatment provided for it), including the following:

- *Stiffness of wrist and adjacent limb joints*: refer for physiotherapy.
- *Malunion and cosmetic problems*: refer to GP/orthopaedic team.
- *Reflex sympathetic dystrophy (Sudeck's atrophy)*: refer for physiotherapy and GP/orthopaedic follow-up.
- *Carpal tunnel syndrome* may occur after Colles' fracture, but also reflect other problems (eg lunate dislocation): check original X-rays.
- *Extensor pollicis longus rupture* may occur some weeks after fractures with minimal displacement: see 📖 Soft tissue wrist injuries/problems, p.447.

Other wrist fractures

Smith's fracture

This is an unstable distal radius fracture (sometimes referred to as a 'reverse Colles' fracture') where the distal fragment is impacted, tilted to point anteriorly and often displaced anteriorly (Fig. 9.24). It usually follows a fall onto a flexed wrist. Give analgesia, immobilize in a backslab POP and refer for MUA (often difficult to hold in position after reduction) or ORIF using a buttress plate (preferred in some orthopaedic centres).

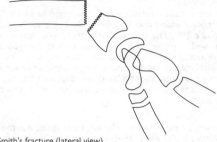

Fig. 9.24 Smith's fracture (lateral view).

Barton's and reverse Barton's fracture (📖 p.498)

An intra-articular fracture involving only the dorsal or volar portion of the distal radius is called a Barton's fracture and reverse Barton's fracture (Fig. 9.25), respectively. The resultant fragment tends to slip, so the fracture is inherently unstable. Provide analgesia, immobilize in a POP backslab and refer. Most patients require ORIF and plating.

Isolated radial styloid fracture

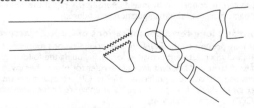

Fig. 9.25 Lateral view of a reverse Barton's fracture.

Caused by similar mechanisms of injury as scaphoid fractures (ie falls onto an outstretched hand or kickback injuries). It is sometimes referred to as a Hutchinson fracture (📖 Eponymous fractures, p.500). Treat with analgesia, backslab POP, elevation sling and fracture clinic. Internal fixation is occasionally required.

Soft tissue wrist injuries/problems

Wrist sprain

Exclude scaphoid or other fracture (or dislocation) before considering the diagnosis of a 'simple wrist sprain'. Relatively minor damage to ligaments around the wrist can occur following hyperextension or flexion of the wrist, causing swelling and tenderness around the joint. Treat with a wrist splint or tubigrip support, analgesia, or NSAIDs, and progressive exercise. Continuing pain and problems arouse suspicions of more significant injury (possibly involving other structures, such as the scapholunate ligament or triangular fibrocartilage complex). Refer for specialist investigation.

TFCC injury

The triangular fibrocartilage complex at the distal end of the ulna may be injured with associated structures. Often, these injuries only become apparent later, when what was diagnosed as a 'simple wrist sprain' fails to settle—pain and tenderness persists over the TFCC. Arrange specialist follow-up for further investigation (eg MRI) and treatment.

Rupture of wrist/hand tendons

Rupture of tendons may occur without penetrating trauma. The most common rupture involves extensor pollicis longus a few weeks after (usually undisplaced) fracture of the distal radius. Rupture of other extensor (and occasionally flexor) tendons occurs in association with OA, rheumatoid arthritis (RA), scaphoid non-union, chronic renal failure (CRF), systemic lupus erythromatosus (SLE). Refer to a hand surgeon.

Radial tenosynovitis ('intersection syndrome')

Typically follows unaccustomed repetitive activity, such as gardening, DIY, or decorating. Over hours to days, a painful fusiform swelling develops over the radial aspect of the distal forearm. Movement of the wrist produces pain and palpable (occasionally audible) crepitus. Immobilize in a simple adjustable wrist splint and unless contraindicated, prescribe NSAID for 7–10days. After this, allow gradual mobilization of the wrist and educate about eliminating the cause. Immobilize severe cases in a forearm POP for 2 weeks before beginning mobilization.

De Quervain's tenosynovitis

Affects the tendon sheaths of abductor pollicis longus and extensor pollicis brevis. Pain, swelling, and crepitus occur over the lateral (dorso-radial) aspect of the radial styloid. Symptoms can be reproduced by thumb or wrist movement. Finkelstein described grasping the patient's thumb and rapidly 'abducting the hand ulnarward', but probably more useful is pain on ulnar movement of the wrist with the thumb clenched in a fist. Treat with NSAID and splintage for 7–10 days. A removable fabric wrist splint (including the thumb) may suffice, but consider a scaphoid type POP for severe pain. Persistent symptoms may respond to steroid injection of the tendon sheath using an aseptic technique.

Forearm fractures and related injury

If one forearm bone is fractured, look for a fracture or dislocation of the other.

Obvious deformity in an adult forearm indicates fracture of the radial and ulna shafts. Initially treat with:

- Analgesia (eg increments of IV morphine + anti-emetic until pain relieved).
- Immobilization in backslab POP.
- If one or both fractures are compound, give IV antibiotics (🔲 p.422), tetanus cover, and dress the wound.

Always check distal pulses and sensation, and examine for associated injuries at the wrist and elbow. Only once this has been done and the patient is comfortable, can he/she be sent for X-ray. Ensure X-rays demonstrate the whole lengths of the radius and ulna, including separate views of both the elbow and wrist joints.

Fractures of both radius and ulna shafts

Adult fractures, unlike those in children, may be markedly displaced with little or no bony contact between the fragments. Rotational deformity is common. Check carefully for clinical evidence of neurovascular injury. Closed reduction is difficult, and often fails or is complicated by late slippage. Treat fractures with analgesia/immobilization as above and refer for ORIF.

Isolated ulna shaft fracture

These usually occur from a direct blow to the outer edge of the forearm (it is typically seen as a defence injury) or from a fall striking the ulna shaft. X-ray the whole ulna and radius to exclude associated fracture or dislocation of the radial head (see below). If undisplaced, treat in an above elbow POP with the elbow flexed to 90° and the forearm in mid-supination. Refer all displaced or angulated fractures for ORIF.

Galeazzi fracture-dislocation (see 🔲 p.499)

Defined as a fracture of the radius associated with dislocation of the distal radio-ulnar joint at the wrist (Fig. 9.26). Always look for subluxation of the ulna in radial fractures. Treat with analgesia and immobilization in a temporary POP backslab. Refer for ORIF.

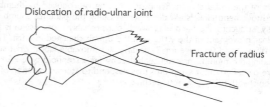

Dislocation of radio-ulnar joint

Fracture of radius

Fig. 9.26

Monteggia fracture-dislocation (see 📖 p.501)

Defined as a fracture of the ulna associated with dislocation of the radial head. Occurs from forced pronation of the forearm (eg fall onto an outstretched, fully pronated forearm). Can also occur by a direct blow or fall onto the proximal ulna, displacing the head of the radius. Treat with analgesia and immobilization in a temporary above-elbow POP backslab. Refer to the orthopaedic team for ORIF (or sometimes in children, for treatment with MUA and POP).

A related injury is the *Hume fracture* (📖 Eponymous fractures, p.500) in which anterior dislocation of the radial head is combined with an olecranon fracture. Refer for ORIF.

Note: Monteggia fracture-dislocations are not infrequently missed at initial presentation, due to attention being distracted by the ulna fracture (Fig. 9.27). To avoid this:
• Request elbow and wrist X-rays in any patient with forearm shaft fracture.
• Check all elbow X-rays carefully to ensure that the radial shaft is normally aligned and that the radial head abuts the capitellum.

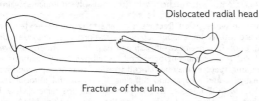

Dislocated radial head

Fracture of the ulna

Fig. 9.27 Monteggia fracture-dislocation.

Isolated radial shaft fracture

These are very uncommon. Always treat and assume that there is some associated damage to the distal radio-ulnar joint at the wrist.

Elbow injuries

In any injured elbow look specifically for:
- Elbow effusion (felt as a tense, bulging swelling halfway between the lateral epicondyle and the point of the olecranon).
- The normal relationship between the olecranon and the lateral and medial epicondyles: all should form an equilateral triangle with the elbow flexed.
- Range of movement: X-ray patients who cannot fully extend the elbow and flex to touch the shoulder tip.

Olecranon fractures

Follow falls onto the point of the elbow. The olecranon fragment may displace proximally due to pull of triceps. Swelling, tenderness, or crepitus are present on examination. In the young, the olecranon epiphysis may cause confusion on X-rays. Treat undisplaced or hairline fractures in an above elbow backslab POP at 90°, provide analgesia and arrange fracture clinic follow-up. Refer fractures that are displaced or involve the elbow joint for ORIF.

Radial head/neck fractures

Follow falls onto outstretched wrist (the radial head impacts against the capitellum) or direct trauma to the elbow. They sometimes occur in combination with a wrist fracture. Examine movements—extension and flexion are usually limited, but supination and pronation may be relatively normal. Look for an elbow effusion and palpate for tenderness over the radial head while supinating/pronating the elbow. X-ray confirms elbow effusion, but fractures may be difficult to see. Treat undisplaced fractures with analgesia, and a collar and cuff sling. If very painful, immobilize in an above elbow POP backslab at 90°. Arrange fracture clinic review. Refer comminuted or displaced fractures as they may require MUA, internal fixation or occasionally excision/replacement of the radial head.

Elbow effusion, no visible fracture

Always assume that a radial head/neck fracture is present: provide analgesia, a collar and cuff sling, and arrange review to ensure that full movement is regained. Extra symptomatic relief may be achieved by aspiration of the elbow joint (via a point midway between the olecranon and lateral epicondyle) under aseptic conditions.

Elbow fat pad sign

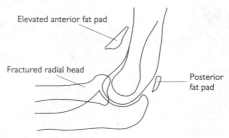

Elevated anterior fat pad

Fractured radial head

Posterior fat pad

Fig. 9.28 Elbow fat pad sign.

Dislocated elbow

Examination reveals loss of the normal triangular relationship between the olecranon and epicondyles. Check distal pulses and sensation as brachial artery, median and ulnar nerves may be damaged. Elbow dislocations may be classified according to the direction of dislocation and the presence of associated fractures (eg fractured coronoid). The most frequent injury is postero-lateral dislocation (ie movement of the distal part in a postero-lateral direction).

After analgesia and X-ray, most dislocations may be reduced in the ED under IV sedation with full monitoring (📖 Sedation, p.308). However, GA is sometimes required.

Reduction Choose between the following techniques for reduction of postero-lateral dislocations:

• Flex the elbow to 60° with countertraction on the upper arm. Pull on the fully pronated forearm at this angle. Slight flexion at the elbow may be necessary.
• Alternatively, lever the olecranon forward with both thumbs while holding the elbow flexed and while an assistant provides traction on the forearm.

Reduction is confirmed by a 'clunk' and restoration of the normal triangular relationship of the elbow landmarks. Once reduced, recheck pulses and sensation, immobilize in an above elbow POP backslab at 90° and X-ray again (looking for associated fractures). Consider admission for analgesia and observation for possible significant limb swelling. If unable to reduce, refer for reduction under GA.

Supracondylar fractures (see 📖 p.722)

Fractures of the distal third of the humerus usually occur from falls onto the outstretched hand. They are most common in children (📖 p.722), but also occur in adults. The elbow may be grossly swollen and deformed, but the normal triangular relationship of the olecranon and epicondyles is characteristically preserved. Check distal pulses and sensation carefully as the brachial artery, ulnar, median, and radial nerves can all be damaged. Immobilize in an above elbow backslab POP and give analgesia. Refer to the orthopaedic surgeon as MUA/ORIF are usually required.

Fractures of the capitellum occasionally occur in isolation. If undisplaced, treat conservatively with analgesia and POP. Refer those with displaced fractures for specialist treatment (possibly ORIF).

Medial collateral ligament injury

Instability on stress testing of the medial (ulnar collateral) ligament implies a significant injury. Treat in backslab POP with the elbow flexed to 90° and supported in a sling. Arrange fracture clinic follow-up.

Other elbow injuries

Elbow injuries are relatively common in children. Specific injuries in children are considered as follows:

• Supracondylar fracture (📖 Paediatric upper limb injuries, p.722).
• Lateral and medial condylar injury—(📖 p.724).
• Pulled elbow—(📖 Paediatric upper limb injuries, p.724).

Soft tissue elbow problems

Injuries to biceps and brachialis

Inflammation of biceps and/or brachialis at the site of attachment at the elbow can cause persistent symptoms: treat with rest and NSAID. Biceps brachii can rupture either at its long head in the bicipital groove or near the elbow insertion. Long head ruptures typically affect the elderly and result in a characteristic abnormal shape and low biceps position on attempted elbow flexion against resistance: unless the patient is young, fit, and active, surgical repair is rarely indicated. Distal ruptures are sometimes treated conservatively, but some may benefit from repair: arrange orthopaedic review to consider this.

Lateral epicondylitis

This is commonly called 'tennis elbow'. It follows repetitive or excessive stress to the origin of the forearm and hand extensor muscles at the lateral epicondyle. It can occur spontaneously, but usually follows repetitive lifting, pulling, or sports (eg as a result of an incorrect backhand technique in tennis). Inflammation, oedema, and microtears occur within the extensor insertion.

Look for localized swelling, warmth or tenderness over the lateral epicondyle and immediately distal to it.

Examine movements: dorsiflexion of the pronated wrist against resistance will reproduce symptoms.

X-ray if the problem follows acute injury. Refer to the orthopaedic surgeon if there is an avulsion fracture.

Treat with analgesia (preferably NSAID) and ice application. Support the arm in a broad arm sling and advise rest, followed by progressive exercise and avoidance of aggravating movements. If symptoms are recurrent or prolonged, refer as steroid injection, forearm clasp, physiotherapy, and occasionally surgery may help. Current evidence suggests that corticosteroid injection may provide short-term relief, but long-term benefit remains unproven.

Medial epicondylitis

Often called 'golfer's elbow', this condition has a similar pathophysiology to lateral epicondylitis: it is frequently seen in racket sports and golf.

Examine for localized tenderness and swelling over the forearm flexor insertion at the medial epicondyle. Flexion of the supinated wrist against resistance will reproduce symptoms. There may be ↓ grip strength and ≈60% of patients have some symptoms of associated ulnar neuritis.

Treat as for lateral epicondylitis.

Osteochondritis dissecans

This can affect the elbow and cause locking of the elbow joint. X-rays may reveal a defect and/or loose body. Refer to the orthopaedic team.

Olecranon bursitis

Inflammation, swelling and pain in the olecranon bursa may follow minor trauma or occur spontaneously. Other causes include bacterial infection (sometimes following penetrating injury) and gout. Elbow movements are usually not limited. Look for overlying cellulitis, wounds, and systemic symptoms and check for ↑T° (these suggest infection). Gout or bacterial infection can be confirmed by aspiration of the bursa under aseptic conditions and immediate microscopy for crystals or bacteria. Aspirate using a small needle at a shallow angle and try to aspirate the bursa completely.

Non-infective bursitis Provide analgesia, NSAID, and rest the arm in a broad arm sling. Symptoms should resolve with rest over a period of weeks. Rarely, persistent symptoms require surgical excision of the olecranon bursa.

Gout bursitis Treat as above. Arrange follow-up through the patient's GP.

Infective bursitis If there is evidence of underlying infection, treat with rest, NSAID and start antibiotics (eg co-amoxiclav or flucloxacillin + penicillin). Occasionally, infection requires referral to the orthopaedic surgeon for surgical drainage.

Olecranon bursa haematoma A history of blunt trauma to the olecranon followed rapidly by 'golf ball-sized' swelling over the olecranon, but with a full range of elbow movement (and no evidence of fracture), implies a haematoma in the olecranon bursa. Treat conservatively: attempts at drainage may result in secondary infection.

Nerve compression

Ulnar nerve entrapment at the elbow ('cubital tunnel syndrome') is the second most common upper limb nerve entrapment (median nerve compression in carpal tunnel syndrome is the commonest. Refer these chronic conditions back to the GP.

Acute radial nerve palsy above the elbow presents with sudden wrist drop following a history of compression (eg crutch use, falling asleep with arm over the back of a chair). The underlying injury is usually a neurapraxia, which has the potential to recover completely given time with conservative measures. It is crucial to ensure that flexion contractures do not develop in the meantime: provide a removable wrist splint, advise regular passive wrist exercises, and refer for physiotherapy and follow-up to ensure recovery.

Anterior shoulder dislocation

This is a common injury, which typically results from forced external rotation/abduction of the shoulder. The humeral head usually dislocates to lie anterior and slightly inferior to the glenoid. Patients often present supporting the affected arm with the uninjured arm.

The diagnosis is usually obvious on examination. Look for:
- Step-off deformity at the acromion with palpable gap below the acromion.
- Humeral head palpable antero-inferiorly to the glenoid.
- Evidence of complications: check especially for distal pulses and ↓sensation over the lateral aspect of the shoulder (the 'badge' area) supplied by the axillary nerve.

Give analgesia and support in a temporary sling. X-ray before reduction to exclude associated fractures. X-rays show loss of congruity between humeral head and the glenoid. The humeral head is displaced medially and inferiorly on an antero-posterior (AP) shoulder X-ray.

Treatment

Reduce under sedation/analgesia with full monitoring, using one of the methods described below/opposite. The choice of technique is personal and depends partly upon familiarity. Apply minimal force to prevent humeral fracture or further soft tissue damage. In patients with habitual recurrent dislocation (and in a significant proportion of other patients as well), reduction may be easily achievable with minimal use of drugs (eg Entonox® alone). Take time and perform the manoeuvre slowly. Note that in situations where IV sedation cannot be used or needs to be avoided, intra-articular lidocaine is an option.

External rotation method

This simple technique has a good rate of success. With the patient reclining at 45°, slowly and gently (without force) externally rotate the shoulder to 90°. If the dislocation has not yet reduced, forward flex (elevate) the shoulder slowly.

Kocher's method

Lie the patient back almost flat, and once sedation and analgesia are adequate:
- With the elbow flexed to 90°, slowly externally rotate the shoulder. Pause if there is any resistance and continue only when muscles relax.
- Slowly adduct the upper arm across the chest with the shoulder still held in external rotation.
- Once adducted as far as possible, internally rotate the shoulder by flipping the forearm towards the opposite shoulder.

Reduction may occur at any time during the manoeuvre: success is more likely if the patient is relaxed (avoid traction) and if initial external rotation reaches 90°. A 'clunk' or return of normal glenoid contour confirms success.

Modified Milch method

Slowly abduct the straight arm to 110°. With the elbow extended, apply gentle steady traction to the arm, while an assistant controls movement of the humeral head back into the glenoid.

Other techniques

Scapular manipulation With the patient lying prone, 'manipulate' the scapula onto the glenoid by pushing the inferior tip of the scapula medially and the superior part laterally.

Stimson's technique A more traditional method with the patient prone. Apply a weight strapped to the forearm/wrist of the affected side as it hangs down and await reduction.

Hippocratic methods Many techniques have been described over many centuries, but are probably of historical interest only.

Post-reduction After reduction, recheck pulses and sensation (including axillary and radial nerves), and obtain a check X-ray. Immobilize in a collar and cuff, and body bandage. Local policy sometimes includes shoulder immobilization webbing or braces as standard. Provide analgesia (eg co-dydramol) and arrange follow-up. If unsuccessful, difficult or if shoulder has been dislocated >24hr, refer for reduction under GA.

Fracture-dislocation of the shoulder

Most involve fractures of the greater tuberosity associated with anterior dislocation of the shoulder (Fig. 9.29). Reduce under sedation as with uncomplicated dislocations—in most cases the fracture will reduce satisfactorily along with the dislocation. However, refer large or complex fracture-dislocations involving the humeral head, neck or shaft.

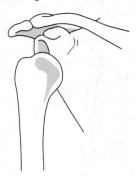

Fig. 9.29 Anterior dislocation of the right shoulder.

Other types of shoulder dislocation

Posterior dislocation

This uncommon injury is easy to miss. It results from a blow onto the anterior shoulder or a fall onto the internally rotated arm. It may also occur during seizures or after an electric shock (when other injuries and medical problems may be partly responsible for it being initially overlooked). The patient presents with the shoulder internally rotated. AP shoulder X-ray may appear normal, but careful inspection reveals an abnormally symmetrical appearance of the humeral head ('light bulb sign') and loss of congruity between the humeral head and the glenoid (Figs 9.30 and 9.31). A modified axial shoulder X-ray (from above) or a translateral view will confirm posterior dislocation of the humeral head. Manipulate under sedation by applying traction and external rotation to the upper limb at 90° to the body. If difficult, refer for reduction under GA. Treat and follow-up as for anterior dislocation.

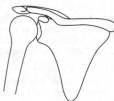

Fig. 9.30 AP view of posterior shoulder dislocation: light bulb sign.

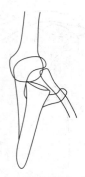

Fig. 9.31 Modified axial view of posterior shoulder dislocation.

Luxatio erecta

This is a rare inferior dislocation of the humeral head. The patient presents with arm held abducted above head. Check carefully for neurovascular complications. Reduce under sedation by traction in line with the abducted upper arm, followed by adduction of the shoulder. May require reduction under GA. Treat and follow-up as for anterior dislocation.

Other shoulder injuries

Acromio-clavicular (AC) joint injury

Common injuries which usually follow falls onto the shoulder or violent sudden movements of the upper limb. Look for local pain, swelling, or a palpable step over the AC joint. X-rays show fractures or AC joint disruption (vertical subluxation of the AC joint >1–2mm) (Fig. 9.32). The diagnosis may be made more obvious by asking the patient to hold a heavy object while the X-ray is taken. AC joint injuries are classified:

- *Grade I*: minimal separation. Only acromio-clavicular ligaments involved.
- *Grade II*: obvious subluxation, but still some apposition of bony ends.
- *Grade III*: complete dislocation of AC joint, indicating rupture of the conoid and trapezoid ligaments, in addition to the acromio-clavicular ligaments.

Treat with analgesia, support in a broad arm sling, and arrange follow-up for grades II and III injuries. These measures allow complete recovery in most cases. Occasionally, selected patients benefit from internal fixation.

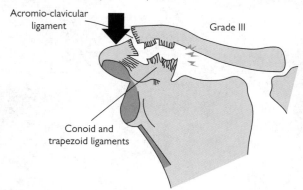

Fig. 9.32

Clavicle fracture

This common injury results from direct trauma or from falls onto the out-stretched hand or point of the shoulder. Check carefully for neurovascular complications (these are rare, but potentially life-threatening).

Treat with analgesia, a broad arm sling and arrange fracture clinic follow-up. The vast majority of fractures unite satisfactorily with conservative treatment. Rarely, grossly displaced fractures are internally fixed.

Scapular fracture

Usually results from direct trauma and implies a forceful mechanism of injury. Check carefully for associated injuries to the thorax, such as rib fractures or haemo-pneumothorax.

Treat isolated fractures with a broad arm sling, analgesia, and arrange follow-up.

Humeral neck/head fracture

These result from direct trauma to the upper arm or from falls onto an outstretched hand. Examine for tenderness or swelling over the proximal humerus. Shoulder movements are usually limited by pain. X-rays typically reveal impacted or oblique fractures, with or without associated fractures of the greater and lesser tuberosities. Fractures may be classified as 2, 3, or 4-part fractures according to the number of fragments resulting (eg a fractured humeral neck combined with a fractured greater tuberosity will be a '3 part fracture').

Treat with a collar and cuff support, analgesia, and follow-up. Warn the patient to expect significant visible bruising to appear, extending down the arm towards the elbow (for this reason, it is helpful to document the lack of any clinical evidence of elbow injury at first presentation). Refer all comminuted, displaced, or markedly angulated humeral neck fractures as MUA and, occasionally, internal fixation/hemi-arthroplasty are indicated.

Shaft of humerus fracture

Results from a fall onto an outstretched hand or onto the elbow. The fracture may be obvious and palpable. Check distal pulses, radial nerve and elbow joint. X-ray reveals a transverse, comminuted, or spiral humeral shaft fracture.

Provide analgesia and support the fracture in a POP U-slab (slab of plaster from the axilla down to and around the olecranon and up the outside of the upper arm). Apply with the elbow flexed to 90° and hold in place with a bandage. Alternative treatment includes a 'hanging cast' POP (above elbow POP at 90°—the weight of POP and arm hold the fracture in a satisfactory position). Refer if displaced, comminuted, or angulated, or if neurovascular complications are suspected. MUA and internal fixation are required in these cases.

Rotator cuff tears

Tears (supraspinatus rupture most commonly) usually follow chronic rotator cuff disease in patients >40years. May follow trauma (eg falls with hyperabduction or hyperextension of the shoulder). Examine for ↓range of movement, weakness, crepitus, and tenderness over the cuff insertions and subacromial area. Examine supraspinatus strength by testing resistance to abduction. Look for bony avulsions on X-ray (tensile strength of the cuff exceeds adjacent bone). Treat conservatively initially with analgesia and support in a broad arm sling, followed by exercises/physiotherapy at ≈10days. Arrange follow-up for patients with significantly ↓range of movement—complete tears (particularly in younger patients) may require surgical repair.

Ruptured biceps

The long head of biceps can rupture at its proximal insertion on lifting or pulling (see 📖 Soft tissue elbow problems, p.452). This may follow little force (and with little pain) in the elderly. Look for the ruptured biceps muscle as a bulge above the elbow. Treat with initial analgesia and support in a sling, followed by later exercises. Surgical repair is rarely indicated.

Soft tissue shoulder problems

The shoulder is vulnerable to degenerative disease and injury, due to its extreme mobility and hence, relative instability. Stability relies mainly on the rotator cuff, a muscle sheath, which wraps around and inserts into the humeral head under the deltoid. The rotator cuff comprises supraspinatus (initiates abduction), infraspinatus and teres minor (externally rotate), and subscapularis (internally rotates). The rotator cuff may be injured acutely or due to a chronic degenerative process (eg impingement syndromes or rheumatoid arthritis).

Impingement syndromes

The acromion process may compress or 'impinge' on the underlying sub-acromial bursa and rotator cuff during repetitive or strenuous shoulder use. Supraspinatus and its tendon are most commonly affected. Minor impingement is associated with inflammation, pain, and loss of function and is reversible with treatment. Rotator cuff tendonitis is more chronic and can lead to degeneration or tearing of the cuff. Although rotator cuff tendonitis and degenerative tears usually occur in later life, acute tears can occur in younger patients.

Examination of the shoulder

Examine both shoulders for comparison with the patient sitting relaxed.

Look for deformity of the clavicle or sternoclavicular joint, AC joint deformity (eg OA or injury), wasting of the deltoid muscle (axillary nerve damage), a step in the deltoid contour, or a gap below the acromion (subluxation or dislocation).

Feel for tenderness over sternoclavicular joint, clavicle, AC joint, subacromial area, rotator cuff insertion, biceps tendon insertion.

Move the shoulder gently in all directions to test passive movements. Test strength of active movements. Test abduction (normal range 0–170°), forward flexion (0–160°), backward extension (0–60°), external rotation (put hand on back of head), internal rotation (put hand behind back to touch shoulder blade).

Examine for crepitus on movement, restriction, pain (note any painful arc) and weakness of particular movements.

Test sensation over the badge area (upper outer arm) supplied by axillary nerve. Examine the cervical spine when shoulder examination does not reveal a cause for symptoms.

In suspected impingement syndromes consider the following:

Neer's impingement test Fully abducting the straight arm will re-create symptoms.

Hawkin's impingement test Hold the arm at 90° abduction and 90° elbow flexion. Rotating the arm across the body will recreate symptoms.

LA injection of 10mL 1% plain lidocaine into the subacromial bursa (approach just under acromion process from behind) should help pain, but will not affect strength or range of movement, aiding assessment. Adding hydrocortisone, methylprednisolone or triamcinolone to LA injection is useful for first presentation of acute impingement. Warn that symptoms may ↑briefly after steroid injection. Avoid repeated injection as it can precipitate tendon rupture.

Differential diagnosis of shoulder pain

Includes referred pain from a degenerative cervical spine, C5/6 disc prolapse, brachial plexus neuritis, axillary vein thrombosis, suprascapular nerve compression, Pancoast's syndrome, or cervical rib.

Subacromial bursitis

Early form of impingement in younger patients. Follows unaccustomed activity or exercise. Look for a painful arc of 60–100° abduction with dull, aching pain, worse on activity. Differential diagnosis includes gout, sepsis, or RA. Treat with analgesia, NSAID, and ice. Demonstrate simple exercises (eg gentle pendulum swings and circling movements of the arm, crawling fingers up a wall). LA injection will improve pain, movement, and help confirm diagnosis. Consider steroid injection if first presentation.

Rotator cuff tendonitis

Usually a longer history, chronic pain (±sleep disturbance), in patients aged 25–40years. Examine for tenderness and crepitus over humeral insertions of the rotator cuff and ↓active and passive shoulder movements. X-ray may show osteophytes or subacromial calcification. LA injection may ↓pain, but usually does not ↑strength or range of movement. Treat as for subacromial bursitis. In more severe cases, consider formal physiotherapy and orthopaedic referral.

Calcific tendonitis

A poorly understood process of calcium deposition and resorption within the rotator cuff tendon. Commoner in women. May be related to degenerative change or follow minor trauma. Most common site is within supraspinatus 1–2cm proximal to humeral insertion. Acute pain (occurs during periods of calcium resorption, granulation, and healing) often starts at rest, worsens on movement and at night. Examine for tenderness at the rotator cuff insertion. There may be crepitus, painful limitation of movement or a painful arc. The calcium deposits may be evident on X-ray.

Most episodes spontaneously resolve in 1–2weeks. Treat with analgesia, NSAID, and ice. Immobilize briefly in a broad arm sling, but start gentle exercises (as above) once symptoms allow. Arrange orthopaedic follow-up; steroid injection and/or physiotherapy and, rarely, surgical treatment, may be required.

Adhesive capsulitis

A misleading term, since it is caused by a generalized contracture of the shoulder capsule, not adhesions. Causes include immobilization, injury, or diabetes. Commoner in women and rare <40 or >70years old. Insidious onset results in diffuse, aching pain (worse at night) and restricted active and passive shoulder movements. The cuff is usually not tender. X-rays exclude posterior dislocation (🕮 p.456). Refer to orthopaedics for MUA, arthroscopy, and capsulotomy.

Soft tissue neck injuries

Neck sprains

Neck injuries that do not involve fractures, dislocations, ligamentous laxity, or spinal cord damage are common. Most follow car crashes involving neck hyperextension. These injuries have been referred to as: 'whiplash' or 'whiplash-type' injuries, 'hyperextension' or 'acceleration flexion—hyperextension' injuries or most simply, 'neck sprains'. Patients with continuing symptoms are often referred to as having a 'whiplash-associated disorder'. MRI (which rarely changes management) reveals many to have significant soft tissue injuries.

History

Neck pain and stiffness may not appear until 12hr after injury—symptoms are typically maximal at ≈48hr. Ask about other symptoms (some are relatively common), which include: headache, shoulder pain, backache, altered limb sensation. A range of other symptoms may also occur, including: dizziness, tinnitus, vertigo, and visual disturbance.

Examination

Perform a neurological examination. In fully alert, neurologically intact patients examine for any midline or paravertebral tenderness, muscle spasm or deformity. If there is no midline tenderness, assess active neck movements. If there is localized bony tenderness, pain on active movements or any neurological symptoms, immobilize fully and X-ray.

X-ray[1]

Arrange cervical X-rays (AP, lateral and odontoid peg views) in the presence of high energy trauma, neurological symptoms or signs, ↓conscious level or serious injury elsewhere. In the absence of these, do not routinely X-ray if the patient is fully conscious, has no midline neck tenderness, and can rotate the neck by 45° to right and left.

Check for evidence of fracture or dislocation. The most common abnormality is loss of the normal cervical lordosis (neck 'straightening')—this implies neck muscle spasm and does not necessarily indicate cervical spine injury. If the patient has severe pain or any abnormal neurology, but the initial plain X-rays are normal, consider requesting a CT scan.

Treatment

If there is any clinical or radiological suspicion of vertebral or spinal cord injury, refer urgently, maintaining cervical spine immobilization.

Treat patients in whom there is no suspicion of spinal cord or vertebral injury with initial analgesia (eg co-dydramol and/or ibuprofen) and advise GP follow-up. Leave referral to a physiotherapist for the GP to decide, based upon progression of symptoms. Avoid the use of a soft collar (the evidence is against it), but instead encourage early mobilization.

Prognosis

The rate of resolution of symptoms after neck sprains is highly variable. Many patients (>40%) continue to complain of pain, stiffness, and other symptoms for many months. It is often difficult to make a long-term prognosis within 12 months of the injury.

1 Available at: www.ohri.ca/emerg/cdr/cspine.html

Non-traumatic neck pain

Neck pain without injury may result from a variety of causes:

- *Cervical disc herniations*: present with neck pain, sensory and motor signs. Even if X-rays are normal, refer for further investigation (such as MRI) and treatment.
- *Acute torticollis* ('wry neck') reflects painful sternocleidomastoid spasm, which may occur on waking or after sudden neck movement. It responds to NSAID, local heat (eg heat pad or hot water bottle), and (in severe cases), physiotherapy.
- *Referred pain*: eg tonsillitis/quinsy (especially in children).
- *Dystonic reactions*: eg drug-induced (see 🕮 Complications of psychiatric drugs, p.619).
- *Cervical arthritis*: including both OA and RA.

Facial wounds

See also the sections on bony facial injuries (📖 pp. 370–376).

Cosmetic considerations

These are very important. The final appearance of a scar depends partly upon the orientation of the wound and its relation to natural skin lines (modified from Langer's description), but also upon initial management. Cleaning is crucial, but do not debride with tissue excision in the ED. Consider suturing facial dog bites (📖 p.414) and non-contaminated facial wounds up to 24hr after injury (get senior advice first). Close facial wounds in layers, using 5/0 Dexon or Vicryl for deeper layers, with knots tied on the deep aspect. Aim to remove skin sutures (interrupted 6/0 non-absorbable monofilament) at 3 days and replace with Steri-Strips™ to minimize scarring. Consider GA to treat facial wounds in children.

Damage to parotid duct/gland and facial nerve

This is particularly likely with incised wounds in the pre-auricular area. The facial nerve emerges through the parotid gland to supply the muscles of facial expression: unrepaired injury results in permanent disfigurement. The parotid duct runs transversely forwards from the anterior portion of the gland, parallel and inferior to the zygomatic arch, before entering the mouth opposite the second upper molar (look for blood here, as this implies proximal duct injury). Refer for exploration in theatre if there is clinical suspicion of involvement of any of these structures.

Associated head injury

Consider the possibility of significant head or neck injury in all patients with a facial wound.

Specific wounds

Lip wounds Oppose the vermilion border accurately (it is often easiest to do this first). Remember that even a 1mm mismatch will result in a permanent visible abnormality. Close in layers if the wound extends into subcutaneous or muscle layers.

Tongue and oral wounds Check the teeth: if any are broken or missing, consider obtaining soft tissue lateral X-rays of the lips in a search for embedded fragments. Small superficial lacerations need not be closed, but close deeper ones in layers, using absorbable sutures (eg 4/0 or 5/0 Vicryl/ Dexon for mucosal surfaces). Close through and through oral lacerations in layers (mucosal, muscle, and subcutaneous tissue, skin).

Eyebrow wounds Do not shave the eyebrows. Exclude an underlying fracture by palpation (and X-rays, as appropriate).

Eyelid wounds Many may be sutured with 6/0 non-absorbable monofilament. Full eye examination, excluding a FB, is necessary. Refer wounds if there is involvement of lid margin, loss of tissue, or if lacrimal duct (medial canthus) or gland (superolateral) injury is suspected.

Ears Involvement of cartilage requires suture with fine absorbable material (by an Ear, Nose and Throat (ENT) specialist) prior to skin closure. Give prophylactic antibiotic cover (eg co-amoxiclav) if there is any contamination.

Langer's lines (Fig. 9.33)

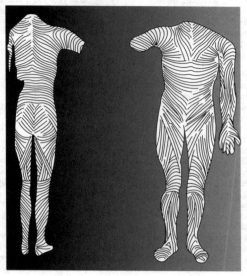

Fig. 9.33 Langer's lines.

Pelvic fractures

Major pelvic fractures result from very high energy trauma and are true orthopaedic emergencies. Associated thoracic or abdominal injuries occur in 10–20%—the principal immediate risk is massive haemorrhage and exsanguination. Compound fractures of the pelvis have a mortality of >50%. Associated bladder or urethral damage is common. Rectal and vaginal injuries occur occasionally.

Assessment

- Resuscitate as for any severely traumatized patient (□ Major trauma: treatment principles, p.320).
- Obtain a pelvic X-ray on all patients with multisystem injury (□ p.322).
- Look carefully for evidence of hypovolaemia and treat appropriately.
- Examine pubis, iliac bones, hips, and sacrum for tenderness, bruising, swelling, or crepitus. Do not try to 'spring the pelvis' to assess stability—this is unreliable, unnecessary, and may cause additional haemorrhage/damage. Similarly, avoid log rolling patients with obvious pelvis fractures—enlist a number of helpers and perform a straight lift.
- Look carefully for wounds especially in the perineum.
- Perform a rectal examination for anal tone, palpable fractures and to detect bleeding, rectal tears, and urethral damage (high riding, boggy prostate).
- Test urine for blood, but do not catheterize if urethral injury is suspected.
- Look at X-rays carefully for disruption of normal pelvic contours (Shenton's lines), asymmetry and widening of the pubic symphysis or sacroiliac joints.

Classification of pelvic fractures (Table 9.3)

Table 9.3 Tile classification of pelvic injuries (see Fig. 9.34)

Type A	(Stable injuries) include avulsion fractures, isolated pubic ramus fractures, iliac wing fractures, or single stable fractures elsewhere in pelvic ring
Type B	Rotationally unstable but vertically stable
B1	'Open book' antero-posterior compression fractures, causing separation of the pubic symphysis and widening of one or both sacroiliac joints
B2	Ipsilateral compression causing the pubic bones to fracture and override
B3	Contralateral compression injury resulting in pubic rami fractures on one side and compression sacroiliac injury on the other
Type C	(Rotationally unstable and vertically unstable) The pelvic ring is completely disrupted or displaced at 2 or more points. Associated with massive blood loss and very high mortality. Subdivided into *C1* (unilateral), *C2* (bilateral) and *C3* (involving acetabular fracture)

Treatment

Stable type A injuries require analgesia and bed rest until able to mobilize (usually 3–6weeks). *Isolated pubic ramus fractures* are common and often missed in the elderly (particularly when the focus is on a potential fractured neck of femur). Refer to orthopaedics for analgesia, initial bed rest, then mobilization.

Unstable type B and C fractures are an orthopaedic emergency

Resuscitate as for any major trauma (📖 p.320). Correct hypovolaemia, anticipate coagulopathy and ensure blood is rapidly available as massive transfusion may be required. If DPL (📖 p.347) is employed, use a supra-umbilical approach, as pelvic haematoma may track up the abdominal wall. Minimize movement, but support an obviously unstable pelvis fracture associated with severe haemorrhage using a pelvic binder or splint (eg SAM sling). Consider reduction and immobilization using an external fixator applied either in the resuscitation room or operating theatre to halt haemorrhage. If this fails, angiography and selective embolization are indicated.

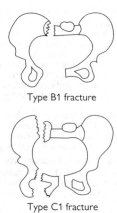

Type B1 fracture

Type C1 fracture

Fig. 9.34 Examples of pelvic fractures.

Avulsion fractures around the pelvis

Avulsion fractures occur at attachments of various muscles as follows:
- *Anterior inferior iliac spine*—rectus femoris (typically results from a miskick into the turf).
- *Anterior superior iliac spine*—sartorius.
- *Ischial tuberosity*—hamstrings.

In most instances, symptomatic treatment based upon rest (consider crutches) and analgesia suffices. Larger avulsions (particularly of the ischial tuberosity) may require internal fixation (to avoid complications such as non-union).

Hip dislocations and acetabular fractures

Acetabular fractures
Often accompany traumatic hip dislocation following violent injury such as falls or blows to the hip. Posterior rim fractures are the most common. Complications include massive haemorrhage, sciatic nerve damage, myositis ossificans, and secondary OA. Resuscitate, give analgesia and deal with priorities first. Additional X-rays (eg 45° oblique 'Judet' views) or CT are often required to make an exact diagnosis. Refer to orthopaedics for traction, protected weight-bearing, or in some cases internal fixation.

Central dislocation of the hip
This injury is essentially a serious pelvic fracture, which involves the head of the femur being driven through the (fractured) acetabular floor following a fall or force directed along the length of the femur (eg car dashboard). The diagnosis is usually obvious on an AP pelvis X-ray. Treat associated injuries and for shock, and give analgesia. Contact the orthopaedic surgeon immediately.

Traumatic posterior dislocation of the hip
Implies major trauma, often with other critical injuries (eg dashboard knee injury in a car crash) or fractured posterior acetabulum. Limb is shortened, internally rotated with hip flexed and adducted. This appearance may be absent if there is also a femoral shaft fracture. Check for sciatic nerve damage—examine foot dorsiflexion and below knee sensation. *Complications:* sciatic nerve injury, avascular necrosis of femoral head (risk ↑ the longer the hip is dislocated), and secondary OA. Diagnosis is usually obvious on AP X-ray, but lateral views may be needed to exclude dislocation. Treat as follows:
- Resuscitate the patient and deal with A, B, C priorities first.
- Give analgesia—posterior dislocation causes severe pain.
- Refer for reduction under GA. In unconscious, multiply injured patients, consider an early attempt to reduce the dislocation.

Reduction technique for posterior dislocation ('Allis technique')
- It is easiest and safest to reduce the dislocation if the anaesthetized patient is placed on the floor. If this is not possible, stand on the trolley. An assistant presses down on the patient's anterior superior iliac spines to hold down the pelvis.
- Flex hip and knee both to 90°, and correct adduction and internal rotation deformities.
- Grip the patient's lower leg between your knees and grasp patient's knee with both hands.
- Lean back and lever the knee up pulling the patients hip upwards. A 'clunk' confirms successful reduction. X-ray to confirm reduction.

Dislocated hip prostheses
Relatively common, follows minor trauma. Confirm posterior dislocation of hip prosthesis by X-ray. Treat with IV opioid and refer to orthopaedics for MUA (and assessment of prosthesis stability) under GA.

Anterior dislocation of the hip
Less common. The leg is held abducted and externally rotated. Complications include damage to the femoral nerve, artery, and vein. Give analgesia and refer for reduction under GA.

Sacral and coccygeal fractures

Fractures of the sacrum

Usually occur from violent direct trauma such as falls. Damage to sacral nerve roots may occur. Check carefully for saddle anaesthesia, ↓anal tone, lower limb weakness, or bladder dysfunction. Refer to the orthopaedic team.

Fracture of the coccyx

Follows a fall onto the bottom. Do not X-ray routinely—the diagnosis is clinical. Perform a rectal examination and check for local coccygeal tenderness, palpable fractures, or evidence of rectal damage. Refer patients with rectal tears to the general surgeon. Refer to the orthopaedic team if the coccyx is grossly displaced, as it may require manipulation under LA or even excision. Treat the remainder symptomatically (eg suggest a ring cushion and provide analgesia).

Hip fractures

Intracapsular fractures of the neck of femur

Can follow relatively minor trauma. Risk ↑ in the elderly, because of osteoporosis, osteomalacia, and ↑rate of falls. These fractures can disrupt the blood supply to the femoral head, causing avascular necrosis.

Fractures around the hip in younger patients imply high energy injury: the incidence of non-union or avascular necrosis may be as high as 20%.

Diagnosis

Usually follows a fall onto the hip or bottom. Pain may radiate down towards the knee. The affected leg may be shortened and externally rotated. Check for hypothermia and dehydration (the patient may have been lying for hours). Look for tenderness over the hip or greater trochanter, particularly on rotation. Suspect hip fracture in an elderly person who:

- Exhibits sudden inability to WB. There may be no history of injury, particularly in the presence of confusion or dementia.
- Is unable to WB and has pain in the knee (the hip may not be painful).
- Has 'Gone off her feet'.

X-rays

Look closely for disrupted trabeculae/cortices and abnormal pelvic contours (Shenton's lines). Fractures of the femoral neck are not always visible on initial X-rays. Repeat X-rays, bone scanning, or MRI may be required if symptoms continue. Intracapsular femoral neck fractures may be graded according to the Garden classification.

Treatment

- Obtain IV access and draw blood for U&E, glucose, FBC, and cross-match.
- Start IV infusion if indicated (eg dehydration or shock).
- Give IV analgesia plus an anti-emetic. Provide all analgesia IV in small increments every few minutes until pain is controlled.
- Obtain an ECG to look for arrhythmias/MI and consider need for CXR.
- Arrange other investigations as indicated by history/examination.
- Admit to orthopaedic ward.

Intertrochanteric fracture

These affect the base of the femoral neck and the intertrochanteric region. Initial management is identical to neck of femur fractures outlined above.

Isolated trochanteric avulsion fracture

Sudden force may avulse insertions of gluteus medius (greater trochanter) or iliopsoas (lesser trochanter). Give analgesia and refer for follow-up for gradual mobilization and symptomatic treatment.

The Garden classification (Fig. 9.35)

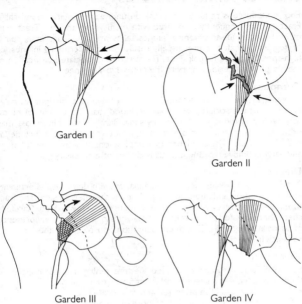

Garden I

Garden II

Garden III

Garden IV

Fig. 9.35 The Garden classification.
Garden I: trabeculae angulated, but inferior cortex intact. No significant displacement.
Garden II: trabeculae in line, but a fracture line visible from superior to inferior cortex. No significant displacement.
Garden III: obvious complete fracture line with slight displacement and/or rotation of the femoral head.
Garden IV: gross, often complete, displacement of the femoral head.

Hip pain after injury, but no fracture

Elderly patients who report hip pain and struggle to walk after a fall, but yet have no fracture of hip or pubic rami on X-ray may need assessment by an occupational therapist or physiotherapist before deciding if they can be safely discharged home with analgesia and appropriate walking aid. A small, but significant, proportion of such patients will turn out to have a hip fracture. Therefore, arrange for all patients to return for further imaging (eg MRI or CT) if pain continues for more than 1 week. In some patients with very significant symptoms, consider requesting MRI or CT scan at the time of initial presentation to show up a hip fracture not identified on plain X-rays.

Shaft of femur fractures

Enormous force is required to break an undiseased adult femoral shaft. Fractures are frequently associated with multisystem trauma. Treatment of immediately life-threatening injuries takes priority. Transverse, spiral, or segmental shaft fractures usually result from falls, crushing injuries, or high-speed road traffic collisions. There is often associated dislocation of the hip or other serious injury to the pelvis, hip, and knee.

Complications

Closed fractures of the femoral shaft, even without obvious vascular injury, may be associated with marked blood loss. Up to 1.5L of blood may be lost without visible thigh swelling. Rarely, gross blood loss may occur from compound femoral fractures. Later complications include fat embolism/ARDS. The incidence of complications is ↓ by early splintage and early definitive treatment (usually closed intramedullary nailing).

Diagnosis

The diagnosis is usually clear on examination with deformity, shortening, external rotation and abduction at the hip on the affected side. The fracture may be felt or even heard on movement of the lower limb. Carefully check for associated pelvic, knee, or distal limb injuries or for the presence of associated wounds. Document sensation and pulses in the limb and re-check frequently.

Treatment

Before X-rays, resuscitate, exclude life-threatening injuries, replace IV fluids, give adequate analgesia, and splint fractures as follows:
- Assess ABCs, establish priorities, and resuscitate.
- Start fluid replacement via 2 large-bore IV cannulae.
- Obtain blood for cross-matching.
- Administer IV analgesia—give small increments of opioid (with an anti-emetic) until pain is controlled,
- Strongly consider femoral nerve block (💭 p.304). As this starts to take effect (≈5–10min), prepare splintage and immobilize in Thomas or other traction splint.
- Arrange X-rays of the femur and contact the orthopaedic team.

Subtrochanteric fractures

Involve the most proximal part of the femoral shaft, at or just distal to the trochanters. Typically involve high-energy trauma in younger patients and are often associated with other serious injuries. They can also occur as isolated injuries following relatively minor trauma in those with osteoporosis or metastatic disease. Treat as for femoral shaft fractures.

Supracondylar fractures

Fractures of the distal third of the femur usually follow violent direct force. They are frequently comminuted and often intra-articular with associated damage to the knee joint. In adults, the distal femoral fragment tends to rotate due to pull from gastrocnemius. Treat as for femoral shaft fractures, but note that femoral nerve block may not be as effective.

Splints for fractured femoral shaft

The Thomas splint is traditional, but other forms of telescopic, metal, or pneumatic traction splints are increasingly being used. These are convenient, and particularly suitable for temporary immobilization in patients going directly to theatre or in transit to hospital. Ensure adequate padding around the groin and the ankle to avoid pressure necrosis of the skin.

Application of a Thomas splint

- Measure circumference of the uppermost part of the uninjured thigh in cm.
- Select splint of appropriate ring size (also have sizes above and below ready).
- Prepare splintage—wrap ring in wool roll.
- Slide sleeve of tubigrip over splint to support leg from ring to distal calf. Secure tubigrip by tying to ring or taping along sides of splint. If the ring has a buckle this should be on the upper half of the ring.
- Prepare the limb for skin traction—gently. If time permits, shave hair from medial and lateral aspects of limb.
- Apply splint (if using femoral nerve block wait until this is effective). Start with adhesive skin traction, making sure the foam part adequately covers the malleoli. Remove backing and apply adhesive tape along sides up limb, extending as far up the limb as possible. Trim off the remaining tape.
- Wrap the leg from ankle to mid-thigh with gauze bandage.
- Apply traction to the leg. Gently pull the ankle with one hand and support the knee with the other. Correct the abduction and external rotation while pulling steadily.
- Slide the Thomas splint over the leg until it is against the perineum. Take care not to snag the skin or genitalia. If the splint does not fit, replace it while maintaining traction.
- Tie the cords from the heel end of the skin traction to the end of the splint while maintaining traction. Insert 2 tongue depressors between the cords and twist them until the cords are reasonably taut.
- Place wool roll padding under the thigh and if necessary, add more padding around the groin.
- Bandage around the whole splint from thigh to lower calf with a broad bandage.
- Support and elevate the leg on a pillow.
- Check distal pulses.
- Arrange X-rays.

Approach to knee injuries

History

Many knee injuries seen in the ED result from sports, particularly football and rugby. Carefully document the exact mechanism of injury as it provides clues to the diagnosis. Valgus or varus stresses can damage the medial and lateral collateral ligaments, respectively. Flexed, twisting knee injuries are frequently associated with meniscal injuries. The anterior cruciate ligament (isolated or associated with medial collateral and/or medial meniscal injuries) may tear during forced flexion or hyperextension. Posterior cruciate ligament injuries may follow falls or dashboard impact where the tibia is forced backwards violently (often associated with medial or lateral ligament injuries).

Rapid onset tense swelling in a knee is usually an *acute haemarthrosis*. Swelling developing more gradually over several days is more likely to represent a reactive effusion. Ask about previous knee problems: swelling, clicking, locking, or giving way (the last two suggest underlying meniscal pathology). Document any previous knee surgery or the presence of other joint problems. In a hot, swollen, painful, and stiff knee without a history of significant trauma consider and exclude septic arthritis.

Examination

Always examine both legs with the patient suitably undressed and lying supine. If there is much discomfort, consider giving oral analgesia and re-examine in 10–15min. Reassure him/her that you will not suddenly pull or move the leg without warning.

Look for bruising, swelling, redness, abrasions, or other wounds.

Feel for warmth, crepitation, or the presence of a knee effusion (patellar tap or ballottable fluid).

Ask the patient to straight leg raise The ability to do this against resistance virtually excludes quadriceps, patellar tendon rupture, or transverse patellar fractures. If unable (possibly due to pain), ask the patient to kick forwards whilst sitting with the affected leg dangling free.

Assess tone and bulk of quadriceps muscle and compare with the other side.

Assess knee movement Gentle encouragement or supporting the limb may be required, but do not use any force.

Assess the cruciate ligaments Try to bring the knee to 90° flexion, sit on the patient's foot and hold the leg with both hands around the upper tibia. Ensure the quadriceps and hamstring muscles are relaxed. Using body weight, gently rock backwards and forwards looking for anterior glide (draw) of the tibia (indicating rupture of the anterior cruciate ligament) or posterior glide of the tibia (indicating rupture of the posterior cruciate ligament). Up to 5mm movement is normal—always compare both legs. If unable to flex to 90°, assess with slight flexion ≈10°. Repeat the procedure with the tibia slightly internally rotated.

Assess the collateral ligaments With the leg straight, gently apply a valgus stress to the knee joint (ie move the lower leg laterally) examining for laxity or pain in the medial collateral ligament. Next apply a varus stress (ie move the lower leg medially) examining for laxity or pain in the lateral collateral ligament complex. Repeat the procedure with the knee in ≈20° flexion as this will relax the cruciate ligaments. Compare both sides.

Palpate around the knee joint examining all the structures around the knee for tenderness, swelling, warmth, or crepitus (eg bony landmarks, ligament insertions, and over the joint line medially and laterally).

X-rays for knee injuries

X-rays form the mainstay of initial imaging for knee trauma: other imaging (eg CT, MRI) may be indicated after specialist consultation. Obtain X-rays following knee injuries where there is suspected fracture or other significant injury. Use the Ottawa knee rules to assist the decision (in those aged between 18 and 55 years) as to whether or not to X-ray:

X-rays are only required if any of the following are present:
• There is isolated bony tenderness of the patella.
• There is bony tenderness over the fibula head.
• The patient cannot flex the knee to 90°.
• The patient could not weight-bear (take at least 4 steps) both immediately after the injury and at the time of examination.

Adopt a lower threshold for obtaining X-rays in those aged <18 or >55years, patients intoxicated with alcohol, those suffering from bone disease (eg RA, documented osteoporosis), and for those who reattend the ED with the same injury (having not been X-rayed initially).

Knee fractures and dislocations

Patellar fracture

This may follow a direct blow or fall onto the patella or sudden violent knee flexion or contraction of the quadriceps muscle. Look for pain, swelling, crepitus, and difficulty extending the knee. Displaced, transverse fractures result in an inability to straight leg raise (this is also a feature of rupture of the quadriceps tendon or patellar tendon—📖 Soft tissue knee injuries, p.478). There may be an associated haemarthrosis.

X-rays may be difficult to interpret as the patella overlies the distal femur on the AP view and can obscure subtle fractures. Do not routinely order 'skyline' views of the patella. Take care not to mistake a bipartite patella for a fracture (the accessory bone is typically in the upper, lateral part of the patella).

Treatment

- Treat vertical fractures with analgesia, immobilize in a non-weight-bearing cylinder POP, supply crutches, and arrange orthopaedic follow-up.
- Transverse fractures tend to displace due to the pull of quadriceps. Treat with analgesia, immobilization in a POP backslab, and refer to the orthopaedic team for probable ORIF (occasionally, the orthopaedic team may decide to treat an undisplaced transverse fracture conservatively).

Dislocation of the patella

The patella typically dislocates laterally. This often follows medial stress to the knee—the dislocation may reduce spontaneously. There may be a history of recurrent dislocation. The patient has a painful knee, held in flexion with obvious lateral displacement of the patella. X-rays are not generally required prior to reduction of the dislocation. Reduction can usually be achieved using Entonox®—IV analgesia is seldom required. Stand on the lateral side of the affected limb and hold the affected knee gently. Using a thumb, lever the patella medially in one smooth, firm movement whilst gently extending the knee at the same time. Successful reduction is obvious and should rapidly relieve symptoms. Once reduced, obtain X-rays, immobilize in a canvas ('cricket pad') back-splint or cylinder cast POP, provide analgesia and arrange orthopaedic follow-up. Surgery is not usually indicated for first time dislocations.

Spontaneous reduction/patella subluxation The patient who has experienced spontaneous reduction and/or subluxation prior to arrival at hospital will typically have maximal tenderness over the medial aspect of the upper patella reflecting damage to the attachment of vastus medialis. There may be 'apprehension' when gentle lateral pressure is applied to the patella. If clinical features are dramatic, rest in a splint (occasionally cylinder POP may be needed), otherwise refer for physiotherapy and orthopaedic follow-up.

Dislocation of the knee

Although rare, this injury indicates severe disruption of the ligamentous structures and soft tissues of the knee. Look carefully for associated injuries (eg femur or lower limb), and document distal pulses and sensation—the popliteal artery or nerve are often injured. Reduction requires adequate (IV opioid) analgesia, and usually GA or sedation with full precautions. Reduce by simple traction on the limb and correcting deformity. Check distal pulses and sensation after reduction, immobilize in a long leg POP backslab, and arrange orthopaedic admission. Check the circulation repeatedly, since popliteal artery damage may not become apparent for some hours—angiography is usually required. Compartment syndrome is another recognized complication.

Tibial plateau fractures

Falls onto an extended leg can cause compression fractures of the proximal tibia. Valgus stresses crush or fracture the lateral tibial plateau. These injuries are commonly seen in pedestrians injured following impact with car bumpers. Varus injuries result in crushing or fracture of the medial tibial plateau and are usually associated with rupture of the opposite collateral ligaments. Examine for tenderness over the medial or lateral margins of the proximal tibia. Look for swelling, haemarthrosis, or ligamentous instability (also try to assess the cruciate ligaments—📖 Approach to knee injuries, p.474). Look carefully on X-rays for breaks in the articular surfaces of the proximal tibia, avulsions from the ligamentous attachments, or loss of height from the medial and lateral tibial plateaux, but beware, this may be subtle.

Treat with immobilization in a long leg POP backslab following adequate analgesia and refer to orthopaedic staff. Fractures of the tibial plateau often require elevation ±ORIF with bone grafting. Admit all patients with an acute haemarthrosis. Treat small, isolated avulsions without haemarthrosis with immobilization, crutches, and analgesia, and arrange orthopaedic follow-up.

Posterolateral corner injuries

The posterolateral corner of the knee is comprised of a group of ligaments and muscles/tendons that add to the stability of the joint. Postero-lateral corner injuries often occur in association with other significant knee trauma (eg dislocations, rupture of anterior or posterior cruciate ligaments, but isolated injuries can occur. Suspect this injury when significant symptoms follow the application of varus force to the anteromedial aspect of the extended knee. Chronic instability can result. X-rays may be normal or show subtle avulsions or widening of the lateral joint space. Urgent MRI and orthopaedic referral will enable prompt treatment.

Soft tissue knee injuries

Acute haemarthrosis

Rapid onset swelling following a knee injury, often warm, tense, and painful. Common causes include cruciate ligament rupture, tibial avulsion, tibial plateau, or other fractures. An acute haemarthrosis indicates serious injury. Refer for orthopaedic appraisal following splintage, analgesia and appropriate X-rays. Aspiration of a haemarthrosis (advocated by some experts to provide analgesia) requires strict aseptic technique.

Cruciate ligament rupture

The combination of considerable pain and swelling can make it difficult to elicit classical physical signs of a fresh cruciate tear. A history of an audible 'pop' at the time of injury is highly suggestive of anterior cruciate rupture.

Anterior cruciate tears often occur in association with tears of the medial collateral ligament and/or medial meniscus. Examine for the presence of haemarthrosis, abnormal ↑anterior glide of the tibia ('+ve anterior draw test') and injuries to the medial collateral ligament or other structures. Look carefully at X-rays for avulsion of the anterior tibial spine (anterior cruciate insertion). Give analgesia and refer to the orthopaedic surgeon.

In *posterior cruciate ligament tears*, the tibia may appear to sag back when the knee is flexed, so the tibia can be pulled into a more normal position causing a 'false +ve' anterior draw. X-rays may reveal the relevant posterior tibial spine to be avulsed. Provide analgesia and refer.

Collateral ligament injuries

Tenderness over the medial or lateral collateral ligament, with pain at this site on stress testing, indicates collateral ligament injury. Most injuries are isolated, and have no associated haemarthrosis and no abnormality on X-ray. Compare the injured knee with the uninjured one. The degree of laxity on stress testing will help to guide treatment:

- Local tenderness with no laxity (or very slight laxity) implies a grade I injury. Treat with analgesia, physiotherapy (±crutches) in the expectation of full recovery in 2–4weeks.
- Local tenderness with minor/moderate laxity, but with a definite end-point implies a grade II injury. Provide analgesia, crutches, instruction on quadriceps exercises and refer for orthopaedic follow-up.
- Major laxity (ie the joint opening up >1cm) with no end-point implies complete rupture. Consider a POP cylinder (or splint), and provide crutches, analgesia, quadriceps exercises, and orthopaedic follow-up.

Ruptured quadriceps

Complete rupture of the distal quadriceps insertion can result from a direct injury or from sudden, violent contraction of the quadriceps muscle. Examination reveals complete inability to straight leg raise—never assume this is just due to pain. There may be a palpable defect in the muscle insertion. Refer to the orthopaedic surgeon for repair.

Ruptured patellar tendon

Examine for complete inability to straight leg raise, a high-riding patella, a palpable defect in the patellar tendon. There is frequently an associated avulsion of the tibial tuberosity. Refer to orthopaedics for repair.

Other knee problems

Acutely locked knee

A springy block to full extension (which varies from just a few degrees to much more) in the knee indicates an underlying meniscal injury or other loose body in the knee joint. Obtain knee X-rays (including a tunnel view), which may show a loose body. Do not attempt to unlock the knee by manipulation as this is usually painful and futile. Give analgesia and refer for arthroscopy.

Prepatellar and infrapatellar bursitis

This results from inflammation of the fluid-filled bursa in front of or just below the patella, respectively, typically from unaccustomed kneeling. Treat with rest (which may involve the use of crutches), a short course of NSAID, and avoidance of the causative activity. Persistent symptoms may necessitate elective excision of the bursa. Infective bursitis may occur (↑T° and cellulitis are clues to this): aspirate fluid for culture and sensitivity, and start antibiotics (eg co-amoxiclav).

Other causes of knee pain

Patients present not infrequently with knee pain of variable duration and no history of trauma.

In adults, causes include Baker's cyst, osteoarthritis (especially in the elderly), and acute arthritic conditions, including septic arthritis (rare but important). Also rare, but worthy of consideration is osteosarcoma, which typically affects teenagers or young adults, producing pain and swelling.

In children, causes include sepsis (including both septic arthritis and osteomyelitis (🕮 The limping child, p.704), Osgood–Schlatter's disease, osteochondritis dissecans, Johansson–Larsen's disease (all in 🕮 Osteochondritis, p.708), chondromalacia patellae, referred pain from the hip, malignancy (eg leukaemic deposits).

Tibial and fibular shaft fractures

Adult tibial fractures are usually a result of direct blows or falls onto the tibial shaft. Spiral fractures of the tibia or fibula follow violent twisting injuries, usually from sports (eg soccer, rugby, skiing). Displaced fractures typically involve both the tibia and the fibula. A large portion of the tibia has relatively little soft tissue covering—compound injuries are common. Displaced tibial shaft fractures may be complicated by injury to the popliteal artery and compartment syndromes (📖 Crush syndrome, p.398). Fractures of the proximal fibula may be associated with injury to the common peroneal nerve. Check (repeatedly) for distal pulses and sensation.

Diagnosis is usually easy. Look for deformity, localized swelling, or tenderness. Regard all wounds near the fracture site as potential compound injuries.

X-rays Ensure X-rays show the whole length of tibia and fibula. Examine closely for the presence of other injuries (eg around the knee or ankle).

Undisplaced stress fractures can occur, particularly in adults involved in sports, and may not be visible on initial plain X-rays. Persisting symptoms suggestive of stress fracture require orthopaedic follow-up (and may eventually require specific coned X-rays or even bone scanning).

Tibial shaft fractures

Treat undisplaced transverse tibial shaft fractures with analgesia and long leg POP backslab. Spiral and oblique fractures also need immobilization, but are potentially unstable, so refer to orthopaedic team for admission. Immobilize displaced fractures in a long leg POP backslab following IV analgesia and refer (to consider MUA or closed intramedullary nailing). Badly comminuted or segmental fractures may require ORIF. Contact orthopaedics immediately if suspected vascular injury, sensory deficit or gross swelling.

Treat compound fractures initially as on 📖 p.422 and refer to the orthopaedic surgeon for urgent wound toilet, debridement, and fixation—see www.boa.ac.uk/en/publications/boast

Fibular shaft fractures

These can occur in combination with a tibial fracture, as a result of a direct blow (eg from a car bumper) or from twisting injuries. The common peroneal nerve may be damaged in proximal fibular injuries. Examine specifically for weakness of ankle dorsiflexion and ↓sensation of the lateral aspect of the forefoot.

Treat undisplaced proximal or fibular shaft fractures with analgesia and elevation. Support in a tubigrip or padded bandage. If unable to WB, use a below knee POP for comfort with crutches until WB is possible. Arrange follow-up in all cases. Refer displaced or comminuted fractures to the orthopaedic team.

Stress fractures of the fibula are relatively common, typically affecting the fibular neck of military recruits and athletes following vigorous training. Treat symptomatically with rest and analgesia.

Maisonneuve fracture (📖 p.501)

Transmitted forces may fracture the proximal fibula following an ankle injury. This usually involves fracture of the medial malleolus, fracture of the proximal fibula or fibular shaft, and implies damage to the distal tibio-fibular syndesmosis. Examine the proximal fibula in all ankle injuries and X-ray if locally tender.

Pretibial lacerations

Common in the elderly following relatively minor trauma. Most pretibial lacerations can be satisfactorily treated in the ED with adhesive strips ('Steri-Strips™'). Clean and irrigate to remove clot, and close using Steri-Strips™ under appropriate anaesthesia. Aim to leave gaps of ≈0.5cm between the Steri-Strips™. Apply a non-adherent dressing and light compression bandage. Instruct the patient to elevate the limb whenever possible (Fig. 9.36). Arrange follow-up (ED or GP) for 5 days' time for wound inspection and dressing change (but leave underlying Steri-Strips™ until the wound is healed). Consider admission for patients with poor social support.

Note Suturing pretibial wounds is not usually recommended as the pretibial skin is friable and undue tension compromises wound healing.

Complications are likely in patients with large, distally based and poorly viable skin flaps, and patients on steroids or anticoagulants (check clotting control). Refer to plastic surgeons large lacerations where skin edges cannot be opposed, or where complications are likely.

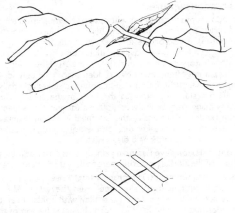

Fig. 9.36 Application of Steristrips.

Calf and Achilles tendon injuries

Calf muscle tears

Acute tears of the gastrocnemius muscle often occur during sports. They can also occur simply from stepping from a bus or kerb, or from a sudden jump. Sharp or burning pain in the calf is followed by ↑stiffness or pain on weight-bearing. Examine for localized tenderness and/or swelling over the calf muscle bellies. The medial head of gastrocnemius is more commonly injured.

Carefully check the Achilles tendon for signs of rupture (see below). Differential diagnosis includes DVT (📖 p.118) or rupture of a Baker's cyst.

Treat with analgesia, NSAID, and initial ice application. Raising the heel with a pad may also help. Advise elevation of the leg and progressive weight-bearing as guided by symptoms. Use of crutches may be required if symptoms are severe (in this case, arrange follow-up and early physiotherapy).

Calf muscle bruising

Direct blunt calf trauma can result in haematoma formation and considerable swelling. Be alert to the possibility of compartment syndrome, particularly where there is a significant mechanism of injury (eg 📖 p.398).

Achilles tendon rupture

Achilles tendon rupture can occur without prior symptoms during sudden forceful contraction of the calf. Usually this occurs during sports (notoriously badminton). It also occurs in other situations (eg running for a bus or missing a step and landing heavily). Patients on ciprofloxacin, oral steroids or with a history of steroid injection of the Achilles tendon area are at ↑risk. The patient often describes a sudden sharp pain behind the ankle like a 'bang' or similar description. Patients often mistakenly initially believe that they have sustained a blow to the back of the ankle. Examination may reveal swelling, pain, bruising, and often a (diagnostic) palpable defect (gap) in the tendon ≈5cm above the calcaneal insertion. Plantar flexion against resistance will be weaker than on the normal (uninjured) side, but do not rely on this when making a diagnosis.

...vare plantar flexion (even standing on tip-toes) may still be possible ...o action of the tibialis posterior, peroneal, and toe flexor muscles.

...ueeze test (Simmonds/Thompson's test) Kneel patient on a chair, ...e back, with feet hanging free over the edge. Alternatively, ...e patient to lie prone on a trolley with ankles over the end. ...ze mid-calf and look for normal plantar flexion of the ankle ...avoid confusion do not describe the result as +ve or −ve, ...ieeze test normal' or 'abnormal'.

...'s controversial, so follow local policy. Treatment

...ment: many ruptures are managed with crutches, ...zation for 6weeks in a long leg plaster with the ...nd knee flexed to ≈45°. This is followed by ...the care of the orthopaedic team and physi-

...employed in young patients and athletes. ...eam to consider this.

Note Sometimes a 'partial' Achilles tendon rupture is suspected. In this instance, the safest initial treatment is immobilization in a non-weight-bearing BKPOP with ankle flexion, crutches, and orthopaedic follow-up. USS can help to determine the state of the tendon.

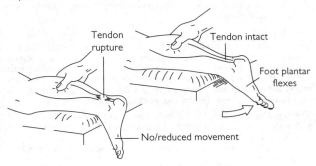

Tendon rupture

Tendon intact

Foot plantar flexes

No/reduced movement

Fig. 9.37 Calf squeeze test to check integrity of Achilles tendon.

Achilles tendonitis/paratendonitis

This frequently follows unaccustomed activity or overuse (eg dancing, jumping, running, or even walking) and may be associated with familial hypercholesterolaemia. There is usually a history of ↑pain, aggravated by ankle movements. Examine for localized pain, swelling, and palpable crepitus over the Achilles tendon (the most common site is ≈5cm from its insertion). The calf squeeze (Simmonds) test is normal. Check lipid profile.

Treat with analgesia, NSAID, and a brief period of rest (eg 1–2 days) before gradually returning to normal activities as guided by symptoms. Occasionally, 1–2 weeks in a BKWPOP may be useful. A heel pad inserted into footwear may help. Athletes may benefit from removal of heel tabs from training shoes if implicated. Avoid local steroid injection, which may ↑risk of tendon rupture by impeding healing or by allowing premature resumption of activity.

Calf/leg pain with no history of trauma

A variety of conditions may be implicated, including:
- *Shin splints*: a variety of pathophysiological processes have been suggested, including tibial periostitis. This condition is characterized by pain over the anterior distal tibial shaft after running on hard surfaces. Advise rest and NSAID.
- *Stress fractures*: can affect the tibia (as well as the fibula—see 📖 p.480). Treat with analgesia and POP with orthopaedic follow-up.
- *Bursitis*: inflammation of the bursae around the insertion of the Achilles tendon responds to conservative measures.
- *DVT*: see 📖 p.118.
- *Cellulitis*: see 📖 p.413.
- *Ischaemia*: see 📖 p.531.
- Ruptured Baker's cyst.

Approach to ankle injuries

Ankle injuries are among the most common problems presenting to the ED. Adopt a logical, consistent approach to identify which patients are likely to have a fracture and to avoid unnecessary X-rays in patients with uncomplicated sprains.

History

Establish the exact mechanism of injury. Most are inversion injuries (where the sole of the foot turns to face medially as the ankle is plantar flexed) causing damage to structures around the lateral malleolus (most notably, the anterior talofibular ligament). Eversion injuries occur less commonly and damage the structures around the medial malleolus. Hyper-dorsiflexion and plantar flexion injuries occur less frequently.

The following are relevant in the initial assessment of ankle injuries:
• A fracture is more likely in patients who are unable to weight bear (WB) immediately following the injury.
• A 'crack' or 'snap' may be heard and is not indicative by itself of a fracture.
• Ice, analgesia, and elevation may influence the appearance of an ankle injury.

Examination

Examine from the knee down for tenderness over:
• Proximal fibula.
• Lateral malleolus and ligaments.
• Medial malleolus and ligaments.
• Navicular.
• Calcaneum.
• Achilles tendon.
• Base of 5th metatarsal (MT).

Is an X-ray required[1]?

Follow the Ottawa ankle rules (Fig. 9.38) for adults and X-ray ankles if patients:
• Were unable to WB for 4 steps both immediately after the injury and at the time of examination.
• Have tenderness over the posterior surface of the distal 6cm (or tip) of the lateral or medial malleolus.

Note that tenderness over the navicular, calcaneum, base of 5th MT or proximal fibula require specific X-rays to exclude fractures.

Adopt a lower threshold for X-ray in the very young, the elderly, and in patients who are difficult to assess (eg intoxicated).

---

1 Adapted from Stiell IG (1993) Decision rules for the use of radiography in acute ankle injuries. Refinement and prospective validation. *J Am Med Ass* **269**: 1127–32.

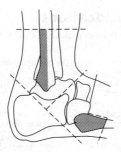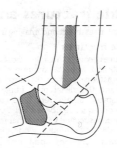

Fig. 9.38 The Ottawa ankle rules.

Guidelines for X-ray in a simple ankle injury. <u>Bony tenderness</u> over the points indicated requires an X-ray. X-ray is also required if the patient is <u>unable to weight-bear immediately after the injury or to walk 4 steps in the ED.</u>

X-ray the *ankle* for malleolar tenderness and the *foot* for metatarsal/tarsal tenderness. If the patient is not X-rayed then they are given <u>instructions to return after 5 days if they have trouble weight-bearing</u>.

Adapted from Stiell IG (1993) Decision rules for the use of radiography in acute ankle injuries. Refinement and prospective validation. *J Am Med Ass* **269**: 1127–32.

Ankle fractures and dislocations

Clinical assessment and imaging after ankle injury is outlined in 📖 p.484.

Ankle fractures

Fractures around the ankle most commonly involve the malleoli—medial, lateral, and what is commonly referred to as the 'posterior malleolus' (the posterior part of the distal tibia). The mortice joint formed by the talus and the distal tibia, fibula, ligaments, and the distal tibio-fibular syndesmosis allows very little rotation or angulation at the ankle joint. As a consequence, forced twisting or angulation of the ankle joint causes fractures associated with ligamentous injuries and in severe cases, disruption of the distal tibio-fibular syndesmosis.

Treatment depends upon a combination of clinical findings and X-ray appearances. Look carefully for talar shift.

- *Small avulsion fractures* essentially reflect ligament/joint capsule damage. Treat with rest, elevation, analgesia, and early mobilization as for sprains.
- *Larger avulsion fractures* may require initial immobilization in BKPOP with crutches and orthopaedic follow-up.
- *Undisplaced, isolated medial or lateral malleolar fractures* are usually stable and do well with conservative measures. Provide analgesia, crutches, and immobilize in a well-padded BKPOP cast. Advise limb elevation and arrange orthopaedic follow-up. Note that an isolated 'high' lateral malleolus fracture may only be apparent on the lateral X-ray and may be associated with deltoid (medial) ligament injury with instability—some require ORIF.
- *Displaced fractures of the medial or lateral malleolus* require ORIF. Give analgesia and, as appropriate, IV sedation to allow reduction of talar shift. Immobilize the limb in a BKPOP slab and refer to the orthopaedic team.
- *Bimalleolar or trimalleolar fractures* are unstable. Having attempted to reduce any significant talar shift (with appropriate sedation), place in a BKPOP, obtain fresh X-rays, and refer to the orthopaedic team.

Ankle dislocation

Dislocation of the ankle is an orthopaedic emergency. Treat promptly on diagnosis. Examination shows gross deformity of the ankle, severe stretching of the skin (resulting in fracture blisters, skin necrosis, or even converting the injury to a compound fracture), and often deficits in peripheral pulses or sensation. The ankle can dislocate in the absence of associated fractures, but this is uncommon.

Treatment Prompt closed reduction and immobilization in POP usually has to precede X-ray (unless available immediately). 'Prompt treatment' does not justify reduction without considering analgesia or sedation.

- Give Entonox®, IV analgesia, or sedation as appropriate with full precautions.
- Warn the patient there may be a brief ↑ in discomfort as the ankle reduces.
- With the knee flexed and supported, gently grasp the heel with one hand and support the patient's calf with the other.
- Pull smoothly on the heel—it may be necessary to slightly exaggerate the deformity in order to obtain reduction. Success is indicated by return of normal ankle contours, relief of skin tension, and often dramatic relief of pain.
- Once reduced, re-check pulses and sensation, immobilize in a POP slab, and arrange check X-rays.
- Refer the patient to the orthopaedic team immediately.

Ankle sprains

Clinical assessment and imaging after ankle injury is outlined in 📖 p.484. The structures most frequently injured in inversion injuries are the lateral joint capsule and the anterior talofibular ligament. Increasing injury causes additional damage to the calcaneofibular ligament and posterior talofibular ligament.

Treatment

Historically, treatment of sprained ankles has been based upon 'RICE' (rest, ice, compression, elevation), but the scientific basis for all the elements of this is distinctly lacking!

Advise initial rest, elevating the ankle above hip level, and to consider applying ice intermittently during the first 2 days for periods of 10–15min. Begin to WB as soon as symptoms allow, but elevate at all other times. An elastic support from toes to knee is traditional, but of no proven value (and may be harmful by ↑pain without speeding recovery). If used, ensure that it is not worn in bed. Advise the patient to gently exercise the ankle in all directions and to use simple analgesia regularly until symptoms improve. Most patients with minor sprains can expect full recovery in ≈4weeks. It may be possible to resume sports gradually within 2weeks, depending on progress.

The inability to WB implies more severe injury. Provide crutches to those completely unable to WB despite analgesia, with advice to elevate the ankle. Arrange review at 2–4days—if still unable to WB, consider 10days' immobilization in a below-knee cast, with subsequent outpatient follow-up. Other approaches include the use of adhesive strapping or pre-formed ankle braces. These may be useful in selected cases. Patients can usually expect good functional recovery and should not regard the ankle as 'weak'. Long-term problems (eg weakness/instability whilst walking over rough ground) are often related to ↓ankle proprioception following immobilization, so aim to mobilize as soon as possible.

Long-term complications

Do not regard ankle sprains simply as trivial injuries: patients may suffer long-term morbidity (which often causes them to return to the ED):

- *Instability* often manifests itself by recurrent ankle sprains. Refer to physiotherapy (to include isometric exercises).
- *Peroneal tendon subluxation* reflects a torn peroneal retinaculum, allowing the peroneal tendons to slip anteriorly. The clinical presentation includes clicking and a sensation of something slipping. Movement of the foot/ankle (especially eversion) reproduces the subluxation. Refer for orthopaedic follow-up—surgery is an option.
- *Peroneal nerve injury* is relatively common, but not frequently sought for. Neurapraxia results from stretching of branches of the peroneal nerve at the time of injury, with subsequent ↓ sensation over part of the dorsum of the foot and ↓ proprioception at the ankle joint (reflecting injury to the articular branches).

Foot fractures and dislocations

Crushing or other violent injuries to the foot can result in significant long-term disability. Multiple fractures or dislocation of the tarsals or MTs are often overlooked in the presence of other severe injuries. Delayed or inadequate treatment result in high rates of post-traumatic OA. Compartment syndromes (🔲 p.398) or vascular injuries may occur. Amputations or severe mangling injuries of the foot are rarely suitable for reconstruction/re-implantation due to poor long-term functional results.

Talar injuries

Falls onto the feet or violent dorsiflexion of the ankle (eg against car pedals in a crash) can result in fractures to the anterior body or articular dome of the talus. Displaced fractures and dislocations frequently result in avascular necrosis.

Treat with analgesia, immobilization in a backslab POP, and refer promptly for orthopaedic treatment (may require MUA and/or ORIF). Dislocations of the talus require prompt reduction under GA.

Upper/midfoot dislocations

These injuries follow violent twisting, inverting or everting injuries of the foot. *Peritalar/subtalar dislocations* involve the articulation between the talus and the calcaneum. Give adequate analgesia and refer to orthopaedics for prompt reduction under GA. *Mid-tarsal dislocations* involve the mid-tarsal joint (comprising the calcaneum and talus posteriorly and the navicular and cuboid anteriorly) and are treated similarly. *Isolated* dislocation of the talus is rare and requires prompt reduction under GA.

Calcaneal fracture

Calcaneal fractures most often follow a fall from height directly onto the heels. Always exclude associated injuries of the cervical and lumbar spine, pelvis, hips, or knees. Examine for swelling, bruising, and tenderness over the calcaneum, particularly over the sides. Examine both calcanei for comparison, remembering that fractures are commonly bilateral. Examine the Achilles tendon for injury (🔲 p.482). Request specific calcaneal X-rays and scrutinize carefully breaks in the cortices, trabeculae or subtle signs of compression (reduction in Bohler's angle—see Fig. 9.39). Refer all fractures to orthopaedic staff. The majority will require admission for elevation, analgesia and in selected cases, ORIF following CT scanning.

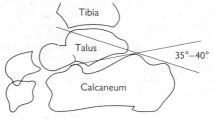

Fig. 9.39 Bohler's angle (normally 35–45°).

Clinically suspected calcaneal fracture, but X-rays normal

Sometimes, clinical suspicion of a calcaneal fracture is not confirmed by X-rays at the time of initial presentation. It is possible that X-rays may initially fail to identify a calcaneal fracture. Therefore, treat clinically with analgesia, rest, elevation, crutches and arrange review at 7–10days, when consideration can be given to further imaging if symptoms persist (eg more X-rays and/or CT scan).

Metatarsal fractures and dislocations

Multiple MT fractures may follow heavy objects falling onto the feet or more commonly, after being run over by a vehicle tyre or wheel. In all such cases, consider the possibility of tarso-metatarsal (Lisfranc) dislocation. This can be easily missed on standard foot X-rays, which do not usually include a true lateral view—look to check that the medial side of the second MT is correctly aligned with the medial side of the middle cuneiform. Check for presence of the dorsalis pedis pulse. Multiple, displaced, or dislocated MT fractures require urgent orthopaedic treatment. Support in a POP backslab following analgesia and refer for MUA, K-wire fixation, or occasionally, ORIF. MT stress fractures are discussed below.

Isolated avulsion fractures of the 5th MT base

These follow inversion injuries of the ankle, the base of the 5th MT being avulsed by the tendon of peroneus brevis. Always examine this area in ankle injuries and request foot X-rays if tender. Do not mistake accessory bones or the epiphysis (which runs parallel, not transverse to the 5th MT base). Treat with analgesia, elevation, and support in a padded crepe bandage or temporarily, in a BKPOP if symptoms are severe. Arrange orthopaedic follow-up.

Jones fracture (of the 5th MT)

This is a transverse fracture of the 5th MT just distal to the intermetatarsal joint. It is a significant fracture as it is prone to non-union. Treat with analgesia, crutches, BKPOP, and orthopaedic follow-up.

Stress fractures of the MTs

Fatigue fractures of the MTs are common. They typically follow prolonged or unusual exercise (hence the term 'march fracture'), but often occur without an obvious cause. The commonest site is the 2nd MT shaft, but the 3rd MT or rarely the navicular or other MTs may be affected. Examine for swelling over the forefoot (there may be none) and localized tenderness over the MT shaft or on longitudinal compression of the MT shaft (do this by pressing on the MT head below the toe—pain will be felt along the MT shaft). X-rays are usually normal initially. Callus or periosteal reaction seen at ≈2–3weeks on X-ray will confirm the diagnosis, but this is not required for treatment.

Treat symptomatically with analgesia, elevation, rest, and modified daily activity as required. A padded insole may help. Firm shoes or boots may be more comfortable than flexible trainers. Expect full recovery in 6–8 weeks. If unable to WB, consider a brief period in a BKPOP (or 'Aircast' boot) until symptoms improve.

Toe injuries

Most toe injuries do not require X-ray

The treatment of isolated closed fractures of the toe phalanges without clinical deformity or other complicating factors is not altered by X-rays.

X-ray the following:
- Obvious deformity, gross swelling or suspected dislocation.
- Suspected compound injuries.
- If any tenderness over the MT head or MTPJ.
- Suspected FB.

Toe fractures

Treat uncomplicated phalangeal fractures with simple analgesia, elevation, and support with padded buddy strapping. Advise the patient to resume normal activities as soon as possible, but explain that some discomfort may be present for up to 4–6weeks. Hospital follow-up is not normally required. Manipulate displaced fractures under LA digital block (as described for fingers on 📖 p.294). Angulated toe phalangeal fractures can be difficult to manipulate—a useful trick is to use a pen (or needle holder) placed between the toes as a fulcrum. Once satisfactorily reduced, buddy strap and confirm the position with X-rays.

Dislocated toes

Untreated, toe dislocations may cause troublesome, persistent symptoms. Reduce promptly under LA digital block and splint by buddy strapping. Always confirm reduction by X-ray, and discharge with analgesia and advice on elevation and gradual mobilization.

Compound toe injuries

Careful wound toilet, debridement, and repair is essential to ensure rapid healing and avoid infective complications. Ensure that there is adequate tetanus prophylaxis. Always clean wounds thoroughly under adequate anaesthesia (usually LA digital block), provide antibiotics and analgesia. Advise the patient to elevate the injured foot and arrange follow-up according to local practice. More severe injuries will require exploration and repair under GA. Refer these cases to the orthopaedic team.

Mangled or amputated toes

Functional results of attempted re-implantation of amputated toes or repair of badly mangled toes are often poor. Provide analgesia and refer to the orthopaedic surgeon for wound management and amputation of unsalvageable toes.

Soft tissue foot problems

Puncture wounds to the foot
- *'Simple' puncture wounds*: see 📖 p.419.
- *Weever fish injuries*: see 📖 p.416.

FBs embedded in the foot
Searching for small FBs in the sole of the foot has been likened to searching for a needle in a haystack. Follow the principles set out in 📖 Further assessment of skin wounds, p.428. Nerve blocks (📖 p.306) can be useful to allow exploration of foot wounds.

Morton's metatarsalgia
A burning discomfort radiating to the toes may result from an interdigital nerve neuroma at the level of the MT heads. The nerve between the 2nd and 3rd MT heads is frequently affected. There is localized tenderness, which is also reproduced on compression of MT heads together. Advise simple analgesia and GP follow-up to consider referral to a foot surgeon.

Plantar fasciitis
Plantar fasciitis can occur spontaneously or as a chronic overuse injury. Inflammation develops in the plantar fascia, typically at its calcaneal insertion. This results in gradually increasing, burning pain in the sole of the foot and heel, which is worse on WB. Examine for localized tenderness over the calcaneal insertion of the plantar fascia and heel pad. X-ray may reveal a calcaneal spur, but this is not a useful diagnostic feature.

Advise NSAID, rest and elevation for 1–2 days, with GP follow-up. A padded shoe insole or sorbothane heel pad may help. Severe, persistent cases are occasionally treated with local steroid injection or even surgical division of the plantar fascia.

Osteochondritis dissecans (📖 p.708)
Osteochondritis of a MT head (usually the 2nd—Freiberg's disease) causes gradual onset pain on WB. The cause is often unclear, but it may follow minor injury. Examination may reveal local tenderness but little else. X-ray for evidence of flattening, widening, or fragmentation of the MT head or narrowing of the MTPJ.

Treat initially with simple analgesia. Refer persistent cases to orthopaedics to consider excision of the MT head or osteotomy.

In-growing toenails
Refer back to the GP for elective treatment, unless there is evidence of infection. In this case, consider oral antibiotics (eg flucloxacillin or co-amoxiclav), or if there is an acute paronychia, incision, and drainage under LA. On occasion, it may be appropriate to excise a wedge of nail under LA.

Low back pain

Low back pain is the commonest cause of lost work days in the UK. The initial ED approach is to identify any patients who may have immediately life-threatening problems (eg leaking aortic aneurysm) and sort the rest into:

- *Simple ('mechanical') back pain*: no investigations or referral required.
- *Nerve root pain*: referral and investigation needed if symptoms persistent or progressive.
- *Possible serious spinal pathology*: referral and investigation required.
- *Suspected cord compression*: immediate neurosurgical/orthopaedic referral mandatory.

Psychogenic back pain is not an ED diagnosis. If in doubt, refer.

History

General Document patient's age, sex and employment. Note onset and duration of symptoms, character, position and radiation of pain, exacerbating or relieving factors. Precipitants include injuries, falls, heavy lifting, or unaccustomed activity.

Past history Detail any previous back problems or surgery, other medical conditions (eg rheumatoid arthritis, OA, osteoporosis).

Drug history Is the patient using analgesia (and has it helped?). Ask about corticosteroids and contraindications to NSAIDs.

Social history Ask about home circumstances, work, and stress.

Systemic enquiry Weakness, altered sensation, weight loss, anorexia, fever, rigors, cough, sputum, haemoptysis, bowel, or urinary symptoms.

Examination

'Unwell' patient Immediately assess airway, breathing, and circulation. Look for shock and a pulsatile abdominal mass, peritonism, evidence of blood loss, radial-femoral pulse discrepancies or asymmetry.

'Well' patient Look for signs of weight loss, cachexia, anaemia, clubbing, or muscle wasting. Inspect the back for muscle spasm, scars, scoliosis, or other deformity. If possible, watch the patient walk, looking for spasm, abnormal posture or limping. Palpate for tenderness over the spine, lower ribs and renal angles. With the patient supine on a trolley, look for muscle wasting in the legs. Examining both sides:

- *Straight leg raise*: note the angle which reproduces pain (lumbar nerve root irritation).
- *Crossed straight leg raise*: nerve root symptoms reproduced by lifting contralateral leg strongly suggests lumbar disc prolapse and nerve root entrapment.

Perform a neurological examination Check tone, power, sensation, and reflexes in the lower limbs:

- L4 covers sensation of medial lower leg; quadriceps power; knee jerk.
- L5 covers sensation of lateral lower leg and great toe; extensor hallucis longus power; hamstrings jerk.
- S1 covers sensation of little toe and lateral foot; foot plantar flexors power; ankle jerk. Always check perineal and perianal sensation.

Perform a rectal examination for anal tone, masses, or blood. Examine the abdomen for masses. Document peripheral pulses and perfusion.

Investigation

Check T° and urinalysis. X-ray is indicated for some patients aged >55years, or those who are systemically unwell, with a history of trauma (except clinical coccyx fracture), or where malignancy, infection, or HIV is suspected. In the latter cases, also check C-reactive protein (CRP), FBC, U&E.

Treatment

Refer urgently patients with lower limb weakness, altered perineal or perianal sensation, sphincter disturbance (this is strongly suggestive of *cauda equina syndrome* due to central lumbar disc prolapse). An MRI scan will confirm this diagnosis—in which case, urgent consultation with a neurosurgeon will allow emergency surgical decompression to be planned as appropriate.

Refer patients with the following: aged <20 or >55years, unremitting or increasing symptoms, widespread neurological signs, weight loss, systemic illness, pyrexia, chronic corticosteroids, osteoporosis, or HIV +ve patients with thoracic pain.

Treat simple 'mechanical' back pain with regular simple analgesia and/or NSAID. Avoid the routine use of opioids. Small doses of benzodiazepines (eg diazepam 2–5mg tds) may be useful, but tend to cause drowsiness. Advise the patient to aim to return to normal activity, even if some discomfort persists. Avoid bed rest. Expect recovery in 4–6weeks. Nerve root symptoms mostly resolve over weeks to months with the above treatment, physiotherapy or manipulation. In all cases, give written and verbal advice for immediate return if limb weakness, numbness, bladder, or bowel problems occur. Advise follow-up with the GP.

Acute arthritis 1

Approach

Whenever a patient presents with a painful joint, try to distinguish whether the source of pain is articular or peri-articular. Painful joints of articular origin produce warmth, tenderness, and swelling about the entire joint, with painful movement in all directions. Pain of peri-articular origin (outside joint capsule), such as bursitis/tendinitis tends to result in tenderness and swelling localized to a small area, with pain on passive movement only felt in limited planes.

Consider a septic cause in every patient who presents with acute arthritis. Useful investigations include white blood cells (WBC), erythrocyte sedimentation rate (ESR), or CRP, and joint aspiration.

Joint aspiration

The most important diagnostic test in patients presenting with acute arthritis is examination of the synovial fluid. When joint aspiration is performed, ensure that an aseptic technique is employed. Avoid joint aspiration through an area of cellulitis. Send fluid for Gram stain, culture, crystal examination, and cell count (Table 9.4). Remember that the absence of bacteria on Gram staining does not exclude septic arthritis.

Table 9.4

	Normal	Reactive	Infectious
Colour	Colourless/pale yellow	Yellow	Yellow
Turbidity	Clear, slightly turbid	Turbid	Turbid, purulent
Cell count/mm	200–1000	3000–10,000	>10,000
Predominant cell type	Mononuclear	Neutrophil	Neutrophil
Gram stain	None	None	+ve
Culture	−ve	−ve	+ve

Causes of polyarthritis

- Rheumatoid arthritis.
- Ankylosing spondylitis.
- Reiter's disease.
- Psoriatic arthritis.
- Arthritis associated with inflammatory bowel disease.
- Viral arthritis.
- Rheumatic fever.
- Gonococcal arthritis.
- Gout.

Septic arthritis

Pyogenic infection usually reaches a joint via the bloodstream, but may also develop from adjacent osteomyelitis or external skin puncture wounds. Sepsis may progress to complete joint destruction within 24hr.

Infective agents Staph aureus, Gonococcus, Strep, TB, Salmonella. Haemophilus was the commonest organism in babies before Haemophilus immunization, but is now rare. There is an ↑ incidence in patients with rheumatoid arthritis, those taking steroids, the immunosuppressed and at the extremes of age. Do not overlook septic arthritis superimposed on a non-infectious joint (eg gout, rheumatoid joints).

Presentation Typically only 1 joint is affected and is red, painful, and swollen. No movement is usually tolerated (but steroids and analgesics can mask many of the common features of septic arthritis). The joint is held in position of most comfort, usually slight flexion. There may be fever, shaking, and rigors. Note that hip joint infection may not produce obvious external findings due to its deep location. Do not overlook a septic joint with signs obscured by concomitant antibiotic use. IV drug abusers may have involvement of uncommon joints of the axial skeleton (eg sacroiliac, vertebral, and sterno-clavicular joints).

Investigation FBC, ESR, or CRP, blood cultures, joint aspiration (see Table 9.4). X-rays may be initially normal or show only soft tissue swelling with displacement of capsular fat planes. Later, features of bone destruction occur.

Treatment Commence IV antibiotics (eg flucloxacillin + benzylpenicillin). Refer urgently to the orthopaedic team for joint irrigation/drainage, analgesia, splintage of the joint.

Note: Prosthetic joint infection can be difficult to detect, but pain is typically constant and present at rest. Early infection (within 3 months of surgery) may cause obvious wound inflammation. This is less likely to be apparent in delayed or later infections. There may be little in the way of systemic symptoms. Suggestive radiological features include widening and lucency of the bone-cement interface by >2mm, movement of the prosthesis, periosteal reaction and fractures through the cement, although X-rays may be normal. Adopt a low threshold for suspecting prosthetic joint infections and referral to the orthopaedic team.

Traumatic arthritis

Joint pain, tenderness, ↓range of movement and haemarthrosis after injury implies intra-articular fracture. Note, however, that septic arthritis may occur in association with trauma, even in the absence of penetrating injury.

Osteoarthritis

Elderly patients with known OA may suffer acute 'flare ups'. Constitutional symptoms are not a feature. X-rays may show asymmetrical joint space narrowing, osteophytes and subchondral cyst formation. Advise NSAID and/or paracetamol, plus graduated exercises.

Acute arthritis 2

Acute gout

Most often affects 1st MTPJ or knee. Precipitated by trauma, diet, diuretics, renal failure, myeloproliferative disease and cytotoxics. Ask about previous renal stones. Look for tophi. Joint aspiration reveals negatively birefringent crystals. Septic arthritis can occur with gout—ensure aspirates are Gram stained and cultured. X-rays initially show soft tissue swelling, later punched out lesions in peri-articular bone. Serum uric acid may be ↑, but can be normal in an attack. Treat with rest and NSAID (eg diclofenac 75mg bd) or if NSAID is contra-indicated, consider colchicine (500mcg bd initially, slowly ↑ to qds as needed to control symptoms, preferably with GP review). Do not alter treatment of patients already on long-term gout therapy. *Note:* oral steroids (eg prednisolone 30mg od for 5 days) may help patients who are unable to tolerate NSAIDs or who are resistant to other treatments.

Acute pseudogout

Typically affects the knees, wrists, or hips of an elderly person with history of arthritic attacks precipitated by illness, surgery, or trauma. Associated with: hyperparathyroidism, haemochromatosis, Wilson's disease, hypothyroidism, diabetes, hypophosphatemia. X-ray shows calcification in joint, menisci, tendon insertions, ligaments, bursae. Aspiration reveals weakly +ve birefringent crystals on polarizing microscopy. Treat symptomatically (with NSAID) and refer.

Rheumatoid arthritis

Presentation Persistent symmetrical deforming peripheral arthropathy typically starts with swollen, painful, stiff hands and feet, which gradually get worse, with larger joints becoming involved. Other modes of presentation are: persistent or relapsing monoarthritis of different large joints, systemic illness with minimal joint problems, sudden onset widespread arthritis, vague limb girdle aches.

Hand signs include MCPJ and PIPJ swelling, ulnar deviation and volar subluxation at MCPJs, boutonnière, and 'swan-neck' finger deformities. Extensor tendon rupture may occur.

Neck problems Degeneration of the transverse ligament of the dens carries the risk of subluxation and cord damage.

Extra-articular features SC nodules, vasculitis, pulmonary fibrosis, splenomegaly, anaemia, pleurisy, pericarditis, scleritis, kerato-conjunctivitis.

Rhematoid factor is +ve in 70% of cases.

X-rays show soft tissue swelling, peri-articular osteoporosis, joint space narrowing, bony erosions/subluxation.

Treatment Refer patients who are systemically unwell. Others may benefit from NSAID, splintage, and rheumatology clinic referral.

Viral arthritis

Rubella, hepatitis B, mumps, Epstein–Barr virus, and enteroviruses may cause arthritis. In hepatitis B, arthritis usually affects PIPJ, MCPJ or knee and precedes the onset of jaundice. Rubella is associated with an acute symmetrical arthritis and tenosynovitis.

Rheumatic fever (see 📖 p.672)

This is a non-infectious immune disease which follows infection with Group A β-haemolytic streptococci. Typically, a migratory or additive symmetrical polyarthritis affects the knees, ankles, elbows, and wrists.

Diagnosis is based on revised Jones criteria: evidence of previous streptococcal infection (ie recent scarlet fever, +ve throat swab, or anti-streptolysin titre >200U/mL) plus 2 *major* or 1 *major* plus 2 *minor* criteria.

Major criteria: carditis (pericarditis, myocarditis or endocarditis), migratory polyarthritis, chorea, SC nodules, rash (erythema marginatum).

Minor criteria: ↑ESR/CRP, arthralgia, fever, history of previous rheumatic fever (or rheumatic heart disease), ↑PR interval on ECG.

Investigations: Throat swab, ESR, CRP, and anti-streptolysin titre.

Treatment Refer for admission, rest, aspirin, benzyl penicillin, and splintage.

Sero-negative spondyloarthropathies

These have the following common features: involvement of the spine and sacroiliac joints, inflammation then calcification of bony tendon insertions, peripheral inflammatory arthropathy, and extra-articular manifestations such as uveitis, aortic regurgitation, and pulmonary fibrosis.

Ankylosing spondylitis

Usually presents with chronic low back pain in men aged 15–30 years. Progressive spinal fusion ultimately results in a fixed kyphotic spine (which is particularly prone to fracture after injury), hyperflexed neck, and restricted respiration. Hips, shoulders, and knees may be involved. Other features are: iritis, apical lung fibrosis, plantar fasciitis, and Achilles tendonitis. There may be normochromic anaemia and ↑ESR. X-rays show 'bamboo spine' (squared vertebrae), eroded apophyseal joints and obliterated sacro-iliac joints.

Reiter's syndrome

Triad of urethritis, conjunctivitis and sero-negative arthritis may follow infection (urethritis, cervicitis, or dysentery). May cause large joint monoarthritis of a WB leg joint. Other features: iritis, keratoderma blenorrhagicum, circinate balanitis, plantar fasciitis, Achilles tendonitis, aortic incompetence.

Joint aspirate yields inflammatory cells, with −ve culture. WCC and ESR are ↑.

Psoriatic arthritis

Arthritis rarely precedes skin involvement.

Enteropathic arthropathies

Inflammatory bowel disease is associated with spondyloarthritis and large joint mono-arthropathy. There may also be a migratory polyarthritis.

Gonococcal arthritis

May present with fever, migratory tenosynovitis and polyarthralgia, arthritis (knee, ankle or wrist) and skin rash. Genital infection may be silent, especially in women. Take swabs with special culture media and refer for investigation.

Eponymous fractures

Correctly applied, the one or two words that comprise an eponymous injury convey succinctly an otherwise involved description of a complex fracture.

Aviator's astragalus

Fractures of the neck of the talus, previously commonly observed amongst World War II pilots who crash-landed their damaged planes on returning from bombing raids. The injuries resulted from the upward thrust of the rudder bar, causing dorsiflexion forcing the talus against the anterior tibia.

Bankart lesion

Avulsion of the joint capsule and glenoid labrum resulting from anterior dislocation of the shoulder joint. It is implicated as a causative factor for recurrent dislocations.

Barton's fracture

First described by Barton in 1839, this complex distal radial fracture is intra-articular. Displacement of the distal radial fragment allows subluxation of the carpal bones. A rare variety is called a Lentenneur's fracture.

Bennett's fracture dislocation

These intra-articular fractures of the base of the first MC are notorious for allowing the main MC fragment to slip into a poor position. If conservative treatment (POP) is preferred to internal fixation, careful follow-up will be needed to ensure a satisfactory outcome.

Boutonnière deformity

Rupture of the central slip of the extensor tendon at the PIPJ allows the base of the middle phalanx to 'button-hole' through. The remaining two parts of the extensor expansion slip along the side of the finger and act as flexors at the PIPJ, whilst still extending the DIPJ. This produces the characteristic deformity.

Boxer's fracture

Fracture of the neck of the little finger MC rarely occurs during formal boxing when gloves are worn. It is much more commonly seen following impromptu street or bar-room brawls: innocuous-looking overlying wounds are often compound human ('reverse fight') bites (🕮 Specific bites and stings, p.416).

Bumper fracture

The height of the average car bumper renders the adult pedestrian (who is unfortunate enough to be knocked down) particularly vulnerable to a fracture through the lateral tibial condyle into the tibial plateau. There is often an associated tear to the medial collateral knee ligament.

Chance fracture

A horizontal fracture through a vertebral body, associated arch, and spinous process may result from an injury involving distraction and flexion. It typically involves the lumbar spine of car passengers restrained only by a lap belt in a road traffic collision.

Clay-shoveller's fracture

Resistance against neck flexion may produce an avulsion of the tip of a spinous process of the lower cervical or upper thoracic spine. The lesion typically affects C7.

Colles' fracture

Abraham Colles, Professor of Surgery in Dublin, described this common distal radial fracture in 1814. The classic dinner fork deformity results from posterior displacement and angulation of the distal fragment (📖 p.444).

Dashboard dislocation

A high speed head-on road traffic collision causing the dashboard to impact upon the flexed knee often results in posterior dislocation of the hip.

Dupuytren's fracture-dislocation

A highly unstable ankle injury in which there is a fracture of the distal fibula shaft, disruption of the medial ankle ligament and posterior tibio-fibular ligament. The result is gross diastasis and dislocation of the talus laterally.

Essex–Lopresti fracture-dislocation

A heavy fall on the outstretched hand may cause a comminuted fracture of the radial head. It is associated with tearing of the interosseous membrane (diastasis), allowing subluxation of the distal ulna.

Galeazzi fracture-dislocation

Describes the combination of a fracture of the distal radial shaft with dislocation of the distal radio-ulnar joint (📖 Forearm fractures and related injury, p.448). A Moore's fracture dislocation is a similar injury, except that the radial fracture involves the distal radius, not the shaft.

Gamekeeper's thumb

Rupture of the ulnar collateral ligament of the 1st MCPJ was originally described as an occupational injury amongst gamekeepers, sustained whilst breaking the necks of wounded rabbits. It is now most commonly seen as a result of skiing injuries, particularly on artificial slopes, when the thumb is caught in the diamond latticework matting. The injury requires prompt diagnosis and treatment in order to avoid the long-term complication of a weak pinch-grip.

Hangman's fracture

Although no longer a part of modern life in the UK, executions were previously achieved by hanging. The victim was allowed to fall several feet before being arrested by a noose. This produced rapid death from severance of the cervical spinal cord. The mechanism of injury is a combination of distraction and extension, causing an unstable (hangman's) fracture of the pedicles of the axis (C2), and disrupting the intervertebral disc between C2 and C3. The fracture may also result from extension and axial compression and may occur without neurological damage.

Hill–Sachs lesion

This is an impacted compression fracture of the humeral head, which occurs during anterior shoulder dislocation. It is produced by the recoil impaction of the humeral head against the rim of the glenoid as the former dislocates. It is believed by some to be an important causative factor for recurrent dislocation.

Horse rider's knee

Frontal impact at the level of the proximal tibio-fibular joint may result in posterior dislocation of the fibular head. Reduction usually requires an MUA.

Hume fracture-dislocation

This refers to the combination of an olecranon fracture with dislocation of the radial head.

Hutchinson fracture

Also referred to as a 'chauffeur' fracture, this is the name sometimes given to a fracture of the radial styloid. It is classically caused by forced radial deviation of the wrist when the starting handle of an old-fashioned motor car 'kicks back'.

Ice skater's fracture

Children aged 2–8years are susceptible to stress fractures of the distal fibula.

Jefferson fracture

An unstable 'blowout' fracture of C1 follows an axial load. One third are associated with a C2 fracture.

Jones fracture

This is a transverse fracture of the base of the 5th MT just distal to the intermetatarsal joint. It is a more significant injury than an avulsion fracture at the insertion of peroneus brevis, as it is prone to non-union (📖 Foot fractures and dislocations, p.489).

Le Fort facial fractures

Experiments by Le Fort in 1901 were followed by descriptions of facial fractures and classification into three anatomical types (📖 Middle third facial fractures, p.372), including the Guérin fracture (Le Fort I).

Lisfranc fracture-dislocation

Fracture dislocation at the tarso-metatarsal joint is a significant injury. It is named after the surgeon who described the surgical operation of partial amputation of the foot at the level of the tarso-metatarsal joint.

Luxatio erecta

First described in 1859, this is an uncommon shoulder dislocation (inferior glenohumeral dislocation). The term is derived from Latin and describes the erect hyperabducted position of the arm after dislocation. The injury follows a hyperabduction force, most often after a fall. Axillary nerve damage occurs in 60%. Reduction of the dislocation may follow overhead traction or conversion to an anterior dislocation to which conventional techniques can be applied.

Maisonneuve injury

An unstable injury in which rupture of the medial ankle ligament is associated with a diastasis and proximal fibula fracture.

Malgaigne's fracture

An unstable injury in which the pelvic ring is disrupted in two places: anteriorly (through both pubic rami) and posteriorly (sacroiliac joint disruption, or fracture of ilium or sacrum).

Mallet injury

Stubbing a finger may rupture the extensor tendon (or avulse its phalangeal attachment) at the DIPJ, causing a 'mallet deformity', in which the DIPJ is held flexed. The mechanism of injury is forced flexion of the extended DIPJ.

March fracture

This refers to a stress fracture of the (usually 2nd) MT shaft after strenuous and unaccustomed exercise. Traditionally, it was observed after heavy marching in new army recruits.

Monteggia fracture-dislocation

Fracture of the proximal ulna shaft is associated with dislocation of the radial head. The latter is relatively easy to miss. Never accept an ulna fracture as an isolated injury without obtaining complete views of both forearm bones, including the elbow and wrist joints.

Nursemaid's elbow

Alternative name for a 'pulled elbow' in a pre-school child (📖 p.724).

Nutcracker fracture

Lateral force applied to the forefoot may cause the cuboid to be fractured as it is compressed between the calcaneum and the base of the 4th and 5th MTs.

O'Donahue's triad

A torn medial meniscus, ruptured anterior cruciate ligament and ruptured medial collateral ligament combine to produce a significant knee injury.

Pelligrini–Stieda's disease

Ossification of the medial collateral knee ligament may follow avulsion of the superficial part from its attachment to the medial femoral condyle.

Pilon fracture

These intra-articular fractures of the distal tibia are uncommon, but may also be subdivided into three types.

Pipkin fracture-dislocation

This refers to a posterior hip dislocation in which part of the femoral head is avulsed by the ligamentum teres and remains attached to it within the acetabulum. The avulsed fragment is rarely large enough to be reattached.

Pott's fracture

This term has come to be applied indiscriminately to any ankle fracture, which may be simply subdivided into 'uni-', 'bi-', or 'tri-malleolar'.

Rolando fracture

Essentially a comminuted Bennett's fracture, the classic description is of Y shaped intra-articular fractures at the base of the 1st MC. Treatment is difficult.

Runner's fracture

Stress fractures of the tibia are particularly common amongst runners who chalk up many miles of running on roads each week.

Smith's fracture

The so-called 'reversed Colles' fracture' was first described by Smith in 1847.

Straddle fracture

Falls astride classically produce bilateral vertical pubic rami fractures.

Tillaux fracture

An avulsion fracture of the distal lateral tibia may occur due to the pull of the anterior tibio-fibular ligament.

Toddler's fracture

Undisplaced spiral fractures of the tibial shaft in children <7 years often follow minimal trauma and not be visible on initial X-ray. Subperiosteal bone formation is usually apparent radiologically by 2 weeks (see 📖 Paediatric lower limb injuries, p.727).

Chapter 10

Surgery

Approach to abdominal pain

First aim to identify patients requiring resuscitation or urgent treatment. The need for resuscitation is apparent in emergencies with associated hypovolaemic and/or septic shock. Less obvious, but equally important, is recognition of patients requiring urgent treatment with no clinical evidence of shock (especially ruptured abdominal aortic aneurysm).

History

The pain Determine details of site, radiation, shift, character, timing, precipitating, and relieving factors.

Vomiting Record anorexia, nausea, and vomiting. Ask about the nature of vomit (blood, bile, etc.). Vomiting that follows the onset of abdominal pain tends to imply a surgical cause, whereas vomiting preceding pain is often non-surgical.

Bowel disturbance Enquire about recent change of bowel habit, particularly any rectal bleeding.

Other symptoms Do not forget that abdominal pain may be due to urological, respiratory, cardiovascular or gynaecological disorders.

Past history Determine the nature of previous surgery, preferably by obtaining old notes.

Examination

Vital signs Pulse, BP, respiratory rate, GCS, and T° may indicate the need for immediate intervention.

Abdomen Note distension and scars from previous surgery. Check the hernial orifices. Palpate gently for areas of tenderness. It is unnecessary and unkind to attempt to elicit rebound tenderness—tenderness on percussion is ample evidence of peritonitis. Perform PR/PV examination.

General Look for evidence of dehydration and jaundice. Examine the respiratory and cardiovascular systems.

Investigations

Assessment of patients with abdominal pain in the ED usually depends upon history and examination rather than sophisticated tests. However, the following investigations may prove useful:

- *BMG:* DKA may present with abdominal pain (Hyperglycaemic crises, p.152).
- *Urinalysis:* abdominal pain may result from urinary stones or infection. Perform a urine pregnancy test on all women of childbearing age.
- *Blood tests:* consider the need for FBC, U&E, amylase, coagulation screen, and cross-matching. If clearly unwell, check ABG, and lactate. Although FBC is frequently requested in patients with abdominal pain, the awaited WCC rarely alters initial patient management.
- *ECG:* especially in patients aged >55 years, who may be suffering from an atypical presentation of an acute medical problem, most notably acute myocardial infarction (MI).

- *Chest X-ray*: a CXR is useful to exclude conditions above the diaphragm, which may mimic abdominal conditions (eg congestive heart failure, basal pneumonia).
- *Abdominal X-ray*: Specific indications for abdominal X-ray include suspicion of intestinal obstruction, toxic megacolon, sigmoid volvulus, GI perforation and urinary calculi (☐ Ureteric colic, p.524). X-rays are not indicated in patients with suspected uncomplicated appendicitis, UTI, 'simple' constipation, gastroenteritis, GI bleeding, acute pancreatitis. They are not 'routinely indicated' in the investigation of abdominal pain. In severely ill patients requiring imaging, CT or USS is usually more appropriate than plain abdominal X-rays.
- *USS*: reveals gallstones, free peritoneal fluid, urinary stones and aortic aneurysms. It is increasingly used in the ED, but needs specific training.
- *CT scan* may have a role in assisting with the diagnosis of certain conditions (eg acute appendicitis).

Treatment

Prompt resuscitation and provision of analgesia are integral components of the management of serious abdominal conditions. Ensure that patients who are very sick and/or hypotensive receive early IV fluids and full monitoring (this includes measuring urinary output via a urinary catheter). Follow the guidelines outlined in ☐ Severe sepsis and shock for patients with suspected sepsis, p.59.

The traditional belief that analgesia should not be given because it might mask a serious diagnosis is incorrect and cruel. Diagnosis is often easier when pain is relieved and the patient can give a better history and co-operate with examination. The most appropriate form of analgesia is usually IV opioid (eg morphine).

It can be difficult to decide if admission is needed for a patient with abdominal pain. Adopt a low threshold for seeking senior help. In general, if doubt exists, refer to the surgeon, who may decide that it is prudent to admit the patient for observation and investigation.

Pitfalls

- Steroids, NSAIDs, or obesity may render physical signs less obvious.
- β-blockade may mask signs of shock.
- Absence of fever does not exclude infection, especially in the very old, the very ill, and the immunosuppressed.
- When severe abdominal pain is out of all proportion to the physical findings, consider mesenteric infarction, aortic rupture/dissection, acute pancreatitis, torsion of ovarian cyst.
- Splenic rupture may occur after relatively trivial trauma in patients with glandular fever or haematological disorders.
- Consider gynaecological causes of abdominal pain in any woman of child-bearing age—always perform a pregnancy test.
- WCC may be normal in established peritonitis/sepsis.
- Amylase may be normal in acute pancreatitis. Conversely, moderate amylase ↑ may occur in acute cholecystitis, perforated peptic ulcer, and mesenteric infarction.

Causes of acute abdominal pain

The cause of abdominal pain is often unclear initially. Indeed, many patients get better without any definite cause being identified ('non-specific' abdominal pain). Remember also that a patient is much more likely to have a common condition (perhaps with an atypical presentation), rather than a very rare condition. Thus, a patient presenting with atypical abdominal pain is more likely to have acute appendicitis than tabes dorsalis, lead poisoning, or acute intermittent porphyria. The following conditions are seen relatively frequently:

Surgical
- Non-specific abdominal pain.
- Acute appendicitis.
- Cholecystitis and biliary colic.
- Pancreatitis.
- Peptic ulcer disease (including perforation).
- Ruptured abdominal aortic aneurysm.
- Mesenteric infarction.
- Diverticulitis.
- Large bowel perforation.
- Intestinal obstruction from various causes.
- Ureteric calculi.
- Urinary retention.
- Testicular torsion.
- Intussusception.
- Cancer (especially of the colon: see below).

Gynaecological
- Ectopic pregnancy.
- Pelvic inflammatory disease (PID).
- Rupture/torsion of ovarian cyst.
- Endometriosis.
- Mittelschmertz.

Medical
- MI.
- Pneumonia.
- Pulmonary embolus (PE).
- Aortic dissection.
- Acute hepatitis.
- DKA.
- Urinary tract infection (UTI).
- Herpes zoster.
- Irritable bowel syndrome.
- Gastroenteritis.

Cancer causing abdominal pain
Unexplained abdominal pain in patients >50 years may be caused by cancer, especially of the large bowel. The pain may result from transient or partial bowel obstruction. Ask about previous episodes of pain, weight loss and change of bowel habit. If there is no indication for admission, consider referral to a surgical clinic for investigation.

Acute appendicitis

This common cause of abdominal pain in all ages is particularly difficult to diagnose in the extremes of age and in pregnancy. However, the diagnosis of acute appendicitis is often missed initially at all ages.

History

The classic presentation is of central colicky abdominal pain, followed by vomiting, then shift of the pain to the right iliac fossa. Many presentations are atypical, with a variety of other symptoms (eg altered bowel habit, urinary frequency) partly depending upon the position of the tip of the inflamed appendix (retrocaecal 74%; pelvic 21%; paracaecal 2%; other 3%).

Examination (see also Table 10.1)

In the early stages, there may be little abnormal; in the late stages the patient may be moribund with septic shock and generalized peritonitis. Between these extremes, there may be a variety of findings, including ↑ T°, tachycardia, distress, foetor oris. There is usually a degree of tenderness in the right iliac fossa (±peritonitis). Rovsing's sign (pain felt in the right iliac fossa on pressing over the left iliac fossa) may be present. PR examination may reveal tenderness high up on the right with inflammation of a pelvic appendix.

Investigations

The diagnosis of acute appendicitis is essentially clinical. CT and X-rays are not routinely indicated, but perform urinalysis ± pregnancy test. Although FBC may reveal an ↑ WCC, this is not invariable.

Differential diagnosis

Depending upon the presentation, the potential differential diagnosis is very wide—remember to consider urinary, chest, and gynaecological causes.

Treatment

- Obtain IV access and resuscitate if necessary. Commence IV fluids if there is evidence of dehydration.
- Give IV opioid and antiemetic (eg slow IV metoclopramide 10mg).
- If acute appendicitis is likely, or even possible, keep 'nil by mouth' and refer to the surgeon. If appendicectomy is required, pre-operative antibiotics (eg cefuroxime + metronidazole) ↓ risk of infective complications.

Appendix mass

Untreated, acute appendicitis may proceed to perforation with generalized peritonitis, or may become 'walled off' to produce a localized right iliac fossa inflammatory mass. There are many causes of such a mass. Refer to the surgeon for further investigation and management.

Table 10.1 Causes of a right iliac fossa mass

• Appendix mass	• Iliac lymphadenitis
• Caecal carcinoma	• Psoas abscess
• Crohn's disease	• Retroperitoneal tumour
• Ovarian mass	• Actinomycosis
• Pelvic kidney	• Common iliac artery aneurysm
• Enlarged gall bladder	• Spigelian hernia
• Iliocaecal TB	

Acute pancreatitis

This is a relatively common serious cause of abdominal pain in the middle aged and elderly, with an incidence of ≈5 per 100,000/year.

Causes

Often due to gallstones and alcohol. Many are idiopathic. Other causes: hypothermia, trauma, infection (glandular fever, mumps, Coxsackie, and infectious hepatitis), hyperlipidaemia, hyperparathyroidism, drugs (steroids, azathioprine, thiazides, and statins), polyarteritis nodosa, pancreatic cancer.

Symptoms

Typically, the complaint is of severe constant epigastric pain radiating to the centre of the back, with associated nausea and vomiting.

Signs

The patient may be distressed, sweating and mildly pyrexial. Look for evidence of shock—there may be a need for urgent resuscitation. Abdominal tenderness is likely to be maximal in the epigastrium ± guarding. The oft-quoted, but uncommon bluish discolouration in the loins (Grey Turner's sign) only develops after several days.

Investigations

- Check BMG and SpO_2.
- Serum amylase is likely to be grossly ↑ to >5 × upper limit of normal range (but if not diagnostically ↑, consider urinary amylase level).
- FBC may reveal ↑ WCC.
- U&E, Ca^{2+}, LFTs, glucose—hypocalcaemia is relatively common.
- Coagulation screen.
- CXR, ECG, ABG; consider lactate if unwell.

Treatment

- Provide oxygen (O_2).
- Obtain IV access and resuscitate with IV fluids as necessary.
- Give IV analgesia (eg morphine titrated according to response— 📖 Approach to abdominal pain, p.504).
- Give an anti-emetic (eg cyclizine 50mg or metoclopramide 10mg slow IV).
- Insert an nasogastric (NG) tube.
- Insert a urinary catheter and monitor urine output.
- Consider early insertion of a central venous line to monitor the central venous pressure (CVP) and guide IV fluid therapy in the seriously ill, particularly the elderly.
- Contact the appropriate specialist(s) and transfer to HDU/ICU.

Complications of acute pancreatitis

Acute pancreatitis has a significant mortality. Early complications include acute renal failure, disseminated intravascular coagulation (DIC), hypocalcaemia, adult respiratory distress syndrome (ARDS). Later, pancreatic abscess or pseudo-cyst may occur. The risk of death may be predicted according to the number of prognostic indicators present (Glasgow scoring system).

3 or more of the following on admission and subsequent repeat tests over 48hr constitutes severe disease:

Age >55yrs; WCC >15 × 10^9/L; fasting glucose >10mmol/L; urea >16mmol/L; arterial partial pressure of oxygen (pO_2) <7.9kPa; Ca^{2+} <2mmol/L; albumin <32g/L; serum LDH >600U/L; AST >100U/L.

Chronic pancreatitis

The term chronic pancreatitis implies permanent pancreatic damage. The condition often results from alcohol excess. Some patients with chronic pancreatitis present frequently to the ED requesting opioid analgesia. This can pose a difficult problem for the doctor who has not treated them previously. Follow the approach shown opposite and request previous hospital case notes early.

Biliary tract problems

The majority of emergency biliary tract problems relate to gallstones. Both solitary cholesterol and multiple mixed gallstones are common amongst the middle aged and elderly. Pigment stones comprise a small proportion—they occur in hereditary spherocytosis, malaria, and haemolytic anaemia.

Complications of gallstones Acute and chronic cholecystitis, biliary colic, obstructive jaundice, ascending cholangitis, mucocoele, empyema, acute pancreatitis, gallstone ileus, carcinoma of the gallbladder.

Acute cholecystitis

History Impaction of gallstones with acute inflammation of the gallbladder usually manifests itself by right hypochondrial pain radiating to the right side of the back ± vomiting.

Examination Look for features of an acute inflammatory process. Fever is frequently present, combined with right hypochondrial tenderness (particularly felt on inspiration—Murphy's sign). There may be a palpable mass—this is also a feature of mucocoele and empyema (the latter causing high fever, extreme tenderness and septic shock).

Management
- Provide IV analgesia and anti-emetic (see 📖 Analgesics: opioids, p.276).
- Check FBC (WCC often ↑), U&E, glucose, amylase, LFTs.
- CXR, ECG (in case pain is due to atypical presentation of MI).
- USS will confirm the diagnosis (tenderness on pressing the USS transducer over the area where the thickened gallbladder containing stones is located is called the ultrasonic Murphy's sign).
- Commence antibiotics (eg cefotaxime 1g IV) and refer to the surgeon.

Biliary colic/chronic cholecystitis

Patients (sometimes with known gallstones) may present with short-lived recurrent episodes of epigastric/right hypochondrial pain ± radiation to the back. This pain of biliary colic/chronic cholecystitis may be difficult to distinguish from other causes, including peptic ulcer disease. If the pain has subsided and there are no residual abnormal physical signs, discharge the patient with arrangements for GP or surgical outpatient follow-up.

Common bile duct stones

Stones within the common bile duct can cause several problems:
- Acute pancreatitis (📖 p.508).
- Obstructive jaundice.
- Ascending infection.

Obstructive jaundice

Biliary obstruction results in ↑ jaundice with pale stools and dark urine (±pain). Acute hepatitis and cholangio-/pancreatic carcinoma may present in a similar fashion. A palpable gallbladder implicates pancreatic carcinoma as the more likely diagnosis (Courvoisier's law: 'In the presence of jaundice, if the gallbladder is palpable, the cause is unlikely to be a stone').

Ascending cholangitis

Biliary stasis predisposes to infection, characterized by Charcot's triad (abdominal pain, jaundice, and fever). The patient may be very ill and require resuscitation for septic shock (📖 p.59).

Peptic ulcer disease

Perforated peptic ulcer

History Perforation of a gastric or duodenal ulcer is usually a severely painful sudden event. It may occur in those without known peptic ulcer disease, as well as those with previously diagnosed problems. However, close questioning may reveal recent symptoms attributed to 'indigestion'. Sudden localized epigastric pain spreads to the remainder of the abdomen—the pain is worse on coughing or moving and may radiate to the shoulder tip.

Examination Although distressed, the patient often prefers to lie still, rather than roll about. However, some patients in extreme pain writhe or roll in agony and are unable to keep still for examination or X-rays until analgesia is given. Absent bowel sounds, shock, generalized peritonitis and fever develop as time passes.

Investigations An erect CXR will demonstrate free gas under the diaphragm in ≈75% of patients with perforated peptic ulceration (if the patient is not fit enough for an erect CXR, obtain a left lateral decubitus X-ray). In those cases where the diagnosis is suspected, but not proven by X-ray, a contrast CT scan may help.

Other relevant investigations are: U&E, glucose, amylase (may be slightly ↑), FBC (WCC typically ↑), SpO_2, ABG, ECG/troponin (ensure symptoms do not reflect MI rather than peptic ulcer disease).

Treatment
- Give O_2.
- Provide IV analgesia (eg morphine titrated according to response).
- Give an antiemetic (eg slow IV metoclopramide 10mg).
- Resuscitate with IV 0.9% saline.
- Refer to the surgeon and give IV antibiotics (eg cefotaxime 1g and in late presentations, metronidazole 500mg as well).

Other GI perforations

Perforations may affect any part of the GI tract, but the chief causes are peptic ulceration, trauma, diverticular disease, and colonic carcinoma. The emergency treatment principles are similar to those of perforated peptic ulcer (described above). Bowel perforation usually results in gas under the diaphragm on an erect CXR, but remember that there are other possible causes, including: recent surgery, peritoneal dialysis, gas-forming infections, and occasionally, vaginal gas insufflation during waterskiing, or oral sex.

Other presentations of peptic ulcer disease

In addition to perforation, peptic ulcer disease may also present with upper or lower GI haemorrhage (p.122), or pain from oesophagitis, gastritis or duodenitis. If the patient's presentation suggests inflammation of the upper GI tract, consider discharging the patient with a supply of antacid and GP follow-up. This course of action is not appropriate if there is any possibility of serious complication. Similarly, it is not usually appropriate to initiate therapy with H_2 blockers or proton pump inhibitors in the ED without an accurate diagnosis.

Intestinal obstruction

Intestinal obstruction may be *mechanical* or *paralytic* in nature.

Paralytic intestinal obstruction is relatively rare in the ED. Causes include postoperative ileus, electrolyte disturbance (eg hypokalaemia) and pseudo-obstruction (see opposite).

Causes of mechanical intestinal obstruction

- Adhesions after previous surgery.
- Obstructed hernia (commonly: inguinal, femoral, para-umbilical, incisional; rarely: obturator, Spigelian, lumbar).
- Tumours (gastric, pancreatic or large bowel carcinoma).
- Volvulus (gastric, caecal or most commonly, sigmoid)—see 🕮 p.516.
- Inflammatory mass (eg diverticular, Crohn's).
- Peptic ulcer disease.
- Gallstone ileus.
- Intussusception.

History

Classic symptoms of intestinal obstruction are: abdominal pain, distension, vomiting, and constipation. The exact presentation depends upon the site of obstruction and the underlying cause. Ask about previous surgery. A history of severe pain suggests strangulation and developing ischaemia in a closed loop. The nature of the vomit (eg faeculent) may give a clue to the site of obstruction.

Examination

Check T°. Look for evidence of dehydration or shock. Carefully examine the hernial orifices (an obstructed femoral hernia is otherwise easily missed). Inspect for scars from old surgery. Note any distension and areas of tenderness (peritonism implies the surgical problem is advanced). Bowel sounds may be tinkling or absent. PR examination may reveal an 'empty' rectum.

Investigations

Blood tests Check U&E, glucose, amylase, FBC, LFTs, clotting, group, and save.

X-rays Request CXR and supine abdominal X-rays. If there is no convincing evidence of obstruction on the supine view, but still a high index of clinical suspicion, consider requesting an erect abdominal film. X-rays may demonstrate distended loops of bowel (with multiple fluid levels visible on an erect abdominal view). The site and nature of the distended bowel loops may suggest the site of obstruction. Note that although gallstone ileus is rare, X-rays may be diagnostic—the fistula between the bowel and gallbladder allows gas into the biliary tree, which shows up as an abnormal Y-shaped gas shadow in the right hypochondrium).

ECG Obtain this if the patient is middle-aged or elderly.

ABG If the patient is shocked, check SpO_2, ABG and lactate.

Old notes Request previous hospital case notes as soon as possible.

Management of mechanical obstruction
- Insert an IV cannula and start IVI 0.9% saline.
- If the patient is shocked, resuscitate with O_2 and IV fluids and insert a urinary catheter. Consider the need to insert a central venous line to guide resuscitation and involve ICU specialists at an early stage.
- Provide analgesia (eg IV morphine titrated according to response— 📖 Analgesics: opioids, p.276).
- Give an anti-emetic (eg cyclizine 50mg).
- Insert a NG tube.
- Refer to the surgical team for ongoing care.

Intestinal pseudo-obstruction

This condition results from chronic impairment of GI motility. Many of the patients affected are elderly and taking tricyclic antidepressants or other drugs with anticholinergic actions. Although pseudo-obstruction may involve any part of the GI tract, it typically presents with colonic distension. On rare occasions, this may be sufficiently severe to rupture the caecum or cause hypotension by compressing the inferior vena cava and blocking venous return. There may be a diagnostic X-ray appearance showing gas in the bowel all the way to the rectum, whereas in a classical, more proximal obstruction, gas will be absent from the rectum. Treatment of acute colonic distension from pseudo-obstruction is by decompression using a colonoscope.

Mesenteric ischaemia/infarction

Acute mesenteric infarction

Abrupt cessation of the blood supply to a large portion of the gut results in irreversible gangrene of the bowel within a relatively short space of time. This is associated with a very high mortality. Unfortunately, however, the diagnosis can be very difficult to make—the challenge therefore lies with making an early diagnosis.

Pathophysiology

One or more of the following processes may be responsible:

- Mesenteric arterial embolism (often associated with AF).
- Mesenteric arterial thrombosis.
- ↓ Mesenteric arterial blood flow (eg hypotension secondary to MI).
- Mesenteric venous thrombosis.

Most cases involve either arterial embolism or thrombosis.

History

Acute mesenteric infarction usually occurs in middle-aged or elderly patients. It is often heralded by severe, sudden onset, diffuse abdominal pain. Typically, the severity of the pain initially far exceeds the associated physical signs. The pain may radiate to the back.

Some patients have a preceding history of chronic mesenteric ischaemia, with pain after meals and weight loss. There is often an associated history of vascular disease elsewhere (eg intermittent claudication).

Examination

Shock, absent bowel sounds, abdominal distension, and tenderness are late signs. Initially, there may be little more than diffuse mild abdominal tenderness. If the diagnosis is suspected, search carefully for evidence of an embolic source (eg AF, recent MI with high risk of mural thrombus, aortic valve disease or valve prosthesis, recent cardiac catheter).

Investigations

- U&E, BMG, and laboratory blood glucose.
- Amylase may be moderately ↑
- FBC may demonstrate ↑ WCC.
- Coagulation screen.
- Group and save.
- ABG typically reveals a severe metabolic acidosis and lactate may be ↑.
- X-rays may show non-specific dilatation of bowel loops and, in advanced cases, gas within the hepatic portal venous system.
- ECG may demonstrate AF.
- Other specialist investigations (USS, CT, angiography) may be helpful, but let the surgeon decide about this.

Management

If the diagnosis is suspected:

- Resuscitate with O_2 and IV fluids.
- Provide analgesia (eg IV morphine titrated according to response).
- Consider broad spectrum IV antibiotics.
- Refer urgently to the surgeon.

Ischaemic colitis

Chronic arterial insufficiency to the bowel usually affects the mucosa and submucosa, typically in the region of the splenic flexure (junction of territory supplied by the superior and inferior mesenteric arteries).

The patient presents with abdominal pain, starting in the left iliac fossa. Loose stools with blood may be passed. The patient may have had previous similar episodes and exhibit evidence of cardiovascular disease. Examination may reveal a low grade pyrexia, tachycardia, and colonic tenderness with blood PR.

Check FBC, U&E, group and save, ECG, CXR. Plain abdominal X-rays may show 'thumb printing' (submucosal colonic oedema), typically at the splenic flexure. Provide analgesia, IV fluids, and refer to the surgical team.

Large bowel emergencies

Volvulus (see bowel obstruction—📖 p.512)

Responsible for ≈10% of large bowel obstruction. Occurs at the caecum or, more commonly, the sigmoid, due to poor fixation in their respective iliac fossae.

Sigmoid volvulus usually occurs in the elderly with initially intermittent cramping lower abdominal pain and progressive abdominal distension, which may be spontaneously relieved by passage of large amounts of flatus/faeces. Some patient's progress to complete obstruction: marked distension progressing to fever and peritonitis suggests strangulation.

Plain abdominal X-ray typically shows a large single dilated loop of colon (a 'bent inner tube') on the left side with both ends down in the pelvis.

Refer to the inpatient surgical team for sigmoidoscopy (if not strangulated) or surgery if strangulated.

Caecal volvulus is most common between the ages of 25–35yr. Patients have symptoms of acute onset small bowel obstruction.

Plain abdominal films usually show one large dilated segment of the colon in the mid-abdomen with distended small bowel loops and empty distal large bowel. Refer to the surgical team.

Diverticular disease

Diverticulosis is common in the middle-aged and elderly, particularly affecting the sigmoid colon. Without significant complications, there may be a change in bowel habit with passage of mucus.

Acute diverticulitis

Results from inflammation/perforation of a diverticulum and may be confined to colonic wall by the serosa. If this perforates, then inflammation may remain localized (pericolic abscess) or spread (frank peritonitis). Symptoms and signs reflect the extent of the infection—there may be lower abdominal dull constant pain, low grade fever with tenderness, rigidity and occasionally a mass in the left lower quadrant. The elderly (the group most at risk of diverticulitis and its complications), and those on immunosuppressants may not manifest the expected pyrexia and signs of peritonitis.

Investigations Check FBC, U&E, CRP, group and save, and blood cultures. Plain abdominal X-rays may show non-specific changes and help to exclude perforation/large bowel obstruction. An erect CXR often shows copious subdiaphragmatic gas in free perforations.

Treatment Give analgesia, IV fluids, keep fasted, and refer to the surgeon. Start broad spectrum antibiotics (eg cefuroxime + metronidazole).

Complications
- Perforation: may be localized and walled off (forming an abscess), or generalized.
- Intestinal obstruction: both large and small (due to adherent loops).
- Massive PR bleeding.
- Fistulae to adjacent structures: small bowel, uterus, vagina, bladder.
- Post-infective strictures.

Ulcerative colitis

Severe acute colitis is characterized by the passage of >6 loose bloody motions per day, together with systemic signs (tachycardia, fever) and hypoalbuminaemia. There is a risk of haemorrhage, perforation and toxic megacolon. The crucial points in management are early recognition and prompt referral to the inpatient gastroenterology service, for aggressive medical therapy (IV and PR steroids, IV fluids) and joint review by medical and surgical teams. Surgery may be required for complications, especially toxic megacolon. Suspect toxic megacolon if the colonic width is >5.5cm on abdominal X-ray (this sign is associated with a 75% risk of requiring colectomy). Refer any patient who presents with suspected new onset ulcerative colitis for investigation and control of the disease.

Mesenteric ischaemia/infarction

See ⊞ p.514.

Crohn's disease

Colonic Crohn's disease may present as colitis with bloody diarrhoea, urgency and frequency, similar to ulcerative colitis.

Fibrosis may cause diarrhoea or obstructive symptoms.

Peri-anal disease with chronic anal fissure may be the first presenting symptom. Emergency surgery is indicated in acute fulminating Crohn's colitis with bleeding, toxic dilatation, or perforation.

Epiploic appendagitis

Primary inflammation of one of the hundreds of appendices epiploicae on the antimesenteric colonic border may present in similar fashion to acute diverticulitis or appendicitis. However, T° and WCC are usually normal. Although often diagnosed at laparotomy, CT scan may be characteristic, allowing conservative treatment (including IV analgesia).

Irritable bowel syndrome

Patients are usually aged 20–40 years with a prolonged history of intermittent symptoms—altered bowel function (diarrhoea, constipation, or diarrhoea alternating with constipation). Typically, the abdominal pain is crampy/aching and localized in the lower abdomen over the sigmoid colon. Pain may be eased by the passage of stool or flatus. Examination fails to reveal any worrying features. The diagnosis is one of exclusion—be vigilant for clues that may point to other organic disease.

Anorectal problems

Any PR bleeding requires surgical follow-up to exclude malignancy.

Complications of haemorrhoids ('piles')

- *Bleeding:* haemorrhoids typically cause painless, bright red PR bleeding, associated with defaecation, but blood is not mixed with the stools. Check the abdomen and inspect the anus—if there is no prolapsed or external haemorrhoid, perform PR and arrange surgical follow-up.
- *Prolapsed piles* are acutely painful—treat conservatively with adequate analgesia (may need admission), bed rest, and stool softeners.
- *Thrombosed external pile* is due to rupture of a tributary of the inferior haemorrhoidal vein, producing a *peri-anal haematoma*. One or more dark blue nodules covered with squamous epithelium may be visible at the anus and a clot palpable. Refer to the surgeon to decide between incision and drainage under LA or conservative management.

Anal fissure

Typically causes severe pain on defaecation and for 1–2hr afterwards. There may be blood on the toilet paper, but usually bleeding is minimal. The fissure is located just inside the anal orifice and is usually associated with the passage of hard stools. Most are located posteriorly in the midline. PR examination may be impossible due to pain, but the fissure is often visible with traction of anal skin.

Treatment Prescribe analgesia and stool softeners. Most heal spontaneously, but the presence of significant ulceration, hypertrophied tissue, or a skin tag suggests chronicity and need for surgical follow-up. Be suspicious of those fissures not in the midline and those that are multiple (the differential diagnosis includes chronic inflammatory bowel disease, anal cancer and adenocarcinoma of the rectum invading the anal canal).

Pruritus ani

Not strictly an emergency problem. There are numerous possible causes:
- Poor hygiene.
- Fissure, prolapsing piles, fistulae, rectal prolapse, anal cancer.
- Contact dermatitis due to local applications (especially local anaesthetics).
- Threadworms.
- Part of a general condition (eg obstructive jaundice, lymphoma, severe iron deficency anaemia, uraemia, diabetes).
- Lichen sclerosis.
- Sexually transmitted disease (herpes, anal warts, HIV).

Treatment requires identification of the underlying problem—refer to the GP. In the meantime, advise avoidance of ointments and creams.

Pilonidal abscess

An infected pit in the natal cleft causes pain and/or offensive discharge.
Treatment Refer to the surgical team. Treatment may involve initial incision and drainage, followed by healing, then elective excision of the sinus.

Note: Fissures, tears or bruising around the anus of a child arouses suspicion of abuse in the first instance. Refer to a specialist and avoid rectal examination.

Anorectal abscesses

Most begin with infection involving an anal crypt and its gland, from which it can spread between the external and internal sphincters to a variety of sites—these determine its symptomatology and mode of presentation.

Peri-anal and ischiorectal abscesses account for ≈80% of cases. In 20%, there is a clear predisposing cause, such as inflammatory bowel disease, anorectal cancer, or anal fissure (Fig. 10.1).

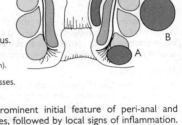

The four types of anorectal abscess—(A) Perianal. (B) Ischio-rectal. (C) Submucous. (D) Pelvi-rectal.

(After W.F.W. Southwood, F.R.C.S., Bath).

Fig. 10.1 Types of anorectal abscesses.

Clinical features Pain is a prominent initial feature of peri-anal and superficial ischiorectal abscesses, followed by local signs of inflammation. Patients complain of persistent dull throbbing pain, made worse by walking and sitting, and prior to defaecation. Such symptoms are less evident with deep infections, which tend to develop slowly with pyrexia and systemic upset. Peri-anal abscesses produce localized fluctuant red tender swellings close to the anus. With ischiorectal sepsis, the findings are more diffuse and fluctuance is a late finding. Deeper infections are less obvious—PR examination may reveal a mass or tender area of induration.

Treatment Provide analgesia and refer to the surgical team for incision and drainage under GA.

Venereal proctitis

The organisms are similar to those transmitted by vaginal intercourse: assume more than one type of organism is present. Patients complain of pain, irritation, discharge, and bleeding. Consider gonococcus, chlamydia, syphilis, herpes simplex. Refer urgently to a genitourinary specialist.

Rectal foreign bodies

X-rays may demonstrate the position and shape of FBs. More especially, look for the presence of any free air—perforation of the rectum or colon is the most frequent and most serious complication, in which case give IV antibiotics (eg cephalosporin + metronidazole). Refer the patient for removal of the FB by the surgical team.

Retention of urine

Causes of acute urinary retention

This more commonly presents in the male:

Common causes in males
- Prostatic hyperplasia/cancer.
- Urethral stricture.
- Post-operative.

Common causes in females
- Retroverted gravid uterus.
- Atrophic urethritis.
- Multiple sclerosis.

Other causes include: acute urethritis, prostatitis, phimosis, urethral rupture following trauma, bladder blood clot, urethral calculus, prolapsed intervertebral disc, drugs (alcohol, antihistamines, anticholinergics, antihypertensives, tricyclics), faecal impaction, anal pain.

Presentation

In most cases, the diagnosis is obvious: the patient complains of inability to pass urine combined with bladder discomfort. Remember, however, to consider the diagnosis in those patients unable to describe their symptoms (eg those unconscious after trauma).

Examination will reveal a tender enlarged bladder, with dullness to percussion well above the symphysis pubis. Search for the causes listed above. In particular, search for evidence of prolapsed disc/cord compression by checking the lower limb power/reflexes and perineal sensation. Perform PR examination to assess anal tone and the prostate.

Initial management

The patient requires urgent bladder decompression. Provided there is no contraindication (eg urinary retention following trauma or as a result of urethral stenosis), achieve this by urethral catheterization. Use an aseptic technique (male catheterization is described opposite). If urethral catheterization is impossible or contraindicated, consider the need for a suprapubic catheter, but this should only be performed by a doctor experienced in the technique.

Further management

After bladder drainage, record the volume of urine obtained, then re-examine the abdomen for pathology that might have been previously masked.

Test the urine for the presence of blood and send a mid-stream specimen of urine (MSU) for culture and sensitivity. Perform investigations appropriate to the likely underlying cause, and then refer to the urology team.

Chronic urinary retention

Patients with chronic retention often have massive, almost painless bladder distension. They are at risk of pressure damage to the upper urinary tract. Following drainage, they may develop haematuria or post-obstructive diuresis, with attendant problems of significant fluid and electrolyte derangements.

Male catheterization

- Prepare the equipment—a Foley catheter size 14G is appropriate for an adult. Ensure that the patient does not have an allergy to latex.
- Check the volume required for the catheter balloon.
- Wash hands and don sterile gloves.
- Clean the external genitalia with antiseptic solution and surround with a sterile field.
- Slowly insert local anaesthetic into the urethra.
- Gently massage the local anaesthetic down the urethra and *wait for a few minutes* for the LA to take effect.
- Holding the penis at right angles to the body, insert the lubricated catheter. The catheter should pass easily into the bladder with drainage of urine. If any resistance or difficulty is encountered, stop and seek senior assistance.
- Once urine appears, advance the catheter a few centimeters further before inflating the balloon.
- Connect the catheter to a closed drainage system and tape the tubing to the upper thigh.
- Ensure that the foreskin is not left retracted—this could result in paraphimosis.

Testicular problems

Remember that any pain of testicular origin may be initially referred to the abdomen.

Testicular torsion

Testicular torsion is most frequently seen in children and young adults. Any suspicion of testicular torsion should prompt immediate referral. The condition is covered fully on 🕮 Inguinal and scrotal swellings, p.700.

Acute epididymitis

Causes

For those aged <35 years, infection with chlamydia or gonococcus is commonly responsible. Acute epididymitis in those aged >35 years is usually secondary to UTI and associated with underlying urinary tract pathology.

Clinical features

There is typically a gradual onset of progressive testicular ache, with subsequent swelling of the epididymis and testis. There may be a history of dysuria or urethral discharge. The patient may be pyrexial. The epididymis is acutely tender, with the testis lying low in the scrotum. Advanced, late cases may have progressed to abscess formation.

Investigations

Send an MSU and take a urethral swab (take lab advice regarding the correct media for chlamydia).

Management

The chief initial concern is to ensure that testicular torsion is not being missed: if there is any possibility of this (🕮 Inguinal and scrotal swellings, p.700), refer urgently. Treatment of acute epididymitis comprises antibiotics (eg ciprofloxacin for 2 weeks), analgesia, and rest. Some patients require admission; others may be managed on an outpatient basis. Urology investigation and follow-up will be required, so involve the urologist early. Patients with suspected chlamydia or gonococcus require appropriate advice and contact tracing of sexual partners.

Orchitis

Orchitis may present as epididymo-orchitis, an extension of bacterial epididymitis (see above). Orchitis of viral origin may also occur—typically mumps, following ≈5days after parotitis. Mumps orchitis may be unilateral or bilateral and can occur in the absence of overt parotitis. Rarely, orchitis is secondary to tuberculosis (TB) or syphilis.

Treatment

All patients with orchitis require analgesia and follow-up. If there is any possibility of bacterial infection, antibiotics are indicated (see above).

Testicular lumps

Patients may present to the ED with scrotal/testicular lumps. Causes are varied and include: hydrocoele, inguinal hernia, epididymal cyst, epididymitis, orchitis, and testicular tumour. Many patients will be managed appropriately by referral back to GP or to an outpatient clinic. Be particularly wary of an apparent epididymo-orchitis which has failed to respond to antibiotics—it could be an atypical presentation of a testicular tumour.

Testicular trauma—See 🕮 p.352.

Penile problems and prostatitis

Paraphimosis

Paraphimosis occurs when the foreskin is left retracted, thereby causing swelling of the glans, which results in difficulty replacing the foreskin to its proper position. Untreated, tissue necrosis may develop. Paraphimosis may be iatrogenic, occurring after urethral catheterization.

Treatment Initially attempt reduction by manual decompression, which may require the use of Entonox®, IV sedation, or LA (a small amount of topical 1–2% lidocaine gel or injection of 10mL plain 1% lidocaine around the base of the penis). Digital pressure may allow the glans to ↓ in size, prior to the foreskin being delivered back into its usual position. If unsuccessful, refer to the surgical team for reduction under GA or dorsal slit of the prepuce followed by later circumcision.

Priapism

Priapism is persistent (and usually painful) penile erection.

Causes

- Iatrogenic (following intra-cavernosal injection of one or more of: papaverine, alprostadil, vasoactive intestinal polypeptide, phentolamine for impotence).
- Others: leukaemia, myeloma, sickle cell disease, spinal injury, drugs (eg sildenafil [Viagra], phenothiazines, cannabis, cocaine), renal dialysis.

Management Priapism is a urological emergency. Refer urgently to the urology team. Initial emergency treatment of a prolonged (>6hr) artificial erection (ie following an intra-cavernosal drug injection or oral sildenafil) is to aspirate 50mL of blood from each corpus cavernosum through a 19G butterfly needle into a 50mL syringe with a Luer lock.

Urethritis

This usually presents with dysuria/urinary frequency, reflecting underlying STD. Refer for appropriate investigation, treatment, and follow-up.

Prostatitis

Inflammation of the prostate may be acute or chronic and present in a variety of ways (fever, urgency, frequency, perineal pain, urethral discharge). PR examination reveals a tender prostate. Urinalysis demonstrates protein. Refer for further investigation and treatment.

Penile trauma

Minor superficial tears

These are relatively common. Most involve the frenulum. The patient complains of pain and bleeding following sexual intercourse. Bleeding usually responds to local pressure (if this is not successful, consider tissue glue or refer to the surgical team). Once bleeding has stopped, advise a period of abstinence from sexual activity (≈10 days) to allow healing to occur and prevent recurrence.

Fracture of the penis

This occurs infrequently. It involves injury to the tunica albuginea of the erect penis. The result is penile tenderness and swelling. Refer to the urologist for urgent surgical exploration, evacuation of haematoma and repair.

Ureteric colic

New onset flank/back pain in the elderly may represent a leaking aortic aneurysm (even if haematuria is present).

Causes

Calculi or blood clots may cause ureteric (or 'renal') colic. Colicky pain is produced by ureteric obstruction, ↑ intraluminal pressure, and muscle spasm. Calculi most commonly consist of calcium oxalate and/or calcium phosphate. Less common are magnesium ammonium phosphate (associated with UTIs and urea-splitting organisms, such as *Proteus*), urate, and cystine stones.

Calculi are associated with hypercalcaemia, hyperoxaluria and hyperuricaemia. 'Staghorn' calculi in the collecting system predispose to infections.

Calculi may form throughout the length of the renal tract. They vary in size from tiny particles to large 'stones' in the bladder. They cause symptoms from local obstruction, infection, and rarely may ulcerate through the wall of the structure in which they are present.

Clinical features

The most common presenting symptoms are pain from obstruction or UTI and/or haematuria. Constant dull, severe, loin discomfort is associated with excruciating colicky pain, spreading to the respective iliac fossa, testis, tip of penis or labia. The pain may cause the patient to move or walk about. Nausea, vomiting, pallor, sweating are common. There is frequently a previous history of stone disease—ask about this and whether there is any past history of renal disease. Ask about urinary and GI symptoms.

Apart from loin tenderness, abdominal examination is usually normal, but check the haemodynamic status, pulses, bruits and the abdominal aorta, as a ruptured aortic aneurysm can present in a similar fashion (📖 p.530). Pyrexia or rigors suggest associated infection. Microscopic (sometimes frank) haematuria is common. Symptoms are usually relieved when the stone passes into the bladder, but larger calculi may then cause obstruction at the bladder neck or the urethra producing acute urinary retention. Bladder calculi may present with symptoms of UTI and/or bladder irritation (frequency, dysuria, strangury, and haematuria).

Investigations

- Urinalysis and MSU: blood on stix testing is present in >80% of patients with proven stones. A pH>7.6 implies associated infection with urea splitting organisms.
- U&E, creatinine, glucose, Ca^{2+}, PO_4^{2-}, urate levels.
- 'KUB' X-ray: 90% of urinary calculi are radio-opaque. X-ray is ≈50% sensitive and ≈70% specific for the diagnosis of ureteric calculi and is a very useful follow-up of patients with known stones. Common sites for calculi include the pelvi-ureteric and vesico-ureteric junctions. Remember that the ureters lie adjacent to the tips of the spinal transverse processes.
- Use USS/Doppler instead in pregnant patients or those with renal disease.
- CT without contrast is ≈95% sensitive and ≈95% specific and has the advantage of assisting diagnosis of other causes of abdominal and/or loin pain.
- Intravenous urography (IVU) is the most accurate investigation when CT is not available or where endoscopic or surgical treatment is contemplated. A delayed nephrogram on the affected side at 5min is common. As contrast enters the collecting system, the site and degree of the obstruction can be assessed.

Treatment

Give IV opioid titrated to effect, together with an NSAID (either IV ketoralac, or oral/rectal diclofenac). Do not use antispasmodics, anticholinergics and 'pushing fluids'.

- Aim to discharge patients (with arrangements for appropriate outpatient investigation) when symptoms have completely resolved, and in whom the CT/IVU shows no obstruction. Note that in some patients the process of becoming pain-free merely represents complete obstruction.
- Admit (for further investigation and treatment) patients whose pain persists, or in whom investigation confirms continued obstruction, infection, sepsis or renal impairment.

Abscesses

An abscess is a localized collection of pus resulting in a painful soft tissue mass that is often fluctuant, but surrounded by firm granulation tissue and erythema. The cause is usually bacterial, resulting from minor trauma to the epithelium/mucosa or blockage of apocrine glands. A history of a previous lump at the site suggests infection of a sebaceous cyst. Check BMG in all patients.

For patients with recurrent abscesses, check for signs of hidradenitis suppurativa, diabetes, inflammatory bowel disease, and malignancy. Ask about steroid use.

Treatment

Incision and drainage A general surgical principle is that a collection of pus requires drainage. On occasions, depending upon local policy, it may be appropriate to do this in the ED. Some abscesses (eg face, breast, perineum, paediatric) require specialist attention. Regional, parenteral, or GA may be needed to supplement LA which works poorly in this situation.

Technique Incise along the length of the fluctuance and deep enough to enter the cavity. An elliptical incision will prevent premature closure and re-accumulation of pus. Send pus for culture. Ensure that loculi in the cavity are gently broken by the use of a curette. Consider inserting a loose antiseptic wick in the cavity to ensure drainage and prevent premature closure.

Antibiotics are not indicated in patients with normal host defences as long as the abscess is localized. Evidence of surrounding or spreading infection may warrant antibiotics (eg co-amoxiclav or penicillin + flucloxacillin) and on occasions, admission (see below).

Refer the following:
- Those who are systemically unwell (pyrexial, tachycardic, rigors), immuno-compromised and those not responding to treatment.
- Abscesses secondary to IV drug misuse.
- Those with infection in certain anatomical sites: face (↑ risk of cavernous sinus thrombosis), those potentially involving the airway (sublingual abscesses, Ludwig's angina), axillary, groin, retropharyngeal, perineal, and breast abscesses.
- Those with extensive or progressing cellulitis/lymphangitis.

These patients may require IV antibiotics (eg co-amoxiclav or flucloxacillin + penicillin), analgesia and surgical drainage. Take blood for FBC, clotting studies and blood culture. Treat sepsis/septic shock where necessary (📖 p.59).

Breast infection

Lactational breast abscess These are usually peripherally located and due to *Staph. aureus*. Local discomfort proceeds to painful swelling. Overlying skin may be red. Extreme cases may undergo necrosis and spontaneous discharge.

Treatment If seen prior to frank abscess formation, consider antibiotic treatment alone—prescribe a penicillinase-resistant antibiotic. If there is any suspicion of an abscess, refer for needle aspiration—if pus is found, drainage will be needed. Encourage the infant to feed from the contralateral breast whilst the affected side is emptied of milk manually or by breast pump.

Non-lactational breast abscess Typically affects the 30–60-year age group, usually peri-areolar, recurrent, and related to duct ectasia/periductal mastitis. Refer for needle aspiration, culture, and antibiotics (metronidazole and flucloxacillin). Note that inflammatory breast cancer may mimic septic mastitis and breast abscess. Incision of neoplastic lesions may have disastrous results.

Perineal abscesses See 📖 Anorectal problems, p.518.

Cellulitis and erysipelas

Cellulitis (see 📖 **Infected wounds and cellulitis, p.413**)

Cellulitis reflects bacterial skin infection (usually streptococcal, occasionally staphylococcal). It can occur in association with a skin wound acting as a portal of entry for infection (eg athlete's foot), but it may also occur without any obvious breach in the skin. Ascertain whether or not there is evidence of systemic upset or any background problems, such as immunodeficiency, diabetes, or steroid therapy.

The area of affected skin is red, warm to the touch with poorly defined margins. Check T° and look for lymphangitis and/or lymphadenopathy.

Treatment depends upon the nature and extent of clinical findings as follows:

- Treat patients who have localized limb infection and no evidence of systemic upset with oral antibiotics (either phenoxymethylpenicillin + flucloxacillin or co-amoxiclav or erythromycin) and arrange follow-up in 24–48hr.
- Admit patients who are systemically unwell or have spreading infection (eg lymphangitis extending above the knee from an area of cellulitis on the foot). Obtain venous access, take blood cultures and start IV antibiotics (either benzylpenicillin + flucloxacillin or co-amoxiclav).

Patients with cellulitis of the face (particularly around the eye) are at risk of significant intracranial complications (notably cavernous sinus thrombosis)—start IV antibiotics and refer for admission to the ophthalmology team.

Erysipelas

This streptococcal infection is limited to the more superficial parts of the skin, resulting in an area of redness and heat with clearly defined margins. Treat with antibiotics as outlined for cellulitis above, except that phenoxymethylpenicillin alone (500mg PO qds for 7 days) suffices in most cases.

Necrotizing fasciitis

See 📖 Streptococcal infections, p.234.

Complications of varicose veins

Occasionally, patients may attend the ED with complications of their varicose veins.

Bleeding from varicose veins

Patients with chronic venous hypertension associated with varicose veins have a significant risk of haemorrhage from the dilated thin-walled veins which commonly surround the area of lipodermatosclerosis at the ankle. Haemorrhages may be profuse and sufficient to cause hypovolemic shock. In extreme cases, this may even cause death.

Treatment

Control bleeding by elevating the leg, applying a non-adherent dressing and pressing firmly. Follow this with appropriate bandaging; unless there is evidence of occlusive arterial disease (varicose veins and arterial disease frequently co-exist in the elderly). Some patients may require resuscitation with IV fluids.

Refer for admission those who were shocked at presentation, those who have subsequently bled through the bandaging, those with occlusive arterial disease, and those who live alone. All patients will require surgical outpatient follow-up—advise patients who are discharged about first aid measures in the event of a rebleed.

Superficial thrombophlebitis

This occurs most frequently in patients with varicose veins or prothrombotic states (eg underlying inflammatory and malignant conditions). It usually manifests itself with redness, tenderness and induration along the course of the involved vein.

Treatment

Bed rest, elevation, and analgesia (NSAID). Pain typically ↓ over 1–2 weeks and the patient is left with a hard thrombotic cord. Superficial thrombophlebitis is only rarely associated with DVT, but occasionally thrombosis spreads from the long saphenous vein to involve the femoral vein. If there is any question of deep vein involvement, request an USS. If the thrombotic process involves the sapheno-femoral junction or the ilio-femoral system, refer for anticoagulation (📖 p.170).

Venous ulcers

Venous (varicose) ulcers tend to be chronic and recurrent. They are typically found on the medial side of the ankle. There is often associated dermatitis with surrounding brown discolouration, thickening of the skin and leg oedema. There is often mixed venous and arterial disease, especially in the elderly. Although ischaemic ulcers tend to lie on the lateral aspect of the ankle, exclude ischaemic ulceration by checking the peripheral pulses (request Doppler in patients with oedematous legs). Look for areas suspicious of malignant change, which may rarely occur in chronic ulcers (Marjolin's ulcer).

Treatment

Clean the ulcer with normal saline and dress it with either paraffin gauze or colloidal dressing. Follow this with firm bandaging (unless there is co-existing arterial disease) and advise leg elevation when the patient rests. Avoid dressings with topical antibiotics and indiscriminate use of oral antibiotics. Prescribe oral antibiotics (eg co-amoxiclav) only if there is cellulitis. Liaise with the GP about the need for surgical outpatient follow-up and to arrange for redressing by the district nurse.

Ruptured abdominal aortic aneurysm

Middle-aged and elderly people frequently develop abdominal aortic aneurysms. Rupture is relatively common and responsible for a large number of deaths, many of which occur suddenly out of hospital. Even when the patient reaches hospital alive, there is a significant mortality. The patient's best chance of survival lies with early diagnosis, prompt resuscitation and rapid transfer to theatre. Most aneurysms are saccular and found in the infrarenal portion of the aorta—haemorrhage after rupture is usually into the retroperitoneum. Aneurysm extension to involve the renal arteries renders surgery more difficult and ↑ risk of post-operative complications.

History

Presentation is highly variable, ranging from PEA cardiac arrest to painless sudden collapse of obscure origin, through to a classical history of central abdominal and lower back pain in a patient with a known aneurysm. Pain is usually a feature: typically sudden in onset and severe in nature.

Examination

The seriously ill patient may present a characteristic picture: distressed, pale, sweating, tachycardic, and hypotensive, with mottled skin of the lower body and a tender pulsatile abdominal mass. One or both femoral pulses may be absent.

Diagnosis

Ruptured aortic aneurysm is not infrequently misdiagnosed as ureteric colic. Adopt a low threshold of suspicion in any middle aged or elderly patient who presents with back pain, abdominal pain or collapse. In some patients (eg the obese), it may be difficult to be certain about the presence of a pulsatile abdominal mass. In such cases, assume that the problem is a ruptured abdominal aortic aneurysm and commence resuscitative measures, whilst appropriate experts are summoned and relevant emergency confirmatory investigations (eg USS or CT scan) are performed. It may be safer and quicker to perform USS in the ED, rather than transfer the patient for CT scan.

Management

- Provide high flow O_2.
- Obtain venous access with 2 large bore venous cannulae.
- Send blood for FBC, U&E, glucose, baseline coagulation screen, LFTs and emergency X-matching (10U red cells + 8U platelets + 8U fresh frozen plasma).
- Provide IV analgesia (eg morphine titrated according to response).
- Provide IV anti-emetic (eg cyclizine 50mg).
- Give IV fluids as necessary, but avoid excessive fluid resuscitation. Treat major hypovolaemia, but accept moderate degrees of hypotension (systolic BP > 90mmHg). In general, patients who are conscious and passing urine require minimal IV fluid therapy until they reach theatre.
- Obtain a CXR.
- Insert a urinary catheter and a radial arterial line and record an ECG.
- Call the vascular surgeon and anaesthetist at an early stage: aortic cross-clamping is the mainstay of resuscitation in the unstable patient.
- Ensure that other relevant staff (eg emergency theatre staff) are informed.

Acute limb ischaemia

Clinical features

Irrespective of the cause, the cardinal features of acute limb ischaemia are summarized by the 6 P's:

- Pain.
- Paraesthesia (later anaesthesia).
- Pallor (later mottled, cyanosed).
- Pulselessness.
- Paralysis (due to muscle damage—this may be irreversible after 4–6hr).
- Perishing cold.

Where an acute arterial occlusion occurs in a previously normal limb, the features of ischaemia will be ↑ because of the absence of a developed collateral circulation. In the absence of a traumatic cause (either direct arterial injury, or indirect injury such as compartment syndrome—📖 Crush syndrome, p.398) the commonest causes are embolism or thrombosis.

Embolic

Cardiac sources account for >80% (AF, post MI, prosthetic valves, atrial myxoma, vegetations, and rheumatic heart disease). Acute embolic events affect the legs much more often than the arms (ratio 5:1). Artery bifurcations are affected most commonly.

Risk factors Diabetes, smoking, hypertension, hypercholesterolaemia.

Past history Ask about previous transient ischaemic attack (TIA), stroke, MI.

Examination A clear demarcation between normal and ischaemic skin suggests an embolic cause of an acutely ischaemic limb. Look for potential sources of emboli (irregular pulse, abnormal heart sounds, murmurs, valve clicks, etc.). Check all pulses in both the affected and contralateral limbs. The presence of normal pulses in the contralateral limb suggests an embolic cause, whereas absent contralateral pulses makes thrombosis more likely (even if a potential embolic source exists).

Investigations ECG, CXR, U&E, CK, FBC, coagulation screen, ABG, urinalysis (checking for myoglobin), cross-match. Cardiac and/or abdominal USS may be required and if thrombosis in situ is suspected, angiography indicated.

Thrombotic

Thrombosis may develop acutely at the site of atheromatous disease. A previous history of intermittent claudication/vascular impairment is likely. The other limb is also likely to have features of chronic vascular insufficiency (muscle wasting, hair loss, ulceration).

Treatment

- Give appropriate pain relief (usually IV opioid).
- Correct hypovolaemia and other causes of low flow states as necessary.
- Re-vascularization is required within 6hr to avoid permanent muscle necrosis (and subsequent need for amputation) and metabolic effects (such as rhabdomyolysis and renal failure). If the cause is embolic, embolectomy is required. If thrombotic, angiography will define the site and extent of the lesion: thrombolysis ± reconstructive surgery is then undertaken.

Ophthalmology

Approach to eye problems

History

Always take a full ophthalmic history. Which eye is affected (are both)? What is the disturbance? Are there flashing lights or floaters? How quickly did the symptoms come on? How does it affect the patient's lifestyle (job, reading, watching TV)? Ask about prior ophthalmic/optician treatment and take a full medical and drug history. Family history of glaucoma may also be relevant.

Always measure visual acuity of patients presenting with eye problems. Patients with potentially serious pathology include those with:
• Sudden visual loss.
• Significantly ↓VA.
• Penetrating eye injuries.
• Chemical burns of the eye (these require immediate treatment and specialist referral).

Have a low threshold for involving an ophthalmologist if a patient who is already blind in one eye, presents with a problem with the 'good eye'.

Examination

Visual acuity (VA) is the key to eye examination: measure this first.
Failure to document VA may constitute negligence

Use a Snellen chart, read at 6m, for each eye separately. Allow patients to use glasses if available, if not employ a pinhole (made using a needle through a piece of card). Use of a pinhole eliminates refractive error.

VA is expressed as:
Distance from chart in m/no. of line on chart (normal vision is 6/6)

For example, a patient whose VA is recorded as Right eye 6/5; Left eye 6/60 can read the bottom line with the right eye, but only the top line with the left eye. If patients read additional letters of the line below, record using + number of extra letters (eg 6/12 + 2).

Bring patients unable to read chart at 6m forward until they can read the chart (eg 3/60 = top line read at 3m). Very poor vision: try counting fingers or detecting hand movement at 1m, or light perception.

A hand-held chart at 30cm is an alternative if a full Snellen chart is unavailable—ability to read small print implies normal VA for that eye. For patients who are illiterate, there is an alternative chart with various different versions of the letter 'E'—ask the patient to state which directions the 3 limbs of the letter point.

Pupils Record pupil size, shape, direct, and consensual responses to light and accommodation.

Eye movements Check full range and ask about diplopia. Look for nystagmus.

Visual fields Check carefully in patients with visual loss.

Fundoscopy In a darkened room, first note the presence of a red reflex. A lost or ↓red reflex is an abnormal finding, typically caused by vitreous haemorrhage, cataracts, or major corneal abrasions. Assess the optic discs, look for retinal haemorrhages and vessel abnormalities.

Direct assessment Under a bright light look for inflammation or FBs.

Subtarsal examination If there is a possibility of FB, evert the upper eyelid by pressing down lightly over the upper lid with a cotton bud or orange stick and rotating the lid upwards over it. Ask the patient to look down throughout.

Slit lamp examination Learn how to use a slit lamp. It allows a detailed view of conjunctiva, cornea, and anterior chamber. Fluorescein staining reveals corneal abnormalities, particularly when viewed under blue light, when abrasions appear green. Fluorescein is available either in drop form or dried onto a strip. Remember that fluorescein can permanently stain clothes and contact lenses.

Intraocular pressure Digital assessment is unreliable. Formal measurement of intra-ocular pressure is useful, but requires training and is left to the eye specialist in many departments.

Temporal arteries Palpate for tenderness if temporal arteritis is a possibility.

LA drops to aid examination

Sometimes, blepharospasm prevents satisfactory examination. Consider LA drops (1 or 2 drops of 1% amethocaine/tetracaine or 0.4% oxybupro-caine. 0.5% proxymetacaine causes less stinging and is useful in children). *Never discharge patients with a supply of local anaesthetic drops.*

Notes on ophthalmological treatments

Antibiotic ointment and drops Apply to the lower fornix (between lower eyelid and sclera) then ask the patient to keep the eye shut for 1–2min. Ointment has the advantage over drops in that it lasts longer: for example, chloramphenicol ointment needs to be given 4 times a day, whereas drops need to be given every 2hr initially. Theoretical concerns about aplastic anaemia are not well-founded (see the *BNF*).

Eye pads Previously recommended following the administration of LA drops and for patients with corneal abrasions, they tend not to be useful unless the pad seals the eyelid shut.

Driving Advise patients not to drive until their vision has returned to normal (this particularly applies after use of mydriatic agents). In addition, advise patients not to drive whilst wearing an eye pad. Document the advice given in the notes.

Ophthalmological trauma

Blunt eye injuries

Blunt injury to the face may result in injury to the orbit or its bony margins. Compression of the eye in an antero-posterior direction (eg squash ball or fist) can cause a *'blow-out' fracture* of the floor of the orbit.

Orbital compartment syndrome and blindness can arise from a *retrobulbar haematoma*. Unless diagnosed and treated as an emergency, optic nerve ischaemia develops and the patient can lose sight in the affected eye within a few hours. Proptosis, reduced eye movements, reduced visual acuity and pain all point to a retrobulbar haematoma. There may be an afferent pupillary defect.

Assessment
- Look for proptosis.
- Check visual acuity.
- Check pupillary reflexes.
- Check for enophthalmos and ↓infra-orbital nerve sensation, both found in a blowout fracture.
- Document range of eye movements, looking in particular for entrapment of the extra-ocular muscles.
- Look for a hyphaema (a horizontal fluid level in the anterior chamber when the patient is upright). It can cause pain, photophobia, blurred vision and can ↑intra-ocular pressure, causing nausea and vomiting.
- Stain the cornea and examine using slit lamp for corneal abrasions.
- Ophthalmoscopic examination may reveal lens dislocation, hyphaema, vitreous, subhyaloid, or retinal haemorrhage. Sometimes retinal oedema ('commotio retinae') may be seen as white patches with diffuse margins on the posterior pole of the eye.

X-ray if there is bony tenderness or clinical evidence of orbital or facial bone fracture.

Treatment
Any patient suspected of a retrobulbar haematoma requires an emergency lateral canthotomy. This should be performed by an ophthalmologist or a trained emergency physician, under local anaesthetic in the ED, and reduces the retro-orbital pressure.

Nurse patients with obvious globe injury head up at 45°. Refer urgently.

Provide prophylactic oral antibiotics (eg co-amoxiclav) for uncomplicated facial or orbital fractures, and arrange for maxillofacial follow-up, with advice to avoid nose-blowing in the meantime.

Penetrating eye injuries

Suspect *intraocular foreign body* if there is a history of hammering or work involving metal on metal. Find out if protective glasses were worn. Ascertain whether a small foreign body travelling at speed may have penetrated the orbit (eg during grinding, hammering, chiselling). Failure to suspect and diagnose these injuries can have serious consequences.

Assessment
- Check visual acuity.
- Look for pupil irregularity.
- Look for puncture/entry wounds on both aspects of the eyelids, the cornea and sclera. Corneoscleral wounds are often situated inferiorly, due to upturning of the eyeball as the patient blinks.
- Examine the anterior chamber. There may be a shallow anterior chamber, air bubbles, a flat cornea, deflated globe and a positive Seidel's test (dilution of fluorescein by aqueous humour leaking from the anterior chamber).
- Look for a hyphaema.
- Look for vitreous haemorrhage on fundoscopy.

X-ray all patients with possible globe penetration (consider also CT or USS)

Give analgesia, tetanus prophylaxis, IV antibiotics (eg 1.5g cefuroxime), and refer all patients with penetrating eye injuries immediately to an ophthalmologist, even if there are other major injuries needing attention at the same time.

Never manipulate or try to remove embedded objects (eg darts).

Corneal trauma

Conjunctival FB

The typical history is of dust or grit blown into an eye by the wind. The FB usually gravitates into the lower fornix—remove with a cotton bud.

Subtarsal FB

FBs may not gravitate into the lower fornix, but may remain stuck under the upper eyelid. The patient reports pain on blinking. Fluorescein staining reveals characteristic vertical corneal abrasions (the cornea has been likened to an 'ice rink'). Evert the upper eyelid and remove the FB with a cotton bud. Discharge with topical antibiotic (eg chloramphenicol ointment qds or fusidic acid eye drops).

Corneal abrasions

Often result from a newspaper or fingernail in the eye. Irritation, photophobia, and lacrimation occur. Use LA drops and fluorescein staining to examine the cornea. Exclude FB or penetrating injury. Prescribe regular antibiotic ointment (eg chloramphenicol) and oral analgesia. An eye patch which seals eyelids closed will aid the symptoms and recovery. If the patient is very uncomfortable, consider instilling a drop of 1% cyclopentolate to dilate the pupil (this reduces iris spasm) or a drop of 0.1% diclofenac. Advise the patient not to drive until vision has returned to normal. Advise also to return for review if symptoms continue beyond 36hr.

Corneal foreign body

Instill LA and attempt removal with a cotton bud. If unsuccessful, remove with a blue (23G) needle introduced from the side (ideally using a slit lamp). Ensure that the patient's head is firmly fixed and cannot move forwards onto the needle: it can help for the operator's hand to rest lightly on the patient's cheek. After complete removal of the FB, check that the anterior chamber is intact, instill and prescribe antibiotic ointment, and advise the patient to return if symptomatic at 36hr. Refer patients with large, deep or incompletely removed FB, or if a rust ring remains.

Arc (welder's) eye/'snowblindness'

Exposure to ultraviolet light can cause superficial keratitis. Climbers/skiers, welders, and sunbed users who have not used protective goggles develop pain, watering, and blepharospasm several hours later. LA drops allow examination with fluorescein staining, revealing multiple punctate corneal lesions. Consider instilling a drop of 1% cyclopentolate or 0.1% diclofenac into both eyes. Discharge with an eye pad, oral analgesia, and advice not to drive until recovered. Anticipate resolution within 24hr. Do not discharge with LA drops.

Chemical eye burns

Chemical burns from alkali or acid are serious. Triage urgently ahead, check Toxbase and provide immediate eye irrigation with lukewarm normal saline for at least 20min, or until the pH of tears has returned to normal (7.4). A 1L bag of 0.9% saline with standard IV tubing is ideal. LA may be needed to enable full irrigation. Identify the substance involved and contact Poisons Unit. Refer alkali and acid burns immediately.

Superglued eyelids

Wash with warm water. The eye will open within 4 days. If the patient reports a FB sensation, this may represent a lump of glue, which may cause an abrasion if left untreated: refer to the ophthalmologist.

Contact lens problems

Contact lenses are of two basic types: hard or soft. Soft lenses, composed of hydrogels, are more comfortable to wear. Avoid using fluorescein with contact lenses, as permanent staining may occur.

'Stuck lens'

Most contact lens users are adept at removing their contact lenses. New users, however, not infrequently experience difficulty in their removal. Moisten soft lenses with saline, then remove by pinching between finger and thumb. Special suction devices are available to help remove hard lenses.

'Lost lens'

Patients may present concerned that they are unable to find their contact lens and cannot remember it falling out. Check under both eyelids carefully (evert the upper lid if the lens is not immediately apparent) and remove the offending lens, if present.

Hypersensitivity and overuse

Preservatives in lens cleaning fluid cause itching and may evoke a reaction. Advise to stop using the lenses, give local antibiotic ointment and arrange ophthalmological follow-up.

Acanthamoeba keratitis

This is a protozoal infection of the cornea which occurs in contact lens users, associated with poor lens hygiene or swimming whilst wearing contact lenses. The eye becomes painful and red. Corneal oedema and ulceration develops. If acanthamoeba infection is suspected, refer immediately for ophthalmological care.

Other problems

Treat and refer conjunctivitis, corneal abrasions, or ulcers apparently related to contact lenses as outlined opposite. Advise avoidance of use of both contact lenses until the problem has resolved.

Sudden visual loss

Sudden visual loss requires emergency assessment and treatment.

Amaurosis fugax

The patient describes temporary loss of vision in one eye, like a 'curtain coming down', with complete recovery after a few seconds to minutes. The cause is usually a thrombotic embolus in the retinal, ophthalmic, or ciliary artery, originating from a carotid atheromatous plaque. Refer urgently to the ophthalmology team.

Central retinal artery occlusion

The central retinal artery is an end artery. Occlusion is usually embolic (check for atrial fibrillation and listen for carotid bruits), causing sudden painless ↓VA to counting fingers or no light perception. The patient may have a history of amaurosis fugax. Direct pupil reaction is sluggish or absent in the affected eye, but it reacts to consensual stimulation (afferent pupillary defect). Fundoscopy reveals a pale retina, with a swollen pale optic disc and 'cherry red macula spot' (the retina is thinnest here and the underlying choroidal circulation is normal). Retinal blood vessels are attenuated and irregular: there may be 'cattle-trucking' in arteries.

Treat by digitally massaging the globe for 5–15sec then release and repeat to dislodge the embolus, whilst awaiting the urgent arrival of an ophthalmologist.

If there is any delay in the patient being seen by the ophthalmologist, consider (and discuss) the following options:
• Giving sublingual glyceryl trinitrate (GTN).
• Giving IV 500mg acetazolamide (to ↓intra-ocular pressure).
• Reconsider the diagnosis. In particular, consider whether or not temporal arteritis is a possibility: ask about jaw claudication, headaches, scalp tenderness.

Central retinal vein occlusion

This is a more frequent cause of sudden painless visual loss than arterial occlusion. Predisposing factors include: old age, chronic glaucoma, arteriosclerosis, hypertension, polycythaemia. Examination reveals ↓VA, often with an afferent pupillary defect. Fundoscopy reveals a 'stormy sunset' appearance: hyperaemia with engorged veins and adjacent flame-shaped haemorrhages. The disc may be obscured by haemorrhages and oedema. Cotton wool spots may be seen. Although the outcome is variable and there is no specific treatment, refer urgently as the underlying cause may be treatable, thus protecting the other eye.

Temporal (giant cell) arteritis

Inflammation of the posterior ciliary arteries causes ischaemic optic neuritis and visual loss. It is relatively common in those aged >50 years and is associated with polymyalgia rheumatica. The other eye remains at risk until treatment is commenced. Rapid and profound visual loss may be preceded by headaches, jaw claudication, general malaise, and muscular pains. The temporal arteries are characteristically tender to palpation. Retinal appearances have been termed 'pale papilloedema': the ischaemic disc is pale, waxy, elevated and has splinter haemorrhages on it. If suspected, give 200mg IV hydrocortisone immediately, check erythrocyte sedimentation rate (ESR) (typically >>40mm/hr, but can be normal) and refer urgently.

Vitreous haemorrhage

Occurs in diabetics with new vessel formation, in bleeding disorders and in retinal detachment. Small bleeds may produce vitreous floaters with little visual loss. Large bleeds result in painless ↓↓VA, an absent red reflex and difficulty visualizing the retina. Refer urgently. Meanwhile, elevate the head of the bed to allow blood to collect inferiorly.

Retinal detachment

Occurs in myopes, diabetics, the elderly and following trauma. The rate of onset is variable: patients may report premonitory flashing lights or a 'snow-storm', before developing cloudy vision. There may be a visual field defect. Macular involvement causes ↓VA. The affected retina is dark and opalescent, but may be difficult to visualize by standard ophthalmoscopy. Refer urgently for surgery and re-attachment.

Optic neuritis

Usually presents in a young woman. Optic nerve inflammation causes visual loss over a few days. Pain on eye movement may occur. An afferent pupillary defect is associated with ↓VA, ↓colour vision (colour red looks faded) and normal/swollen optic disc. Most recover untreated, later some develop multiple sclerosis. Refer to the ophthalmologist.

Other causes

Patients with chronic visual loss due to a variety of conditions may present acutely (senile macular degeneration, glaucoma, optic atrophy, cataract, choroidoretinitis). Drugs which can cause painless visual loss include methanol (p.202) and quinine (in overdose). Refer immediately all patients in whom an acute visual loss cannot be excluded.

The red eye

Patients commonly present with a red eye with no history of trauma, but it is critical not to miss certain diagnoses. Refer all patients with new findings of ↓VA, abnormal pupil reactions, or corneal abnormalities.

Orbital and preseptal cellulitis

This is a major infection of the orbital tissues. The infection is most frequently spread from the paranasal sinuses (ethmoid sinusitis), facial skin or lacrimal sac. Occasionally, the infection follows direct trauma to the orbit or from haematogenous spread. Patients present with fever, eyelid swelling, erythema, and proptosis. Always assess patient for signs of severe sepsis (🕮 Severe sepsis and shock, p.59) and resuscitate as necessary. Obtain venous access, take blood for cultures, commence intravenous antibiotics (eg co-amoxiclav) and fluids. Refer urgently to the ophthalmologist. Some aggressive infections may require surgical treatment. Cavernous sinus thrombosis and meningitis are potential complications.

Acute iritis (acute uveitis)

A relapsing condition of the young and middle-aged associated with ankylosing spondylitis, ulcerative colitis, sarcoid, AIDS, and Behçet's syndrome.

Symptoms include Acute onset pain, photophobia, 'floaters', blurred vision and watering.

Signs ↓VA, tender eye felt through the upper eyelid, circumcorneal erythema, small pupil (may be irregular due to previous adhesions). Shining a light into the 'good' eye causes pain in the other. Pain ↑ as eyes converge and pupils react to accommodation (Talbot's test). Slit lamp may reveal hypopyon and white precipitates on the posterior cornea.

Refer urgently to the ophthalmologist for steroid eye drops, pupil dilatation, analgesia, investigation, and follow-up.

Acute closed angle glaucoma

Long-sighted middle-aged or elderly with shallow anterior chambers are at risk. Sudden blocked drainage of aqueous humor into the canal of Schlemm causes intra-ocular pressure to increase from 10–20mmHg up to 70mmHg. This may be caused by anticholinergic drugs or pupil dilatation at night (reading in dim light).

Symptoms include preceding episodes of blurred vision or haloes around lights due to corneal oedema. Acute blockage causes severe eye pain, nausea/vomiting.

Signs ↓VA, hazy oedematous cornea with circumcorneal erythema and a fixed semi-dilated ovoid pupil. The eye feels tender and hard through the upper eyelid. Measure intraocular pressure if this facility is available.

Treatment Instill a 4% pilocarpine drop every 15min to produce ciliary muscle contraction and aqueous humor drainage. Apply prophylactic 1% pilocarpine drops into the other eye also. Give analgesia (eg morphine IV with anti-emetic). Arrange an emergency ophthalmology opinion: consider giving acetazolamide 500mg IV (to ↓intra-ocular pressure) meantime and/or mannitol 20% up to 500mL intravenous infusion over 1hr.

Conjunctivitis

Caused by bacteria (*Strep. pneumoniae* or *H. influenza*), viruses (adenovirus), or allergy. The sensation of a FB may involve both eyes. The conjunctiva is red and inflamed, sometimes with eyelid swelling. VA and pupils are normal. Bacterial infection classically produces sticky mucopurulent tears, viral infection copious watery tears (associated with photophobia and pre-auricular lymphadenopathy in the highly contagious adenoviral 'epidemic keratoconjunctivitis'). Prescribe antibiotic eye drops or ointment (eg fusidic acid, chloramphenicol, or gentamicin) regularly for 5 days. Advise not to share towels or pillows. Most cases settle relatively quickly: advise patients to return if symptoms do not improve within 4 days.

Ulcerative keratitis

Corneal ulceration causes pain with photophobia. It is apparent on fluorescein staining under a slit lamp.
- Hypopyon (pus in the anterior chamber) implies bacterial infection.
- Vesicles in the ophthalmic division of the trigeminal nerve occur with herpes zoster infection.
- A dendritic branching ulcerative pattern suggests herpes simplex. If this is misdiagnosed and steroid eye drops given, ulceration can be disastrous. As a non-specialist, do not prescribe steroid eye drops—leave this to the ophthalmologist.

Whatever the infective agent, refer corneal ulceration immediately.

Episcleritis

Inflammation beneath one area of the conjunctiva is usually associated with a nodule and a dull aching discomfort. VA, pupils, and anterior chamber are normal. Prescribe oral NSAIDs and advise outpatient follow-up to consider steroid eye drops if there is no resolution.

Blepharitis

This chronic problem is quite common. Eyelashes are matted together and itchy. Ensure that there is no associated corneal ulceration, provide topical antibiotics (eg chloramphenicol) and refer for GP follow-up.

External hordeolum (stye)

Treat staphylococcal infections of eyelash roots with antibiotics drops.

Internal hordeolum (chalazion)

A chalazion is an inflammatory reaction in a blocked meibomian gland, which may become secondarily infected. Treat infected tarsal (meibomian) glands with topical antibiotics (eg chloramphenicol) together with oral antibiotics (eg co-amoxiclav). Refer patients who develop an abscess or nodule affecting vision.

Dacrocystitis

Acute infection of the lacrimal sac may follow nasolacrimal duct obstruction. Treat early infections with oral antibiotics (co-amoxiclav); later, refer for drainage.

Subconjunctival haemorrhage

This usually presents as a painless, well-defined area of haemorrhage over the sclera. May result from vomiting or sneezing. Following trauma, consider orbital or base of skull fracture and treat accordingly.

Ear, nose and throat

Ear, nose, and throat foreign bodies

Ear foreign bodies

All sorts of FBs may become lodged in the external auditory canal, including insects, vegetable matter, and various inert objects. The patient may present with pain, deafness, discharge or, in the case of live insects, an irritating buzzing in one ear.

Diagnosis depends upon direct visualization with the auriscope. In children, remember that, as with FBs elsewhere, there may be no history of FB available.

Removal
- Many FBs can be removed under direct vision with hooks. Manipulate gently to avoid causing damage or further impaction.
- Drown live insects in 2% lidocaine first.
- Do not try to syringe out vegetable matter with water, as this may cause swelling and pain.
- If there is some difficulty (eg ball bearing or bead in an uncooperative child), refer to ear, nose, and throat (ENT) department to consider removal under GA. Removal of beads using an orange stick with a tiny amount of superglue on the end has been described, but carries some obvious dangers and requires complete patient co-operation.

Embedded ear-rings The 'butterfly' piece of an ear ring may become embedded in the posterior part of the ear lobe, causing inflammation or infection. The ear-rings are usually easily removed once adequate analgesia has been established: render the ear anaesthetized with a greater auricular nerve block (🕮 Nerve blocks of forehead and ear, p.300), or directly infiltrate local anaesthetic into the lobe, remembering that this is a highly sensitive area. The butterfly is released by applying pressure in a posterior direction. Occasionally, forceps and a small posterior skin incision may be required to open up the track. If there is evidence of infection, prescribe antibiotics (eg co-amoxiclav) and arrange GP follow-up. Advise the patient not to wear ear-rings until the symptoms have settled.

Nasal foreign bodies

Usually affects children, who present with offensive unilateral nasal discharge. Also occurs in adults with psychotic illness or learning disabilities.

Removal Remove easily accessible, anterior nasal FBs in ED. However, there is a risk of aspiration with any nasal FB, particularly in uncooperative patients. Refer such patients to an ENT surgeon for removal with airway protection. Instruct the patient to blow their nose whilst occluding the unaffected nostril. If unsuccessful, consider attempting removal with a nasal speculum, hook, and forceps, as appropriate. A fine bore tracheal suction catheter attached to wall suction can also work. One technique which has been reported in cooperative children is to ask a parent to blow into the child's mouth ('parent's kiss'), having first ensured a good seal and also occluded the normal nostril.

Nasal button, batteries, or magnets (🕮 p.213) can cause significant damage, so refer to ENT.

Inhaled foreign bodies

Aspiration causing complete upper airway obstruction is an emergency, requiring immediate intervention (📖 p.324). FBs lodged in the larynx or tracheobronchial tree cause persistent coughing. There may not be a clear history—a coughing/spluttering episode in a child should arouse suspicion of an inhaled FB. Auscultation of the chest is often normal, but may reveal wheezes or localized absence of breath sounds.

CXR may be normal or show a radio-opaque FB with distal consolidation or hyperinflation (FB acting as a ball valve). A CXR in expiration may show this more clearly. Refer to a cardiothoracic surgeon.

Ingested foreign bodies

Various FBs, both radio-opaque (eg coins, rings) and non-radio-opaque (eg plastic pen tops, aluminium ring pulls) are frequently swallowed by children and by adults with psychiatric disorders. Provided the FB reaches the stomach, it is likely to pass through the remainder of the gastrointestinal tract without incident. An exception is button battery ingestion (📖 p.213). For radio-opaque FBs, confirm with lateral neck X-ray and CXR that it is not impacted in the oesophagus. A metal detector may confirm a swallowed coin has reached the stomach. Refer patients who are symptomatic, have impacted FBs, or who have swallowed potentially dangerous items (button batteries, razor blades, open safety pins). Note that magnets can be dangerous if two or more are ingested, since they can attract each other through tissues and cause pressure necrosis/perforation of bowel. Only discharge patients who are asymptomatic (with advice to return if they develop abdominal pain and/or vomiting), and arrange suitable follow-up. Unless the ingested FB is valuable or of great sentimental value, examination of the stools by the patient for the FB is unnecessary. It may take weeks to pass.

Impacted fish bones

Fish bones often become stuck in the pharynx or oesophagus. Direct visualization with a good light (a head torch can be useful) and wooden spatula acting as tongue depressor may reveal fish bones lodged in the tonsils or base of the tongue—remove with Tilley's forceps. If no FB is seen, obtain soft-tissue lateral neck X-rays (look for prevertebral soft tissue swelling and fish bone, bearing in mind not all are radio-opaque), then refer to ENT for endoscopy. Depending on local policy, the ENT team may decide to see the patient immediately, or (provided the patient can swallow) the following day (in which case discuss the need for prophylactic antibiotics). A fish bone can scratch the pharynx causing sensation of a FB to persist after it has gone.

Oesophageal food bolus obstruction

Usually involves a lump of meat. Patients with complete obstruction present unable to swallow solids or liquids (including their own saliva). There may be retrosternal discomfort. Refer to the surgical team for endoscopy. Glucagon (1mg IV) relieves some episodes of food bolus obstruction, but endoscopy is still advisable to look for oesophageal stenosis or malignancy.

Ear examination

Scope of the examination

Full ear examination includes assessment of the vestibulocochlear nerve and auroscope examination. Check for mastoid or pinna tenderness. Look at the external ear canal for discharge, or swelling and examine the tympanic membrane for colour, translucency, bulging, and the cone of light.

Assessing hearing

Hearing can be assessed by asking the patient to place one finger in their ear. Stand a foot behind the patient's unoccluded ear and whisper a two syllable word. Ask the patient to repeat the word.

Weber's and Rinne's tests

Weber's test—strike a 512Hz tuning fork and place in the centre of the forehead. In conductive deafness, the sound localizes to the deaf ear, with sensorineural deafness, the sound localizes to the good ear.

Rinne's test—strike a 512Hz tuning fork and place it on the mastoid process. Ask the patient to tell you when they no longer hear the sound, then immediately place in front of the auditory meatus. In a normal ear, air conduction is heard for twice as long as bone conduction. In conductive deafness, bone conduction is heard for longer than air conduction. In sensorineural deafness, air conduction is heard longer than bone conduction.

Nystagmus

To complete assessment of the vestibulocochlear nerve, examine for nystagmus. All forms of nystagmus can be associated with intracranial lesions, as well as peripheral causes; however, downbeat and upbeat nystagmus in particular, signify a central cause. Tinnitus or deafness tends to suggest a peripheral cause. Peripheral nystagmus is exacerbated by gazing towards the side of the fast phase (Alexander's Law). Central nystagmus may change direction, depending on the side of gaze.

Vertigo

Vertigo is the impression or illusion of movement when there is none. Take care to distinguish vertigo from the more general term of 'dizziness', which is often used to describe a feeling of light-headedness.

Causes

- Benign positional vertigo. Diagnosed with Hallpike's test which induces positional vertigo. Mostly caused by posterior semicircular canal canalithiasis. Medications are ineffective.
- Ménière's disease: a disorder of the inner ear. Patients have recurrent vertigo, tinnitus and deafness and should be managed by ENT.
- Acute labyrinthitis: Caused by reactivation of herpes simplex virus. Some have an upper respiratory tract prodrome. Some individuals are unable to work or perform normal daily duties because of vertigo and vomiting.
- Otitis media.
- Acoustic neuroma (or vestibular schwannoma). This presents with slow onset deafness and tinnitus. Dizziness is less common.
- Cholesteatoma.
- Stroke or transient ischaemic attack.
- Trauma.
- Wax or FB in the ear.

Take a careful history and examine for causes of vertigo. Manage patients who present with vertigo according to the underlying cause. The cause may be unclear, in which case refer to the medical/ENT team as appropriate.

Cochlear implants

Cochlear implants consist of an implanted radio receiver and decoder package containing a magnet (above and behind the ear), together with a removable external microphone/radio transmitter. X-rays and CT do not damage this device, provided that the external microphone/transmitter is first removed and switched off. MRI can cause significant damage to the device and the patient. If there are concerns relating to a cochlear implant, refer to ENT. In particular, refer patients with:

- Significant direct trauma, including exposure by a scalp wound.
- Suspected otitis media of the implanted ear.

Earache

Otitis externa

Often caused by *Pseudomonas, Staph. aureus, Strep. pneumoniae, E. coli*. Common in swimmers/surfers and after minor trauma. This causes intense itching and pain, which gradually increases. Discharge and hearing loss may be present (profuse discharge implies middle ear disease). On examination, the external canal is inflamed and oedematous. Oedema and debris may obscure the tympanic membrane. Pain is induced by pressing on the tragus or pulling the pinna.

Management Prescribe topical antibiotics and topical steroids, advise against swimming, and arrange GP follow-up. In severe cases (eg if the drum is not visible), refer to an ENT surgeon for aural toilet to remove debris from the auditory canal.

Cellulitis or furunculosis of the ear canal

Cellulitis of the ear canal may be caused by scratching or by infection of hair follicles (furunculosis). *Staph. aureus* is the usual organism. Itching and a feeling of pressure are followed by pain in the ear, with deafness if the ear canal is occluded by swelling. Examination shows swelling and inflammation of the ear canal, with tenderness over the tragus and pain on movement of the ear.

Treat with analgesia (eg NSAID) and antibiotics (eg flucloxacillin 500mg PO qds for 5 days). Arrange follow-up by a GP (or ENT in severe cases).

Acute otitis media

Most common in children aged 3–6 years and may follow an upper respiratory tract infection. Commonest pathogens are *Strep. pneumoniae* and *H. influenzae*.

Presentation Earache may be accompanied by fever, deafness, irritability and lethargy. Typically, hearing loss precedes pain. Examination of the tympanic membrane shows evidence of inflammation with loss of the light reflex and bulging of the drum. Eventual perforation results in purulent discharge with some relief of pain. Look for associated swelling/tenderness over the mastoid—this implies secondary mastoiditis (see below).

Treatment Prescribe oral analgesia. The use of antibiotics remains very controversial. Oral antibiotics (eg 5-day course of amoxicillin or clarithromycin) are of questionable value, but are frequently given. Consider oral antibiotics if no improvement within 72hr, or earlier if there is deterioration or perforation. If perforation has occurred (often heralded by a sudden ↑ pain), arrange ENT follow-up and advise not to swim. Otherwise, arrange GP follow-up.

Acute mastoiditis

This is an uncommon, but important diagnosis to make, because of the risk of intracranial spread of infection. Mastoiditis follows an episode of acute otitis media—consider it if there is no response to therapy (eg discharging ear for >10 days). Suspect it if there is pain, redness, swelling or tenderness over the mastoid process. The pinna may be pushed forwards/outwards—swelling may mean that the drum is not visible. Refer urgently to the ENT surgeon for admission and IV antibiotics.

Cholesteatoma

This erosive condition affects the middle ear and mastoid. A cholesteatoma can result in life-threatening intracranial infection. There may be an offensive discharge, with conductive hearing loss, vertigo or facial nerve palsy. Tympanic membrane examination shows granulation tissue and/or perforation with white debris. Refer to the ENT surgeon.

Traumatic tympanic membrane rupture

This may result from direct penetrating injury, blast injury (📖 p.389) or basal skull fracture (📖 p.361). Pain is associated with ↓ hearing. Perforation is visible on examination.

Treatment Most heal spontaneously with conservative measures and advice to keep out of water. Arrange ENT follow-up and give prophylactic oral antibiotics according to local policy. Note that gentamicin or neomycin eardrops may cause sensorineural deafness because of ototoxicity when the tympanic membrane is ruptured.

Barotrauma

Sudden changes in atmospheric pressure with a blocked Eustachian tube can result in pain and hearing loss. This usually affects aircraft passengers and divers, especially if they have a cold (viral upper respiratory tract infection). Pain is often relieved by the Valsalva manoeuvre (breathing out with the mouth closed, while pinching the nose). Decongestant nasal spray may help if the problem does not resolve spontaneously. Give analgesia (NSAID). Arrange ENT follow-up if the pain persists.

Epistaxis

Nasal bleeding may be idiopathic or follow minor trauma (eg nose picking). When it occurs in patients with hypertension and coagulation disorders haemorrhage can be severe with significant mortality. Epistaxis may follow isolated nasal fracture and more major facial injury.

Site of bleeding

Most nasal bleeding is from the anterior nasal septum in or close to Little's area. A few patients have posterior nasal bleeding, which may be brisk.

Equipment

Direct visualization of the anterior nasal cavity is aided by a headlamp (eg battery-operated head torch), fine soft suction catheter, and nasal speculum. Wear goggles to avoid blood splashes in the eyes.

Initial approach

Associated facial injury Assess ABC (especially pulse and BP) and resuscitate as necessary. Treat hypovolaemia vigorously.

No associated injury Check airway patency, pulse, and BP. Treat hypovolaemia aggressively. Check coagulation status of patients on anticoagulants and treat appropriately (📖 p.170). Sit the patient up and instruct them to compress the fleshy part of their nose between finger and thumb for 10min. If this stops the bleeding, the patient may be discharged after 30min observation.

Continuing bleeding after pressure

Adults Apply a cotton wool pledget soaked in 4% lidocaine with 1 in 1000 adrenaline. Then, with a headlamp and nasal speculum, try to identify the bleeding point. Treat small anterior bleeding points with cautious cautery by applying a silver nitrate stick for 10–15sec. Avoid excessive cautery and never cauterize both sides of the septum—this may cause septal necrosis. If cautery stops the bleeding, observe for 15min, and discharge with GP follow-up. Advise avoidance of sniffing, picking or blowing the nose meantime.

Children Applying nasal antiseptic cream (eg Naseptin®) is as effective as cautery in stopping bleeding. The cream is relatively easy to apply.

Continuing bleeding despite cautery

Insert a nasal pack. A specialized compressed surgical sponge nasal tampon (eg Merocel® or Rapid Rhino) is ideal: gently insert a lubricated tampon (horizontally) and 'inflate' with a 10mL syringe of saline. Alternatively, pack the nose in a traditional way with 1.25cm wide ribbon gauze soaked in oily paste (eg bismuth iodoform paraffin paste). Once packing has stopped the bleeding, refer to ENT for admission: observation is advisable (especially in the elderly). The pack may dislodge and obstruct the airway.

Continuing bleeding despite packing

Refer to the ENT surgeon. The bleeding site is likely to be posterior and can cause hypovolaemic shock. In this situation, insert 2 large bore venous cannulae, send blood for FBC, coagulation screen, cross-matching, and commence an IVI.

Posterior nasal bleeding usually responds to tamponade with a Foley catheter. Remove the nasal tampon and insert a lubricated, uninflated Foley catheter through the bleeding nostril into the nasopharynx. Inflate the balloon with air and gently withdraw the catheter, thus tamponading the bleeding site. Secure the catheter to the cheek with tape, and then re-insert the anterior nasal tampon.

Nasal fracture

The prominent exposed position of the nose, combined with the delicacy of its bones, render it relatively prone to injury.

Remember that the nose is part of the head, so nose injury = head injury (and potentially cervical spine injury also).

History

The nose is commonly broken by a direct blow (eg from a punch) or following a fall onto the face. Nasal fracture is usually accompanied by bleeding. Search for a history of associated facial/head injury (diplopia, loss of consciousness, etc.).

Examination

This is a clinical diagnosis based upon a history of injury with nasal swelling and tenderness. Having made the diagnosis, assess whether there is nasal deviation: it is useful to ask the patient to look in a mirror. Check and record whether the patient can breathe through each nostril. Look for an associated septal haematoma—this will appear as a smooth bulging swelling, which may obstruct the nasal passage. Children are at particular risk of septal haematoma, which predisposes to secondary infection and septal necrosis.

Assess for additional injuries to the head or face (eg tender mandible, diplopia, tender maxilla). Injury to the bridge of the nose may result in persistent epistaxis and/or cerebrospinal fluid rhinorrhoea.

Investigation

Do not X-ray to diagnose a nasal fracture—the diagnosis is a clinical one. Obtain appropriate X-rays (eg orthopantomogram (OPG) or facial views) if there is clinical suspicion of other bony injuries. Nasal fractures are often apparent on facial X-rays or CT scans.

Treatment

- Resuscitate and treat for associated head injury.
- Continuing nasal haemorrhage is uncommon—refer to an ENT surgeon to consider urgent manipulation under anaesthetic (MUA) to stop the bleeding: meanwhile, insert a nasal tampon.
- Refer urgently to an ENT surgeon if there is a septal haematoma—this will require incision and drainage in order to prevent septal necrosis.
- Clean and close overlying skin wounds: steristrips often allow good skin apposition. If there is significant contamination of the wound, start a course of prophylactic oral antibiotics (eg co-amoxiclav: one tablet PO tds for 5 days).
- Provide oral analgesia (eg ibuprofen 400mg PO tds).
- If the nose is deviated/distorted, or if there is too much swelling to judge, arrange for ENT follow-up at 5–7 days, so that MUA may be performed within 10 days. It is particularly important to ensure accurate reduction of fractures in children.
- Discharge with head injury instructions to the care of a relative.

Sore throat

Tonsillitis

Causes Acute pharyngo-tonsillitis may result from infection with a variety of viruses or bacteria:

- *Viral:* Epstein–Barr virus (EBV), *herpes simplex virus, adenoviruses.*
- *Bacterial:* group A *β-haemolytic streptococcus* (most common bacterial cause), *mycoplasma, Corynebacterium diphtheriae.*

Features Sore throat is frequently accompanied by fever, headache, and mild dysphagia. Inspection of the tonsils reveals inflammation—the presence of pus on the tonsils suggests bacterial infection. Enlarged cervical lymph nodes are found in a variety of infections, but generalized lymphadenopathy (sometimes also with splenomegaly) is indicative of glandular fever (infectious mononucleosis—see 📖 p.241).

Diagnosis Despite the clinical pointers described above, it is usually impossible to distinguish clinically bacterial from viral causes.

Investigation Consider throat swabs and anti-streptolysin titre in severe cases. If glandular fever is suspected, send blood for FBC and Paul–Bunnell (or Monospot) test.

Treatment Unless contraindicated, give paracetamol (1g PO qds PRN) or ibuprofen (400mg PO tds PRN) and discharge to GP. Although frequently prescribed, oral antibiotics are rarely of benefit: a sensible approach is to limit their use for patients with any of the following: a history of valvular heart disease, immunosupression, diabetes, marked systemic upset, peritonsillar cellulitis, known β–haemolytic streptococci. In this case, prescribe penicillin 500mg PO qds for 5 days (or clarithromycin 500mg PO bd for 5 days if allergic). Avoid ampicillin, amoxicillin, and co-amoxiclav, which cause a rash in patients infected with EBV.

Occasionally, patients with acute tonsillitis may be unable to swallow fluids (this is more commonly a feature of peritonsillar or retropharyngeal abscess). In this case, refer for IV antibiotics and IV fluids.

Complications Otitis media, sinusitis, retropharyngeal abscess, peritonsillar abscess.

Peritonsillar abscess (quinsy)

Typically, preceded by a sore throat for several days, the development of a peritonsillar abscess is heralded by high fever, pain localized to one side of the throat, and pain on swallowing. Difficulty swallowing can result in drooling. Trismus may make inspection difficult, but if visualized there is tense bulging tonsil, pushing the uvula away from the affected side. Group A β-haemolytic streptococci are frequently implicated.

Treatment Insert an IV cannula and give IV benzyl penicillin 1.2g (clarithromycin 500mg if allergic to penicillin), and refer immediately to an ENT surgeon for aspiration or formal drainage.

Retropharyngeal abscess

Spread of infection from adjacent lymph nodes may occasionally cause a retropharyngeal abscess, particularly in children aged <3 years.

It is characterized by a sore throat, difficulty swallowing, fever, and dehydration. In children, cough is typically absent from the history (unlike in croup and other viral causes of upper airway obstruction). There may be evidence of airway compromise (stridor, neck hyperextension, signs of hypoxia). The differential diagnosis includes acute epiglottitis (📖 p.677). Lateral X-rays of the neck show soft tissue swelling (obtain these in the resuscitation room, rather than moving the patient to the X-ray department).

Treatment Get senior ED, ENT, and anaesthetic help. If the patient is a child with evidence of respiratory distress, do not upset them further. Airway obstruction may be precipitated by examination of the throat, so avoid this until appropriate staff and equipment are ready to cope with airway problems. The child can sit on mum's knee in the resuscitation room. On suspicion of a retropharyngeal abscess in an adult, insert an IV cannula, take bloods and blood cultures, give IV fluids and IV co-amoxiclav 1.2g, and refer immediately to an ENT surgeon.

Pharyngeal burns after cocaine use

Smoking cocaine can result in dangerous burns of the throat, since the drug acts as a local anaesthetic. Swelling of the epiglottis may result in airway obstruction.

Paranasal sinusitis

Bacterial infection may result from direct spread from infected tooth roots or (more usually) be secondary to viral upper respiratory tract infection (URTI).

Clinical features
- Clear nasal discharge becoming purulent.
- Pain in (and often also tenderness over) the affected sinus.
- Fever.
- Headache and/or toothache.

Management
Provide analgesia. Despite a lack of convincing evidence, oral antibiotics (eg amoxicillin, doxycycline or erythromycin) and nasal decongestant (eg 1% ephedrine) are commonly given. Advise GP follow-up. In severe cases, refer to ENT.

Facial nerve palsy

The facial (VII) nerve supplies the muscles of facial expression. Clinical examination reveals whether facial nerve palsy is of upper motor neurone or lower motor neurone type.

Upper motor neurone paralysis is usually due to a stroke (p.144), resulting in unilateral facial muscle weakness, but with sparing of the muscles of the forehead. If stroke is the cause, there may be additional evidence elsewhere (eg hemiparesis affecting the limbs).

Lower motor neurone paralysis of the facial nerve results in weakness of the muscles of one side of the face. The facial nerve arises from its nucleus in the pons, emerges from the pons to travel past the cerebello-pontine angle, through the petrous part of the temporal bone, to emerge from the stylomastoid foramen and thence into the parotid gland, where it divides into branches. During its passage through the petrous temporal bone, the facial nerve is accompanied by the *chorda tympani* (carrying taste fibres from the anterior 2/3 of one half of the tongue) and gives off the *nerve to stapedius*. Lesions of the facial nerve in the temporal bone therefore produce loss of taste and hyperacusis (noise is distorted and sounds loud) on the affected side.

Causes of lower motor neurone facial palsy

- Bell's palsy: the commonest cause (see below).
- Pontine tumours and vascular events: usually associated with other signs.
- Acoustic neuroma: usually with evidence of other nerve involvement (V, VI, VIII nerves) at the cerebello-pontine angle.
- Ramsay–Hunt syndrome (herpes zoster infection—see below).
- Trauma.
- Middle ear infection and cholesteatoma (see Earache, p.550).
- Sarcoidosis.
- Parotid gland tumours, trauma and infection.
- Human immunodeficiency virus (HIV).

Bell's palsy

Bell's palsy is the commonest cause of sudden onset isolated lower motor neurone facial nerve palsy. It is believed to result from viral infection, producing swelling of the facial nerve within the temporal bone: there may be associated hyperacusis and loss of taste of the anterior two-thirds of one half of the tongue. The absence of involvement of other cranial nerves is a reassuring feature, helping to secure this clinical diagnosis.

Treatment Most patients recover completely over several months without treatment—a small percentage are left with permanent weakness. Recovery is quicker if prednisolone is started within 72hr of the onset of symptoms (prednisolone 60mg daily for 5 days, then 10mg less each day; total of 10 days of treatment). Antiviral drugs do not seem to be helpful. Advise the use of artificial tears and an eye patch at night, to prevent corneal drying, and refer for ENT follow up.

Ramsay–Hunt syndrome

This is due to herpes zoster infection of the geniculate ganglion. Clinical features of Bell's palsy are present, together with (painful) herpetic vesicles present in the external auditory meatus and occasionally also, the soft palate. Refer to an ENT specialist for aciclovir and follow up.

Salivary gland problems

Saliva is a mixture containing water, various ions, mucin, and amylase, produced by the parotid, submandibular, and sublingual salivary glands. The problems most commonly affecting the salivary glands are infection and calculous disease.

Acute bilateral parotitis

Painful swelling of both parotid glands in children is most frequently due to mumps infection (p.222). In adults, painless bilateral parotid swelling may be due to Sjögren's syndrome, sarcoidosis, hypothyroidism, lymphoma, drugs (eg oral contraceptive). In each of these cases, there are often other features, which will help in diagnosis.

Acute unilateral parotitis

Painful unilateral parotid swelling may occur as part of mumps infection, but also in other circumstances (eg poor oral hygiene, post-operatively). Refer to an ENT surgeon for admission and IV antibiotics. Chronic painless unilateral parotitis is often neoplastic (mostly benign) in origin.

Calculous disease

Mechanical obstruction of the flow of saliva is most commonly due to salivary gland stones, affecting the submandibular gland. Obstruction may also occur from neoplasms or strictures.

Features Blockage of a salivary duct causes pain and swelling of the affected gland on eating. Bimanual palpation of the floor of the mouth may reveal a stone—occasionally this may be visible intra-orally at the duct orifice. If there is superimposed infection, it may be possible to express pus from the duct.

Investigation Obtain X-rays of the floor of the mouth. If the patient presses down with the tongue when the X-ray is taken the stone may be seen more easily below the mandible on a lateral view or OPG.

Treatment Refer to an oral or ENT surgeon. If an immediate consultation is not available, discuss the use of antibiotics in the meantime (these are often reserved for situations where there is evidence of salivary gland infection).

Dental emergencies: 1

Dental anatomy (Figs. 12.1 & 12.2)

The primary teeth erupt between 6 months and 2 years—they are replaced by permanent teeth which first start to appear at ≈6 years (Table 12.1). There are 20 primary and 32 permanent teeth. The permanent teeth are made up of 4 quadrants of 8 teeth: right upper, left upper, right lower, left lower. Each quadrant comprises (from medial to lateral): central incisor, lateral incisor, canine, first premolar, second premolar, first molar, second molar, and third molar ('wisdom tooth').

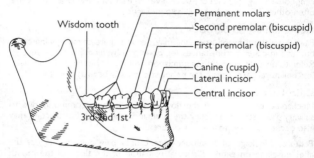

Fig. 12.1 Dental anatomy: lower jaw lateral view.

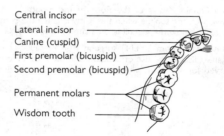

Fig. 12.2 Dental anatomy: upper jaw—view from below.

Table 12.1 Tooth eruption

	Deciduous	Permanent
Incisors	6–10 months	7–8 years
Canine	16–20 months	11 years
Premolars		11–13 years
Molars	10–24 months	6–25 years

Dental emergencies: 2

Damaged teeth

Chipped teeth and crowns which have become dislodged do not require immediate attention: redirect the patient instead to their dentist. Specialist 'sensitive teeth' toothpaste rubbed over the broken area of tooth may ↓ pain.

Tooth fractures which involve the pulp present with a small area of bleeding and are exquisitely tender to the touch. Refer to the on-call dentist.

Mobile teeth after trauma need to be stabilized as soon as possible—advise the patient to avoid manipulating the tooth and to refer to the dentist.

Simple classification of tooth fractures

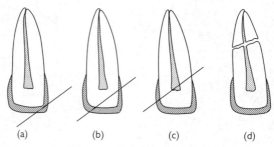

(a)   (b)   (c)   (d)

Fig. 12.3 Simple classification of tooth fractures (a) enamel only; (b) enamel and dentine; (c) enamel, dentine, and pulp; and (d) root fracture.

Avulsed teeth

Missing teeth need to be accounted for (especially in the unconscious patient) in order to exclude the possibility of aspiration. Obtain a postero-anterior (PA) and lateral CXR to search for both the tooth and secondary problems, such as pulmonary collapse and air trapping distal to the obstruction. Ensure that there is adequate tetanus prophylaxis.

Avulsed permanent teeth brought to the ED may be suitable for re-implantation. Avulsed primary teeth are usually not suitable. A history of rheumatic fever, valvular heart disease, or immunosuppressive treatment are contraindications to re-implantation. Milk is the best easily available transport medium to advise a patient to bring a tooth in. The best chance of success lies with early re-implantation (within the first few hours). Handle the tooth as little as possible. Hold it by the crown to clean it gently with 0.9% saline. Orientate the tooth, and then replace it within the socket using firm pressure (this may be easiest after LA—see Dental anaesthesia 📖 p.302). Refer immediately to the on-call dentist for stabilization and prophylactic antibiotics (eg clarithromycin). Ensure tetanus prophylaxis.

Post-extraction problems

Haemorrhage after tooth extraction may respond to simple measures. Ask the patient to bite on a rolled up piece of gauze placed over the socket for 10min. If this is unsuccessful, consider stopping the bleeding by inserting a horizontal mattress suture (eg using 'Vicryl'), placed under LA using lidocaine with adrenaline (Fig. 12.4). If bleeding continues despite these measures, apply direct pressure, send a coagulation screen and refer to the on-call dentist.

Dry socket pain may follow tooth extraction (typically 3–8 days later) when bone is exposed in the empty socket. Gently irrigate the socket with warm saline. Prescribe oral antibiotics (eg penicillin or erythromycin) and analgesia and refer to the dentist.

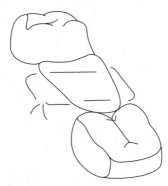

Fig. 12.4 Horizontal mattress suture in tooth socket.

Dental infection

Toothache without associated local or systemic symptoms/signs usually responds to analgesia (eg ibuprofen 400mg PO tds with food). Add antibiotics (eg penicillin or clarithromycin) if there is a suspicion of local infection. Advise follow-up with a dentist.

Toothache with associated swelling, trismus, dysphagia, or systemic evidence of infection requires immediate referral to a maxillofacial surgeon for IV antibiotics and surgical drainage.

Obstetrics and gynaecology

Gynaecological problems

The history

For gynaecological problems, always take a proper gynaecological history. This involves asking personal and sometimes sensitive questions so privacy and confidentiality are of utmost importance. Interview the patient without other family members being present:

- Ask about the presenting problem. Always ask about abdominal pain, dyspareunia, and vaginal discharge.
- Take a detailed menstrual history including the date of the last menstrual period, length of cycle, and description of the bleeding.
- Obtain a full obstetric history asking about children, pregnancies, miscarriages, terminations, and infertility treatment.
- Do not forget to ask about sexual activity, type and number of partners in past year. Also establish what form of contraception has been used.
- Has she ever been treated for a sexually transmitted disease (STD)?
- When was the last smear test and what was the result?

Examination procedure

Prior to performing a vaginal examination, explain the procedure to the patient and ensure you are in a private room. Allow the patient privacy to undress. Wearing gloves, examine the patient in an unhurried manner, in the presence of a chaperone, who might usefully 'guard' the door to prevent sudden inadvertent interruption. Use a chaperone even when the patient is being examined by female member of staff. Document the name of the chaperone in the medical record. Full examination includes digital and speculum vaginal examination to inspect the vagina and cervix, and taking swabs. This is followed by digital bimanual palpation. In certain circumstances (eg patients with painful vulval ulcers), this may not be appropriate in the ED. Vaginal examination in young children may require GA and should be undertaken by an expert. Adopt a low threshold for referring such patients.

Vulvovaginal pain

Distinguish between dysuria, dyspareunia (pain on vaginal penetration), and constant vulvovaginal pain/irritation. The latter is often associated with infection or ulceration. Enquire about other symptoms (abdominal pain, vaginal discharge and bleeding).

Vulval ulcers

- *Herpes simplex virus* is sexually transmitted and usually due to type II, but is increasingly due to type I virus (responsible for cold sores). Primary infection is extremely painful, lasting up to 3 weeks and sometimes causing urinary retention. Look for shallow yellow vulvovaginal or perineal ulcers with red edges. Cervical ulcers may also be present, although pain may prevent speculum examination. Refer primary infections immediately for aciclovir, analgesia and to exclude co-existing infection. Recurrent infections are less severe, but may last up to a week. Treat with topical and oral aciclovir (200mg five times a day for 1 week) and arrange genitourinary (GU) follow-up, with advice to avoid sexual contact meantime. Do not prescribe aciclovir in pregnancy, but arrange for an obstetric opinion.
- *Other sexually transmitted diseases* may cause ulceration: syphilis (non-tender indurated ulcers ('chancres') and lymphadenopathy), chancroid, lymphogranuloma venereum, and granuloma inguinale (📖 p.238). Refer to GU clinic and advise to abstain from sexual contact until treated.
- *Squamous carcinoma* causes indurated ulcers with everted edges especially in the elderly. Refer.
- *Consider also*: Behçet's syndrome (arthritis, iritis, genital/oral ulceration), tuberculosis (TB), Crohn's disease.

Painful lumps

- *Bartholin's abscess*: infection of vestibular (Bartholin's) cyst/gland at the posterior part of the labium majus is usually due to *Staph.*, *Strep.*, or *E. coli*, but may be due to *N. gonorrhoea*. Refer for incision and drainage (under GA) and a full GU screen.
- *Infected sebaceous cysts* may also require incision and drainage.
- *Urethral carbuncle*: this small, red, painful swelling at the external urethral meatus is due to urethral mucosal prolapse. It may cause dysuria. Refer to an appropriate clinic to consider excision or diathermy.

Pruritis vulvae

Vulval irritation may be caused by a generalized pruritic skin disorder (eg eczema), infection (particularly candidiasis) and other causes of vaginal discharge (📖 p.566), urinary incontinence, threadworms, and vulval warts. Genital warts (including condylomata accuminata) are usually sexually transmitted and caused by human papillomavirus 6. Other STDs may coexist. Refer to GU clinic.

Vaginal discharge

May be physiological or due to atrophic vaginitis, infections including STDs, cervical and endometrial carcinoma, a variety of fistulae, and FBs.

Physiological

A creamy/white discharge is normal. Variation in its consistency and amount occurs with puberty, pregnancy, oral contraceptive pill (OCP) use, ovulation, and immediately prior to menstruation.

Atrophic vaginitis

A profuse, sometimes bloody, yellow discharge may result from vaginal epithelial thinning due to ↓ oestrogen levels associated with the menopause. This responds well to local topical or oral oestrogens, most appropriately prescribed by the patient's GP.

'Thrush'

Candida albicans is the commonest vaginal infection. A white discharge accompanies a red painful vulvovaginitis. Occurs in pregnancy, after oral antibiotics, and with HIV and diabetes: check for glycosuria. Treatment options include clotrimazole pessaries, oral fluconazole, and topical application of live yoghurt. Advise GP for follow-up of any continuing symptoms.

Other infections

Refer patients suspected of the following STDs to GU clinic and advise abstinence from sexual contact in the meantime:

- *Neisseria gonorrhoea* may be asymptomatic, cause urethritis (dysuria), cervicitis (vaginal discharge), or pelvic inflammatory disease (PID; 📖 Gynaecological pain, p.573).
- *Trichomonas vaginalis* infection results in a smelly profuse yellow discharge.
- *Chlamydia trachomatis* causes chronic cervicitis, Reiter's syndrome, and PID. It may be present asymptomatically.
- *Gardnerella vaginalis* produces a brown offensive discharge.

Cervical and endometrial carcinoma

Classically presenting with bleeding between periods, these may cause discharge. Refer to a gynaecologist.

Fistulae

Colovaginal fistulae may follow diverticulitis or locally invasive colorectal carcinoma. Other fistulae (including vesicovaginal and ureterovaginal) may occur after pelvic surgery. Refer for admission and investigation.

Foreign bodies

Tampons, condoms, and various other items may be 'lost' or forgotten about in the vagina. Removal with forceps under direct vision should cure the offensive vaginal discharge. If a condom has been removed, ascertain whether or not post-coital contraception is required (📖 Contraceptive problems, p.568). Consider hepatitis B/HIV prophylaxis and GU referral for STD screen, depending upon the circumstances. Vaginal tampons (particularly highly-absorbent ones which have been left in situ for many hours) are associated with 'toxic shock syndrome'.

Toxic shock syndrome

Tampons used during menstruation have been implicated in many cases of the 'toxic shock syndrome'. First described in 1978, it is caused by exo-toxin produced by *Staph. aureus* (usually TSS toxin 1), or occasionally, *Strep*. Multi-organ failure may follow.

Features High fever, headache, vomiting, diarrhoea, myalgia, altered conscious level, hypotension, and a widespread erythematous macular rash (with subsequent desquamation one week later, especially of palms and soles).

Diagnosis Based upon clinical findings. Recent menstruation and the above features should prompt suspicion.

Investigation Includes vaginal examination. U&E, LFTs, clotting screen, FBC, blood lactate, blood and vaginal cultures, ECG, CXR.

Treatment Manage the patient in the resuscitation room. If due to a tampon: remove it. Follow guidelines for severe sepsis (📖 p.59). Obtain venous access, give intravenous antibiotics and start crystalloid. If hypotension is refractory, consider measuring central venous pressure, placing an arterial line, and starting inotropic support. The patient may require intensive care treatment.

Contraceptive problems

Missed pill

Advice will depend on the type of OCP the patient takes (combined, combined low dose oestrogen, or progesterone only). However, as a general rule, if the combined pill is delayed for more than 12hr, the patient should be advised to take the forgotten pill and use barrier contraception for 7 days. If there are less than 7 days of pills left in the pack, she should run two packs together. The same applies if they have diarrhoea. If the patient has had unprotected sexual intercourse and may require emergency contraception, it is worth referring to the NHS website (http://www.nhs.uk), which gives specific advice for each type of pill. This provides comprehensive patient advice that could also be printed and given to the patient.

Post-coital contraception

Women may attend the ED requesting post-coital contraception after:
- Isolated unprotected sexual intercourse.
- Burst or lost condom.
- Missed OCP.
- Complete or partial expulsion of intrauterine contraceptive device (IUCD).
- Rape.

The risk of pregnancy following unprotected intercourse is greatest during 5 days around ovulation, but exists at other times also. Patients given post-coital contraception require assessment and treatment including counselling and follow-up: usually this will be with the GP and/or family planning clinic. Options include levonorgestrel and insertion of IUCD. Levonorgestrel must be given within 72hr of intercourse (95% effective if taken <24hr, 58% effective at 72hr). An IUCD must be inserted within 5 days of intercourse. Both levonorgestrel and IUCD act principally to render the endometrium hostile to implantation.

Levonorgestrel (previously called 'the morning after pill')
In the UK, pharmacists can sell this without prescription to women aged over 16 years. It is usually the preferred option if patient presents within 72hr of unprotected intercourse. Exclude contraindications (acute porphyria, pregnancy, focal migraine), then give levonorgestrel 1.5mg (Levonelle® 1500) as soon as possible. Advise the patient to return if she vomits shortly after taking the medication: give a replacement dose if vomiting occurs within 3hr of taking it. Explain that there is a chance of failure. Arrange follow-up (usually with the GP) in 3 weeks to confirm that menstruation has occurred. Advise alternative contraception (eg condoms) meantime and discuss future contraception plans. Advise also about the theoretical risk of ectopic pregnancy: instruct her to return if she develops abdominal pain. Document that this advice has been given.

Note: hormonal emergency contraception is less effective if the patient is already taking enzyme-inducing drugs: take specialist advice. Options include an IUCD or ↑ dose of levonorgestrel to 3mg (see *BNF*).

IUCD

This may be useful for patients unable to take the OCP (eg previous pulmonary embolus), patients who wish to use IUCD long-term and for those presenting between 3 and 5 days after unprotected intercourse. Failure is very rare. Insertion is uncomfortable and requires appropriate training: refer to the gynaecology team. Note that IUCD should not be used with a history of recent PID.

Prescribing to patients on OCP

Both progestogen-only oral contraceptives and (combined) OCP may fail if enzyme inducing drugs are prescribed. These include: rifampicin, rifabutin, carbamazepine, phenytoin, topiramate, griseofulvin, phenobarbital, and primidone. Patients need alternative or additional contraception if these drugs are started. Rifampicin and rifabutin are such potent enzyme-inducing drugs that contraceptive precautions should continue for at least 4 weeks, even after a short course of rifabutin or rifampicin (as used for prophylaxis of meningococcal infection).

Antibiotics and the OCP (refer to BNF)

Broad spectrum antibiotics commonly prescribed in the ED may interfere with oestrogen absorption and cause contraceptive failure. Before prescribing antibiotics to a female of childbearing age, ask whether she is taking the OCP. Advise additional contraceptive precautions (eg condoms), whilst taking the antibiotics and for 7 days after. If these 7 days run beyond the end of a packet, start the next packet immediately without a break. Document in the notes that this advice has been given.

Genital injury and assault

The history may be misleading. Combine a high index of suspicion with a full examination to exclude significant injury.

Blunt genital injury may result from falls astride. Most resultant vulval haematomas settle with rest and ice packs. Refer very large haematomas for evacuation in theatre.

Penetrating injury may follow assault, FB insertion, or migration/perforation of an IUCD (particularly during insertion). Abdominal pain associated with a vaginal wound may be due to peritonitis. Obtain venous access, erect chest X-ray (for free gas), abdominal X-ray (for FB), group and save, give antibiotics, and refer for exploration and repair. Refer other vaginal tears without peritonitis for repair.

Rape and sexual assault

Rape is defined in the UK as vulval penetration by the penis without consent. Rape and other forms of sexual assault are believed to be grossly under-reported. Those who do report it have special requirements. Privacy is essential: ideally, a specially equipped room will be devoted to assessment of women who have been sexually assaulted. Ensure that a female member of staff is present throughout. Documentation must be legible and meticulous. An established protocol will allow prompt and thorough investigation and treatment. Usually, ED staff provide emergency treatment and resuscitation, but most of the other aspects, including collection of forensic evidence are dealt with by a forensic physician (police surgeon), ideally in a specialized Sexual Assault Referral Centre. Sometimes, women initially decline police involvement: full assessment and documentation may prove useful if there is a change of mind.

First exclude life-threatening or serious injuries.

History
Establish the type, date, time, and place of the assault. Ask what occurred (vaginal/anal penetration), oral sexual activity, other injuries). Ask about contraception use and enquire about LMP. Find out what is known about the assailant(s), and their risk of HIV and hepatitis B. In particular are they injecting drug users, do they originate from sub-Saharan Africa, are they homosexual?

Examination
Look for evidence of vaginal, oral or anal injury (the forensic physician will take swabs). Record any other injuries, such as bites, bruising, or skin wounds (photographs of non-genital injuries may be useful—taken by the police with the patient's consent).

Investigation
Obtain written informed consent. The police will be keen to retain clothing, loose hairs, fingernail clippings, and tampons for evidence. Similarly, the forensic physician will take appropriate swabs (vaginal, oral, anal). Perform a pregnancy test. Take and store blood for future DNA and viral testing.

Treatment

- Resuscitate as necessary. Refer urgently the 1% of patients who have significant genital injuries (eg vaginal tears) requiring surgical intervention.
- Consider the need for post-coital contraception (see ▢ p.568).
- If the patient is not immunized, give hepatitis B immunoglobulin and start an active immunization course.
- Assess the risk of HIV. If the assailant is known to have HIV or is from an at risk group, discuss the risk of disease transmission with the patient. Involve a local expert such as a virologist or infectious disease specialist prior to offering HIV prophylaxis (▢ Needlestick injury, p.418).
- Assess tetanus vaccine requirements.
- Arrange follow-up to exclude STD. Consider antibiotic prophylaxis against STD if the patient is unlikely to attend follow-up: liaise with the GU team.
- Provide initial counselling and ensure a safe place to stay (a social worker may arrange this).
- Arrange future counselling. Inform the patient about independent local advice available (eg Rape Crisis Centre).
- Ascertain from the patient if she wishes her GP to be informed.

Telephone advice

Women may telephone the ED for advice after being raped. Advise them to inform the police immediately, and then attend the police station or the ED. Discourage them from washing, changing clothes, using a toilet or brushing teeth before being examined.

Gynaecological pain

Gynaecological disorders presenting to the ED with abdominal pain may be difficult to distinguish from other disorders. Obtain a full history of the pain: sudden onset of severe colicky pain follows ovarian torsion and acute vascular events; more insidious onset and continuous pain occur in infection and inflammation. Radiation of the pain into the back or legs suggests gynaecological origin. Other clues in the history include co-existing symptoms of vaginal discharge, vaginal bleeding, or missed last menstrual period (LMP).

Abdominal and pelvic pain in early pregnancy may be due to ectopic pregnancy or threatened abortion (印 p.584): both occur in patients who do not realize that they are pregnant or who deny the possibility of pregnancy due to embarrassment.

Pain related to the menstrual cycle

Consider first: could any associated vaginal bleeding be from ectopic pregnancy or threatened abortion?

Physiological dysmenorrhoea Pain regularly preceding menstruation and peaking on the first day of a period may be physiological. Suggest NSAID and refer to the GP.

Endometriosis Growth of functional endometrial tissue in the pelvis outside the uterus may produce cysts and adhesions. Patients often present age ≈30 years with dysmenorrhoea and menstrual problems, infertility and dyspareunia. Symptoms are usually chronic and recurrent in a cyclical fashion, and are appropriately followed up by the GP. Occasionally, an endometrial cyst may rupture and bleed severely into the pelvis, presenting in similar fashion to ruptured ectopic pregnancy. Resuscitate for hypovolaemia and refer urgently.

Rupture of a corpus luteum cyst Occurs premenstrually, but may also cause significant haemorrhage, requiring resuscitation.

Mittelschmerz Mid-cycle extrusion of an ovum from a follicular cyst can cause abdominal pain, which seldom requires admission or investigation.

Uterine problems

Perforation is seen especially in the presence of IUCD.

Leiomyomas ('fibroids') may undergo torsion (sudden severe colicky pain with tender uterus), or may infarct ('red degeneration') particularly during pregnancy. Refer such suspected problems for specialist investigation.

Ovarian problems

Torsion causes sudden onset sharp unilateral pain and usually involves an already enlarged ovary (cyst, neoplasm). Abdominal and per vagina (PV) tenderness may be present. Clinical diagnosis is difficult: if suspected, refer for USS and/or laparoscopy.

Bleeding into an ovarian cyst may present similarly and require investigation.

Pelvic inflammatory disease

This term includes infection which has spread from the cervix to the uterus (endometritis), Fallopian tubes (salpingitis), ovaries (oophoritis), or adjacent peritoneum (peritonitis). Severity ranges from chronic low grade infection (with relatively mild symptoms) to acute infection (with severe symptoms) which may result in abscess formation.

Causes 90% are sexually transmitted: sexually active women aged 15–20 years are at particular risk. Most of the remaining 10% follow pregnancy terminations or dilatation and curettage.

Organisms *Chlamydia trachomatis* commonest. Also: *Neisseria gonorrhoea, Mycoplasma hominis, Ureaplasma urealyticum.*

Features Bilateral lower abdominal tenderness, vaginal discharge, fever >38°C, abnormal vaginal bleeding, deep dyspareunia, cervical motion tenderness, and adnexal tenderness all point to PID.

Management Resuscitate with IV fluids if shocked. Check urinalysis and send high vaginal swab and cervical swab, FBC, ESR. Refer all suspected cases to the gynaecologist: even though not all will require admission, they will require antibiotics (eg oral ofloxacin 400 mg twice daily plus oral metronidazole 400mg twice daily for 14 days) and follow-up.

Sequelae Ectopic pregnancy (5 × ↑ risk) or infertility, therefore have a low threshold for empirical treatment. (See http://www.rcog.org.uk).

Vaginal bleeding

See 📖 Vaginal bleeding in pregnancy, p.582.

Triage ahead patients with severe bleeding or evidence of hypovolaemic shock. Resuscitate first (O_2, cross-match and obtain Rhesus status, start IV fluids) and ask questions later. Most patients with vaginal bleeding, however, do not require resuscitation. Take a careful menstrual history and ask about associated symptoms. Attempt to assess the amount of bleeding. Interpretation of a patient's description is notoriously difficult, but useful pointers are the presence of clots and the rate of tampon use. Always consider the possibility of pregnancy: remember that ruptured ectopic pregnancy can present before a period is missed (📖 p.586). Examine for evidence of hypovolaemia and abdominal masses/tenderness. Depending upon the circumstances, speculum and bimanual vaginal examinations may be required: local policy will determine who should perform this.

Menorrhagia

Dysfunctional uterine bleeding Heavy and/or irregular periods without obvious pelvic pathology may result from hormonal imbalance. It is particularly common at menarche. Most settle without treatment or with simple measures (eg mefenamic acid 500mg PO tds after food). Refer to the GP, unless the bleeding is very heavy.

Uterine leiomyomas (fibroids) Often cause menorrhagia. May present with a painful complication, such as torsion or infarction.

Other causes Endometriosis, PID, IUCD, polyps, vaginal carcinoma, hypothyroidism.

Bleeding unrelated to pregnancy or periods

Trauma The history may be elusive.

Post-operative Significant bleeding is a risk of any gynaecological operation. Resuscitate and refer.

OCP problems Breakthrough bleeding on the OCP may be due to endometrial hyperplasia. Exclude treatable vaginal/cervical lesions, arrange a cervical smear and refer to GP.

Cervical erosion Replacement of stratified squamous epithelium by columnar epithelium may produce a mucoid discharge with a small amount of post-coital or intermenstrual bleeding. The cervix appears red. Obtain a cervical smear and arrange follow-up.

Cervical polyp Causes post-coital bleeding. Refer to the gynaecologist.

Cervical cancer 90% are squamous carcinoma. Strongly associated with human papilloma virus, some consider it an STD. Suspect in anyone presenting with post-coital or intermenstrual bleeding. Speculum examination reveals nodules, ulcers, or erosions, which may bleed to touch. Advanced disease may present with pyometra, ureteric obstruction, rectovaginal fistula. Arrange urgent gynaecology follow-up for any patient with an abnormal looking cervix.

Uterine carcinoma Mostly adenocarcinoma. Classically presents with heavy and frequent post-menopausal bleeding, but normal examination. Arrange assessment and diagnostic curettage with the gynaecologist.

Other causes Thrombocytopenia, other coagulation disorders and anti-coagulant drugs.

The pregnant patient

Pregnant patients presenting with emergency problems create understandable anxiety. There are two patients: one may be suffering unseen. Maintaining foetal oxygenation is crucial: call the obstetrician early.

Terminology

The 40 weeks of pregnancy are divided into 3 trimesters. Traditionally, problems in the first trimester are considered 'gynaecological'.

- *Gravidity* = total number of pregnancies (eg a woman in first pregnancy is a 'primigravida').
- *Parity* = number of pregnancies after 24 weeks + number before (eg a woman who has had 1 child and 2 spontaneous abortions is described as 1 + 2; gravidity = 3).
- *Abortion* is foetal death before 24 wks; *stillbirth* is foetal death after 24 wks.

Progression of pregnancy (see also Fig. 13.1)

Peristalsis and ciliary action carries the fertilized ovum to the uterus, which it reaches as a blastocyst ≈5 days after ovulation. The blastocyst implants in the endometrium: the inner part forms the embryo, the outer part membranes and placenta. Trophoblastic tissue produces human chorionic gonadotrophin (HCG), (peaks in first trimester) acting on the corpus luteum, (essential until the placenta produces oestrogen and progesterone). HCG then ↓, whereas oestrogen and progesterone ↑.

Symptoms of pregnancy Amenorrhoea, breast tenderness and fullness, polyuria, tiredness, nausea (appear by ≈6 weeks). Vomiting is common, occasionally severe enough to cause dehydration and weight loss ('hyperemesis gravidarum'). Refer for admission and rehydration.

Signs of pregnancy Not obvious in early pregnancy: uterine enlargement (see opposite), breast changes.

Pregnancy testing see p.582.

Maternal physiological changes

Cardiac output ↑ by 30%, peripheral vascular resistance ↓: BP (especially diastolic) ↓ slightly. Blood vol ↑ by 30%, plasma vol ↑ by 45%, Hb ↓ slightly. Systolic flow murmurs are common. Water retention occurs, causing ankle oedema and carpal tunnel syndrome. Ventilation ↑: the patient may feel dyspnoeic. Backache is common.

↓ Lower oesophageal pressure causes heartburn; ↓ gut motility causes constipation; ↑ venous pressure in pelvis may cause varicose veins and haemorrhoids. Platelets, ESR, cholesterol, fibrinogen ↑; albumin ↓.

See Table 13.1 for normal values in pregnant and non-pregnant women.

Diagnostic imaging in pregnancy

Try to avoid X-rays and CT scans. Excessive radiation exposure risks congenital malformation, growth retardation, and neoplasia. However, do not withhold necessary X-rays in life-threatening illness. Most head, neck, and extremity X-rays can be obtained without foetal risk by appropriate lead screening. When requesting X-rays, ensure the radiographer is aware the patient is pregnant. USS has not been shown to have adverse effects. If in doubt, discuss imaging requests with a radiologist.

Prescribing in pregnancy and during breast-feeding

Consult the *BNF* before prescribing drugs in pregnancy or during breast feeding. The following are generally considered safe in pregnancy: penicillin, cephalosporins, nystatin, paracetamol, chlorphenamine, cimetidine.

Avoid the following: trimethoprim, tetracyclines, streptomycin, warfarin, thiazides.

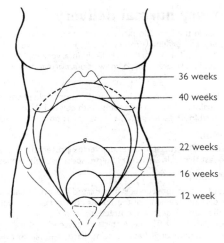

Fig. 13.1 Uterine size in pregnancy.

Table 13.1 Normal values in pregnant and non-pregnant women

Value	Non-pregnant	Pregnant
Haematocrit	0.37–0.47	0.32–0.41
Haemoglobin (g/dL)	11.5–16.0	11.0–15.0
White cell count (/L)	$4.0–11.0 \times 10^9$	$5.0–16.0 \times 10^9$
Platelets (/L)	$150–400 \times 10^9$	$134–400 \times 10^9$
ESR (mm/hr)	(age in years + 10)/2	44–114
Fibrinogen (g/L)	2–4	4–6
Albumin (g/L)	35–50	28–40
Urea (mmol/L)	2.5–6.7	1.6–6.0
Creatinine (mmol/L)	<110	38–90
pCO_2 (kPa)	4.5–6.0 (34–46mmHg)	3.6–4.2 (27–32mmHg)
pO_2 (kPa)	>10.6 (>80.6mmHg)	>10.6 (>80.6mmHg)
HCO_3^- (mmol/L)	24–28	18–23

'All pregnant women attending (accident and) emergency departments with anything other than minor complaints should be seen quickly and in conjunction with an obstetrician or senior midwife.' (See http://www.cmace.org.uk/).

Emergency normal delivery

Sometimes even the best laid plans for controlled delivery in the labour ward go awry and patients present in an advanced stage of labour and deliver in the ED. This is particularly likely in a very rapid ('precipitate') labour. ED staff therefore need to know about normal delivery.

Labour

At onset of labour, painless and irregular (Braxton Hicks) contractions are replaced by painful uterine contractions with cervical dilatation (>3cm) ± 'show' (mucus/blood discharge). There may be rupture of membranes.

Presentation

In the ED only 'OA' (occiput anterior) vertex presentations are likely to proceed so fast that delivery occurs before specialist help arrives.

Stages of labour

First Onset of labour until cervix is fully dilated (10cm). Usually lasts >6hr. The upper part or 'segment' of the uterus contracts, the lower segment (including the cervix) dilates. Contractions ↑ in frequency (every 2min) and duration (last 1min). The head starts to descend.

Second Full dilatation until baby is born. Lasts ≈40min in primigravida, ≈20min in multigravida. Contraction of upper segment, abdominal muscles and diaphragm cause head to descend then rotate (usually to lie occiput anterior). An overwhelming desire to push helps expel the baby.

Third Placenta and membranes deliver and uterus retracts (≈15min).

Assessment of a patient in labour

Check pulse, BP, and palpate the abdomen. Listen for foetal heart sounds with fetal stethoscope or Doppler probe (rate should be 120–160/min). Gently examine the perineum. Do not fully examine the vagina unless the head is crowning and birth is imminent. Instead, transfer to labour ward.

Management of delivery (see Fig. 13.2)

- Call obstetric/paediatric/anaesthetic help and encourage partner to stay.
- Offer Entonox® (50:50 mixture of nitrous oxide and O_2).
- Don sterile gloves and stand on the patient's right.
- As head crowns discourage bearing down: advise rapid shallow breaths.
- Use left hand to control escape of head (to prevent perineal tearing).
- Press gently forwards with right thumb and fingers either side of anus.
- Once head is delivered, allow it to extend.
- Feel for cord around neck: slip it over head, or if impossible, clamp, and divide.
- Allow anterior shoulder to deliver first (mother pushing if necessary).
- Give 5U oxytocin and 500mcg ergometrine IM (Syntometrine®).
- Deliver the baby, wrap him/her up and resuscitate as necessary (📖 p.642).

Management of the cord

Once baby cries and cord pulsation ceases, hold baby level with mother and clamp the cord twice (15cm from umbilicus). Divide between clamps. Place a plastic Hollister crushing clamp 1–2cm from umbilicus and cut 1cm distally. Check that 2 normal arteries are present in the cord.

Management of the third stage

A few minutes after delivery, regular contractions begin again, causing the placenta to detach. The cord may be seen to move down accompanied by a small gush of blood. The placenta may be felt in the vagina. The Brandt–Andrews technique helps removal: apply gentle downwards traction on the cord whilst exerting upward pressure on uterus (preventing inversion). Examine placenta carefully. Give Rhesus anti-D immunoglobulin if Rh –ve (📖 p.582). Immediate post-partum problems are the domain of the specialist and include: post-partum haemorrhage, amniotic fluid embolism, uterine rupture, or inversion.

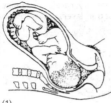

(1)
1st stage of labour. The cervix dilates. After full dilatation the head flexes further and descends further into the pelvis.

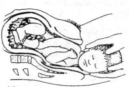

(4)
Birth of the anterior shoulder. The shoulders rotate to lie in the anteroposterior diameter of the pelvic outlet. The head rotates externally. Downward and backward traction of the head by the birth attendant aids delivery of the anterior shoulder.

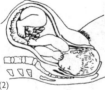

(2)
During the early second stage the head rotates at the level of the ischial spine so the occiput lies in the anterior part of pelvis. In late second stage the head broaches the vulval ring (crowning) and the perineum stretches over the head.

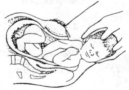

(5)
Birth of the posterior shoulder is aided by lifting the head upwards whilst maintaining traction.

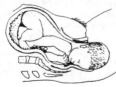

(3)
The head is born. The shoulders still lie transversely in the midpelvis.

Fig. 13.2 Management of pregnancy.

Difficulties in normal delivery

Meconium-stained liquor
See 📖 Cardiopulmonary resuscitation of the newborn, p.644.

Imminent perineal tear
The risk of perineal tearing may be minimized by controlled delivery. An extensive tear risks the integrity of the external anal sphincter. If a tear is imminent, perform an episiotomy (Fig. 13.3). Infiltrate 5–10mL of 1% lidocaine postero-laterally from the posterior fourchette. Cut the perineal tissues postero-laterally using straight scissors with blunt points (see diagram below), avoiding large veins. After delivery, carefully examine the episiotomy wound which needs to be closed in layers using absorbable sutures.

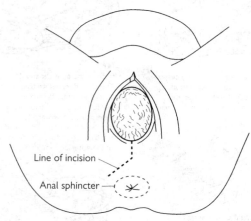

Line of incision

Anal sphincter

Fig. 13.3 Performing an episiotomy.

Difficulty in delivering the shoulders (shoulder dystocia)
After delivery of the head, the shoulders usually rotate to lie in an antero-posterior (AP) direction, so the first one can be delivered anteriorly. If this does not occur, apply gentle digital pressure to obtain rotation. Try to help delivery of the anterior shoulder by gently bending the baby's neck towards the mother's anus. The reverse action may then deliver the posterior shoulder. If these manoeuvres are unsuccessful, hook a finger into the axilla of the anterior shoulder to bring it down.

Vaginal bleeding in pregnancy

Vaginal bleeding in pregnancy produces understandable maternal distress. It may indicate serious illness that is a threat to the life of both the foetus and mother.

Causes

An indication of possible causes of vaginal bleeding related to pregnancy is apparent from gestation (see opposite). Bleeding may, of course, be unrelated to pregnancy.

Pregnancy testing

Even if the patient denies pregnancy and there is no history of amenorrhoea, consider pregnancy. Most pregnancy tests look for β-HCG produced by the developing trophoblast. Serum β-HCG levels rapidly ↑ so that pregnancy may be confirmed by serum tests within days of implantation and remain +ve until 20 weeks. Urine tests have improved considerably in recent years, but do not rely upon them to definitely exclude pregnancy.

USS easily demonstrates most pregnancies by 5 weeks after LMP.

Principles of treating blood loss in pregnancy

- Give O_2.
- Obtain venous access with large bore cannulae and replace fluids aggressively.
- Consider coagulopathy: obtain FBC and clotting screen.
- Consider prophylaxis against Rhesus haemolytic disease of the newborn.

Anti-D immunoglobulin

A Rhesus −ve mother exposed to Rh +ve foetal blood during pregnancy may develop antibodies. These IgG antibodies may cross the placenta during subsequent pregnancies and cause Rhesus haemolytic disease of the (Rh +ve) newborn. The production of maternal antibodies may be prevented by appropriate use of anti-D Ig. Consider this every time that there is possible foeto-maternal bleeding (ruptured ectopic pregnancy, spontaneous abortion, trauma, antepartum haemorrhage, labour, and delivery). Guidelines have been produced for the use of anti-D Ig (see www.rcog.org.uk). Check the Rhesus and antibody status of all women with bleeding in early pregnancy and give 250U anti-D Ig IM to those that are Rh −ve and non-immune. After delivery or bleeding occurring in later pregnancy, Rh −ve mothers are likely to require larger doses of anti-D Ig (see *BNF*). Therefore, check the Rhesus and antibody status and also perform a Kleihauer test. This will give an indication of the extent of any foeto-maternal haemorrhage: Blood Transfusion Service will advise.

Causes of vaginal bleeding in pregnancy

Table 13.2 Causes of vaginal bleeding in pregnancy

Pregnancy related			Non-pregnancy related
1st trimester	Spontaneous abortion	At any stage	Infection
	Ectopic pregnancy		Vaginal ulcers
	Trophoblastic disease		Vaginal inflammation
			Cervical erosions
			Cervical polyps
			Coagulation disorders
			Trauma
2nd trimester	Spontaneous abortion		
	Trophoblastic disease		
	Abruptio placentae		
	Placenta praevia		
3rd trimester	Abruptio placentae		
	Placenta praevia		
	'Show' of pregnancy		
	Vasa praevia		

Spontaneous abortion

Terminology

Use the term 'miscarriage' (not 'abortion') with patients. Both refer to foetal loss before 24 weeks. Spontaneous abortion affects >20% pregnancies. *Threatened abortion* refers to vaginal bleeding through a closed cervical os. 50% proceed to miscarry. If the cervix dilates or products of conception are passed, abortion is inevitable. *Inevitable* abortion becomes *complete abortion* if all products are passed. Retained products of conception in an *incomplete abortion* may become infected, causing a *septic abortion*. Alternatively, products may be retained as a *missed abortion*, which carries a risk of disseminated intravascular coagulation (DIC).

Aetiology

Mothers may feel guilty, but the causes are largely beyond their control. Risk factors include:
- Chromosomal anomalies (>50%).
- First pregnancy, maternal disease, and age >30 years.
- Uterine abnormalities.
- Drugs (especially isotretinoin).
- Cervical incompetence, immunological factors, and trauma.

Approach

Establish the gestation. Think: is this a ruptured ectopic pregnancy? Vaginal bleeding in spontaneous abortion ranges from light to severe. Severe bleeding with hypovolaemia may occur in inevitable abortion. Abdominal pain is associated with a lower chance of fetal survival. Any pain with threatened abortion tends to be light and crampy. Severe pain and bleeding with hypotension and bradycardia implies 'cervical shock', where products of conception are stuck in the cervical os. Abdominal or cervical tenderness suggests an alternative diagnosis (ectopic pregnancy or septic abortion). Vaginal examination provides other important clues: look for cervical dilatation (remember that the external os of a multigravida usually accepts a fingertip) and products in the os.

Investigation

USS may exclude ectopic pregnancy and indicate foetal viability: local policy will determine who performs this. Urine pregnancy tests remain +ve for several days after foetal death. Check Rhesus status and baseline serum β-HCG. Cross-match and obtain FBC if shocked.

Treatment

Resuscitate if significant pain or haemorrhage and refer urgently. If cervical shock is present, remove products of conception from the cervical os using sponge forceps. If severe bleeding continues, give 500mcg ergometrine IM. Unfortunately, no intervention appears to alter foetal survival in threatened abortion. Patients with light bleeding, no abdominal pain, and a closed os (threatened abortion) may be allowed home after USS and gynaecology review. Reassure, emphasize that it is not her fault, advise bed rest and abstinence from sexual intercourse until gynaecology follow-up in 2 days. Provide Rhesus anti-D Ig 250u IM if Rh –ve and non-immune.

Septic abortion

Sepsis may follow spontaneous, surgically induced or 'backstreet' abortion.

Organisms S. aureus, C. welchii, Bacteroides, E. coli, streptococci, Clostridium sordelli.

Features vaginal bleeding, offensive discharge, ↑ T°, ↓ BP, uterine tenderness, peritonitis. Note that pyrexia is not invariable—particularly with *Clostridium sordelli* which can result in a severe infection with high mortality.

Obtain FBC, clotting screen, blood cultures, blood lactate, vaginal swabs, X-match, Rhesus status, erect CXR (to look for free gas).

Resuscitate with IV fluids, give co-amoxiclav 1.2g IV, follow the severe sepsis guidelines (📖 p.59) and refer urgently. Monitor urine output and consider central and arterial lines.

Missed abortion

Very occasionally presents several weeks or months after foetal death with no expected features of pregnancy, a –ve pregnancy test and DIC. Resuscitate, and involve senior obstetrician and haematologist.

Ectopic pregnancy

Gestational sac implantation outside the uterus has ↑ and now occurs in ≈1 in 100 pregnancies in the UK. 96% implant in the Fallopian tube, 2% in the interstitial part of uterus, 1.5% intra-abdominally. The risk of heterotopic pregnancy (combined intrauterine and ectopic pregnancy) is ≈1 in 4000.

Importance

Ectopic pregnancy is the commonest cause of maternal mortality in the first trimester. The diagnosis is frequently missed. Consider it in any young woman presenting with abdominal pain or vaginal bleeding, especially when combined with an episode of syncope.

Risk factors

These include anything which delays or limits normal transit of the fertilized ovum to the uterus: PID, pelvic surgery/adhesions, previous ectopic, endometriosis, assisted fertilization, IUCD, progesterone only pill, congenital anatomical variants, ovarian and uterine cysts/tumours. Note that although pregnancy is unusual after tubal ligation, when it does occur there is a relatively high chance (≈1 in 6) of it being an ectopic pregnancy.

Pathology

Implantation of the gestational sac in the Fallopian tube may have three results:
• Extrusion (tubal abortion) into the peritoneal cavity.
• Spontaneous involution of pregnancy.
• Rupture through the tube causing pain and bleeding.

Implantation in a uterine horn is particularly dangerous: pregnancy may reach 10–14 weeks before rupture. Exceptionally, intraperitoneal pregnancies may proceed almost to term.

Symptoms

Ectopic pregnancy may present with sudden severe lower abdominal pain with collapse or fainting, and vaginal bleeding. There is usually (but not always) a history of amenorrhoea (often 8 weeks). Haemorrhage may cause shoulder tip pain (from blood irritating the diaphragm) and features of hypovolaemia. Nausea and vomiting are common.

Many patients have more chronic symptoms, with recurrent abdominal pain and slight irregular vaginal bleeding, which may be fresh or dark (like 'prune juice'). Pain may have continued for > 1week before presentation, occasionally as long as 4 weeks. The pain may be worse on defecation. Some patients have no vaginal bleeding.

Enquire about symptoms of pregnancy (eg breast tenderness) and possible risk factors for ectopic pregnancy.

Signs

Look for hypovolaemic shock. If present, volume replacement must accompany full assessment. Abdominal tenderness is variable, ranging from mild to severe with peritonism. Cullen's sign (discolouration around the umbilicus) is of historical interest only. Bimanual vaginal examination reveals tender adnexa and sometimes a mass, but may be better deferred to a specialist (risk of ↑ bleeding). Speculum inspection usually shows vaginal blood.

Investigation

Must not delay resuscitation and referral.

Pregnancy test is almost always +ve, but serum β-HCG levels are lower than expected for normal pregnancy.

Transabdominal USS is useful if it demonstrates an intrauterine pregnancy, free fluid in the pouch of Douglas and/or an adnexal mass. Frequently it is inconclusive. Transvaginal USS may be better.

Differential diagnosis

- *Threatened abortion*: bleeding is usually more severe (📖 p.584).
- *Ruptured corpus luteum cyst*: the corpus luteum supports pregnancy for the first 6–8 weeks. Rupture causes sudden peritoneal irritation, but rarely bleeds significantly.
- *PID* (📖 p.573): Note that ectopic pregnancy can cause mild pyrexia and a raised WCC, which may easily be misinterpreted as evidence of pelvic infection.
- *Trophoblastic disease* (📖 Vaginal bleeding in later pregnancy, p.588).

Treatment

Give O_2, insert two large (12 or 14G) cannulae, cross-match 6U of blood, request Rhesus status. Resuscitate initially with crystalloid IV fluids as necessary. If suspected, refer urgently to the gynaecology team since sudden deterioration may occur. Significant haemorrhage requires urgent surgery. Alert the anaesthetist and theatre team early. Check Rhesus and antibody status: anti-D immunoglobulin may be needed (📖 p.582).

Vaginal bleeding in later pregnancy

Gestational trophoblastic disease

Occasionally, a fertilized ovum may form abnormal trophoblastic tissue, but no fetus. The pathological spectrum ranges from benign hydatidiform mole to invasive choriocarcinoma. Choriocarcinoma is relatively rare, affecting ≈1 in 40,000 pregnancies.

Presentation Usually vaginal bleeding at 12–16 weeks, with passage of tissue, which may resemble frogspawn. Often accompanying abdominal pain and sometimes pre-eclampsia or eclampsia. The uterus may be much larger than expected for dates. DIC may occur.

Investigations USS shows 'snowstorm' and no foetus. Serum HCG is grossly ↑.

Management Obtain venous access, serum HCG, FBC, group and save, IV fluids/resuscitation, and refer.

Antepartum haemorrhage

Bleeding after 20 weeks occurs in 2.5% of pregnancies. Abruptio placentae and placenta praevia are most likely causes, although other cervical or vaginal lesions may be responsible.

Abruptio placentae

Premature separation of the normally situated placenta affects ≈1% of pregnancies. It causes haemorrhage which may risk the foetus, depending on the extent of placental involvement, and rapidity of separation.

Risk factors Pre-eclampsia, previous abruption, trauma (📖 p.594), smoking, ↑ parity, cocaine.

Presentation There is usually some vaginal bleeding ('revealed haemorrhage'), but occasionally bleeding is limited to the confines of the uterus ('concealed haemorrhage'). In either case, there may be much more utero-placental bleeding than is immediately apparent. There may be abdominal pain and tenderness or back pain. Abruptio placentae may precipitate labour. A large bleed can cause DIC or absent foetal heart sounds.

Placenta praevia

The placenta is situated wholly or partly over the lower uterine segment and cervical os.

Risk factors Mother aged >35 years, high parity, previous placenta praevia, twins, uterine abnormalities (including previous Caesarian section).

Presentation Most present with bright red painless vaginal bleeding in the third trimester. 15% present in labour.

If placenta praevia is a possibility, do not perform digital or speculum vaginal examination.

Vasa praevia

Rarely, an abnormal foetal blood vessel may be attached to the membranes over the internal os. Haemorrhage may cause foetal exsanguination, usually during labour.

Management of antepartum haemorrhage
- Call an obstetrician immediately.
- Give O_2.
- Obtain venous access (2 large bore cannulae) and resuscitate with IV fluids as necessary.
- Send U&E, FBC, blood glucose, cross-match, Rhesus and antibody status, Kleihauer test, clotting screen.
- Monitor the foetus (cardiotocography).
- USS locates the placenta, demonstrates the foetus and may show concealed haemorrhage.
- Give anti-D immunoglobulin as advised by Blood Transfusion Service if Rh −ve (📖 p.582).

Abdominal pain in pregnancy

Approach

Attempting to deduce the cause of abdominal pain can ordinarily be quite difficult: in pregnancy it is even more so. Some possible underlying diseases may be causing unseen foetal distress and can produce rapid maternal deterioration. Therefore, triage ahead, contact the obstetrician, and resuscitate vigorously. Initial investigations usually include BMG, urinalysis, blood tests, and USS. Vaginal bleeding accompanying abdominal pain implies a gynaecological or obstetric problem. Remember, however, that the reverse is not necessarily true: ruptured ectopic pregnancy and concealed haemorrhage in abruptio placentae may present without vaginal bleeding. In later pregnancy, even if there is doubt as to whether the principal problem is obstetric or not, involve the obstetrician at an early stage.

Pregnancy related causes of abdominal pain

The following are considered elsewhere:

- Ectopic pregnancy (📖 p.586).
- 'Red degeneration' of a fibroid (📖 Uterine problems, p.572).
- Gestational trophoblastic disease (📖 Vaginal bleeding in later pregnancy, p.588).
- Abruptio placentae (📖 p.588).
- Onset of labour (📖 Emergency normal delivery, p.578).

Torsion, rupture, or haemorrhage into an ovarian cyst

This may involve the corpus luteum of pregnancy. Sudden onset lower abdominal pain results. USS may demonstrate the problem.

Acute polyhydramnios

Excessive amniotic fluid may complicate pregnancy involving uni-ovular twins. Pain and vomiting is accompanied by a large abdomen for gestation and an unusually mobile foetus.

Pre-eclampsia

Abdominal pain (particularly right upper quadrant pain) in pregnancy may reflect pre-eclampsia (see 📖 p.592). Check BP and urinalysis and refer urgently.

Non-obstetric causes of abdominal pain

Urinary tract infection

UTI is relatively common in pregnancy due to urinary stasis. Women are at particular risk if they have had previous UTI. Abdominal/loin pain and pyrexia with rigors indicate acute pyelonephritis. Send MSU, FBC, and blood cultures, and refer for IV antibiotics. Treat patients with asymptomatic UTI or cystitis without evidence of pyelonephritis with oral antibiotics (eg amoxicillin 250mg PO tds or a cephalosporin) and arrange GP follow-up when the MSU result will be available. When prescribing antibiotics in pregnancy, take care to avoid those drugs which are contra-indicated (eg trimethoprim, tetracyclines—see *BNF*).

Acute appendicitis

Presentation in early pregnancy may be as classically described, but can be confused with ectopic pregnancy or rupture/torsion of an ovarian cyst. In later pregnancy, the point of maximal tenderness in acute appendicitis rises towards the right hypochondrium. Check BMG, serum amylase, and urinalysis. Give analgesia and refer if suspected.

Gallstones

Pain from gallstones not infrequently presents for the first time in pregnancy. The presentation of biliary colic and cholecystitis is similar to that in the non-pregnant patient (📖 Biliary tract problems, p.510). USS reveals stones and associated pathology. Give analgesia and refer: if possible, the patient will be treated conservatively.

Acute pancreatitis

This is usually related to gallstones. There is a significant risk to mother and fetus. Presentation and treatment are as described in 📖 p.508.

Perforated peptic ulcer

If suspected, obtain erect CXR with lead shield for the fetus. Resuscitate and refer (📖 p.511).

Intestinal obstruction

Often follows adhesions from previous surgery. The diagnosis may not be immediately obvious: pain, vomiting, and constipation may be initially attributed to pregnancy. These symptoms, together with abdominal tenderness and high pitched bowel sounds suggest the diagnosis. An erect abdominal X-ray will confirm it, but this should only be requested by a specialist.

Medical complications of pregnancy

Pre-eclampsia and eclampsia

This poorly understood vasospastic uteroplacental disorder affects 7% of pregnancies. It results in widespread systemic disturbance involving the liver, kidneys, coagulation, and cardiovascular systems. Placental infarcts may occur and compromise the foetus.

Pre-eclampsia 2 or more of: hypertension (>140/90), proteinuria and oedema. Variant presentation: haemolysis, elevated LFTs, low platelets (HELLP syndrome) particularly affects multigravida.

Progression to eclampsia is heralded by: confusion, headache, tremor, twitching, ↑ reflexes. Visual disturbance and/or abdominal pain may occur.

Eclampsia The onset of fits after 20 weeks (or fits in association with pre-eclampsia). Maternal mortality is 2%, perinatal mortality 15%.

Management
See www.rcog.org.uk
- Refer all patients with BP>140/90, or proteinuria and oedema.
- Obtain FBC, uric acid, U&E, LFTs, clotting screen, ECG, foetal monitoring.
- Restrict fluids to a total of 80mL/hr or 1mL/kg/hr (because of the risk of pulmonary oedema).
- If there is evidence of impending eclampsia or the patient starts to fit: call the obstetrician and anaesthetist, check BMG, control airway, consider left lateral position, give O₂ and 4g magnesium sulphate slowly IV over 10min, followed by a maintenance magnesium sulphate 1g/h IVI. Treat recurrent fits with a further 2g magnesium sulphate IV over 10min.
- Follow local advice regarding control of hypertension (eg labetalol 10mg slow IV bolus, followed by an IVI starting at 1–2mg/min, ↑ as required).
- Urgent delivery is a priority in eclampsia, both for mother and foetus.

Disseminated intravascular coagulation

DIC may complicate a variety of obstetric problems: abruptio placentae, intrauterine death, missed abortion, amniotic fluid embolism, eclampsia, sepsis, trophoblastic disease.

Clinical picture Widespread haemorrhage and microvascular occlusion.

Obtain FBC, cross-match, clotting screen, fibrin degradation products, fibrinogen, U&E, and LFTs.

Treatment Resuscitate with O₂, IV fluids (according to CVP), blood transfusion, and FFP. Refer urgently and consider urgent delivery and treatment of underlying disease.

Diabetes mellitus

Pregnancy encourages hyperglycaemia. IDDM in pregnancy may be more difficult to control and is associated with an ↑ insulin requirement. DKA occurs relatively easily (📖 Hyperglycaemic crises, p.152).

Thromboembolic disease

Pregnancy carries an ↑ risk and is a significant cause of maternal mortality. The exact risk in each trimester is as yet unclear, as little research has involved pregnant women. However, it would seem that the more gravid the woman, the greater the risk of DVT and PE. Caesarian section, previous DVT/PE, a family history and bed rest all increase the risk.

Clinical probability scoring for DVT or PE is difficult as all derived scores excluded pregnant women. Therefore, pregnant women should have imaging, rather than D-dimer and clinical probability assessment.

USS is the safest initial investigation for DVT. Remember that to exclude DVT with ultrasound requires either one normal complete scan (calf, popliteal fossa and thigh) or two normal thigh and popliteal scans, one week apart (📖 p.118).

Pulmonary embolism presents with pain or dyspnoea (📖 p.120). Unfortunately, these are not infrequent symptoms during pregnancy. A normal SpO$_2$ in air will not exclude PE. Always request a CXR as this will reveal other life threatening causes (pneumothorax) and is required for VQ reporting. Investigation for PE starts with *bilateral leg ultrasound scans* (no risk to foetus). If these are normal, the patient should have a *VQ scan* (📖 Pulmonary embolism, p.120). If the VQ scan cannot diagnose or exclude PE, arrange a *CT scan*.

During investigation for DVT or PE it is standard practice to commence thrombosis treatment with low molecular weight heparin (LMWH). Thrombolysis has been used successfully in peri-arrest pregnant women with a clear clinical picture of PE. If the patient is not peri-arrest, always endeavour to obtain diagnostic imaging.

Warfarin is teratogenic in the first trimester and may cause fetal or placental bleeding in later pregnancy, so avoid it in pregnancy.

Other problems

Thyrotoxicosis presents not infrequently in pregnancy.
Pre-existing heart disease worsens as blood volume and cardiac output ↑: involve a specialist early.

Although rare, consider aortic dissection in any pregnant patient with unexplained, severe chest, back or neck pain (📖 p.92).

Trauma in pregnancy

Background
Principal causes are similar to those in the non-pregnant: road traffic collisions, falls and assaults. Contrary to popular opinion, the use of seat belts does ↓ risk of serious injury in pregnancy. The 'lap' belt should lie over the anterior superior iliac spines.

Anatomical considerations
The following are worthy of consideration:
- As the uterus enlarges it rises out of the pelvis with the bladder—both are at ↑ risk of injury.
- The size of the uterus and stretching of the peritoneum make abdominal assessment difficult.
- The bony pelvis is less prone to fracture, but retroperitoneal haemorrhage may be torrential due to ↑ vascularity.
- The pregnant uterus may obstruct the inferior vena cava, causing supine hypotension and increased bleeding from lower limb wounds.
- The diaphragm is higher in pregnancy.
- The pituitary doubles in size and is at risk of infarction in untreated hypovolaemic shock.

Physiological considerations
Pregnancy is associated with dramatic changes in physiology:
- Pregnant patients may tolerate up to 35% loss of blood volume before manifesting classic signs of hypovolaemic shock, largely at the risk of uteroplacental circulation.
- The ↓ functional residual capacity and ↑ O_2 requirement result in hypoxia developing more quickly.
- There is an ↑ risk of regurgitation of gastric contents.
- Coagulation may be deranged or rapidly become so.

Injuries to the uterus, placenta, and foetus
Foetal injury Both blunt and penetrating trauma may damage the foetus. It is, however, more likely to suffer as a result of maternal hypoxia/hypovolaemia or placental abruption.

Placental abruption Deceleration forces in blunt trauma may shear the inelastic placenta from the elastic uterus. Haemorrhage (maternal and foetal) may be significant and result in DIC. This may present with vaginal bleeding (much may be concealed internally), uterine tenderness, or foetal distress.

Uterine rupture This is relatively uncommon. Major rupture causes severe bleeding. The uterus and foetus may be felt separately.

Amniotic fluid embolism Rare and carries a poor prognosis. Presents with sudden collapse, dyspnoea, ↓ BP, fitting, and bleeding (from DIC).

Approach to the injured pregnant patient

Follow that outlined in 📖 Major trauma, p.319, with the additional specific points.

History
Determine gestation and any problems in this and previous pregnancies.

Examination
- Involve an obstetrician early: examine vagina for bleeding or rupture of membranes.
- Palpate for fundal height (mark skin), abdominal tenderness, uterine contractions.
- Listen for foetal heart sounds and rate using a foetal stethoscope (Pinard) or Doppler probe.
- Remember that head injury may mimic eclampsia and vice-versa.

Investigation
- Check BMG, coagulation screen, Rhesus/antibody status, and Kleihauer test.
- Consider CVP monitoring (remembering the CVP is lower in pregnancy).
- Monitor foetal heart (cardiotocograph)—the rate should be 120–160/min.
- USS investigates foetal viability, placental injury, gestational age, and free peritoneal fluid.
- Do not withold essential X-rays, but do consider early USS to look for free intra-abdominal fluid and foetal viability. Seek senior advice. Remember that the greatest risks from X-rays to the foetus are in early pregnancy. In later pregnancy, risks to the foetus may be outweighed by failure to identify injuries by not obtaining X-rays.
- DPL has been largely superceded by USS (FAST scan)—but if indicated, use a supra-umbilical open approach (see 📖 p.347).

Treatment
- Give O_2 and summon senior obstetric, ICU, and surgical help early.
- If chest drains are required insert 1–2 intercostal spaces higher than usual.
- Decompress the inferior vena cava by manually displacing the uterus to the left or by using a 15° right lateral (Cardiff) wedge, or if neck injury has been excluded, by nursing in left lateral position.
- Treat fluid losses with aggressive IV fluid replacement.
- An NG tube ↓ risk of regurgitation and aspiration.
- Remember tetanus prophylaxis (📖 p.410).
- Consider anti-D immunoglobulin if the patient is Rh –ve.
- Even if there is no overt maternal injury refer for foetal monitoring for 4hr.
- Abdominal tenderness, hypovolaemia or foetal distress may require urgent laparotomy.
- If the patient has a cardiac arrest, perform emergency Caesarian section if the patient is >24wks pregnant and 5mins has elapsed without output (see 📖 p.596).

Cardiac arrest in pregnancy

Rate Estimated in late pregnancy at ~1 in 30,000.

Causes stroke, PE, uteroplacental haemorrhage, amniotic fluid embolism, eclamptic fits and haemorrhage, anaesthetic problems, and drug reactions, underlying heart disease. Ischaemic heart disease is rarely implicated: the underlying rhythm is more commonly pulseless electrical activity than ventricular fibrillation. Unfortunately, this is reflected in the poor prognosis.

Remember the following physiological factors

- The airway is difficult to control (large breasts, full dentition, neck oedema and obesity). Ventilation may be difficult and intubation technically challenging.
- ↑ aspiration risk (↓ lower oesophageal pressure, ↑ intragastric pressure) therefore securing definitive airway early is essential.
- ↑ O$_2$ requirements in pregnancy, yet harder to ventilate (↓ chest compliance).
- Chest compression is awkward (flared ribs, raised diaphragm, obesity, breast hypertrophy).
- Gravid uterus compresses inferior vena cava diminishing venous return.
- There are 2 patients: mother and foetus.

Approach to resuscitation

Follow Resuscitation guidelines for managing adult cardiac arrest (📖 p.46). The special situation of pregnancy means some additional points apply. If there is advanced warning, think ahead. In addition to the usual team needed for airway control, IV access and chest compressions, organize:

- An anaesthetist for the airway, an obstetrician to perform a Caesarian section and a paediatrician to resuscitate the baby.
- The neonatal resuscitation equipment (overhead warmer, suction, airway equipment and oxygen).
- A member of staff to apply cricoid pressure at the beginning of resuscitation and until the airway is secured.
- A member of staff to manually displace the uterus to the left until a left lateral tilt has been established with a Cardiff wedge.

It may take time for help to arrive and there may be no warning prior to patient arrival. In the meantime, proceed as follows:

- Call the obstetrician, paediatrician, and ED consultant immediately.
- Apply cricoid pressure (Sellick manoeuvre) at the beginning of resuscitation and until the airway is secured.
- Aim to secure the airway with a cuffed tracheal tube at an early stage.
- Decompress the inferior vena cava by either manual displacement of the uterus to the left, or the use of sandbags or a special 15° right lateral ('Cardiff') wedge.
- Consider and treat the cause (eg remember that hypovolaemic shock from unseen haemorrhage may respond to a large IV fluid challenge).
- If there is no return of spontaneous circulation within 5min perform a Caesarian section (providing the patient is >24 weeks pregnant).

Emergency Caesarian section

Rationale After several minutes of maternal cardiac arrest the best chance of survival for the foetus is to be removed from the now hostile hypoxic environment of the uterus. Caesarian section also benefits the mother by decompressing the inferior vena cava, resulting in ↑ venous return.

Procedure Continue closed chest compression and ventilation. Make a midline skin incision from pubic symphysis to epigastrium. Incise the underlying uterus vertically, starting 6cm above the bladder peritoneal reflection. Continue the uterine incision upwards to the fundus, through an anteriorly placed placenta if necessary. Speed is essential. Deliver the baby, holding it head down and below the level of the mother's abdomen. Clamp and cut the umbilical cord. Resuscitate the baby (📖 p.642).

Post-partum problems

Physiology of the puerperium

Within 24hr of delivery uterine involution results in the fundus being level with the umbilicus. By 2 weeks the uterus should be impalpable. Uterine discharge ('lochia') gradually ↓, but may last up to 6 weeks. An initially bloody discharge becomes yellow within 2 weeks. The external cervical os gradually closes so that after 1 week it no longer accepts a finger. Speculum examination will now reveal the typical parous os (see Fig. 13.4).

Post-partum haemorrhage

Primary Haemorrhage >500mL in the first 24hr is often related to retained placenta/clots. This, together with uterine inversion and amniotic fluid embolism are principally problems of the labour ward.

Secondary Excessive fresh vaginal bleeding between 1 day and 6 weeks after a delivery affects ≈1% pregnancies. The most common cause is retained products of conception: uterine involution may be incomplete and USS may reveal the retained products. Other causes include intrauterine infection (see below), genital tract trauma, trophoblastic disease. Resuscitate appropriately for blood loss and refer. Severe bleeding may respond to IV oxytocin.

Pyrexia

Treat according to the underlying cause, which include the following:
• Pelvic infection (see below).
• UTI.
• Mastitis.
• Chest infection.
• DVT or PE.
• Illness apparently unrelated to pregnancy/delivery.

Pelvic infection

Involves a significant threat: may be complicated by septicaemia, necrotizing fasciitis, DIC or septic PE. There is an ↑ risk with: surgical procedures in labour, prolonged membrane rupture, internal foetal monitoring, and repeated examinations.

Features Uterine tenderness and subinvolution, pyrexia, offensive lochia, peritonitis.

Send Vaginal swabs for culture, FBC, group and save, clotting screen and blood cultures.

Resuscitate with O_2 and IV fluids and refer. For septic shock, follow severe sepsis guidelines, give IV co-amoxiclav (1.2g) and IV metronidazole (500mg), monitor CVP, consider inotropes and ventilation.

Infected episiotomy wound

Refer to obstetrician.

Mastitis and breast abscess

Mastitis is commonly due to *Staph.* or *Strep.* Send milk for culture and commence oral antibiotics (eg co-amoxiclav). Instruct patient to express and discard milk from the affected breast, but to continue breast-feeding from the other. Arrange GP follow-up.

Refer patients with abscesses for surgical drainage by incision or the now preferred aspiration.

Psychiatric illness

Rapid hormonal swings are responsible for elation being frequently replaced by tearfulness and anxiety ('fourth day blues'). Less commonly (0.5% pregnancies) puerperal psychosis occurs. Those with a previous psychotic illness are at particular risk. Exclude sepsis and refer for psychiatric help. The patient may need to be compulsorily detained (□ Compulsory hospitalization, p.628).

Thromboembolic disease

A major cause of maternal mortality throughout pregnancy and the puerperium. Adopt a high index of suspicion and refer for investigation (□ Pulmonary embolus, p.120).

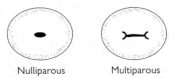

Nulliparous   Multiparous

Fig. 13.4 Appearance of the cervical os.

Psychiatry

Approach to psychiatric problems

Psychiatric presentations comprise ≈1–2% of ED new attendances. These patients are sometimes considered unwelcome because they are seen as complex, heavy consumers of staff time and energy, and not infrequently exhibit aggressive and/or disturbed behaviour. A careful systematic approach to patients presenting with psychiatric emergencies produces an accurate diagnosis in most cases. If this is not possible, the information gained will at least assist referral to the appropriate service, allowing management of the problem.

Liaison psychiatry service

Many EDs have close links with liaison psychiatrists and specialist psychiatric nurses. These individuals are used to managing a variety of psychiatric problems, including overdose and deliberate self-harm. In an emergency situation, they can act as an important source of advice.

Potential points of conflict

The ED is not an ideal environment for the assessment of potential psychiatric illness. Remember the following:

- The vast majority of aggressive, violent or bizarrely behaving patients in the ED are not suffering from a formal psychiatric illness. Many require the police, rather than psychiatric services.
- Admission is not mandatory simply because a psychiatric illness has been diagnosed.
- The presence of alcohol or drug intoxication makes any assessment of mental state very difficult and in many cases impossible—do not assume that this in itself reflects an acute psychiatric problem.
- Acute alcohol withdrawal is a medical emergency with a significant mortality—refers to the medical team, not acutely to the psychiatric service.
- Acute confusional states are usually organic rather than psychiatric in origin – investigate with this in mind.
- An emergency Section form must be signed by the examining doctor, but this does not have to be a psychiatrist.

Similarly, *psychiatric staff within the ED* need to consider the following:

- EDs are under pressure to manage large numbers of patients in a timely fashion, so it may be difficult for ED staff to spend large amounts of time with any single patient.
- Lack of appropriate interview facilities may make it necessary to compromise patient privacy rather than the safety of staff.
- A psychiatric referral can be appropriate in a patient who has consumed alcohol, if there is a significant psychiatric history ('Dual Diagnosis').

General approach to psychiatric problems

Adopt the same approach of history taking and examination as with other general medical problems. Do not dismiss psychiatric patients as 'mad, therefore the psychiatrist can sort them out'—this can result in misdiagnosis and inappropriate referral.

Glossary of psychiatric terms

Concrete thinking Impairment of abstract, or symbolic thinking (eg interpretation of proverbs, explanation of similarities).

Delirium An organic syndrome characterized by rapid onset global disturbance of cognition, and disturbed consciousness.

Delusion A firm, usually false, belief unshakeable by logical argument or contrary experiences and which is out of keeping with the patient's social or cultural norms.

Flight of ideas Thoughts rapidly cycle linked by chains of ideas or verbal associations or sounds resulting in disjointed, or in extreme cases, incomprehensible speech.

Hallucination A false perception not due to a sensory distortion or misinterpretation, but which occurs at the same time as real perceptions. Hallucinations can occur in each of the sensory modalities. Auditory hallucinations are most commonly associated with psychiatric illness. Visual and other hallucinatory phenomena suggest organic aetiology.

Ideas of reference A feeling that others are talking about or looking at the patient for some reason. Insight is usually retained, which is not the case in delusions of reference.

Obsession Recurrent, persistent, and intrusive thoughts, impulses or mental images that the individual usually tries to resist, finds unpleasant and recognizes as senseless.

Passivity An experience of being under external control either physically, emotionally or intellectually. Suggests schizophrenia.

Perseveration Repetition of an idea, thought, speech or an action beyond the point of relevance (eg giving the answer of an initial question in response to subsequent unrelated questions). Pathognomonic of organic brain disease.

Pressure of speech Rapid or hurried speech, often occurs with flight of ideas.

Psychosis Extreme disorders of thinking and perception, often involving delusions and hallucinations, with loss of insight.

Thought blocking A feature of schizophrenia in which a train of thought stops abruptly and, following a pause, a new line of conversation begins.

Thought broadcasting More than simply feeling others can read personal thoughts. An experience of thoughts spilling out beyond personal control or that, thoughts are being relayed from external sources.

Thought insertion Thoughts that are not the patient's own are put in his mind from outside.

Thought withdrawal The feeling that thoughts have been removed or stolen by an external influence.

The psychiatric interview

Setting and safety

Conduct the interview in a quiet, relatively private and preferably less clinical setting. Many EDs have specific facilities designed for this purpose (following specific joint guidance from the Royal College of Psychiatrists and British Association for Emergency Medicine – Council Report CR118, 2004). Irrespective of this, *do not* under any circumstances allow the need for privacy to compromise your safety! Ensure that other staff are easily available and can be summoned *immediately* if necessary. If this is not possible, either conduct the interview within the main ED (in a cubicle or side-room) and/or ensure that other staff are present during the interview. Position yourself between the patient and the exit.

Approach

In the initial interview, focus upon the following:
- Listen in supportive fashion and obtain an accurate history of the presenting problem.
- Assess the mental state, emotions, and attitudes of the patient.
- Make a formulation (identify the key factors of the present illness, list probable causes, explain why the patient became ill, and plan treatment).

Initial history

Take a rapid, thorough history, concentrating upon the following questions:
- What is the presenting complaint?
- What factors have caused the patient to present here and now?
- Is there a past history of psychiatric illness or medication?
- What does the patient want (advice, treatment or admission)?
- Are the patient's wishes appropriate?

Ethnic minorities

Be aware of the different communities living within the vicinity and take special care to remain sensitive to their needs. Assessment of mental health problems needs to take into account the relevant cultural and religious issues.

Language

It can be particularly challenging to assess the mental health of patients who do not speak English. The following solutions may be explored:
- Assessment may be performed by an ED or mental health professional who speaks the patient's language (the ideal result).
- A health professional from another discipline acts as an interpreter.
- An interpreter who is not a health professional, but who is trained in mental health issues may be used.

Note that children should not be used as interpreters. Similarly, it is not good practice to rely upon family members to interpret.

Taking a full psychiatric history

The extent to which a detailed psychiatric history is required in the ED varies according to the circumstances. The key features of a psychiatric history are:

Presenting complaint List the principal complaints and try to detail the course and severity of each. Ask about the effect of each problem on the person's life and work. Carefully determine how he came to be referred or why he presented here and now. When was he last well?

Past psychiatric history Ask about previous psychiatric or physical illness, hospital admissions (particularly if compulsory) and any outpatient contact (eg community psychiatric nurse), day hospital, day centres, or crisis intervention groups. Record psychiatric or other medications as accurately as possible.

Personal and family history Obtain an outline of the patient's life history: birth, childhood, circumstances of upbringing (including parental relationships—marital disharmony, separation, violence, adoption, single parent, brought up by a grandparent, etc.). Ask about education, academic achievements, and relationships with family or friends. Ask if there has been any recent bereavement and what effect this has had.

Work history Is the patient employed? If not, ask about any previous jobs. Ask about the impact of any loss, change, or failure in work on the patient's life or mental status, and conversely determine if psychiatric or other illness has had any effect on employment.

Sexual/marital history Gently enquire about relationships and sexual experiences only where relevant. This may reveal important information about the patient's personality and relationships to others. It may form a major part of the presenting complaint (eg recent ending or change in a relationship or a history of sexual abuse). A more detailed account of sexual aberration or fantasy may be required in a forensic examination.

Substance misuse Try to estimate alcohol, tobacco, drug, or other substance misuse by the patient. Although it may be difficult to obtain accurate information, do not assume that patients always underestimate their consumption of such substances.

Forensic history Record any previous criminal charges, convictions or contact with the police, including the dates on which they occurred. Ask if the patient has any present charges or court actions pending against him.

Social circumstances Determine where the patient lives and if he shares accommodation with others. Enquire about income and how he is coping financially. Ask if there are any dependents, any outstanding debts, and if he is receiving any form of social support or monetary assistance.

Personality Try to describe the patient's usual and present mood. How does he feel about himself and about other people? How does he enjoy himself and how does he react to good, bad or stressful events?

Corroboration Extremely important information can be gathered from close relatives, GPs, community, or social services, and should be sought to verify or enhance information obtained directly from the patient.

Mental state examination

Having taken an appropriately thorough history, make an assessment of the patient's mental state. If the patient is violent, disturbed, or for some other reason unable to provide background history, the information or observations gathered, whilst assessing mental state become even more crucial to diagnosis.

Appearance and behaviour

Gather information from the moment the interview begins. Is the patient appropriately dressed; is he clean and tidy, or neglected? Does his general posture, body movement, and facial expression suggest fear, anxiety, aggression, withdrawal, detachment, or low mood? Does he maintain eye contact? Does he respond appropriately to external stimuli or is he easily distracted? Does he appear to be hallucinating or responding to no obvious stimuli? Are there any abnormal movements, tics, grimaces, or dystonic movements? Note whether behaviour is steady and consistent, or labile and unpredictable.

Speech

Describe the rate, volume, intonation, and spontaneity of speech. Note the presence of dysarthria or dysphasia. Record any examples of invented new words (neologisms), unusual phrases, perseveration, or garbled speech verbatim. Note vagueness, over-preciseness, or sudden switching to new themes or subjects (flight of ideas).

Mood

Taking cues from appearance and behaviour, enquire about the patient's prevailing mood, opinion of himself, and view of the future. Enquire about suicidal thoughts and thoughts of harm to others. Ask about disturbances in sleep, appetite, libido, concentration, and mood variations during a typical day. Ask about irritability or memory disturbance (particularly of short-term memory).

Thought abnormalities

These are best recorded as they are found during the interview (eg thought blocking or flight of ideas). Test for concrete thinking by asking the patient to interpret a simple proverb. Ideas of reference or persecutory delusions may require direct enquiry to be revealed (eg asking about neighbours, electrical devices). Similarly, passivity phenomena may require specific questioning to be elicited (eg Is anyone making you think or move without you wanting to?)

Hallucinations

Record the presence of any hallucinations including their nature and specific content. Visual, olfactory, gustatory and tactile hallucinations should prompt suspicion of organic, rather than psychiatric disease.

Insight and mental capacity

Does he believe he is ill, does he think he requires treatment and would he be willing to accept it? Does he have mental capacity (📖 p.615)?

Assessment of risk

Consider whether the patient and/or others are at any risk of harm. Ask if the patient has any thoughts of self-harm and/or harm to other individuals. Establish if there is any past history of self-harm or violence. Try to decide if the patient is at risk of abuse/neglect and consider whether he may be a 'vulnerable adult'—such concerns should trigger a Safeguarding Alert.

Children at risk

Find out if there are any children in the patient's household and, if so, whether or not there are satisfactory arrangements in place to care for them. Concerns should prompt consideration of involvement of Social Services and/or Child Protection referral.

Physical examination

A physical examination completes any psychiatric evaluation. Specifically check for evidence of those physical illnesses which can be associated with psychiatric disturbance (eg thyroid disease, substance withdrawal, head injury, epilepsy, cerebrovascular disease, or other intracranial pathology). Carefully examine for focal neurological signs, meningism, organic confusional states, intoxication, and injury. In acute psychological disturbance, perform and record the following basic observations and investigations (this may prove to be very difficult in violent or aggressive individuals):

- Baseline pulse, respiratory rate, BP and SpO_2.
- Temperature (T)°.
- BMG/blood glucose.
- Urinalysis.
- Breath alcohol.

Undertake other investigations such as U&E, FBC, CXR, or CT scanning if clinically relevant. Urine drug screening, TFTs or electroencephalogram may be indicated in some situations, but are rarely available acutely.

Cognitive assessment

Although the psychiatric interview will, in general, reveal information about a patient's cognitive abilities, a formal evaluation of higher mental function is essential. Failure to do this can lead to organic brain disease being falsely labelled as a 'functional' or purely psychiatric illness, resulting in inappropriate treatment. Assess the following:

- Level of consciousness (eg alert, hyperalert, withdrawn, or comatose).
- Orientation.
- Attention and concentration.
- Registration of new information.
- Recall of recent and distant memories.
- Ability to interpret instructions and carry out tasks.

The Mini-Mental State Examination

The Mini-Mental State Examination was designed as a screening tool for the assessment of cognitive function in the elderly. It is in widespread use, but note that as with many psychological tests, it is subject to copyright.

The aggressive patient: background

A significant (albeit small) proportion of patients exhibit aggressive behaviour towards staff (and others) who are attempting to help them. Sometimes this amounts to physical violence. It is vital that all ED staff receive appropriate training in this area, bearing in mind that recognition and prevention of aggression is just as important as knowing how to manage it when it occurs.

Underlying causes

Medical illness

Recognize that a patient's agitation or aggression may be because of an underlying treatable acute medical condition. Such conditions may be compounded (as well as being potentially caused) by the use of *alcohol and/or illicit drugs*:

- Hypoglycaemia (📖 p.150).
- Head injury.
- Hypoxia (any cause).
- Distended bladder.
- Post-ictal confusional states (epilepsy or drug overdose).
- Organic brain syndromes (eg acute confusional states—📖 p.134).

Psychiatric illness

Most violent, aggressive, or bizarre patients in the ED are not mentally ill. Violence resulting directly from psychiatric illness, which needs urgent treatment is relatively uncommon. It is restricted to a small number of patients and tends to be associated with the following:

- A past history of violent behaviour.
- Schizophrenia and other psychoses (eg mania or paranoid disorders), especially when there are delusions or hallucinations that focus upon one particular individual.
- Personality disorder, particularly sociopathic, impulsive, or explosive disorders.
- Learning disability.

Warning signs of impending violence

Violent episodes can frequently be predicted and often prevented. The experienced practitioner may be able to spot the signs of approaching trouble at an earlier stage. Warning signs include the following:

- Angry facial expressions, gestures, and posture (aggressive body language).
- Restlessness, overt irritation, discontentment, pacing about, over-arousal (dilated pupils, tachycardia, increased respiratory rate).
- Prolonged eye contact.
- Loud speech and changes in tone of voice.
- Verbally threatening and/or reporting feelings of anger/violence.
- Repeating behaviour, which has previously preceded violent episodes.
- Blocking escape routes.

Safe consultations with potentially violent patients

Planning before the consultation

Physical design issues

Many departments have specially designed facilities with the interview room door designed to open outwards in order to allow rapid, easy exit.

It is important to regard any loose items as potential weapons (eg telephones, chairs, lamps).

Safety first

Safety comes first—ensure that patients are not allowed to harm themselves, other patients, or staff. Aim to conduct the consultation in a quiet, comfortable and, preferably, non-clinical area. However, compromise privacy, rather than safety, so if there are concerns, it may be necessary to undertake the consultation in a standard cubicle. Consider having another member of staff present during the consultation. Before consulting with any potentially violent patient ensure the following:

- Other staff know where you are and who you are with.
- You know how to get help (a 'panic button' or other personal alarm).
- Staff know to respond immediately.
- Staff know what to do if there is a problem.

Information gathering

Obtain as much information as possible beforehand. Useful sources of information may include relatives, police, social services, GP, and other health professionals.

The consultation

The outcome of the consultation depends heavily upon how it is conducted:

- Ensure that your own body language does not provoke the situation.
- Remain calm and sympathetic, maintaining a reassuring and non-judgmental manner.
- Listen to any immediate complaint or grievance with a minimum of interruption.
- Engage in conversation, with continuing reassurances that you are there to help.
- Adopt an attentive, but relaxed posture.
- Speak slowly and clearly, keeping your voice low.
- Avoid excessive eye contact.
- Sit between the patient and the door and not directly facing the patient (as this may appear confrontational and will provide a larger target for attack).
- Never turn your back on the patient, particularly when leaving the room.

Managing aggression

Violent behaviour is unusual if a calm, sensible approach is followed. If violence does occur, focus upon preventing the patient from harming other patients/relatives, staff, or themselves. See www.nice.org.uk

Approach to the aggressive patient

Get immediate help from police/security officers and other staff. Avoid physical confrontation, and ensure that you position yourself within the examination room or cubicle with no block to your escape. Take note of where the alarm buttons are situated. Continue de-escalation techniques.

- Find out what the problem is, establish a rapport and encourage reasoning.
- Show concern and stay attentive.
- Avoid patronizing comments. Never insult the patient, or make promises or commitments that cannot be kept.
- Direct body contact can be misinterpreted.
- Do not engage in prolonged eye contact.
- Remember that psychotic patients have different perceptions of personal space and may feel threatened by staff coming into what would otherwise be a normal and non-threatening distance.
- Try to maintain a calm atmosphere with a non-critical, non-domineering approach.

Management of physical violence

If physical violence occurs, safety of staff, other patients, and relatives takes priority. Concern for property is secondary—it can be replaced. Even during a violent act, a calm approach with talking and listening often prevents escalation of the event and the need for physical confrontation.

Physical restraint Avoid physical intervention if at all possible. Where physical restraint is required, use the minimum degree of force, applied for the minimum length of time in order to control the episode. Apply it in a manner that attempts to calm, rather than provoke, further aggression. This will require sufficient members of staff to control the event without injury to anyone involved.

Restrain the patient by holding clothing rather than limbs. If limbs have to be grasped, hold near a major joint in order to reduce leverage and the possibility of fracture or dislocation. Remove the patient's shoes or boots. In exceptional circumstances (eg when a patient is biting) the hair may have to be held firmly. Never apply pressure to the neck, throat, chest, back, pelvis or abdomen. Do not deliberately inflict pain.

Do not attempt restraint unless sufficient staff/expertise is available. Put one person in charge to ensure airway and breathing are not compromised and vital signs are monitored. Only ↓ restraint once it is certain that the risk has ↓—this may mean use of medication.

Weapons Ask for any weapon to be placed in a 'neutral' position, rather than handed over. Do not attempt to remove a weapon from an aggressor.

Emergency sedation of a violent patient

Pharmacological restraint using sedative drugs is a last resort, and should only be given on the advice of senior and experienced staff. Emergency sedation carries significant dangers. Sedative drugs may mask important signs of underlying illness, eg an intracranial haematoma requiring urgent treatment. The normal protective reflexes (including airway reflexes, such as gag and cough response) will be suppressed. Respiratory depression and the need for tracheal intubation and IPPV may develop. Adverse cardiovascular events (eg hypotension and arrhythmias) may be provoked, particularly in a struggling, hypoxic individual. Finally, staff need to be aware of medicolegal implications of carrying out any restraint.

Oral tranquillization

If possible sedative drugs should be given orally, rather than by injection, but oral treatment may not be feasible in a violent and disturbed patient.
- Give *lorazepam* (1–2 mg PO) if there is no psychotic context.
- Give *lorazepam* (1–2 mg PO) + antipsychotic (eg *haloperidol* 1.5–3mg PO) if there is a psychotic context.
- Allow sufficient time for response before considering a second dose.

IM tranquillization

If oral therapy inappropriate (refused, failed or not indicated).
- Give *lorazepam* (2–4 mg intramuscular (IM) in non-psychotic context).
- Give *lorazepam* (2–4 mg IM) + antipsychotic (eg *haloperidol* 5–10mg IM) if there is a psychotic context. When using haloperidol ensure procyclidine is immediately available to treat acute dystonia or other extrapyramidal side-effects.
- Allow sufficient time for response before considering a second dose.
- Avoid IM diazepam, chlorpromazine or thioridazine.

IV tranquillization

Only in truly exceptional circumstances, when immediate tranquillization is essential, IV drugs may be used (ideally after senior consultation):

Consider IV benzodiazepine or IV haloperidol.

Avoid parenteral clomethiazole, barbiturates, and paraldehyde, as they are associated with a significant risk of respiratory depression.

See NICE Clinical Guideline 25 on '*Violence*'

http://guidance.nice.org.uk/CG25/QuickRefGuide/pdf/English

After the violent episode

Following any episode of verbal aggression or physical violence, ensure that the staff involved record full detailed notes and that standard local incident forms are completed. Report the episode to the senior member of staff and to the police (as appropriate), if they are not already involved. Subsequently, when dealing with the violent patient, do not purposely avoid the patient or treat him obviously differently, since this will merely emphasize concepts of his own unacceptability and may lead to further aggression.

Deliberate self-harm

Deliberate self-harm (DSH) accounts for ≈20% of acute medical admissions in the UK. Psychiatric symptoms are often associated with DSH, but tend to be transient and predominantly related to social or emotional factors. Psychiatric illness is relatively uncommon (≈5–8% of cases, mostly depression). ≈90% of DSH involve self-poisoning, the remainder physical self-injury (eg cutting). Most DSH episodes are impulsive (considered for <1hr beforehand). Associated alcohol consumption is common and may have precipitated the event. However, assess carefully—1% of DSH patients do commit suicide within a year. Some hospitals admit DSH patients to an ED observation ward, allowing alcohol to wear off until the situation can be properly assessed. Useful guidance on the treatment and management of self-harm in EDs has been published by NICE (www.nice.org.uk).

Triage

Patients who present following an episode of physical self-harm and/or overdose require rapid initial assessment (triage) in order to establish the degree of urgency of the situation, mental capacity, and willingness to stay, distress levels, and presence of mental illness. Factors that may render the situation more urgent include:
- Need for urgent treatment for physical injury and/or overdose.
- Immediate risk of violence to others.
- Immediate risk of further self-harm.
- Need for treatment, but patient threatening to leave.

Australian Mental Health Triage Scale

This combined physical and mental health triage scale is recommended by NICE and can be adapted for easy use (see www.rcpsych.ac.uk). Some features are summarized in the Table 14.1.

Table 14.1 The Australian Mental Health Triage Scale

Triage category	Features
1 Extremely urgent	Violent, possessing a weapon, or further self-harm in the ED
2 Very urgent	Extremely agitated/restless, aggressive, confused/unable to cooperate, or requiring restraint
3 Urgent	Agitated/restless, bizarre behaviour, psychotic symptoms, severe depression and/or anxiety
4 Less urgent	Symptoms of anxiety and/or depression without suicidal ideation
5 Least urgent	Compliant, cooperative and communicative

There should be a system in place so that self-harm patients are checked upon at least every hour—a change in triage category may require more urgent assessment.

Management plan

All patients who present to the ED after self-harm should be offered a psychosocial assessment of needs and risk by an appropriately trained individual. Some units continue to admit all patients with DSH for psychiatric appraisal once medically fit, but sheer numbers can make this difficult. A selective approach distinguishes patients with underlying psychiatric pathology and/or true suicidal intent—both requiring formal psychiatric evaluation. Many centres have developed psychiatric liaison services with medical and nursing mental health specialists who can offer timely and expert input.

Assessment

Involve family/carers whenever possible, with the patient's consent.

Focus upon:
- Events and circumstances leading up to the episode of self-harm.
- Preparation, concealment, and true intention of a DSH act.
- Outcome of DSH act (eg unintended danger or accidental discovery).
- Current stresses, financial, legal, or interpersonal problems.
- Alcohol or substance misuse.
- Previous self-harm or psychiatric illness.

Decide about psychiatric referral using this information. If in doubt, refer. Also refer immediately any child or adolescent who presents with DSH. Many EDs have a system whereby patients who are not deemed to be at immediate risk can return the following day for an appointment with a psychiatric liaison nurse/specialist for psychosocial assessment. In the absence of such a system, ensure that the patient's GP receives written communication about the patient's ED attendance and discharge.

Factors suggesting suicidal intent

- Careful preparation (eg saving tablets) and/or significant premeditation.
- Final acts (eg organizing finances, insurance or a will).
- Carrying out DSH alone, secretly or when unlikely to be discovered.
- Not seeking help following DSH.
- A definite, sustained wish to die.

Suicide notes can be important, but are sometimes left for dramatic effect and so are not always reliable indicators.

Consider all self-harm acts by individuals aged >65 years to be evidence of suicidal intent until proved otherwise.

Risk of further self-harm

Recurrence is most likely if there have been repeated previous episodes (eg habitual self-cutters or recurrent overdoses).

Socio-demographic predictors include being single or separated, aged 25–54 years, being unemployed or social class V.

Other factors include drug or alcohol dependence, a history of criminal behaviour, previous psychiatric treatment, or the presence of a personality disorder.

Assessment of suicide risk

Prevention of suicide is a primary aim in assessing DSH. Certain factors are common among completed suicides and are significant if found in a DSH patient:

- Male.
- Elderly (particularly female).
- Living alone.
- Separated, divorced, or widowed.
- Unemployed or retired.
- Physical illness (eg painful, debilitating, or terminal conditions).
- Psychiatric illness (especially schizophrenia and depression).
- Alcoholism.
- Sociopathic personality disorder.
- Violent method of DSH (eg hanging, shooting, drowning, or high fall).

Modified Sad Persons Scale

It can be difficult for clinicians without a psychiatric background to make an assessment of the suicide risk. The modified 'Sad Persons Scale' attempts to assist non-psychiatrists with this task. It may serve as a guide regarding the need for referral or admission (Table 14.2).

Table 14.2 Modified Sad Persons Scale

	Score
Sex male	1
Age <19 or >45 years.	1
Depression or hopelessness	2
Previous suicide attempts or psychiatric care	1
Excessive alcohol or drug use	1
Rational thinking loss (psychotic or organic illness)	2
Separated, widowed, or divorced	1
Organized or serious attempt	2
No social support	1
Stated future intent (determined to repeat or ambivalent)	2

Interpretation of total score

Score <6 may be safe to discharge (depending upon circumstances).

Score 6–8 probably requires psychiatric consultation.

Score >8 probably requires hospital admission.

Mental health assessment issues

Patients who present with deliberate self-harm can present difficult problems that are not often a feature of patients who do not have mental health problems. The management of some of these issues is addressed by NICE (www.nice.org.uk) and summarized below.

Timing of psychosocial assessment

The ideal is to offer psychosocial assessment of patients with DSH as soon as possible. There are occasions when this assessment needs to be delayed, including the following:

- Life-saving treatment for physical injuries is needed.
- The patient is unconscious and/or significantly under influence of alcohol/drugs and, therefore, not capable of being properly assessed.

Patient threatening to leave the department

Not infrequently, patients state that they wish to leave the department before psychosocial assessment. Very often, it is possible to persuade them to stay. Perform an assessment of the patient's mental capacity and mental illness to decide whether it is necessary to detain him/her under the Mental Capacity Act or Mental Health Act if he/she attempts to leave.

Diminished mental capacity and/or significant mental illness

If there is diminished mental capacity and/or significant mental illness, refer for urgent mental health assessment and prevent the patient from leaving the department. If the patient does manage to leave the department despite best efforts, contact the police in order to try to bring him/her back.

No reduction in mental capacity and no significant mental illness

If there is no reduction in mental capacity and no significant mental illness and the patient leaves the department, pass information on to his/her GP and to the relevant mental health services as soon as possible, to enable rapid follow up.

Physical treatments

Management of poisoning is the focus of Chapter 4. Note that it is sensible to measure paracetamol levels in any patient who presents with a history of overdose of paracetamol and/or other drugs.

Superficial skin wounds <5cm long are often managed satisfactorily with tissue adhesive strips. Deeper skin wounds, or those >5cm in length require standard assessment and treatment (📖 Wound management, p.406).

Repeat self-harmers

There may be local organizations to help self-harmers, as well as national organizations, such as the Samaritans (a listening service). Specific advice for people who repeatedly self-injure includes advice and instruction on harm minimization issues, self-management of superficial injuries, and dealing with scar tissue.

Depression

Everyone experiences low mood at times. It needs treatment when prolonged, unrelenting, inappropriate or disabling. Lifetime risk of depression is ≈10% for men and ≈20% for women. General population prevalence is 3–6% (↑ with age). Co-existing psychiatric or physical illness can make the diagnosis of depression difficult. Conversely, depression may be the presenting feature of physical illness (eg hypothyroidism, Cushing's syndrome, or malignancy). ≈15% of those with recurrent affective disorder eventually commit suicide. Persisting suicidal ideation or recent DSH, even if trivial, is highly significant in the presence of a diagnosis of depression.

Aetiology

Complex, with genetic, social, environmental, and neurochemical factors. Mood disorders are more common in relatives of depressives. Life events involving loss (partner, friend, health, job, status) can precipitate depression (risk ↑ to 6× normal in 6 months after such an event). Loss of a parent in childhood, unemployment, and lack of confiding relationship with a partner ↑ vulnerability. Neurochemical mechanisms are involved ('amine theory'). Effective antidepressants ↑ brain availability of serotonin and noradrenaline.

Presentation and symptoms

Depressed patients almost always have persistent low mood, loss of interest and enjoyment (anhedonia) and lack of energy. Mood is unaffected by circumstances. Look for common features (Table 14.3).

Table 14.3 Common features indicating a person's mood

Common symptoms	Somatic or vegetative symptoms
↓ Self-esteem and self-confidence	Sleep disturbance
↓ Concentration and attention	↓ Appetite
Memory disturbance (esp short-term)	Weight loss
Bleak and pessimistic views of the future	Constipation
Ideas of self-harm or suicide	Amenorrhoea
Feelings of guilt or worthlessness	Loss of interest or enjoyment

Look for self-neglect. Does the patient exhibit psychomotor retardation (slow movements and speech) or is he agitated? Is eye contact maintained? Are there deficits of short-term memory and cognition that improve with ↑ effort? Psychotic symptoms occur in very severe cases (eg hallucinations or delusions). These are mood congruent: derogatory voices, ideas of poverty, guilt, nihilism (patient believes he has no bowel, no clothes, no life, etc.). Anxiety can be a feature of depression.

Atypical depression can involve reversal of usual somatic symptoms leading to ↑ appetite, ↑ weight, hypersomnia, and reversed diurnal mood variation.

Treatment

Arrange psychiatric assessment for patients with *severe depression*, suicidal ideation, or psychotic features. Most respond to antidepressants, but do not start these in the ED. Some patients also require antipsychotics or ECT. In cases with psychotic features or where there is a high risk of death from suicide or profound self-neglect, ECT is effective.

Mild/moderate cases may respond to psychological therapy. Counselling can help specific problems (eg bereavement or marital difficulties).

Mania

Mania and hypomania are less common than other mood disorders, but more often require compulsory hospital admission. Pathologically elevated mood combines with over-activity, irrationality, poor judgement and lack of insight (see Table 14.4 for primary and other features). This leads to severe disruption of relationships, employment or finances. Untreated, high rates of divorce, debt, violence, or suicide occur. Onset may be acute or insidious. Manic disorders can arise spontaneously or follow depressive illness, stress, surgery, infection, or childbirth. Antidepressant medication, ECT, steroids, and amphetamines can all precipitate mania, as can lithium withdrawal.

Table 14.4 Primary and other features of mania

Primary features	Other features
Over-cheerfulness	Irritability
Over-talkativeness	Flight of ideas
Over-activity	Distractibility
	Grandiosity
	↓ Requirement for sleep
	Delusions (mood-congruent)
	Hallucinations
	Impaired judgement
	Irresponsibility and impetuousness
	Gambling and promiscuity

Hypomania denotes an intermediate state without delusions, hallucinations or complete disruption of normal activities.

Differential diagnosis

Schizophrenia can present with disorganized behaviour, violent excitement, delusions, and incomprehensible speech. The content of delusions (ie bizarre, rather than mood-congruent), will help distinguish this from mania.

Approach to the patient

Stay calm and non-confrontational. Beware infectious optimism, which can easily lead to underestimating the severity of illness or the requirement for admission. Seek additional information from relatives. Irritability can be the dominant symptom of mania and may be expressed as a savage, highly detailed catalogue of the interviewer's shortcomings. Irritable patients can become angry or violent in the face of even minor frustrations.

Treatment

Overt manic illness is best managed in hospital to avoid behaviour harmful to the patient or others. Insight is often ↓ or absent, so compulsory admission may be required. Liaise with the psychiatrist before commencing definitive drug treatment as this may adversely affect assessment. Lithium carbonate is traditional and effective in most cases, both to treat the acute episode and as prophylaxis against recurrent mania. However, it usually takes some days to work, so an antipsychotic (eg olanzapine) or benzodiazepine may be needed initially.

Schizophrenia

This affects all areas of personal function, including thought content and process, perception, speech, mood, motivation and behaviour. A common pattern is acute exacerbation with ↑ residual handicap between episodes. 30% of those who suffer a first episode never have another. Another 30% develop chronic symptoms requiring frequent admission or long-term care. The lifetime risk is 1/100.

Clinical features

No single symptom is pathognomonic: hallucinations or delusions simply confirm psychosis.

Schneider's First Rank Symptoms originally suggested schizophrenia in the absence of organic disorder. It is now acknowledged that they can occur in mania and other conditions:

- *Auditory hallucinations* ≥2 voices discussing the subject in the third person or giving a running commentary on his/her thoughts/behaviour.
- Thought withdrawal, insertion, or broadcasting.
- *Somatic passivity* sensations, emotions, or actions are externally imposed or controlled.
- *Delusional perception* a genuine perception takes on abnormal significance for the subject and is the basis of their delusional system.
- *Gedankenlautwerden* voices repeating the subject's thoughts out loud or anticipating the subject's thoughts.

Diagnosis

Mental state examination will help to exclude organic and affective disorders, remembering:

- Non-auditory hallucinations are more common in organic conditions.
- Delusions in depression and mania are mood-congruent.

Differential diagnoses
Organic causes: temporal lobe epilepsy, drug-induced states, alcoholic hallucinosis, cerebral tumour, encephalitis, head injury.

Psychiatric: affective psychoses, schizo-affective disorder, psychogenic psychosis, delusional disorder (eg infestation), personality disorder.

Management

Patients not known to have schizophrenia
Refer to the psychiatric team who will advise about the need for urgent antipsychotic treatment.

Patients known to have schizophrenia
Schizophrenics frequently present to the ED with mental health issues and problems. It can be difficult to formulate a management plan unless relevant background information is available. Liaise with relevant individuals (including community psychiatric nurse and psychiatrist) to decide whether to treat in hospital or in the community and what form any treatment should take.

Complications of psychiatric drugs

Antipsychotic drugs

Acute dystonic reactions (grimacing, facial, and masseter spasm, deviated gaze, torticollis, limb rigidity, and behavioural disturbances) frequently present to EDs. They follow ingestion of antipsychotics (eg phenothiazines or haloperidol) and/or other drugs (eg metoclopramide), even in therapeutic dosages. Reactions can occur up to 1 week after ingestion. Acute dystonia can dislocate the mandible. Dystonia can be mistaken for malingering, as symptoms can be briefly interrupted by voluntary actions. Once diagnosed, *treat with*:

Procyclidine 5 mg IV bolus, repeated as necessary after a few minutes.

Dramatic resolution of symptoms occurs within minutes, confirming the diagnosis. Symptoms may recur—treat with oral procyclidine 5mg every 8hr. Large doses of procyclidine cause euphoria and fixed dilated pupils, hence, its abuse by some patients. Diazepam also works, but is less specific and carries risks of excessive drowsiness or respiratory depression.

Clozapine

An atypical antipsychotic used in treatment-resistant schizophrenia. Agranulocytosis occurs in 3% of patients. For this reason, all patients are enrolled with the Clozaril Patient Monitoring Service (telephone 0845 769 8269) who supervise regular blood screening. Check FBC for neutropenia in any patient presenting with fever, sore throat, or other infection.

Monoamine oxidase inhibitors (MAOIs)

MAOIs (eg phenelzine, tranylcypromine), irreversibly block enzymes responsible for oxidative metabolism of 5HT, noradrenaline, tyramine, and other amines. Once discontinued, enzyme inhibition continues for up to 2 weeks, during which time other drugs should not be introduced. Newer, reversible MAOIs ('RIMAs'—eg moclobemide) cease to have effects after 24–48hr. MAOIs cause postural hypotension, but acute hypertensive reactions follow ingestion of amine rich foods (eg Bovril™, Marmite™, cheese, red wine). Noradrenaline release causes vasoconstriction, tachycardia, and hypertension that can, in severe cases, lead to intracerebral or subarachnoid haemorrhage. Similar hypertensive crises can be caused by concurrent use of L-dopa, sympathomimetics, amphetamine, or drinking certain low-alcohol beers or wines.

Lithium

Lithium toxicity presents with severe nausea, vomiting, cerebellar signs, or confusion. SSRIs (eg fluoxetine), anticonvulsants, antipsychotics, diuretics, methyldopa, and calcium channel blockers can all precipitate toxicity. *Look for* tremor, cerebellar ataxia, muscular twitching (myoclonus), spasticity, choreiform movements, up-going plantar responses, incoordination, slurred speech, impaired concentration, drowsiness, coma. *Check serum lithium* (plain, not lithium heparin tube!) and U&E immediately. Serum lithium levels correspond poorly with clinical signs (toxicity can occur within therapeutic range), so diagnosis of toxicity is based on clinical observations. Stop lithium and treat according to severity of toxicity (☐ p.197).

Munchausen's syndrome

Also known as 'hospital hopper', this is characterized by recurrent hospital admissions with factitious symptoms and signs of physical illness. Other basic components are a morbid attraction to the sick role, pathological lying and pleasure from deceiving medical staff. The incidence is unknown, but it is probably underestimated. It is believed to be commoner in men with peak onset at 30–40 years. There may be an underlying personality disorder, but true psychiatric illness is rare. Origins are uncertain: excessive dependency, inability to form trusting relationships, attention-seeking, childhood hospitalization, and resentment of doctors for previous treatment have all been suggested.

Presentation

Common presentations involve detailed and convincing descriptions of cardiac chest pain, abdominal pain (especially pancreatitis), haematemesis, haemoptysis, rectal bleeding, haematuria, or pyrexia. More rarely, patients present with artefactual dermatitis or with a dramatic history of trauma (eg fall or pedestrian knockdown). Distinguish Munchausen's from:

- *Malingering:* fabricating illness for definite gain (eg stealing drugs, avoiding court appearance, faking symptoms to obtain opioids).
- *Somatoform disorders:* physical symptoms or signs without organic cause, but not under voluntary control.
- *Fabricated and induced illness:* see 📖 p.733.

Suspicious features

- Incomplete or inconsistent disclosure of personal details and past history.
- Patient a long way from home area for unclear reasons.
- Recent dramatic history of myocardial infarction (MI), surgery, or complications elsewhere.
- Excellent knowledge of finer details of past treatment and/or complications.
- *Multiple scars:* laparotomies, sternotomy, venous cutdowns.
- Elaborate history of allergy (eg allergic to all painkillers except pethidine).
- Unconvincing claims of medical or paramedical occupation.
- Unusual/demanding behaviour and/or avoidance of eye contact.
- No ascertainable organic cause for the symptoms.

Management

Early recognition is important, but first exclude genuine illness. There may be no alternative to admission and observation to make the diagnosis, even though this achieves the patient's aim. If suspicions are aroused, discreetly check past history. Once discovered, most patients self-discharge, often noisily, but rarely violently.

Avoid a 'showdown' Simply state that deception is at an end, that no retribution is planned and offer to help the patient with their problem.

Do not use placebos to uncover fabricated illness—they can work equally well on genuine symptoms!

Once discovered, record events carefully, particularly the medical history given, background details, appearance, scars. Circulate details to other EDs.

Factitious disorder in health care workers

The Clothier report (Department of Health, 1994) advised that patients with severe personality disorder (by inference, factitious disorder) should be prevented from working in health-related disciplines. Detection of factitious disorder in health care workers has serious implications. If suspected, discuss immediately with the ED consultant.

Medically unexplained symptoms

Background

A significant proportion of patients who attend the ED have symptoms for which no cause is found. Some of these patients manage to build up a significant volume (or volumes!) of medical records.

Terminology

There is a potentially confusing range of terms in use.

Somatization
Physical symptoms with presumed psychological origin.

Somatoform pain disorder
Persistent, severe unexplained pain, which is attributed to psychological disorders.

Conversion (dissociative) disorders
Loss or disturbance of normal motor or sensory function, which is attributed to a psychological origin (thoughts/memories to the conscious mind are 'converted' into physical symptoms (eg amnesia).

Factitious symptoms
Symptoms which are intentionally produced, with the aim of receiving a medical diagnosis—when there is secondary gain (eg legal compensation, obtaining opioid drugs), it is known as *malingering*.

Medically unexplained symptoms
This is an umbrella term, which makes no assumptions about the cause of the symptoms.

Differential diagnosis

Patients who present acutely with medically unexplained symptoms may be suffering from a range of problems, including: anxiety, depression, psychosis, 'functional somatic illness', conversion disorders, factitious disorders, malingering, and uncommon medical syndromes that have not yet been diagnosed.

Approach to patients with medically unexplained symptoms

The Royal College of Psychiatrists (www.rcpsych.ac.uk) has published some useful recommendations. Consider the following:

- Try to obtain past medical and psychiatric records/summaries (computerized records may assist in this process) and/or speak to the GP.
- If the patient's medical complaints are known to be unexplained (or part of a psychiatric illness), then further investigations may be inappropriate.
- Investigate judiciously—do not underestimate the ability to cause iatrogenic harm.

Alcohol abuse

Alcohol-related problems account for up to 15% of the ED workload in the UK. Alcoholics have ↑ rates of heart disease, malignancy, and stroke, but often succumb to injuries. Excessive alcohol consumption is a feature of 30% of road traffic fatalities, 25% of fatal work injuries, 30% of drownings and 50% of burn deaths. Alcohol is involved in ≈30% of suicides, ≈60% of homicides and most assaults. Suspicion is the key to detecting alcohol problems.

Units

The number of 'units' (10mL of pure alcohol) is included on packaging. A bottle of wine contains ≈10U and a bottle of spirits ≈30U. Current advice is a 'safe' limit of 21U/week (males) and 14U/week (females).

Alcohol absorption, metabolism, and elimination

Alcohol is absorbed from the small intestine and to a lesser extent, the stomach. The rate of absorption depends on the nature of the drink and any associated food consumed. Alcohol is absorbed more slowly from dilute drinks (eg wine) compared with more concentrated fortified sherry or port. Alcohol is water soluble, so distributes throughout the body. It is mostly metabolized in the liver by an enzymatic process involving alcohol dehydrogenase, which converts it to acetaldehyde and then acetic acid. A relatively small amount of alcohol is excreted unchanged in the urine (and to a lesser extent, in breath and sweat).

Clearance of alcohol The rate of clearance of alcohol from the blood varies enormously between individuals, with typical quoted values of 10–20mg/dL/hr in most adults, although higher values occur in some chronic alcoholics.

Assessing alcohol problems

A history of alcohol consumption is notoriously unreliable when taken from heavy drinkers and chronic alcoholics, who may significantly under-report the extent of their drinking and its effect upon their lives. The actual amount of alcohol consumed is less important than the consequences of drinking to the patient. Cover the following areas:
Biological GI upset/bleeding, withdrawal fits, blackouts, peripheral neuropathy.
Psychological Low mood, hallucinations, delusions, memory problems.
Social Marital, work, driving, debt, criminality.
Significant features include compulsion to drink and loss of control.

The CAGE questionnaire

• Have you ever felt you should *Cut down* your drinking?
• Have people *Annoyed you* by criticizing your drinking?
• Have you ever felt *Guilty* about your drinking?
• Have you ever had a drink first-thing in the morning to steady your nerves or to get rid of a hangover *(Eye-opener)*?

Any single, +ve answer is significant and >1 +ve answer is probably diagnostic of chronic alcohol dependence.

Acute alcohol intoxication

Effects of intoxication

Alcohol depresses the nervous system—initial euphoric effects are due to suppression of inhibition by the cerebral cortex. Effects vary between individuals and Table 14.5 is a very rough guide. Behaviour, including propensity to violence, is influenced by environment and social setting. Although death may occur at levels >350mg/100mL, the risk of a harmful or fatal event increases at *any* level: especially road traffic collisions, work and home accidents and assaults (including sexual assault). The current UK blood alcohol legal limit for driving is 80mg/mL.

Table 14.5 Effects of various concentrations of alcohol

Blood alcohol concentration (mg/100mL = mg/dL)	Effects
30–50	Measurable impairment of motor skills
50–100	Reduced inhibitions, 'excitant effect'
100–150	Loss of co-ordination and control
150–200	'Drunkenness', nausea, ataxia
200–350	Vomiting, stupor, possible coma
350+	Respiratory paralysis, possible death

Alcohol intoxication is characterized by slurred speech, incoordination, unsteady gait, nystagmus, lethargy, and facial flushing. The differential diagnosis is extensive: head injury, hypoglycaemia, post-ictal confusional states, hepatic encephalopathy, meningitis, encephalitis, or intoxication with other drugs. In most patients these conditions can be excluded by examination and simple investigations (although some not infrequently coexist with acute alcohol intoxication—especially head injury and hypoglycaemia).

Management

Aim to discharge conscious, ambulant patients who exhibit uncomplicated acute alcohol intoxication if accompanied by a responsible adult.

Violent patients who appear intoxicated require examination prior to escort from the ED by police. As a minimum, perform a brief neurological examination, simple observations and BMG.

Comatose patients are a medical emergency. Protect the airway and anticipate vomiting (recovery position may be useful). Exclude hypoglycaemia and other metabolic causes of coma. Exclude head or neck injury, and adopt a low threshold for X-ray and/or CT scanning. Close observation is mandatory.

Alcohol-induced hypoglycaemia particularly affects chronic alcoholics and children. It also occurs in binge drinkers who present with alcoholic ketoacidosis. Hypoglycaemia can occur during intoxication and up to 24hr after. In children, fits may result.

Coagulation disorders often occur in chronic alcoholics with liver damage. Consider this in patients presenting with GI haemorrhage or head injury.

Alcohol withdrawal

'Simple' alcohol withdrawal

Uncomplicated alcohol withdrawal is common, usually starting within 12hr of stopping (or reducing) alcohol intake. Withdrawal symptoms often commence before alcohol is completely cleared from the blood. Features include anxiety, restlessness, tremor, insomnia, sweating, tachycardia, and ataxia. Simple withdrawal can be managed on an outpatient or day patient basis. It may be appropriate to commence treatment in the ED for uncomplicated withdrawal (eg diazepam 5–10mg PO or chlordiazepoxide 10–30mg), but continuing treatment should not be prescribed by ED staff. Inpatient detoxification is indicated for those with a history of withdrawal seizures, delirium tremens or with withdrawal symptoms who are being admitted for other problems. The revised Clinical Institute Withdrawal Assessment for Alcohol (CIWA-Ar) Score assesses 10 clinical signs of withdrawal and may help to guide treatment (www.agingincanada.ca/CIWA.HTM). Note: alcoholics admitted with 'simple' withdrawal may be thiamine deficient, and need parenteral and/or oral thiamine.

Delirium tremens

Occurs in a small minority of alcoholics who undergo withdrawal and carries a significant mortality. It typically starts >48hr after stopping drinking. As well as 'simple' withdrawal, there may be significant autonomic hyperactivity, with tachycardia, hyper-reflexia, hypertension, fever, visual or tactile hallucinations, sinister delusions, disorientation, and confusion. Deaths occur from arrhythmias (secondary to acidosis, electrolyte disturbance, or alcohol-related cardiomyopathy), infection, fits or cardiovascular collapse. Monitor closely, check BMG, give IV diazepam as appropriate (especially for fits) and refer to the medical team/HDU.

Alcohol withdrawal fits

These typically comprise self-limiting grand mal seizures which occur hours or days after the last alcoholic drink. Check BMG and treat fits in a standard fashion (📖 Seizures and status epilepticus, p.149). Examine carefully for possible head injury.

Alcoholic ketoacidosis

This can occur when an alcoholic stops drinking, vomits repeatedly and does not eat. Ketoacidosis develops from fatty acid breakdown, complicated by dehydration from vomiting. The patient usually presents 1–2 days after the last binge with vomiting, signs of chronic alcohol abuse and a high anion gap metabolic acidosis. Arterial blood gas (ABG) may reveal ↓ pCO_2, ↓ HCO_3^-, normal pO_2. pH is variable because metabolic acidosis may be altered by metabolic alkalosis from vomiting and possibly respiratory alkalosis. Plasma ethanol is low or absent. Differential diagnosis includes salicylate, methanol and ethylene glycol poisoning (📖 p.203). Give IV 0.9% saline with 5% glucose and thiamine supplementation, whilst monitoring U&E, glucose. Refer to the medical team and consider HDU/ICU.

Alcohol-related brain injury

Wernicke Korsakoff syndrome develops in problem drinkers who are thiamine deficient. Autopsy analysis suggests that the syndrome may occur in as many as 12.5% of chronic alcohol misusers. A presumptive diagnosis of the Wernicke Korsakoff syndrome may be made in patients with a history of alcohol misuse and one or more of the following unexplained symptoms: ataxia, ophthalmoplegia, nystagmus, confusion, memory disturbance, reduced conscious level, hypotension, and/or hypothermia.

Wernicke's encephalopathy

This is characterized by degenerative changes surrounding the third ventricle and aqueduct, particularly the mammillary bodies. It presents with an acute confusional state, nystagmus, ophthalmoplegia, ataxia, and polyneuropathy. Ataxia typically affects the trunk and lower extremities. Clinical abnormalities may develop acutely or evolve over several days.

Initial treatment involves parenteral thiamine (eg Pabrinex® 10mL as an IV infusion in 100mL 0.9% saline over 30min). Note that this may occasionally cause anaphylaxis, so ensure that resuscitation facilities are available. Subsequent treatment involves oral thiamine.

Korsakoff's psychosis

This is an amnesic state with profound retrograde and anterograde amnesia, but relative preservation of other intellectual abilities. It typically develops after Wernicke's encephalopathy, but some patients develop a combined syndrome from the outset with memory loss, eye signs and unsteadiness but without confusion.

Treat with parenteral thiamine and admission as for Wernicke's encephalopathy.

Help for alcoholics

The relatively regular contact between those with alcohol problems and EDs may be viewed as an opportunity to offer intervention. There is good evidence to suggest that brief interventions may reduce alcohol consumption and the risk of physical harm. Consider the 1min Paddington Alcohol Test to help patients who present with alcohol-related problems (http://alcalc.oxfordjournals.org/cgi/reprint/44/3/284).

The following organizations may help:

Alcoholics Anonymous (www.alcoholics-anonymous.org.uk), plus local networks and telephone numbers.

Al-Anon for relatives telephone number 020 7403 0888 (and websites www.al-anonuk.org.uk and www.al-anon.alateen.org).

Drug and substance abuse

Drug users present to the ED at times of crisis (eg acute intoxication, overdose, withdrawal or other medical complications of drug use). Do not assume all drug users present to the ED simply to obtain drugs. Find out about local addiction services and how referrals are made. Direct those seeking help with a drug problem to the appropriate services. Know local preferred drugs of abuse and the preferred methods of taking them. Find out what terminology is used locally for each substance.

Do not supply drugs of dependence to addicts. Prescriptions are carefully controlled by addiction services and pharmacists. Elaborate tales of lost or stolen drugs/prescriptions are invariably false.

Manage painful conditions in drug addicts as for other patients. Do not withhold analgesia if in obvious pain. For minor complaints, simple analgesia is as effective as in non-drug users. Do not dismiss symptoms simply because the patient is a drug user. Even drug abusers get acute appendicitis and other common acute illnesses.

Intoxication

As with alcohol, mild cases require little intervention. Observation by a responsible adult or briefly in a ward usually suffices. Discharge patients when ambulant and fully orientated, having excluded serious problems.

Glue and solvents Users may smell of substances or have them on their clothes or skin. There may be a perioral rash. Intoxication produces euphoria, agitation or drowsiness, slurred speech, and unsteady gait.

Benzodiazepines and CNS depressants Mild intoxication is similar to that with alcohol. ↑ intoxication produces nystagmus, diplopia, strabismus, hypotonia, clumsiness, and moderately dilated pupils.

Amphetamines, ecstasy, cocaine and mephedrone Produce hyperstimulation, restlessness, pyrexia and sympathomimetic effects. Cocaine effects occur more rapidly. Severe cases exhibit paranoia, violent behaviour or seizures. Cocaine may also cause chest pain, arrhythmias or even MI. Ecstasy can cause an idiosyncratic reaction similar to malignant hyperthermia (see 📖 Illicit drugs, p.214).

Overdose

Protect the airway, provide oxygen (O_2) as required and exclude hypoglycaemia or serious injury in all cases.

Opioid overdose is often inadvertent, either from use of unusually pure drugs or after a period of abstinence (tolerance is ↓). Characteristic signs are coma with pinpoint pupils and respiratory depression (see 📖 p.188). Pulmonary oedema, hypothermia and rhabdomyolysis can occur. Hypoxia may cause dilated pupils. If opioid overdose is suspected, give naloxone 0.4–0.8mg IV, repeated according to response. See 📖 Antidotes to poisons (📖 p.186) for further detail regarding treatment. Remember to ensure that the patient is observed for at least 6h after the last dose of naloxone.

Intentional overdose requires assessment of suicide risk (📖 p.614) and mental capacity in case the patient threatens to leave against advice.

Skin complications

SC drug injection ('skin popping') can cause cellulitis, abscesses, extensive skin necrosis, necrotizing fasciitis, tetanus, botulism and anthrax. Refer for formal exploration, drainage and follow-up by the surgical team for all but the most minor infections. Apparently 'simple' abscesses may extend deeply into muscle or form part of a false aneurysm! Needle fragments rarely require removal unless they embolize (eg to the lungs).

Anthrax in drug users

After an outbreak of anthrax in heroin users in Scotland in 2010, Health Protection Scotland (www.hps.scot.nhs.uk) advised doctors to suspect anthrax in a drug user presenting with any of the following:

- Severe soft tissue infection and/or signs of severe sepsis/meningitis.
- Clinical features of inhalational anthrax (📖 p.233).
- Respiratory symptoms + features of meningitis or intracranial bleeding.
- GI symptoms (eg pain, bleeding, nausea, vomiting, diarrhoea, ascites).

Approach

Get expert help early to advise on management (ICU, surgeons, microbiology, Public Health, hospital infection team). Start IV antibiotics according to advice (eg combination of ciprofloxacin, clindamycin + penicillin or if there is soft tissue infection: ciprofloxacin, clindamycin, penicillin, flucloxacillin + metronidazole). Experts will advise on whether to use anthrax immune globulin intravenous (human) antitoxin.

Vascular complications

IV injection ('mainlining') of drugs causes phlebitis, DVT, and bacterial endocarditis. Chronic injectors may resort to neck or groin vessels (the femoral artery being commonly damaged). Arterial injection can cause false aneurysms, fistulae, or peripheral emboli. Occasionally, IV drug users present with massive and devastating blood loss from an injection site (particularly the groin): apply firm pressure, resuscitate with IV fluids ± blood and call for the surgical team.

Inadvertent arterial injection of poorly soluble preparations causes severe limb pain, skin pallor and mottling with paraesthesiae in the presence of palpable (often bounding) peripheral pulses. Diffuse soft tissue damage may result in compartment syndromes, rhabdomyolysis, renal failure, and irreversible limb damage necessitating amputation.

Orthopaedic complications

Injecting drug users who present with acutely painful joints (especially hip joints) may have septic arthritis. Clinical and radiological evidence may be minimal, so adopt a high index of suspicion. Provide analgesia, take blood cultures, and FBC, and admit for joint aspiration and IV antibiotics.

Drug withdrawal states

Sometimes drug users present to hospital with overt evidence of drug (±alcohol) withdrawal. It can be difficult to judge whether the problem is due to drug intoxication, drug-related (eg stimulant induced psychosis, 'panic reaction'), drug withdrawal, or to coexistent disease. Observe and monitor closely—treat symptomatically (eg with small doses of oral benzodiazepines as necessary) and refer to the medical team.

Compulsory hospitalization

Compulsory detention of patients in the UK requires the patient to be *both*:
- Suffering from a mental disorder (mental illness or handicap).
- Requiring emergency hospital admission to protect the health or safety of the patient or for the protection of others.

Emergency detention under mental health legislation does not allow treatment for psychiatric illness. Emergency treatment of psychiatric or physical illness is carried out under *common law*. In this situation, there must be an immediate threat to life or serious danger to the patient or others, if treatment is not given. For this reason, mental health legislation cannot be used to impose emergency treatment without patient consent. Note that ED patients are not legally inpatients until they go to a ward.

Detention of psychiatric emergencies in the ED

England and Wales
Section 2 is used most commonly in the ED. It requires recommendations from 2 doctors to be accepted by an approved social worker and allows detention for up to 28 days for assessment and treatment.

Scotland
The Mental Health (Care and Treatment) (Scotland) Act 2003 came into effect in 2005—see www.nes-mha.scot.nhs.uk/. Part 5 of the Act enables a fully registered medical practitioner to grant an *emergency detention certificate* that authorizes managers of a hospital to detain someone for 72hr. Before granting an emergency detention certificate, the medical practitioner also needs to consult and gain the consent of a mental health officer, unless impracticable. The patient is then examined by an approved medical practitioner (psychiatrist), who if not satisfied that the relevant criteria are met, cancels the certificate.

Northern Ireland
Mental Health (Northern Ireland) Order 1986, Part II.

Article 4—Admission for assessment of mental disorder.
- Requires 2 or 3 doctors including the responsible medical officer (RMO) —in charge of patient's treatment.
- Application by nearest relative or an approved social worker.
- Lasts 7 days, renewable up to 14 days.
- Lasts until discharge by RMO board or nearest relative or until detained under article 12.

Section 136 (England)
This allows a police officer to detain someone in a public place when he/ she appears to be mentally disordered and is causing a disturbance. The police officer's responsibility is to take the detained person to a 'place of safety' (usually a police station or psychiatric ward) where he/she is assessed by a psychiatrist and approved social worker.

The *Mental Health Act (Scotland) 2003* provides police officers in Scotland with similar powers: a police constable may remove a person to a place of safety from a public place, if a mental disorder is suspected and it is also suspected that the person needs immediate care and treatment.

Mental Capacity Act

The Mental Capacity Act 2005 (MCA) offers a comprehensive framework for decision-making on behalf of adults aged >16 years lacking capacity to make decisions on their own behalf. It only applies in England and Wales.

Defining capacity

A person lacks capacity if, when a decision needs to be made, they are unable to make or communicate the decision because of an 'impairment or disturbance of the mind or brain'. There is a 2-stage test of capacity:

- Is there an impairment of, or disturbance in the functioning of, the person's mind or brain? If so,
- Is the impairment or disturbance sufficient that the person lacks the capacity to make that particular decision?

Five statutory principles

- Capacity must be assumed unless it is established to be lacking.
- A person is not being treated as unable to make a decision unless all practicable steps to help him do so have been taken without success.
- A person should not be treated as unable to make a decision merely because he makes an unwise decision.
- A decision made, or action performed, for or on behalf of a person who lacks capacity must be taken in his/her best interests.
- Before a decision is made or an action performed, consideration must be given to whether the purpose for which it is needed can be as effectively achieved in a way that is less restrictive of the person's rights and freedom of action.

Assessment of capacity

A person lacks capacity if he/she fails:

- To understand the information relevant to the decision.
- To retain the information relevant to the decision.
- To use or weigh the information.
- To communicate the decision (by any means).

Admission and treatment

Patients can be admitted and treated under the Mental Capacity Act 2005 only if 6 qualifying safeguards are met:

- The person is at least 18 years old.
- The person has a mental disorder.
- The person lacks capacity to decide whether to be in hospital or care home for the proposed treatment or care.
- The proposed deprivation of liberty is in the person's best interests and it is necessary and proportionate response to the risk of harm.
- The person is not subject, or potentially subject, to specified provisions of the Mental Health Act in a way that makes them ineligible.
- There is no advance decision, or decision of an attorney or deputy which makes the proposed deprivation of liberty impossible.

In other circumstances, consider using the Mental Health Act 1983 to admit mentally disordered patient who lack capacity to consent.

Chapter 15

Paediatric emergencies

Paediatric emergencies

The paediatric environment

Dealing with children

Children are not little adults. They differ from adults anatomically, physiologically, emotionally, and in the spectrum of pathological conditions to which they are susceptible. It is natural for those hospital staff who have not previously dealt with children to be slightly apprehensive about treating them, particularly when they are distressed or seriously unwell. Be guided by more experienced staff, who are often adept at dealing with children as patients (and very often as parents as well). Such staff are particularly good at recognizing children who are seriously unwell—listen carefully to what they have to say. There is no substitute for experience, but practical courses aimed at managing emergencies in children (eg Advanced Paediatric Life Support (APLS)) are highly recommended. These courses deservedly devote much time to the recognition of seriously ill or injured children, according to whether or not they are physiologically deranged. Consider each child according to expected 'normal' physiological values (see Table 15.1).

Children do not always respond in the same way to illness as adults. They are particularly likely to be frightened of doctors, nurses, and hospitals. Do not waste the opportunity to make important observations (respiratory rate, pattern, and effort, behaviour, conscious level, colour, and parental interaction). Spend time talking to children to reassure them and win their confidence before starting any examination or performing any procedure (unless, of course, they require emergency resuscitation). Lowering yourself to their physical level will make you less intimidating. Involve the parents from the start (see below). Where appropriate, allow children to relax and play with toys. Play therapists can be particularly helpful providing distraction during procedures.

Dealing with parents

Parents are patients too. They are likely to be understandably upset and worried. Take time to explain to the parents exactly what is happening to their children at all stages. Obtain appropriate consent, but do not delay life-saving measures. For the sake of both parents and children, try to allow parents to remain with their children as much as possible. This is especially important during resuscitation where an experienced member of the nursing staff should be allocated to look after and explain to parents what is happening. If the presence of the parents is impeding the progress of the resuscitation, gently ask them to leave.

Analgesia

Differences between adults and children do not diminish the need to provide adequate analgesia for children. Reassurance is often an important component, but be honest and do not be tempted to tell to a child that a painful procedure (eg emergency insertion of an intravenous (IV) cannula) will not produce any pain or discomfort—this will simply cause the child to lose confidence.

Weight estimation

All children should be weighed when they require treatment in the ED. This is as important as the vital signs in children. In an emergency, use a Broselow tape or one of the formulae for estimating children's weight. The following formula estimates a child's weight based upon age (between 1 and 10 years):

$$\text{weight in kg} = (\text{age in years} + 4) \times 2$$

so a 6-year old child will weigh:

$$(6+4) \times 2 = 20\text{kg}$$

This formula often underestimates the weight of many children in the UK or other developed countries but it may overestimate the weight of children from other regions. A formula using mid-arm circumference (MAC) has been developed in Asia[1] and is:

$$\text{weight in kg} = (\text{mid-arm circumference in cm} - 10) \times 3$$

so a child with a 15cm MAC will weigh: $(15 - 10) \times 3 = 15\text{kg}$.

Drug doses

Do not estimate 'rough doses' of drugs for children based on knowledge of adult doses. Instead, use the weight and age of a child, together with a reference source (eg *BNF for Children* http://bnfc.org/bnfc) to determine the appropriate dose.

Preparation for resuscitation

Find out where the paediatric resuscitation equipment is kept and how it works. Learn the paediatric resuscitation guidelines and practice basic life support (BLS) and other procedures on manikins. Ask your local resuscitation officer for help with training. Knowledge of normal (expected) physiology at various ages will help you to evaluate sick children in the ED.

Table 15.1 Normal (expected) physiological values at different ages[*]

Age (years)	Respiratory rate	Heart rate	Systolic BP
<1	30–40	110–160	70–90
1–2	25–35	100–150	80–95
2–5	25–30	95–140	80–100
5–12	20–25	80120	90–110
>12	15–20	60–100	100–120

Expected systolic BP = 80 + (age in years × 2) mmHg.

[*]Adapted from APLS.

1 Cattermole GN *et al.* Mid-arm circumference can be used to estimate children's weights. Resuscitation. 2010. Available at: http://dx.doi.org/10.1016/j.resuscitation.2010.05.015. PMID: 20619953.

Primary assessment and resuscitation of the sick child

Caring for a sick child is a daunting task. Get experienced help early; call for senior ED, paediatric, and ICU/PICU help if you are alerted that a sick or injured child is being brought to the ED.

Perform a primary assessment of Airway, Breathing, Circulation, and Disability to identify and treat life-threatening problems as they are found in order to maintain vital functions before disease specific therapies are started. Early recognition and treatment is essential to avoid cardio-respiratory arrest with its poor outcome.

Airway

Assess patency by looking, feeling, and listening.

Resuscitate: if there is no air movement, perform chin lift or jaw thrust. If there is still no evidence of air movement, give rescue breaths using an appropriately-sized bag-valve-mask device. If the child is breathing, listen for stridor, and look for recession.

Breathing

Assess the effort of breathing by measuring the respiratory rate, looking for intercostal recession and accessory muscle use, and listen for gasping, stridor, wheeze, and grunting.

Assess the efficacy of breathing by looking for chest expansion, auscultation of the chest, and measuring SpO_2.

Assess the effects of respiratory failure by assessing mental status and by measuring the heart rate (increases with hypoxia, but bradycardia is a pre-terminal sign) and examining skin colour (hypoxia causes pallor, cyanosis is a late sign). Reduced breathing effort may indicate exhaustion (a pre-terminal sign), cerebral depression, or neuromuscular disease.

Resuscitate: give high flow O_2 to any child with respiratory difficulty or hypoxia. If respiration is inadequate, support with basic airway care and bag valve mask ventilation and get senior ED/ICU/PICU help to provide a definitive airway (tracheal intubation and IPPV).

Circulation

Assess heart rate (bradycardia is a late sign of cardiovascular failure) pulse volume, capillary refill, BP (hypotension is a pre-terminal sign), skin temperature. Look for the effects of circulatory failure: tachypnoea, mottled cold skin, poor urine output, agitation, and drowsiness.

Resuscitate: give high flow oxygen (O_2) to all shocked patients. Gain IV/IO access, take blood samples and give 20mL/kg of crystalloid. Re-assess and repeat if necessary.

Disability

Any problem with 'ABC' can affect 'D'.

Assess conscious level. Initially, categorize according to AVPU scale:

A—Alert

V—responds to Voice

P—responds to Pain

U—Unresponsive

Check pupil size, reaction and equality.

Assess GCS (or children's equivalent—see 📖 Head injuries in children, p.716) and posture (floppy, decerebrate, decorticate, etc.). Check BMG.

Resuscitate: a child who does not respond to voice has an urgent need to secure the airway. Treat hypoglycaemia and fits, and get senior help urgently.

After initial evaluation and intervention, a more detailed approach to identify specific problems should follow. Re-assess ABCD frequently to assess progress and detect deterioration. Undertake a secondary assessment by obtaining a full history (from parents, paramedics, teachers and witnesses) and undertaking a detailed physical examination.

Standard immunization schedule

The UK Department of Health actively encourages immunization for children according to the standard schedule shown below.[1] The recommended timing of the early immunizations is a compromise between trying to protect children whilst they are at most risk and delaying it until immunization is likely to be most effective. Children who have completed a course of immunization against a particular disease are obviously less likely to present with that disease. Unfortunately, a significant proportion of children are still not receiving standard vaccines (Table 15.2). Carefully enquire exactly which immunizations the child has received (information is often available from the child's GP or health visitor). Failure to follow the recommended schedule may result in the child presenting with an otherwise unusual disease.

Table 15.2 Standard childhood vaccines

Age	Vaccine
2 months	Diphtheria, tetanus, pertussis, polio, Hib, pneumococcal
3 months	Diphtheria, tetanus, pertussis, polio, Hib, meningitis C
4 months	Diphtheria, tetanus, pertussis, polio, Hib, pneumococcal, meningitis C
12 months	Hib, meningitis C
13 months	Measles, mumps, rubella, (MMR), pneumococcal
3–5 years	Diphtheria, tetanus, pertussis, polio, MMR
13–18 years	Tetanus, diphtheria, polio

*May also be given in infancy, if appropriate.

The Hib vaccine

Haemophilus influenzae, a small Gram –ve bacillus, has been responsible for the deaths of many young children. Type b has been implicated most frequently in serious paediatric disease, causing meningitis, pneumonia, cellulitis, and most, particularly, acute epiglottitis. The *Haemophilus B* ('Hib') vaccine has dramatically reduced the incidence of epiglottitis.

Pneumococcal vaccine

This was introduced as routine in the UK in 2006.

---

1 Department of Health. *Immunization against infectious disease - 'The Green Book'*. HMSO, London, 2007. Available at: http://www.dh.gov.uk/en/Publicationsandstatistics/Publications/PublicationsPolicyAndGuidance/DH_079917. See also: *BNFC*.

Reactions to immunizations
Vaccination is frequently wrongly blamed for symptoms caused by incidental viral illness. However, mild reactions, such as swelling and erythema at the injection site, are relatively common following administration of a variety of immunizations. These respond to symptomatic treatment and an expectant approach. Severe anaphylactic reactions, involving airway obstruction or circulatory collapse are uncommon, but require prompt and aggressive treatment (📖 Anaphylaxis, p.42).

Immunization in other countries

If a child who normally lives outside the UK attends the ED, enquire carefully about their vaccination history. Likewise, if you are working outside the UK, make sure you know the local immunization schedule as this can have a significant impact on the type of communicable disease seen, particularly in children.

Immunization in the ED

If a child attending the ED has not been immunized against diphtheria, tetanus, and pertussis and needs tetanus immunization, give the 'triple vaccine' (DPT) to avoid repeated injections. Inform the GP about any immunizations given.

Table 15.3 Paediatric milestones[1] (after allowance for preterm delivery)

2 months	Eyes follow movement. Smiles and makes noises when talked to
3 months	Holds object placed in hand
3–4 months	Turns head to sound
6 months	Sits on floor with hands forwards for support
	Transfers object from one hand to the other
9–10 months	Crawls
12 months	Walks with one hand held; says 2 or 3 words with meaning
13 months	Walks unaided
18 months	Makes tower of 2 or 3 bricks
21–24 months	Joins 2 or 3 words together to make sentence
2 years	Can build a tower of 6 or 7 bricks
2½ years	Knows full name and gender; can stand on tiptoes

1 See: Illingworth RS. *The Normal Child.* 10th edn. Churchill Livingstone, Edinburgh, 1991.

Venous access and venepuncture

Venepuncture

Needles frighten children. Topical anaesthetic cream (eg tetracaine—
📖 p.288) is useful whenever the need for blood sampling is not urgent. 4%
tetracaine (Ametop®, amethocaine) anaesthetizes the skin and ↓ pain, but
should be applied for 30min before venepuncture and for 45min before cannulation. Identify prominent veins at 2 separate sites, apply cream and cover
with an adhesive film dressing, then let the child play.

As in adults, if an IV cannula is inserted, it should be possible to obtain
samples of blood via this: even if aspiration fails, blood will often drip out.
The amount of blood sampled depends upon the size of the child and
laboratory requirements, remembering that total blood volume is only
80mL/kg. Check requirements and obtain the appropriate bottles before
attempting venepuncture.

Neonates FBC and U&E can be performed on capillary samples obtained
from heel pricks. Ask an assistant to hold the foot and ankle firmly to
encourage venous engorgement, then smear white soft paraffin on the
heel and prick it with a lancet. Collect drops of blood into prepared
capillary sample tubes.

Toddlers and infants Aspirate via a 23G butterfly needle in the hand or
forearm. This allows the needle to stay in the vein, despite the child
moving. Samples of 1mL are usually required.

Older children Use a 21G butterfly needle.

IV cannulae

The route chosen to obtain venous access will depend upon the available
veins and urgency of the problem. First attempt to insert an IV cannula
percutaneously into an upper limb vein. Once inserted, flush the cannula,
then secure it with adhesive tape, a splint, and bandage. In general, the following sizes of cannulae are appropriate:
- 24G (orange/yellow): neonates and infants.
- 22G (blue): toddlers and small children.
- 20G (pink) or 18G (green): older children.

Smaller cannulae are designed so the needle does not protrude much
beyond the end of the cannula. This means that once a 'flashback' is
obtained, the tip of the cannula may already be within the vein: advancing
the needle further may puncture the other side of the vein and exit it. If
attempts to insert a cannula into the hand or arm fail, it may be possible
to use veins in the feet, ankle, or in the scalp (useful in neonates, but first
ensure that the intended target is not the superficial temporal artery). In
an emergency, allow a maximum of 90sec and if still unsuccessful then gain
intra-osseous access (📖 p.640), which is quick, easy, and reliable. Other
venous access routes (eg central, femoral) require specialist training, are
time-consuming and are associated with significant complications (see
opposite). Give fluids by infusion pump or paediatric infusion set to avoid
over-transfusion.

Other routes of venous access

Femoral lines The femoral vein lies medial to the artery in the groin. It allows rapid venous access to be obtained and is particularly useful in cardiac arrest where physical constraints (eg several resuscitating staff) restrict access to the neck. Complications include sepsis (use strict aseptic technique), ↑ risk of thrombosis and damage to other structures including the hip joint.

External jugular vein cannulation is an option in children in whom spinal injury is not a concern. Place the child 15–30° head down and turn the neck to one side. The vein runs superficially and caudally over the sternocleidomastoid at the junction of its middle and lower third. Ask an assistant to compress the vein distally to distend and immobilize it.

Central venous access The techniques (and complications) are similar to those in adults (📖 p.56), except that smaller equipment is needed. The safe insertion of central lines in children requires considerable experience and training, and often requires ultrasound guidance, which is sometimes unavailable in a resuscitation situation. Other routes are usually more appropriate during resuscitation.

'Cut downs' (eg long saphenous vein at the ankle) may be performed during resuscitation, but can be time-consuming. In infants, the long saphenous vein is located half a finger breadth superior and anterior to the medial malleolus. For children it is one finger breadth superior and anterior to the medial malleolus.

Umbilical venous access can useful in newborn resuscitation (📖 p.645).

Intra-osseous infusion

If urgent venous access is required, but not obtained within 90sec by percutaneous venous puncture, strongly consider using the intra-osseous route. Fluid and drugs given into the medullary cavity of long bones rapidly reach the central venous circulation. Gaining intra-osseous access is reasonably easy and can be performed quickly. It is particularly useful in young children, but may be used in all ages, including adults.

Indications include major burns and trauma, cardiac arrest, and septic shock.

Contraindications include infection or fracture at (or proximal to) the insertion site, ipsilateral vascular injuries, multiple unsuccessful attempts, osteogenesis imperfecta, osteopetrosis.

Equipment Intra-osseous needles are usually of 16–18G and have a central metal stylet attached to a handle. A battery powered mechanical driver (EZ-IO) with paediatric or adult intra-osseous needles is available and can be used to insert the needle to a specific depth, possibly reducing complications such as compartment syndrome. It can be used in children weighing more than 3kg.

Site of insertion First choice is the proximal tibia 2.5cm below the tibial tuberosity on the flat anteromedial surface (thus avoiding the epiphyseal growth plate). If this route is not available, because of local infection or trauma, use the distal tibia (proximal to the medial malleolus), distal femur (3cm above the lateral lower femoral condyle on the anterolateral surface), or the anterolateral proximal humerus at the greater tuberosity (Fig. 15.1).

Manual intra-osseous needle insertion technique

- Support the limb on a pad or blanket.
- Sterilize the skin and use an aseptic technique. A small skin incision may be needed.
- Firmly grasp the handle and use a twisting motion to advance the needle and stylet through the cortex of the bone. (Note that some intra-osseous needles are designed with a thread and so require a rotatory, not an oscillatory, action).
- Aim at 90° to the bone surface, or slightly away from the epiphyseal growth plate. Stop when the slight 'give' of the medullary cavity is felt.
- Remove the stylet and try to confirm correct placement by aspirating bone marrow (use this to check BMG or cross-match).
- If aspiration is not possible, the needle may still be correctly positioned: attach a primed 3-way tap with extension set and flush the needle and 3-way tap with 10mL of 0.9% saline, and ensure that there is no swelling of the surrounding soft tissues.
- Although connecting it to IV tubing and a pressurized infusion bag may work, it is often much more effective in children to give drugs and fluid by boluses using 20mL syringes and the 3-way tap).
- If necessary, immobilize with a plaster of Paris (POP) backslab applied carefully to the posterior leg (eg for transport to a PICU).

Mechanical intra-osseous needle insertion technique

- Support the limb on a pad or blanket.
- Use a 15mm needle for patients weighing 3–39kg; a 25mm needle for patients more than 39kg; and a 45mm needle for obese adult patients.
- Identify the insertion point and place the needle, loaded into the mechanical driver (drill), at the insertion point.
- Insert the needle, perpendicular to the skin, up to the 5mm line.
- Remove the driver and stylet, attach a primed 3-way tap with extension set and flush the needle and 3-way tap with 10mL of 0.9% saline.
- Attach the giving set and secure as for manually inserted intra-osseous needles.

Use the blood taken from an intra-osseous needle for BMG or cross matching, but not for FBC (automated blood counters may give spurious results). If using an intra-osseous needle in responsive patients, infiltrate 1% lidocaine into the skin before insertion, and consider administering 1–2mL of 2% lidocaine slowly into the needle before beginning the infusion to minimize pain (maximum 3mg/kg lidocaine in children).

Complications of intra-osseous access

- Extravasation of fluid and compartment syndrome.
- Infection (cellulitis or osteomyelitis).
- Iatrogenic fracture.
- Fat or bone micro-emboli.
- Fractures and/or epiphyseal growth plate injury.

Intra-osseous needles must be removed within 24hr to minimize the risk of infection and other complications. Conventional IV access should be secured as soon as possible after intra-osseous needle insertion.

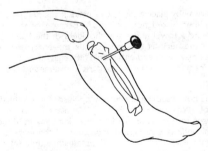

Fig. 15.1 Tibial intra-osseous access.

Resuscitation of the newborn

Neonatal resuscitation is usually undertaken by paediatricians, but unexpected deliveries require other personnel to initiate resuscitation. Fortunately, most newborn babies do not need resuscitation. The discomfort of being born into a hostile environment provides the major initial stimulus to breathe. Ideally, any baby requiring resuscitation should be treated in a warm room with an overhead heater. Call urgently for experienced help.

Approach (see Fig. 15.2)

Make sure the cord is securely clamped and then dry the baby, remove the wet towels and wrap the baby in dry towels. Very preterm babies (<28 weeks) should be wrapped in food grade plastic as rapidly as possible without drying. Assess colour, tone, breathing by chest movement (auscultation at birth is unreliable), and heart rate (best assessed by stethoscope placed over the apex). Repeat assessments every 30sec during resuscitation. Traditionally, an Apgar score (ranging from 0–10, based upon assessment of heart rate, respirations, muscle tone, reflex irritability, and colour) at 1 and 5min is calculated, and used to assess newborn babies. However, do not delay resuscitation to calculate the score.

A healthy baby will have good tone, will cry within a few seconds of delivery and have a heart rate of 120–150/min, and will become rapidly pink during the first 90sec.

Less healthy babies will have poorer tone, slower heart rates, and may not establish adequate respiration by 90–120sec. The most sick will be pale, floppy, apneic, and bradycardic.

Airway

Open the airway by placing the baby's head in the neutral position (with the neck neither flexed nor extended). Because of the large occiput, this will require a towel under the shoulders of the baby. Avoid hyper-extension of the neck as this can occlude the pharyngeal airway. Very floppy babies may also need either chin lift or jaw thrust. Remove visible meconium or secretions using a paediatric Yankauer sucker.

Breathing

If the baby is not breathing adequately by 90sec, give 5 inflation breaths (pressures of 30cm water for 2–3sec). Ventilate a term baby with air, but use oxygen for premature and/or hypoxic neonates. If the heart rate increases, this indicates successful ventilation of the lungs. If the baby is apnoeic, continue ventilation at 30–40 breaths/min until self-ventilating. If the heart rate does not increase, then the most likely cause is that the lungs have not been inflated. Recheck head position and consider a jaw thrust and longer inflation time. If the airway is obstructed, consider an oropharyngeal airway, laryngoscopy and suction. Repeat the 5 inflation breaths. If the heart rate remains <60/min or absent despite good chest movement, start chest compressions.

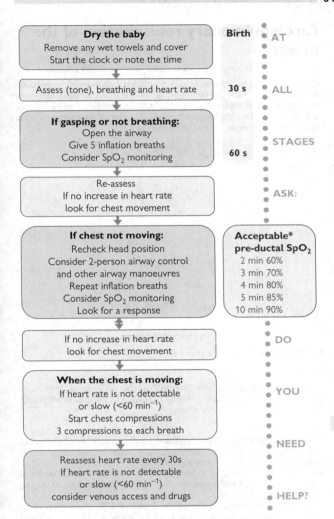

Fig. 15.2 Algorithm for newborn life support. From Resuscitation Council (UK). *Newborn Life Support*, 2010. See www.resus.org.uk

Cardiopulmonary resuscitation of the newborn

Chest compression (only to be started after successful lung inflation).

Grip the chest in both hands in such a way that two thumbs can press on the lower third of the sternum, (just below the intermammary line) with the fingers over the spine at the back (Fig. 15.3). Aim for a rate of 100/min, and to depress the antero-posterior (AP) diameter of the chest by a third. Use a chest compression to inflation *ratio of 3:1*.

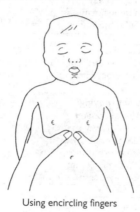

Using encircling fingers

Fig. 15.3 Method of CPR in the newborn.

Tracheal intubation

Treat continuing apnoea with tracheal intubation using a 3mm tube (2.5mm in premature babies). Precede intubation by pre-oxygenation with bag valve mask ventilation for 30sec.

Drugs

Only use drugs if there is no significant cardiac output despite effective lung inflation and chest compression. Give drugs intravenously via an umbilical vein catheter or intra-osseous needle.

- *Give adrenaline* 10mcg/kg (0.1mL/kg of 1 in 10 000) if there is no initial response. If this is ineffective the dose may be increased to 30 mcg/kg (0.3mL/kg of 1 in 10 000).
- *Give sodium bicarbonate* 1–2mmol/kg (2–4mL of 4.2% solution/kg) when there is no cardiac output despite all resuscitative efforts or in profound or unresponsive bradycardia.
- *Hypoglycaemia* is a potential problem for all newborns and BMG is unreliable when reading <5mmol/L. Take blood sample to confirm and treat immediately with a bolus of 2.5mL/kg of 10% glucose.

- *Suspect hypovolaemia if*: very pale baby, pulseless electrical activity (PEA), history of antepartum haemorrhage, placenta praevia, or vasa praevia, or unclamped cord. Give 10mL/kg 0.9% saline followed by O −ve blood, repeated as necessary.
- *Atropine* and *calcium* have no role in newborn resuscitation.

Venous access—the umbilical vein

The easiest and fastest method of obtaining venous access in the newborn is to cannulate the umbilical vein. Identify the umbilical vein in the cut umbilical stump: it is the single large dilated vessel adjacent to the two constricted arteries (Fig. 15.4). Prepare a 5F gauge catheter with 0.9% saline and insert it 5cm into the umbilical vein. Suture and secure in place.

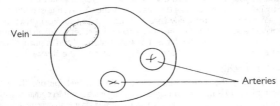

Vein

Arteries

Fig. 15.4 Diagram of a cross-section of the umbilicus.

If there are no signs of life after 10min of continuous and adequate resuscitation efforts, then discontinuation of resuscitation may be justified; involve senior ED and neonatal staff in this decision.

Meconium aspiration

In the presence of meconium, do not attempt to aspirate the nose and mouth of meconium as the head presents. If a baby is delivered with thick meconium and is unresponsive at birth (absent or inadequate respiration, heart rate <100/min or hypotonia), perform laryngoscopy and clear meconium under direct vision using a wide bore catheter. Aim to intubate the larynx and apply suction to the tracheal tube which is then withdrawn.

However, if intubation cannot be achieved immediately, clear the orophyarynx and start bag-valve-mask inflation. If while attempting to clear the airway the heart rate falls <60/min, stop airway clearance, give inflation breaths and start ventilating the baby with a bag-valve-mask device.

If meconium staining is present, but the infant is vigorous at birth, no special treatment is required immediately, but the infant should be closely observed.

Paediatric basic life support

Follow the algorithm (Fig. 15.5). Note that the approach to choking is considered on 🔲 p.648.

Evaluate responsiveness

Check the child's responsiveness—gently stimulate and ask loudly 'are you alright?' Do not shake if you suspect cervical spine injury. If the child does not respond, shout for help ± get someone to go for assistance.

Open airway

Open the airway by head tilt and chin lift. Desirable degrees of tilt are neutral <1 year and 'sniffing the morning air' >1 year. Do not press on the soft tissues under the chin as this may block the airway. If it is still difficult to open the airway, try a jaw thrust. If there is any suspicion that there may have been a neck injury, instruct a second rescuer to manually immobilize it, and use either chin lift or jaw thrust alone. If this is unsuccessful, add the smallest amount of head tilt needed to open the airway.

Check breathing

Whilst keeping the airway open, look listen and feel for breathing for 10sec. If the child is not breathing or is making infrequent irregular breaths, carefully remove any obvious obstruction, give 5 initial rescue breaths (with the rescuer taking a breath between each rescue breath).

Rescue breaths

For children >1 year, whilst maintaining head tilt and chin lift, give breaths mouth to mouth, pinching off the nose. Blow steadily for 1–1.5sec watching for the chest to rise. Take your mouth away, watch the chest fall and repeat this sequence 5 times.

For the infant (<1 year) ensure the neutral position of the head and apply chin lift. Give mouth to mouth and nose breaths, ensuring a good seal. Blow steadily for 1–1.5sec watching for chest rise. Take your mouth away, watch the chest fall and repeat this sequence 5 times.

Difficulty achieving an effective breath suggests airway obstruction. Open the mouth and remove visible obstruction (no blind finger sweep), ensure appropriate head tilt/chin lift and neck position. Try a jaw thrust if head tilt/chin lift has not worked. Try up to 5 times to give effective breaths. If still unsuccessful, move to chest compression.

Check pulse

Over the next 10sec check for signs of life: any movement, coughing or normal breathing and check for a pulse (use carotid for >1yr and brachial for those <1 year). If there are no signs of life and/or no pulse or pulse <60/min with poor perfusion or you are unsure: start chest compression.

Chest compression

For infants, perform chest compressions (100–120/min) by placing both thumbs flat side by side on the lower third of the sternum with the tips pointing towards the infant's head. Encircle the rib cage with tips of fingers supporting the infant's back. Press down with thumbs at least one third of the depth of the chest.

In children >1 year using the heel of one hand, compress the lower half of the sternum by at least one-third of the depth of the chest at a rate of 100–120/min. Use two hands if necessary to achieve the depth required.

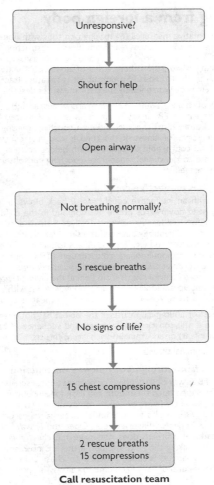

Fig. 15.5 Paediatric basic life support (healthcare professionals with a duty to respond). Resuscitation Council (UK). *Paediatric basic life support*, 2010. See www.resus.org.uk

Choking from a foreign body

Despite preventative measures (eg making pen tops with holes in them), children continue to die each year from airway obstruction due to FB impaction. FB aspiration produces a sudden onset airway problem and must be distinguished from other causes of airway obstruction (epiglottitis, bacterial tracheitis see 📖 Stridor: upper respiratory tract infections, p.677), which may be worsened by the basic measures described below.

The majority of choking events in children are witnessed and occur during play or whilst eating. FB airway obstruction is characterized by sudden onset of respiratory distress associated with coughing, gagging or stridor with no other signs of illness. If the child is coughing effectively (fully responsive, loud cough, able to take a breath before coughing, crying or verbal response to questions), encourage coughing and observe for the cough becoming ineffective.

Conscious, but ineffective cough

If conscious with an ineffective cough, give 5 back blows. In the infant, support in a head downwards prone position and in the child aim for a head down or forward leaning position. Deliver 5 sharp *back blows* with the heel of one hand centrally between the shoulder blades. If ineffective, turn to supine position and give 5 *chest thrusts* to infants (using the same landmarks as for cardiopulmonary resuscitation (CPR), but thrusts are sharper and delivered at a slower rate) and *abdominal thrusts* to children >1 year. Perform *abdominal thrusts* from behind the child, placing your fist between the umbilicus and xiphisternum, and grasping it with your other hand, then pulling sharply inwards and upwards—repeat up to 5 times.

Following chest or abdominal thrusts, if the object has not been expelled and the victim is still conscious then repeat the sequence of back blows and chest (for infant) or abdominal (for children) thrusts.

Do not use abdominal thrusts for infants.

Unconscious from foreign body airway obstruction

If a child with FB airway obstruction is or becomes unconscious, place him on a flat surface, then open the mouth and look for any obvious object. If one is seen, use a single finger sweep to remove it. It may be possible to remove the FB with Magill's forceps under direct laryngoscopy. Do not attempt blind or repeated finger sweeps. Open the airway and attempt 5 rescue breaths. If a breath does not make the chest rise, reposition the head before making the next attempt. If there is no response whilst attempting the 5 rescue breaths, proceed to chest compression with ventilation using a ratio of 15:2. Each time the airway is opened, check for a foreign body and if visible, try to remove it (Fig. 15.6).

If it appears that the obstruction has been relieved, open and check the airway. If the child is not breathing, deliver rescue breaths. If initial measures prove unsuccessful and the child is hypoxic, oxygenate via a *surgical airway* until senior help arrives. Perform needle cricothyroidotomy in children aged <12 years, surgical cricothyroidotomy in older children (📖 Airway obstruction: surgical airway, p.326).

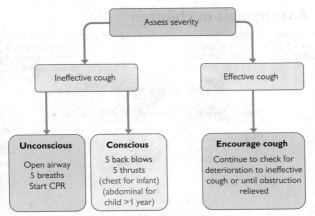

Fig. 15.6 Paediatric foreign body airway obstruction treatment. Resuscitation Council (UK). *Paediatric FB airway obstruction*, 2010. See www.resus.org.uk

Anaphylaxis in children

The background, causes and pathophysiology of anaphylaxis in children is similar to that in adults—see p.42. Treat according to the 2008 UK Resuscitation Council algorithm, shown in Fig. 15.7. After initial treatment, admit the child for observation in case of a delayed or biphasic reaction.

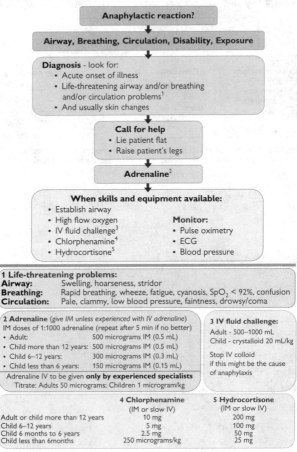

Anaphylactic reaction?

Airway, Breathing, Circulation, Disability, Exposure

Diagnosis - look for:
- Acute onset of illness
- Life-threatening airway and/or breathing and/or circulation problems[1]
- And usually skin changes

Call for help
- Lie patient flat
- Raise patient's legs

Adrenaline[2]

When skills and equipment available:
- Establish airway
- High flow oxygen
- IV fluid challenge[3]
- Chlorphenamine[4]
- Hydrocortisone[5]

Monitor:
- Pulse oximetry
- ECG
- Blood pressure

1 Life-threatening problems:
Airway: Swelling, hoarseness, stridor
Breathing: Rapid breathing, wheeze, fatigue, cyanosis, SpO_2 < 92%, confusion
Circulation: Pale, clammy, low blood pressure, faintness, drowsy/coma

2 Adrenaline *(give IM unless experienced with IV adrenaline)*
IM doses of 1:1000 adrenaline (repeat after 5 min if no better)
- Adult: 500 micrograms IM (0.5 mL)
- Child more than 12 years: 500 micrograms IM (0.5 mL)
- Child 6–12 years: 300 micrograms IM (0.3 mL)
- Child less than 6 years: 150 micrograms IM (0.15 mL)
Adrenaline IV to be given **only by experienced specialists**
Titrate: Adults 50 micrograms; Children 1 microgram/kg

3 IV fluid challenge:
Adult - 500–1000 mL
Child - crystalloid 20 mL/kg

Stop IV colloid
if this might be the cause of anaphylaxis

	4 Chlorphenamine (IM or slow IV)	5 Hydrocortisone (IM or slow IV)
Adult or child more than 12 years	10 mg	200 mg
Child 6–12 years	5 mg	100 mg
Child 6 months to 6 years	2.5 mg	50 mg
Child less than 6months	250 micrograms/kg	25 mg

Fig. 15.7 UK Resuscitation Council algorithm 2008.

1 See http://www.resus.org.uk/pages/reaction.pdf for details. Notes are shown opposite.

Notes for anaphylaxis algorithm opposite

1 Intramuscular (IM) adrenaline is the agent of choice in anaphylaxis and should be administered without delay.

2 If profound shock is judged immediately life-threatening, consider giving a slow bolus of 1mcg/kg of intravenous (IV) adrenaline as a *1 in 100,000* solution (= 10micrograms/mL solution). *This is hazardous* and is recommended *only* for experienced specialists who can also obtain IV access without delay. Note that a different dilution of adrenaline is required for IM compared to IV use. Adrenaline can also be given via the IO route in the same dose as the IV route.

3 An inhaled β_2-agonist such as salbutamol may be used as an adjunctive measure if bronchospasm is severe and does not respond rapidly to other treatment.

4 For children who have been prescribed an EpiPen®, 150 mcg can be given instead of 120 mcg, and 300 mcg can be given instead of 250 mcg or 500 mcg.

5 Crystalloid may be safer than a colloid.

6 Do not use the subcutaneous route for adrenaline. It has no role in anaphylaxis because its absorption is appreciably slower than IM adrenaline.

Consider taking blood samples for mast cell tryptase testing as soon as possible after starting treatment if the cause is thought to be venom-related, drug-related or idiopathic (see www.nice.org.uk/cg134):

• A sample as soon as possible after emergency treatment has started.
• A second sample ideally within 1–2 hours (but no later than 4 hours) from the onset of symptoms.

Paediatric advanced life support

Overall, cardiac arrest in children has a worse outcome than in adults, because the underlying causes are different. However, the situation is likely to be far from hopeless if a child arrests within the ED or other areas of the hospital. Effective immediate resuscitation is important to minimize hypoxic organ damage. Early recognition of the child presenting with impending cardio-respiratory arrest may allow prompt intervention and prevent secondary cardiac arrest (Fig. 15.8).

Follow the guidelines shown opposite. Establish BLS (📖 p.646) and use a ratio of 15:2 while ventilating with a bag-valve-mask. Aim for tracheal intubation by a highly skilled operator as soon as possible, then ventilate at a rate of 10–12/min with compressions uninterrupted at 100–120/min.

Non-shockable rhythm: PEA and asystole

Give BLS with high concentration O_2. Give adrenaline IV/IO 10mcg/kg (0.1mL/kg of 1 in 10,000). If no other access is present, consider giving 100mcg/kg adrenaline via the trachea, but this is the least satisfactory route. Give IV/IO adrenaline every 3–5min (every other loop). As in adults (📖 p.51), PEA may reflect a correctable underlying cause.

In particular, exclude tension pneumothorax and consider hypovolaemia. Haemorrhage, septic shock, and dehydration are implicated relatively frequently, so consider an initial IV fluid bolus of 20mL/kg 0.9% saline early in the resuscitation. Follow this with further IV fluid/blood if hypovolaemia is still present or suspected. If circulation returns, ventilate at 12–20breaths/min to achieve a normal pCO_2 and monitor ETCO$_2$ to confirm correct tracheal tube placement.

Shockable rhythm: VF/pulseless VT

VF is uncommon in children, but is more likely in witnessed and sudden collapse. It occasionally occurs in children with congenital heart disease, hypothermia or electrolyte disturbance. Follow the 'VF/VT' treatment algorithm shown opposite. Give one shock of 4J/kg if using a manual defibrillator. These energy levels are appropriate for both monophasic and biphasic defibrillators. When selecting the energy level to use during defibrillation, if the defibrillator can only deliver certain predetermined 'stepped' shocks, choose the nearest higher 'step' to that required. Pads or paddles for children should be 8–12cm in size and 4.5cm for infants. Resume CPR immediately without reassessing rhythm or feeling for a pulse. Continue CPR for 2min and if still in VF/VT, give a second shock and resume CPR immediately for 2min. Consider reversible causes. If still in VF/VT at this time, give a third shock. Give adrenaline 10 mcg/kg and amiodarone 5mg/kg (diluted in 5% glucose) once chest compressions have restarted and give a fourth shock after 2min CPR. Continue giving shocks every 2min and adrenaline immediately before every other shock (ie every 3–5min), until a return of spontaneous circulation. Amiodarone 5mg/kg can be repeated once after the fifth shock. Uninterrupted good quality CPR is vital—only interrupt chest compressions and ventilation for defibrillation.

See 📖 Paediatric advanced life support notes, p.654.

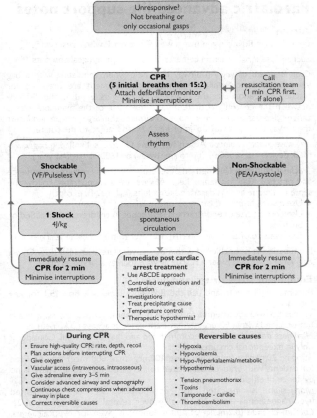

Fig. 15.8 Paediatric advanced life support. Resuscitation Council (UK). *Paediatric advanced life support guidelines*, 2010. Available at: www.resus.org.uk

Paediatric advanced life support notes

Airway

O₂ Give high flow oxygen (use a well-fitting mask with a reservoir).

Suction Use a rigid suction catheter to aspirate pharyngeal contents.

Oropharyngeal airway An airway may help when ventilating with a bag valve mask device while personnel and equipment are prepared for tracheal intubation. Size the airway by matching its length to the distance between the central incisor teeth and the angle of the mandible. Use a tongue depressor or laryngoscope to displace the large tongue and insert the airway the 'right way up' in order to avoid trauma to the palate.

Bag-valve-mask ventilation Attach high flow O_2 to a self-inflating bag-valve-mask device. Use a 500mL (up to age 1 year) or 1600mL bag (>1 year).

Tracheal intubation This method of securing the airway requires experience and practice. Call for senior help. Always use a capnograph. Follow the same technique as that described for adults (📖 p.324), except:

- Use a straight-bladed laryngoscope in infants (<1 year).
- Use correct size of endotracheal (ET) tubes in children, either cuffed or uncuffed.
- Correct size of ET tube: internal diameter (mm) = (age in years/4) + 4

If intubation is not achieved within 30sec, ventilate with high flow O_2 via bag-valve-mask. Consider a rescue airway, such as a laryngeal mask.

Equipment sizes, drugs, and doses

Become familiar with and use the Broselow tape. See Box 15.1 for key formulae

Venous access First attempt to secure peripheral venous access. If this is not obtained within 90sec, attempt intra-osseous access (📖 p.640).

High dose adrenaline is not recommended and may be harmful. Consider it only in exceptional circumstances.

Atropine 20mcg/kg (minimum dose 100mcg, max 600 mcg) may be used for patients with bradycardia related to increased vagal tone. There is no evidence of efficacy for atropine.

Magnesium is indicated for polymorphic VT or documented hypomagnesaemia—give 25–50mg/kg over several min to a max of 2g.

Calcium chloride (0.2mL/kg of 10% solution) is given for hypocalcaemia, hyperkalaemia and clinically severe overdose of calcium channel blocking drugs. Do not give in the same IV/IO line as bicarbonate.

Sodium bicarbonate is not recommended routinely, but consider it in prolonged arrest, hyperkalaemia, and arrhythmias associated with tricyclic antidepressant overdose. The dose is 1–2mL/kg of 8.4% solution IV/IO. Ensure adequate flushing after giving it. Avoid mixing with other agents (it inactivates adrenaline and precipitates out calcium).

Glucose Treat hypoglycaemia with IV glucose (0.5g/kg).

IV fluids Give a 20mL/kg IV normal saline bolus where cardiac arrest is secondary to hypovolaemia or sepsis.

Discontinuing resuscitation

Resuscitation efforts are unlikely to be successful if there is no return of spontaneous circulation at any time after 30min of life support and in the absence of recurring or refractory VF/VT. Prolong resuscitation for patients who are hypothermic or who may have been poisoned.

Paediatric resuscitation chart (Fig. 15.9)

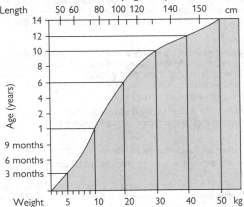

Fig. 15.9

Box 15.1 Key resuscitation formulae

Assume birth weight of 3.5kg, reaching 10kg by the end of the first year

Weight in kg = (age in years + 4) × 2 {works for ages 1–10 years}

Tracheal tube internal diameter in mm = (age/4) + 4

Tracheal tube length (oral) in cm = (age/2) +12

Laryngeal mask sizes for children:
- Size 1 for weight up to 5kg.
- Size 1.5 for weight 5–10kg.
- Size 2 for weight 10–20kg.
- Size 2.5 for weight >20kg.

IV fluid challenge 20mL/kg

Defibrillation for VF/pulseless VT = 4J/kg

Drug doses
- *Glucose in hypoglycaemia*: 5mL/kg of 10% (2.5mL in neonates).
- *Adrenaline IV in cardiac arrest*: 0.1mL/kg of 1 in 10,000.
- *Lorazepam IV for seizures*: 0.1mg/kg.
- *Diazepam PR for seizures*: 0.5mg/kg.
- *Midazolam buccal for seizures*: 0.5mg/kg.
- *Phenytoin IVI for continuing seizures*: 18mg/kg IVI over 30min.
- *Morphine for pain*: IV 0.1–0.2mg/kg (titrated according to pain).

Children with abnormal heart rates or rhythms

Background

Arrhythmias are uncommon: *obtain expert advice* at an early stage. Children may present with poor feeding, heart failure, shock or palpitations. Sinus tachycardia may be as fast as 220/min in infants and 180/min in children. Consider undiagnosed congenital heart disease in infants.

Bradycardia

Heart rates of <60/min are usually pre-terminal events in response to profound hypoxia and ischaemia, but can be due to ↑ ICP or poisoning. Treat the underlying cause and if the child is shocked and <60/min start CPR, give O_2 and ventilate as necessary. Give IV 20mL/kg fluid bolus. If this is ineffective, give adrenaline 10mcg/kg IV.

If the bradycardia is due to vagal stimulation (eg tracheal intubation or tracheal suctioning), give atropine 20mcg/kg (minimum dose 100mcg, max 600mcg).

Ventricular tachycardia in children

Until proved otherwise, initially consider wide complex tachycardia in children to be VT.

- *Causes of VT:* hyperkalaemia, long QT syndrome. Tricyclic poisoning (p192) often produces a tachycardia and wide QRS resembling VT.
- *Children with VT and who are clinically shocked* but conscious require urgent anaesthesia followed by synchronized shocks starting at 1J/kg (followed if necessary by 2J/kg).
- *If the child is not clinically shocked*, involve a (paediatric) cardiologist and consider amiodarone 5mg/kg IVI over 60 min.
- *Torsades de pointes* is treated with magnesium sulphate IVI 25–50mg/kg (up to a maximum of 2g); seek expert guidance.

SVT in children

Distinguish SVT from sinus tachycardia (where heart rate is <200/min, P waves are upright in ECG leads I and AVF, there is beat to beat variation in rate, and history consistent with shock).

If *clinically shocked*, but responsive, obtain expert help to give synchronized shocks (starting at 1J/kg, increasing if unsuccessful to 2J/kg) under anaesthesia. If there is any delay, try adenosine IV as outlined for haemodynamically stable patients.

In the *absence of clinical evidence of shock*, try *vagal stimulation*: immersion of the face in iced water, or Valsalva manoeuvre or unilateral carotid massage. If this is unsuccessful, give adenosine 100mcg/kg rapid IV followed by a saline flush, followed if still unsuccessful by further dose(s) at 200mcg/kg, then 300mcg/kg. If this fails, seek expert help and consider IV amiodarone.

Sudden infant death syndrome (SIDS)

Sudden infant death syndrome (SIDS)

SIDS (also called SUDI—sudden unexplained death in infancy; previously known as 'cot death' or 'crib death') is decreasing in incidence, but each death is a tragedy. A senior doctor (consultant) should manage distressed parents (and staff). It remains a leading cause of infant death (1 in 2000 live births), 90% occurring between 1 and 6 months of age. Most hospitals now have detailed SUDIC (Sudden Unexpected Death in Infancy and Childhood) protocols, which should be followed in this situation.

Definition Sudden death in infancy with no cause identified after autopsy.

Aetiology Although the aetiology is unknown, a variety of theories have been proposed, including prone sleeping position, airway obstruction, apnoea, viral illness, and overheating.

Risk factors Passive smoking, males, winter months, sleeping prone, premature babies, twins, apnoeic spells in first week of life, lower socio-economic groups, maternal illicit drug abuse in pregnancy, sibling with SIDS.

Prevention
- Avoid overheating (aim for ambient T° of 16–20°C).
- Avoid duvets and excess bedding in infancy.
- Place infant's feet at cot end to prevent migration under blankets.
- Sleep supine (unless Pierre–Robin, scoliosis, or oesophageal reflux).
- Consider apnoea alarm.
- Avoid infant sharing bed with parent.

Approach
- Take the infant into the resuscitation room and continue resuscitation as for cardiac arrest unless there is post-mortem staining or rigidity.
- Call the ED consultant and consultant paediatrician.
- Ensure that a named senior nurse stays with the parents.
- Immediately death is declared, prepare yourself, then inform the parents in the presence of the senior nurse. Use the techniques described in 📖 Breaking bad news, p.24. Refer to the child throughout by their first name.
- Some hospitals have dedicated bereavement counsellors—involve them early.
- Allow the parents to see and hold the baby, and suggest that they keep a lock of their hair.
- Take digital or polaroid photographs of the baby: give them to the parents and file copies in the notes.
- Explain further procedures (eg autopsy) to the parents and provide written information eg 'A guide to the post mortem examination procedure involving a baby or child' (DoH ref 29768/A).
- Offer to request a minister of religion and involve a social worker.
- Careful documentation including general appearance, state of nutrition, weight, rectal temperature (T°), marks from procedures, rashes, any visible injuries, and appearance of the retinae.
- Inform GP to arrange to visit parents and discuss whether to suppress lactation with bromocriptine if mother is breast-feeding.

- Retain clothes and bedding (stored in a paper bag, not polythene) and inform police and coroner (Procurator Fiscal in Scotland) in all cases.
- Ensure blood, urine, and skin specimens will be obtained (looking for infection and inborn errors of metabolism).
- Arrange a further appointment for the parents with the same consultant paediatrician.
- Suggest the Foundation for the Study of Infant Deaths, which has various leaflets and a 'Cot Death Helpline' (Telephone 0870 787 0554).
- Advise about preventative measures for siblings. If the baby was a twin, recommend admission of the surviving twin with the mother for monitoring and investigation.
- Cancel any hospital outpatient appointments and vaccination appointments for the child.
- Inform the parents that the police will visit them as a matter of course.
- Finally, consider yourself and your colleagues.

Staff have feelings too

All staff involved with the child and family (ambulance staff, police, GP, nurses and doctors—including you) will be traumatized by the experience. Those who are themselves parents with young children may be particularly distressed. At the very least, a debriefing session over a cup of coffee will be required.

'Near miss sudden infant death syndrome' (apparently life-threatening event)

Refer to the paediatrician for admission and monitoring any infant whose parents report an apparently life-threatening event ('ALTE'): apnoea, colour change, tone change, cyanosis, choking, gagging. The patient may appear well at the time of presentation. Liaise with the paediatric team and take blood (to include FBC, U&E, glucose, calcium, magnesium, phosphate) and admit for apnoea monitoring.

The *differential diagnosis* includes arrhythmias and congenital heart disease, child abuse, gastro-oesophageal reflux, meningitis and sepsis, seizures and metabolic disorders. In 50% of cases, no cause is found. Despite parental anxiety, short apnoeic episodes (<15sec) may, in fact, be entirely normal. Theophylline, home monitoring devices, and counselling have all been used for infants believed to be at risk.

Problems of neonates and infants

Neonatal cephalhaematoma

This haematoma results from birth trauma and overlies a single skull bone (usually parietal). It resolves spontaneously: do not attempt to aspirate.

Umbilical cord sepsis

The dried cord separates at 1 week. If the stump develops signs of infection (becoming moist and red), refer to the paediatrician.

Breast swelling

Neonatal breasts commonly swell, due to exposure to maternal hormones. Occasionally, these breasts lactate ('witch's milk') and very occasionally become infected, requiring parenteral antibiotics.

Neonatal jaundice

Jaundice within 24hr of birth is highly abnormal. Neonates who develop jaundice after 24hr mostly have 'physiological jaundice' (typically in the first week, especially premature babies) or 'breast milk jaundice' (typically in second week: self-limiting, breast feeding can usually continue). Refer all patients to exclude serious underlying disorders: Rhesus haemolytic disease; ABO incompatibility; congenital spherocytosis; glucose-6-phosphate dehydrogenase (G-6-PD) deficiency; CMV infection; hypothyroidism; biliary atresia. The paediatrician will check: serum bilirubin (including ratio of conjugated: unconjugated), FBC; blood film; U&E; LFTs; direct antiglobulin test; TFTs; and infection screen.

Neonatal conjunctivitis

A watery/sticky eye in the first few days of life may be due to an unopened tear duct, or occasionally to gonococcal or chlamydial infection acquired from the mother's genital tract. Therefore, take a swab for Gram staining for gonococci and culture for chlamydia. Refer the baby and mother if organisms are demonstrated, otherwise arrange GP follow-up.

Sepsis

Potentially life-threatening sepsis (eg meningitis) may present in a non-specific manner in infants (this is especially true of neonates). Classic presentations are replaced by: feeding problems, irritability, drowsiness, jaundice, hypotonia, poor weight gain, petechiae or skin rash, apnoea, bradycardia, and cyanotic episodes. Neonates at ↑ risk are those with low birth weight, those previously ventilated and those with congenital abnormalities.

Treatment Give O_2 and IV fluids (20mL/kg). Refer for admission and urgent investigation: BMG, urine culture, FBC, blood cultures, TORCH screen (Toxoplasma, Rubella, CMV, Herpes), CXR, abdominal X-ray (if necrotizing enterocolitis suspected), LP. Commence 'blind' antibiotics (see *BNFC*).

Crying babies

It is quite normal for babies to cry. The amount of crying varies enormously, as does the ability of parents to cope with it. With more acute onset of irritability and crying exclude an acute cause (eg otitis media, incarcerated hernia, testicular torsion, intussusception, fractured limb), before reassuring and counselling the parents. Parents who are driven to despair may benefit from a self-help group (eg CRY-SIS 020 7404 5011 www.cry-sis.com) or follow-up with a paediatrician.

Feeding difficulties

Parents bring their babies to the ED with a variety of feeding problems. The underlying causes vary widely and range from acute life-threatening sepsis to chronic parental anxiety or overfeeding. Obtain a careful history and watch the baby feed. Babies normally require at least 15mL of milk/kg/day at day 1, increasing to ≈150mL/kg/day by day 7. Plot weight, height, and head circumference on centile charts. Take weight loss or failure to satisfactorily gain weight seriously—it may be due to a significant underlying disorder (eg pyloric stenosis). Remember that newborn babies lose up to 10% of their birth weight in the first week, but should regain it by 2 weeks. Arrange for the health visitor to advise. Refer chronic feeding problems to GP or paediatrician.

Bilious vomiting

Occasionally neonates and infants present with bilious vomiting, a sign of serious pathology. The most important differential diagnosis is intestinal malrotation (volvulus) secondary to peritoneal bands, which requires emergency laparotomy to avoid total small bowel infarction (📖 Abdominal pain in children, p.698). Consult a paediatric surgeon urgently. Other differential diagnoses include an obstructed hernia, Hirschsprung's disease or sepsis.

Metabolic diseases (inborn errors of metabolism)

Occasionally neonates present to the ED days after birth with coma or seizures with no obvious cause (infection, trauma, hypoglycaemia, etc.). These infants may have an inborn error of metabolism (e.g. maple syrup urine disease, urea cycle disorders, and hyperammonaemia) and they require urgent specialist paediatric care, often at a tertiary children's hospital. If an older child presents to the ED with a previously diagnosed metabolic disease, seek expert advice by referring to the paediatricians early. Remember the parents will know more about the disease than you.

Treatment Give O_2 and IV fluids (20mL/kg) and treat hypoglycaemia, and sepsis. Refer for admission and urgent investigation by a paediatrician. Emergency treatment protocols for this challenging group of patients are available at the British Inherited Metabolic Disease Group website (http://www.bimdg.org.uk/protocols/documents.asp?o=1&tid=1).

Skin problems in infants

Minor skin problems are common in infants. The combination of a skin rash and an ill infant should arouse suspicion of serious illness (eg 📖 Meningococcal disease, p.666) and prompt urgent referral. *Do not discharge an infant with an undiagnosed rash*—obtain an expert opinion.

Neonates

Multiple tiny white papules (*milia*) seen on the face of neonates are superficial epidermal inclusion cysts. Erythematous lesions with central white vesicles are common in the first days of life—*erythema toxicum* ('neonatal urticaria'). Both are harmless and disappear spontaneously within days.

Peeling skin

Peeling skin is a common feature of post-mature babies and should be distinguished from scalded skin syndrome and Kawasaki disease (📖 p.672).

Scalded skin syndrome ('toxic epidermal necrolysis')

This staphylococcal infection results in red peeling skin, sometimes with blistering. Refer for admission and IV antibiotics.

Eczema

Usually managed most appropriately by GP and outpatient department with emollients ± topical corticosteroids, but if very severe, refer for a period of inpatient treatment. Sometimes the scratched skin becomes secondarily infected, requiring admission for IV antibiotics.

Impetigo

Any breach in the skin (eg eczema, nappy rash, scabies) may develop impetigo. Staphylococcal or streptococcal infection results in an ulcerative erythematous area, which forms a golden brown crust that spreads rapidly. If the infection is localized and the child is well, treat with topical fucidic acid (if extensive—oral penicillin and flucloxacillin), arrange GP follow-up and advise the parents to isolate the child from other children until it has resolved. If the child is unwell, refer for IV antibiotics.

Nappy rash ('ammoniacal dermatitis')

Erythema with some ulceration in the nappy area, but sparing the flexures, is usually the result of excessive moisture contact with the skin. Treat by exposure to fresh air as much as practicable and frequent changing of nappies. Consider barrier creams (see BNFC).

Monilial infection

Nappy rash may become infected with *Candida albicans*, leading to erythema of the flexures. Give nystatin cream and advise regular changing.

Seborrhoeic dermatitis

This erythematous greasy rash commonly involves the nappy area, the occipital region and behind the ears. It may become infected with *Candida albicans*—treat with nystatin and refer to GP.

The febrile child

Febrile illness is extremely common in childhood and many parents will bring their child to the emergency department, rather than to a primary care team for assessment, particularly when they feel the child is very unwell. Primary care teams will also refer febrile children to hospital for assessment when the child is seriously ill or the diagnosis is in doubt.

Approach

- Assess the airway, breathing and circulation of the child to identify and treat life-threatening problems as they are found in order to maintain vital functions before disease specific therapies are started (Primary assessment and resuscitation of the sick child, p.634).
- Involve senior ED staff, PICU, and senior paediatric staff as soon as you suspect the child is critically unwell.
- Measure and record the temperature (electronic thermometer in axilla if <4 weeks old, can also use tympanic thermometer if older than 4 weeks).
- Specifically look for an impaired conscious level and lack of recognition of parents/carers. Check BMG in all sick children.
- Early recognition and treatment of respiratory failure and shock is essential to avoid cardiorespiratory arrest.
- Administer oxygen to maintain SpO_2>94%.
- Give a bolus of IV/IO 0.9% saline 20mL/kg if any signs of shock (tachycardia, CRT>2sec, mottled skin, purpuric rash, ↓ conscious level).
- If there is any suspicion or sign of meningococcal disease, administer parenteral benzylpenicillin or cefotaxime as soon as possible.
- If the child is <3 months old, check FBC, blood cultures, CRP and urine; if unwell, or WCC <5 or >15 × 10^9/L, or <1 month old, perform lumbar puncture (LP) and give parenteral antibiotics. If <1 month old, add ampicillin to cover *Listeria*.
- If the child is >3 months old, check FBC, blood cultures, CRP and urine; get CXR if T°>39°C or WCC>20 × 10^9/L or clinically unwell.
- Check U&E, ABG, and lactate if clinically unwell or drowsy.
- Consider LP if clinically unwell and febrile at any age, especially <1 year.
- If drowsy or ↓ conscious level, consider adding IV acyclovir to cover possibility of herpes simplex encephalitis.
- Resuscitate aggressively with repeated IV fluid boluses, inotropes and early ventilation for children with ↓ conscious level.
- In older children, do not forget rarer causes of fever and impaired conscious level, including illicit drugs such as MDMA ('Ecstasy') or other amphetamines, or ketamine.
- Get a detailed history of the illness from parents and carers at the earliest opportunity; remember the vaccination history and any recent travel, or recent illness in the child's family or school.

---

1 See the 'NICE Guidance on Feverish Illness in Children'. Available at: http://www.nice.org.uk/ nicemedia/live/11010/30524/30524.pdf

Purpuric rashes

The development of a purpuric rash in a child is often greeted with considerable and understandable parental alarm, due to the well-publicized association with meningococcal disease. History, examination, and FBC will help to identify the cause.

Causes of purpuric lesions

- Meningococcal disease.
- Henoch–Schönlein purpura.
- Thrombocytopenia.
  - Idiopathic thrombocytopenic purpura;
  - Leukaemia;
  - Septic shock;
  - Aplastic anaemia.
- Some viral illnesses.
- Trauma.
- Forceful coughing or vomiting may cause petechiae of the face.

Meningococcal disease (see 📖 p.666)

Presume that an ill child (particularly an infant) who develops a purpuric rash has meningococcal meningitis/septicaemia and treat urgently for this.

Henoch–Schönlein purpura

This vasculitic process affects small arteries in the kidneys, skin, and GI tract. It is relatively common in 4–11-year olds and appears to follow a viral or bacterial infection. Erythematous macules develop into palpable purpuric lesions, which are characteristically concentrated over the buttocks and extensor surfaces of the lower limbs, although the distribution can be atypical in younger children. Associated symptoms include abdominal pain, testicular pain and joint pains (arthritis in ankles and knees). Nephritis may occur, producing micro- or macroscopic haematuria, proteinuria. Very occasionally, this progresses to renal failure.

Check BP, urinalysis, urine microscopy, FBC (platelets are normal), U&E.

Refer to the paediatrician.

Idiopathic thrombocytopenic purpura

Probably results from autoimmune reaction to preceding viral infection. Presents with a purpuric rash, mucous membrane bleeding, conjunctival haemorrhage and occasionally, GI bleeding. Check FBC (platelets are <30 × 10^9/L). Refer for investigation and follow-up. In the presence of lymphadenopathy or splenomegaly, consider alternative diagnoses.

Treatment is usually expectant, since the natural course is for most cases to resolve spontaneously over 3 months. Occasionally, life-threatening haemorrhage occurs: obtain expert help, resuscitate with O_2 and IV fluids and give platelets.

Acute leukaemia

This may present acutely to the ED with purpura associated with thrombocytopenia. Look for hepatomegaly, splenomegaly and lymphadenopathy. FBC/blood film reveals anaemia with blast cells, ↓ platelets, and ↑ WBC).

Refer for admission.

Meningococcal disease

See algorithm Fig. 15.10 ⬚ p.668–9.

Meningococcal disease is unpredictable. Most children present acutely febrile and may not have a rash in the early stages.

Septicaemia

Children presenting with septicaemia may have:
- A history of fever/rigors but be afebrile at the time of presentation.
- Isolated severe limb pain in the absence of any other physical signs.
- Abdominal pain, diarrhoea and vomiting are common in septicaemia.
- Alertness until late in the illness.

Patients presenting in septic shock without meningitis have the worst prognosis.

Meningitis

Young children may present with fever, vomiting, irritability and confusion. Those aged <2 years are less likely to have neck stiffness or photophobia. Take parental concerns about a child's responsiveness and alertness seriously. Older children typically present more classically with fever, vomiting, headache, stiff neck and photophobia. Teenagers may present with a change of behaviour (eg confusion, aggression), which may be falsely attributed to alcohol or drugs.

Rash

Underlying meningococcal disease may be very advanced by the time a rash appears. This may initially be blanching, macular, or maculopapular. Children without a rash or with a blanching rash can still have meningococcal disease. The classic rapidly evolving petechial or purpuric rash may be a very late sign and can carry a poor prognosis.

Urgent treatment and experienced help are essential. CT scanning of the brain should be undertaken if there is impaired conscious level or focal neurological signs or signs of ↑ ICP. CT scans must not delay treatment. LP has no immediate role in the ED care of the critically ill child and can be fatal. LP is contraindicated if there is extensive purpura, shock, impaired consciousness, coagulopathy, local infection or ↑ ICP on CT or clinically.

Give antibiotics (IV ceftriaxone or cefotaxime) immediately to:
- All children with a fever and petechial/purpuric rash.
- Children in shock with or without a rash.
- Children with clinical meningitis, but LP contraindicated.

Take any haemorrhagic rash in a febrile child very seriously. Although many children with fever and petechiae have viral illnesses, there is no room for complacency. Ensure that all have their vital signs measured, and are carefully checked for signs of meningitis or septicaemia.

Airway and ventilation

Intubate and ventilate:
- If impaired conscious level or ↑ ICP clinically.
- Prior to CT scanning if critically ill.
- If fluid resuscitation requirement is >40mL/kg.

Seek expert help for rapid sequence induction/intubation (RSI)—haemodynamic collapse is common. Consider using IV ketamine for induction if experienced in its use.

Fluid resuscitation

Vast quantities of IV fluids are required in meningococcal septicaemia—often up to 100mL/kg. Many UK authorities recommend 4.5% human albumin solution (HAS) for fluid resuscitation, but give crystalloid (0.9% saline) if HAS is not immediately available.

Inotropes

- Dopamine or dobutamine at 10–20mcg/kg/min. Make up 3× weight (kg) mg in 50mL 5% glucose and run at 10mL/hr = 10mcg/kg/min.
- These dilute solutions can be used via a peripheral vein.
- Start adrenaline via a central line only (seek expert help) at 0.1mcg/kg/min. Make up 300mcg/kg in 50mL of saline at 1mL/hour = 0.1mcg/kg/min.

Hypoglycaemia (glucose <3mmol/L)
5mL/kg 10% glucose bolus IV and then glucose infusion at 80% of maintenance requirements over 24 hrs.

Correction of metabolic acidosis (pH <7.2)
1mmol/kg $NaHCO_3$ IV = 1mL/kg 8.4% $NaHCO_3$ over 20min or 2mL/kg 4.2% $NaHCO_3$ in neonates.

If K^+ <3.5mmol\L
Give 0.25mmol/kg KCl diluted in saline or glucose over 30min IV with ECG monitoring. Caution if anuric.

If total calcium <2mmol/L or ionized Ca^{2+} <1.0mmol/L
Give 0.1mL/kg 10% calcium chloride (0.7mmol/mL) over 30min IV (max 10mL) or 0.3mL/kg 10% calcium gluconate (0.22mmol/mL) over 30min (max 20mL).

If Mg^{2+} <0.75 mmol/L
Give 0.2mL/kg of 50% $MgSO_4$ over 30min IV (max 10mL).

See: Meningitis Research Foundation (www.meningitis.org) and 'NICE Guidance on Bacterial meningitis and meningococcal septicaemia'. Available at: http://www.nice.org.uk/nicemedia/live/13027/49341/49341.pdf

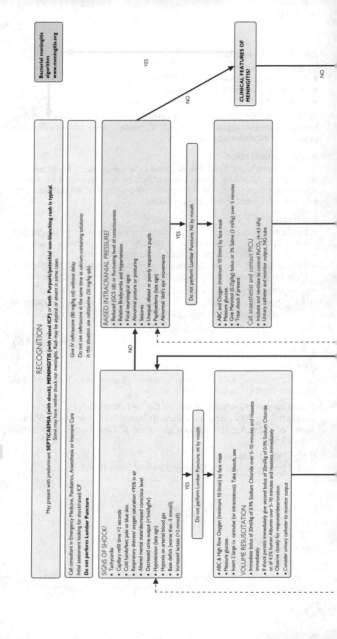

RECOGNITION

May present with predominant **SEPTICAEMIA (with shock)**, **MENINGITIS (with raised ICP)** or both. **Purpuric/petechial non-blanching rash is typical.**
Some may have neither shock nor meningitis. Rash may be atypical or absent in some cases.

Call consultant in Emergency Medicine, Paediatrics, Anaesthesia or Intensive Care
Initial assessment looking for shock/raised ICP
Do not perform Lumbar Puncture

Give IV ceftriaxone (80 mg/kg od) without delay
Do not use ceftriaxone at the same time as calcium-containing solutions;
in this situation use cefotaxime (50 mg/kg qds)

SIGNS OF SHOCK?
- Tachycardia
- Capillary refill time >2 seconds
- Cold hands/feet; pale or blue skin
- Respiratory distress oxygen saturation <95% in air
- Altered mental state/decreased conscious level
- Decreased urine output (<1ml/kg/hr)
- Hypotension (late sign)
- Hypoxia on arterial blood gas
- Base deficit (worse than –5 mmol/l)
- Increased lactate (>2 mmol/l)

YES → Do not perform Lumbar Puncture; nil by mouth

- ABC & High flow Oxygen (minimum 10 l/min) by face mask
- Measure glucose.
- Insert 2 large i.v. cannulae (or intraosseous); Take bloods, see

VOLUME RESUSCITATION
- Immediate bolus of 20ml/kg of 0.9% Sodium Chloride over 5–10 minutes and reassess immediately
- If shock persists immediately give second bolus of 20ml/kg of 0.9% Sodium Chloride or of 4.5% human Albumin over 5–10 minutes and reassess immediately
- Observe closely for response/deterioration
- Consider urinary catheter to monitor output.

NO

RAISED INTRACRANIAL PRESSURE?
- Reduced (GCS ≤8) or fluctuating level of consciousness
- Relative Bradycardia and Hypertension
- Focal neurological signs
- Abnormal posture or posturing
- Seizures
- Unequal, dilated or poorly responsive pupils
- Papilloedema (late sign)
- Abnormal 'doll's eye' movements

YES → Do not perform Lumbar Puncture; Nil by mouth

- ABC and Oxygen (minimum 10 l/min) by face mask
- Measure glucose.
- Give Mannitol (0.25g/kg) bolus or 3% Saline (3 ml/kg) over 5 minutes
- Treat shock if present

Call anaesthetist and contact PICU
- Intubate and ventilate to control PaCO₂ (4–4.5 kPa)
- Urinary catheter and monitor output. NG tube

CLINICAL FEATURES OF MENINGITIS?

YES

NO

Bacterial meningitis
algorithm
www.meningitis.org

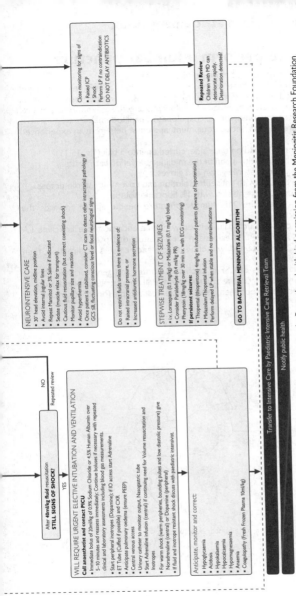

Close monitoring for signs of
• Raised ICP
• Shock
Perform LP if no contraindication
DO NOT DELAY ANTIBIOTICS

Repeated Review
Children with MD can
deteriorate rapidly.
Deterioration detected!

NEUROINTENSIVE CARE
• 30° head elevation, midline position
• Avoid internal jugular lines
• Repeat Mannitol or 3% Saline if indicated
• Sedate (muscle relax for transport)
• Cautious fluid resuscitation (but correct coexisting shock)
• Monitor pupillary size and reaction
• Avoid hyperthermia
• Once patient is stabilised, consider CT scan to detect other intracranial pathology if GCS ≤8, fluctuating conscious level or focal neurological signs

Do not restrict fluids unless there is evidence of:
• Raised intracranial pressure, or
• Increased antidiuretic hormone secretion

STEPWISE TREATMENT OF SEIZURES
• i.v. Lorazepam (0.1 mg/kg) or Midazolam (0.1 mg/kg) bolus
• Consider Paraldehyde (0.4 ml/kg PR)
• Phenytoin (18mg/kg over 30 min i.v. with ECG monitoring)

If persistent seizures:
• Thiopental (thiopentone) 4mg/kg in intubated patients (beware of hypotension)
• Midazolam/Thiopental infusion
Perform delayed LP when stable and no contraindications

GO TO BACTERIAL MENINGITIS ALGORITHM

NO

Repeated review

After 40ml/kg fluid resuscitation
STILL SIGNS OF SHOCK?

YES

WILL REQUIRE URGENT ELECTIVE INTUBATION AND VENTILATION
Call anaesthetist and contact PICU
• Give a bolus of 20ml/kg of 0.9% Sodium Chloride or 4.5% Human Albumin over 5–10 minutes and reassess immediately; Continue boluses if necessary with repeated clinical and laboratory assessments including blood gas measurements.
• Start peripheral inotropes (Dopamine), if IO access start Adrenaline
• ET Tube (Cuffed if possible) and CXR
• Anticipate pulmonary oedema (ensure PEEP)
• Central venous access
• Urinary catheter to monitor output, Nasogastric tube
• Start Adrenaline infusion (central) if continuing need for Volume resuscitation and Inotropes
• For warm shock (warm peripheries, bounding pulses and low diastolic pressure) give Noradrenaline (central) or Dopamine (peripheral)
• If fluid and inotrope resistant shock discuss with paediatric intensivist.

Anticipate, monitor and correct:
• Hypoglycaemia
• Acidosis
• Hypokalaemia
• Hypocalcaemia
• Hypomagnesaemia
• Anaemia
• Coagulopathy (Fresh Frozen Plasma 10ml/kg)

Transfer to Intensive Care by Paediatric Intensive Care Retrieval Team

Notify public health

Fig. 15.10 Management of meningococcal disease in children and young people. Reproduced with kind permission from the Meningitis Research Foundation www.meningitis.org

Take blood for glucose, FBC, coagulation screen, U&E, Ca^{2+}, Mg^{2+}, PO_4^{3-}, blood cultures, ABG, lactate, cross-match, and PCR for *N. meningitidis*.

How to perform a lumbar puncture

- Take senior advice before performing a LP.
- Confirm that there is no contra-indication to LP (eg prolonged or focal seizure, focal neurological signs, purpuric rash, GCS<13, pupillary dilatation, impaired oculocephalic reflexes, abnormal posture, hypertension, bradycardia, coagulopathy, papilloedema).
- Prepare parents, set up equipment, and enlist help from an experienced nurse.
- Position the child on their side, curled up into a ball (Fig. 15.11).
- Mark the skin with a pen in the midline at level of iliac crests.
- Scrub and don sterile gown and gloves.
- Clean the skin with antiseptic solution and cover with sterile drapes.
- Consider LA for the skin with 1% lidocaine solution.
- Slowly insert the 21G lumbar puncture needle aiming towards the umbilicus.
- If this causes much pain, withdraw needle and use more lidocaine LA (but <3mg/kg—📖 Analgesia in specific situations, p.280).
- If no CSF is obtained, withdraw needle and reassess its direction, then try again.
- Collect 4 drops of CSF in each of 3 bottles and send for: microscopy and Gram stain, culture and sensitivity; cell counts; glucose and protein.
- If bloody tap is obtained, send the clearest sample for cell counts.

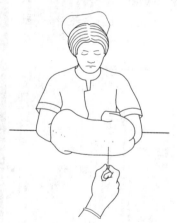

Fig. 15.11 Positioning for a lumbar puncture.

Skin lesions in multisystem disease

The appearance of the skin may provide a valuable clue to an underlying disease process. If suspected, refer all of the following diseases to a paediatrician.

Kawasaki disease (mucocutaneous lymph node syndrome)

This disease, believed to be related to a viral infection, was first reported in Japan in 1967 and has now spread worldwide. Most cases affect children <5 years. Extensive skin and mucosal changes occur, including an erythematous rash, which may affect palms and soles and desquamate. Conjunctivitis, uveitis, fissured lips, and a strawberry tongue may be seen.

Other features: fever, acute cervical lymphadenopathy, arthritis, and diarrhoea. Coronary artery aneurysm (and subsequent thrombosis) is a significant complication.

If Kawasaki disease is suspected check FBC, erythrocyte sedimentation rate (ESR), and viral titres, and refer to a paediatrician.

Dermatitis herpetiformis

This is the skin manifestation of coeliac disease. Vesicles and papules occur over the knees, elbows and buttocks. The lesions are very itchy and produce much scratching. Dapsone is effective treatment: refer to a paediatrician.

Erythema multiforme

Target lesions often with pale blistered centres are symmetrically distributed, particularly over the extensor surfaces of the limbs, sometimes including the hands and feet. The skin lesions combined with fever, systemic illness, oral and genital ulceration comprise the Stevens–Johnson syndrome.

Causes include infection (herpes, mycoplasma, tuberculosis TB) and drugs (sulphonamides, barbiturates).

Erythema nodosum

Painful red skin nodules or plaques on the anterior surfaces of both shins with associated fever, lethargy and arthralgia. It may be due to streptococcal infection, TB, sulphonamides, ulcerative colitis, or sarcoid.

Erythema marginatum

A transient erythematous rash with raised edges occurs in 20% of cases of *rheumatic fever* (□ p.496). Rheumatic fever is an autoimmune disease which follows infection with group A streptococci. Once common, it is now unusual in the UK.

Diagnose using the revised Duckett–Jones criteria (2 or more major; or 1 major and 2 minor, plus evidence of preceding streptococcal infection eg throat swab, ↑ ASO titre):

Major criteria Erythema marginatum, carditis, polyarthritis, Sydenham's chorea, subcutaneous nodules.

Minor criteria Fever, arthralgia, ↑ ESR, ↑ WBC, previous rheumatic fever, prolonged PR interval.

Erythema chronicum migrans (see 📖 Infestations, p.230)

The characteristic skin rash of Lyme disease begins as a red papule, which spreads to produce erythematous lesions with pale centres and bright edges. Lyme disease is a multisystem disorder resulting from tick-borne infection. It initially manifests with one or more of a variety of symptoms, including fever, headache, malaise, arthralgia, myalgia. The rash is present in most cases. The diagnosis can be elusive, but consider it if there has been any history of travel to an affected area.

Identifying skin lesions (Table 15.4)

Description
- Impalpable coloured lesion <1cm diameter = macule.
- Impalpable coloured lesion >1cm diameter = patch.
- Palpable lump <0.5cm diameter = papule.
- Palpable lump >0.5cm diameter = nodule.
- Palpable fluid-filled lesion <0.5cm diameter = vesicle.
- Palpable fluid-filled lesion >0.5cm diameter = bulla

Table 15.4 Skin lesions and possible causes

Feature	Causes
Peeling skin	Toxic epidermal necrolysis ('scalded skin syndrome'), Kawasaki disease.
	Streptococcal infection
Blistering lesions	*Staphylococcus* (impetigo and toxic epidermal necrolysis), scabies, chickenpox, herpes zoster, herpes simplex, Stevens–Johnson, pompholyx, coxsackie A16 (hand, foot and mouth disease), dermatitis herpetiformis, epidermolysis bullosa, drugs
Lesions on palms and soles	Coxsackie A16, Kawasaki disease, erythema multiforme, scabies, pompholyx
Pruritis	Eczema, urticaria, psoriasis, chickenpox, scabies, lice, insect bites, dermatitis herpetiformis

Paediatric ENT problems

Background

Due to frequent infections and large concentrations of active lymphoid tissue, certain ear, nose, and throat (ENT) problems are very common in paediatric practice. For example, acute suppurative otitis media (📖 Earache, p.550) has an incidence of 20% amongst pre-school children; secretory otitis media ('glue ear') has a prevalence of 5% amongst all children. Rhinorrhoea from coryza and rhinitis is even more common.

Approach

Although many ENT diseases are usually considered as primary care problems, children often present to the ED suffering from them. It is obviously important to examine the ears and throat of any child presenting with a fever. Remember, however, that the ill, septic child with large red tonsils may also have a significant septic focus elsewhere (eg meningitis or pneumonia).

Examination

Examination of the ears and throat is generally disliked by children and as a result, can prove to be rather a struggle. It is therefore sensible to leave this part of the full examination of a child until last. Parental help can be invaluable in allowing examination of the slightly uncooperative toddler or younger child. Sit the child on a parent's lap for examination of the ears and throat, as shown in Fig. 15.12.

The difficult examination

Despite various manoeuvres, it can be very difficult to adequately visualize the throat of a child who adamantly refuses to open their mouth. A useful trick is to draw the face of a 'Smiley Man' on the end of a wooden spatula. The child may then consent to the 'Smiley Man' having a look at their throat (preferably with the ink side up!).

Presentation and treatment

The presentation, diagnosis and treatment of specific ENT diseases in both children and adults are described in Chapter 12.
- 📖 Ear, nose, and throat foreign bodies, p.546.
- 📖 Earache, p.550.
- 📖 Epistaxis, p.552.
- 📖 Nasal fracture, p.553.
- 📖 Sore throat, p.554.

Examining a child's ear In an infant pull the pinna back and down (rather than up) for the best view.

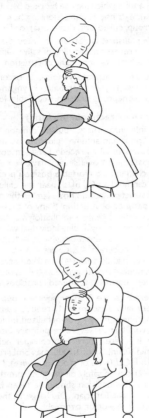

Fig. 15.12 Examining a child's throat.

Stridor: upper respiratory infections

The upper airway is a tube which may be blocked by: distortion (eg tongue falling back in coma), extrinsic compression (eg haematoma), swelling of its wall (eg burns, croup, epiglottitis, diphtheria), or FB within.

Signs of upper airway obstruction Stridor, marked dyspnoea, drowsiness, subcostal/suprasternal recession, drooling of saliva, difficulty speaking, and cyanosis. Any of these warn of impending obstruction.

Stridor is a high pitched inspiratory noise. It occurs in croup, acute epiglottitis, inhaled FB, laryngeal trauma, laryngomalacia ('congenital laryngeal stridor'), angioneurotic oedema. See Table 15.5.

Acute croup (laryngotracheobronchitis)

Viral in origin (para-influenza virus in >80%). Common between 6 months, and 5 years of age. Spring and autumn epidemics occur. Illness lasts ≈3–5 days. Coryzal symptoms usually precede harsh stridor, a barking cough ('seal's bark') with hoarseness ↑ over several days. Temperature (T)° is only mildly ↑. Leave the child in a comfortable position preferably in the arms of the parent, who can hold an O_2 mask near the child. Look for signs of significant airway obstruction, but do not examine the pharynx as this may precipitate laryngospasm or obstruction. If any of these signs are present, or if SpO_2 <92% in air refer urgently—intubation may be required. Use the modified Westley croup score by adding individual values as follows:

- *Stridor*: none = 0, only when upset or agitated = 1, at rest = 2.
- *Retractions*: mild = 1, moderate = 2, severe = 3.
- *Air entry*: normal = 0, mild decrease = 1, marked decrease = 2.
- *SpO_2 <92% on air*: none = 0, with agitation = 4, at rest = 5.
- *Level of consciousness*: normal = 0, altered conscious level = 5.

Children with moderate (score 3–5) or severe croup (score 6–11) and impending respiratory failure (score >11) require admission to hospital. Give oral dexamethasone 0.15mg/kg or nebulized budesonide (1–2mg in 5mL 0.9% saline) if vomiting or severe respiratory distress and refer to the paediatric team. If severe (score >5), consider nebulized adrenaline driven by O_2 at 8L/min (0.5mL/kg of 1:1000, max 5mL; repeat as required). Refer severe cases to PICU (<1% of croup is severe). Many children with mild croup (score 0–2) can be safely discharged from the ED after a brief period of observation. This decision should be taken by an experienced emergency physician or paediatrician. Discharge in the evening may be inadvisable, since croup can worsen overnight.

Diphtheria

Although rare in the UK, the exotoxin of *Corynebacterium diphtheriae* may produce serious organ damage (especially myocarditis) and upper respiratory tract obstruction. The non-immunized child may present with pyrexia, sore throat, and dysphagia due to an adherent pharyngeal exudate. Cervical lymphadenopathy causes a 'bull neck' appearance. (Note that infectious mononucleosis may present similarly—🔲 p.241).

Treat with O_2, obtain ECG and venous access, send blood for FBC, blood culture, and obtain a throat swab. Refer for antitoxin (20,000U IM after a test dose) and IV erythromycin.

Acute epiglottitis

Increasingly uncommon, due to widespread Hib vaccination. Rapidly progressive airway obstruction may result. Children aged 2–7 years are most usually involved, although it does occur in older children and adults. Unlike croup, stridor is usually soft and may even be absent. Onset is typically acute. The child is systemically unwell with pyrexia >38.5°C, but little or no cough. In severe cases, the child may be ominously quiet, unable to speak, sitting upright drooling saliva in a 'sniffing position'.

Management Do not attempt to visualize the throat as this may precipitate total airway obstruction. Let the child adopt the most comfortable position, give humidified O₂ and call urgently for anaesthetic, ICU and ENT help. Nebulized adrenaline (0.5mL/kg of 1:1000, max 5mL) may 'buy time'. Defer doing blood tests (FBC, blood cultures) and treatment with IV cefotaxime until an anaesthetist has assessed the child. Lateral neck X-rays are unnecessary and potentially hazardous. Intubation, if required, may be very difficult to perform. A safe approach is for an experienced anaesthetist to use a gaseous induction in the presence of a surgeon who is prepared for a surgical airway. Airway swelling may require a smaller than expected diameter (and thus uncut) ET tube. Let the anaesthetist know the number of adrenaline nebulizers given, as halothane induction could precipitate arrhythmias. If visualization of the tracheal orifice is difficult at laryngoscopy due to oedema, ask an assistant to squeeze the chest and look for an air bubble emerging from the trachea.

Loss of the airway—if this happens, summon help and attempt to ventilate with O₂ using bag and mask. If ventilation proves impossible, obtain a surgical airway (needle cricothyroidotomy if <12 years, surgical cricothyroidotomy if ≥12 years)—see 📖 p.326.

Bacterial tracheitis

May be due to *Staph. aureus, Strep.*, or *H. influenzae*. The presentation of 'croup', plus moderate/severe pyrexia, and production of copious secretions suggests the diagnosis. If suspected, refer and treat as for acute epiglottitis (intubation is often required). Bacterial tracheitis can cause rapid onset of septic shock.

Table 15.5 Clinical presentations of upper airway obstruction

	Croup	Epiglottitis	Bacterial tracheitis	Foreign body
Age	1–2 years	2–6 years	Throughout childhood	Throughout childhood
Onset	1–2 days	<24hr	<24hr	<24hr
History	Coryza, barking cough	Sore throat, dysphagia	Rattling cough, sore throat	
Signs	T°<38.5 non-toxic, harsh stridor, hoarseness	T°>38.5 toxic, upright position	T°>38.5 toxic, mucopurulent secretions, soft/absent stridor	Afebrile, non-toxic

Severe acute asthma in children

Assess conscious level, degree of breathlessness, degree of agitation, use of accessory muscles, amount of wheezing, pulse rate and respiratory rate. Attempt to measure peak flow if age >5 years (See Fig. 15.13 for normal peak flow).

Follow the 2011 British Thoracic Society/Scottish Intercollegiate Guidelines Network (BTS/SIGN) Guidelines based on age and severity (http://www.sign.ac.uk/pdf/sign101.pdf). Investigations, including blood gas estimations, rarely alter immediate management.

Cautions Children with severe asthma attacks may not appear distressed. Wheeze and respiratory rate correlate poorly with severity of airway obstruction. Increasing tachycardia denotes worsening asthma, a fall in heart rate in life-threatening asthma is pre-terminal.

Assessment in the very young (<2 years) may be difficult—get expert help.

Normal peak expiratory flow in children aged 5–18 years.

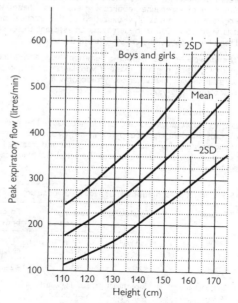

Fig. 15.13

Management of acute asthma in children aged >2 years (Figs 15.14 and 15.15)

- Summon senior ED/PICU/paediatric help if asthma is severe.
- Provide high flow O_2 via face mask (or nasal cannulae).
- Give an inhaled β-agonist. In mild or moderate asthma use a metered dose inhaler with a spacer, and 2–4 puffs of 100mcg salbutamol every 10–20min.
- In severe or life threatening asthma use an O_2-powered nebulizer with salbutamol 2.5–5mg or terbutaline 5–10mg.
- Give oral prednisolone (20mg for children aged 2–5 years; 30–40mg if aged >5 years). If already taking maintenance steroids, give 2mg/kg (max 60mg). In children who vomit, repeat the dose of prednisolone and consider IV hydrocortisone 4mg/kg.
- Add ipratropium bromide 0.25mg every 20–30 min if there is poor initial response to nebulized β-agonist.
- Consider salbutamol (15mcg/kg) given IV over 10min in severe cases with a poor response to initial nebulized salbutamol and ipratropium bromide. Refer to PICU urgently and check K^+ levels.
- Aminophylline is not recommended in children with mild to moderate asthma. In severe or life-threatening asthma unresponsive to maximal doses of bronchodilators and systemic steroids, take specialist advice and consider IV aminophylline (5mg/kg over 20min; maintenance IV infusion at 1mg/kg/hr; omit loading dose if already receiving oral theophyllines).
- Consider an IVI of magnesium sulphate 40mg/kg over 20min, but evidence of benefit is limited.
- Do not give 'routine' antibiotics.

Notes If possible, repeat and record peak flow 15–30min after starting treatment. If the patient is not improving, give further nebulized β-agonist. Pulse oximetry is helpful in assessing response to treatment. An SpO_2 ≤92% in air after initial bronchodilator therapy usually indicates the need for more intensive in-patient care usually in PICU. CXR is indicated for severe dyspnoea, focal chest signs, or signs of severe infection.

Consider need for anaesthesia/intubation/IPPV and PICU transfer
- Deteriorating peak flow or worsening or persistent hypoxia or normal/increased pCO_2 levels on ABG.
- Exhaustion, feeble respiratory effort, confusion, or drowsiness.
- Coma or respiratory arrest.

Management of acute asthma in children aged <2 years

Assessing acute asthma in early childhood is difficult: get specialist help (see www.sign.ac.uk). Intermittent wheezing attacks are usually due to viral infection. Differential diagnosis includes: aspiration and other pneumonias, bronchiolitis, tracheomalacia, complications of underlying conditions (eg congenital abnormalities, cystic fibrosis). If there is no response to inhaled bronchodilators, review the diagnosis:
- Use a metered dose inhaler with spacer to give β-agonist therapy.
- Consider systemic steroids early in the management of moderate to severe asthma in infants (10mg of soluble prednisolone).
- Consider adding inhaled ipratropium bromide (0.25mg) to inhaled β-agonists for more severe symptoms.

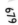

Age 2–5 years

ASSESS ASTHMA SEVERITY

Moderate asthma	Severe asthma	Life threatening asthma
• SpO_2 ≥92% • No clinical features of severe asthma NB: If a patient has signs and symptoms across categories, always treat according to their most severe features	• SpO_2 <92% • Too breathless to talk or eat • Heart rate >140/min • Respiratory rate >40/min • Use of accessory neck muscles	SpO_2 <92% plus any of: • Silent chest • Poor respiratory effort • Agitation • Altered consciousness • Cyanosis

Oxygen via face mask/nasal prongs to achieve SpO_2 94–98%

• β_2 agonist 2–10 puffs via spacer ± facemask [given one at a time single puffs, tidal breathing and inhaled separately] • Increase β_2 agonist dose by 2 puffs every 2 minutes up to 10 puffs according to response • Consider soluble oral prednisolone 20 mg **Reassess within 1 hour**	• β_2 agonist 10 puffs via spacer ± facemask or nebulized salbutamol 2.5 mg or terbutaline 5 mg • Soluble prednisolone 20 mg or IV hydrocortisone 4 mg/kg • Repeat β_2 agonist up to every 20–30 minutes according to response • **If poor response** add 0.25 mg nebulized ipratropium bromide	• Nebulized β_2 agonist: salbutamol 2.5 mg or terbutaline 5 mg **plus** ipratropium bromide 0.25 mg nebulized • Oral prednisolone 20 mg or IV hydrocortisone 4mg/kg if vomiting **Discuss with senior clinician, PICU team or paediatrician** • Repeat bronchodilators every 20–30 minutes

ASSESS RESPONSE TO TREATMENT
Record respiratory rate, heart rate and oxygen saturation every 1–4 hours

RESPONDING
• Continue bronchodilators 1–4 hours prn
• Discharge when stable on 4 hourly treatment
• Continue oral prednisolone for up to 3 days

At discharge
• Ensure stable on 4 hourly inhaled treatment
• Review the need for regular treatment and the use of inhaled steroids
• Review inhaler technique
• Provide a written asthma action plan for treating future attacks
• Arrange follow up according to local policy

NOT RESPONDING
• **Arrange HDU/PICU transfer**
Consider:
• **Chest X-ray and blood gases**
• **IV salbutamol** 15 mcg/kg bolus over 10 minutes **followed by** continuous infusion 1–5 mcg/kg/min (dilute to 200 mcg/ml)
• **IV aminophylline** 5 mg/kg loading dose over 20 minutes (omit in those receiving oral theophyllines) **followed by** continuous infusion 1 mg/kg/hour

Fig. 15.14 Management of acute asthma in 2–5-year-olds.
See: www.brit-thoracic.org.uk and www.sign.ac.uk

Age >5 years

ASSESS ASTHMA SEVERITY

Moderate asthma
- SpO_2 ≥92%
- PEF >50% best or predicted
- No clinical features of severe asthma

NB: If a patient has signs and symptoms across categories, always treat according to their most severe features

Severe asthma
- SpO_2 <92%
- PEF 33–50% best or predicted
- Heart rate >125/min
- Respiratory rate >30/min
- Use of accessory neck muscles

Life threatening asthma
SpO_2 <92% plus any of:
- PEF <33% best or predicted
- Silent chest
- Poor respiratory effort
- Altered consciousness
- Cyanosis

Oxygen via face mask/nasal prongs to achieve SpO_2 94–98%

- β_2 agonist 2–10 puffs via spacer
- Increase β_2 agonist dose by 2 puffs every 2 minutes up to 10 puffs according to response
- Oral prednisolone 30–40 mg

Reassess within 1 hour

- β_2 agonist 10 puffs via spacer or nebulized salbutamol 2.5–5 mg or terbutaline 5–10 mg
- Oral prednisolone 30–40 mg or IV hydrocortisone 4 mg/kg if vomiting
- **If poor response** nebulized ipratropium bromide 0.25 mg
- Repeat β_2 agonist and ipratropium up to every 20–30 minutes according to response

---

- Nebulized β_2 agonist: salbutamol 5 mg or terbutaline 10 mg **plus** ipratropium bromide 0.25 mg nebulized
- Oral prednisolone 30–40 mg or IV hydrocortisone 4mg/kg if vomiting

Discuss with senior clinician, PICU team or paediatrician

- Repeat bronchodilators every 20–30 minutes

ASSESS RESPONSE TO TREATMENT
Record respiratory rate, heart rate, oxygen saturation and PEF/FEV every 1–4 hours

RESPONDING
- Continue bronchodilators 1–4 hours prn
- Discharge when stable on 4 hourly treatment
- Continue oral prednisolone 30–40 mg for up to 3 days

At discharge
- Ensure stable on 4 hourly inhaled treatment
- Review the need for regular treatment and the use of inhaled steroids
- Review inhaler technique
- Provide a written asthma action plan for treating future attacks
- Arrange follow up according to local policy

NOT RESPONDING
- **Continue 20–30 minute nebulizers and arrange HDU/PICU transfer**
- Consider: Chest X-ray and blood gases
- **Consider risks and benefits of:**
- **Bolus IV salbutamol** 15 mcg/kg if not already given
- Continuous **IV salbutamol** infusion 1–5 mcg/kg/min (200 mcg/ml solution)
- **IV aminophylline** 5 mg/kg loading dose over 20 minutes (omit in those receiving oral theophyllines) **followed by** continuous infusion 1 mg/kg/hour
- **Bolus IV infusion of magnesium sulphate** 40 mg/kg (max 2 g) over 20 minutes

Fig. 15.15 Management of acute asthma in children aged less than 2 years.
See: www.brit-thoracic.org.uk and www.sign.ac.uk

Acute bronchiolitis[1]

Viral infection of the small airways results in inflammation, oedema, and excessive secretions, presenting with signs of obstructive airways disease. Acute bronchiolitis is common, particularly in the winter months and predominantly involves infants (typically 3–6 months). Those at particular risk are the very young (aged <6 weeks), the premature (born <35 weeks) and those with chronic respiratory, congenital heart disease, immunodeficiency, or neurological problems. Parental smoking increases the risk of bronchiolitis. Breast feeding for more than two months appears to have a protective effect. Most infants recover completely within 2 weeks.

Agents responsible

75% are caused by respiratory syncytial virus (RSV). Other causes include influenza, para-influenza, adeno-, and enteroviruses.

Presentation

Coryza, rhinorrhoea, and mild fever progress to respiratory distress with dyspnoea, dry cough, feeding difficulties, and wheeze (variable). Some children may present with apnoea. Inspection may reveal cyanosis, dehydration, tachypnoea (>50/min), nasal flaring, grunting, subcostal and intercostal recession. The chest is usually visibly hyperinflated in bronchiolitis. There may be tachycardia and prolonged expiration (±wheeze) with fine end-inspiratory crepitations.

Complications

Feeding difficulties, apnoeic spells, and respiratory failure (hence, adopt a low threshold for admission). Secondary bacterial infection can occur, but is uncommon. Long-term airway damage may occasionally occur (obliterative bronchiolitis).

Investigations

- Apply a pulse oximeter, and check the pulse and CRT.
- Do not do routine blood tests unless the infant is febrile or an alternative diagnosis, such as pneumonia or sepsis is more likely.
- Consider CXR and ABG/capillary gas only for those with progressive, atypical or severe illness. Do not do CXR routinely.
- Fluorescent antibody tests on nasopharyngeal aspirate to demonstrate the presence of RSV are recommended; these help with cohorting and isolation arrangements on the wards (see opposite), particularly during the annual epidemic season in winter.
- Assess feeding difficulties by offering a bottle feed.

CXR shows hyperinflation with downward displacement of the diaphragm due to small airway obstruction and gas trapping. There may also be collapse or consolidation (usually upper lobe) or perihilar infiltrates hard to distinguish from pneumonia.

Differential diagnoses for bronchiolitis include congenital heart disease, asthma, pneumonia, cystic fibrosis, inhaled foreign body and septicaemia.

Treatment

Refer all infants with respiratory distress, feeding difficulties (<50% usual fluid intake in previous 24 hr), SpO_2 <94% on air, apnoeic episodes, or dehydration. Emergency treatment is largely supportive, comprising humidified O_2 (aiming to keep SpO_2 >92%), NG or IV fluids and sometimes CPAP or IPPV. Dehydration may be severe enough to warrant an IV fluid bolus of 20mL/kg. Treatment with inhaled bronchodilators may achieve short-term (30–60min) clinical improvement in a minority, but there is no convincing evidence of efficacy. Nasal suction may help those in respiratory distress. Ribavirin is of no value and should not be used. Do not give antibiotics for bronchiolitis, but consider for severe illness suggestive of co-existing pneumonia or septicaemia. There is no benefit from using ipratropium, oral or inhaled steroids, or nebulized adrenaline. Do not use these therapies in acute bronchiolitis.

PICU referral and ventilatory support is indicated for those with recurrent apnoea, persistent acidosis pH <7.25, infants with ↓ conscious level, poor chest wall movement, and low SaO_2 (<92%) despite FiO_2 >60%, and those with hypercapnoea.

Cross infection is a serious problem during epidemics. Ensure all persons entering a cubicle containing a child with bronchiolitis clean their hands before and after seeing the patient, and use gloves and plastic aprons.

Prevention

Palivizumab is a humanized monoclonal RSV antibody, which is used as a prophylactic agent to reduce the severity of RSV disease in at risk infants. It can be considered for use on a case-by-case basis in infants who:
• Were born prematurely (<35 weeks gestation).
• Have acyanotic congenital heart disease.
• Have chronic lung disease.
• Have severe congenital immunodeficiency.

Infants should be selected for this treatment by a local lead paediatric specialist.

1 See the SIGN *Guideline on Bronchiolitis in Children*. Available at: http://www.sign.ac.uk/pdf/sign91.pdf

Whooping cough[ND]

Caused by Bordetella pertussis, whooping cough is a notifiable disease with an incubation period of 5–14 days (□ p.220). It is common (particularly in the autumn) in children not immunized against it. A similar disease may also occur with other viral infections (*Bordetella parapertussis* and adenoviruses).

Presentation

Coryza is followed by increasing cough (typically worse at night, and tending to occur in bouts, often culminating in vomiting). Severe coughing bouts may result in conjunctival haemorrhages. The characteristic 'whoop' is an inspiratory noise produced after a coughing bout. It is not present in all infants with whooping cough. The cough may persist for several weeks.

Complications

Illness is often prolonged. There is a risk of neurological damage and bronchiectasis. Infants are at particular risk of death from apnoeic episodes.

Investigations

Send blood for viral titres, mycoplasma antibodies and FBC (usually reveals markedly ↑ lymphocytes). CXR may be normal or show 'shaggy' right heart border.

Treatment

Refer infants aged <6 months (risk of apnoea) and any acutely unwell child. Discharge others (having informed the Infectious Diseases consultant) with PO erythromycin (12.5mg/kg qds) and advice to avoid contact with other children for 5 days. Arrange GP follow-up and give PO erythromycin (12.5mg/kg qds) as prophylaxis to unimmunized infant siblings.

Prevention

Encourage immunization.

TBND and cystic fibrosis

Pulmonary TB

TB is being seen increasingly again (📖 p.232). It is more common in visitors from overseas or HIV +ve children. TB may present in a variety of ways in children: persistent cough and fever, growth retardation, meningitis, pleural effusion, monoarticular arthritis, lymphadenopathy, back pain, hepatosplenomegaly.

Investigation CXR.

Treatment Refer suspected cases for specialist evaluation, including Mantoux (0.1mL intradermal tuberculin) and treatment.

Cystic fibrosis

Recurrent respiratory infections in neonates and infants raise the possibility of cystic fibrosis, tracheo-oesophageal fistula, cleft palate, or a defect in immunity. Cystic fibrosis is an autosomal recessive disorder affecting 1 in 2000 children. It may present neonatally with meconium ileus or later with respiratory infections (±finger clubbing), failure to thrive, rectal prolapse and steatorrhoea. Once diagnosed, a child will remain closely monitored and treated by both GP and a specialist CF respiratory team. Involve this team at an early stage if a child with cystic fibrosis presents with respiratory infection.

Pneumonia

Pneumonia is relatively common at all ages, but the infective agents responsible vary (Table 15.6). Viruses are most commonly found as a cause in younger children. In older children, when a bacterial cause is found, it is most commonly *Strep. pneumoniae*.

Table 15.6 Infective agents responsible for pneumonia

Age	Common causes
Neonates	*E. coli*, β-haemolytic Strep., *Chlamydia trachomatis*, *Listeria monocytogenes*, CMV
Infants and toddlers	RSV, para-influenza viruses, *Strep pneumoniae*, *H. influenzae*, *Mycoplasma*
Older children	*Strep pneumoniae*, *H. influenzae*, *Mycoplasma*

Symptoms

Often an URTI is followed by ↑ fever, cough, dyspnoea, lethargy, feeding difficulties, and dehydration. Pleuritic chest pain, abdominal pain, and neck stiffness may occur. The presence of headache, abdominal pain, maculopapular rash, and joint pains suggests *Mycoplasma* infection.

Signs

The child is usually dyspnoeic, pyrexial, and unwell. Classic signs of consolidation (📖 p.114) are often absent, especially in infants and younger children. Look for evidence of infection elsewhere (ears, throat) and dehydration. If wheeze is present in a pre-school child, bacterial pneumonia is unlikely, although it does occur occasionally with mycobacteria in older children.

Investigations

- Take throat swabs.
- Obtain blood for FBC, cultures, viral titres, and mycoplasma antibodies.
- Check SpO_2.
- Obtain urine for culture.
- CXR may demonstrate widespread bronchopneumonia or lobar consolidation. Cavitation suggests Staphyloccocal pneumonia or TB.

Treatment

If SpO_2<92%, give O_2. Treat dehydration with IV fluids. Refer for admission and antibiotics. IPPV is rarely required.

The choice of antibiotic will depend upon the likely infective agent and local/national protocols (see British Thoracic Society guidelines: www. brit-thoracic.org.uk and see Box 15.2).

Refer to ICU those unable to maintain SpO_2 >92% with 60% O_2, those with signs of shock, increasing respiratory rate/pulse rate with respiratory distress and exhaustion, those with slow irregular breathing or recurrent apnoea.

Box 15.2 Antibiotic treatment for suspected bacterial pneumonia

Uncomplicated community acquired pneumonia

- *Neonate*: benzylpenicillin and gentamicin.
- *Neonate and child under 6 months*: cefuroxime or co-amoxiclav (or benzylpenicillin if lobar pneumonia or S. pneumoniae suspected).
- *Child 6 months to 5 years*: oral amoxicillin or oral erythromycin.
- *Child 5–18 years*: oral erythromycin (or oral amoxicillin if S. pneumoniae suspected).

Add flucloxacillin if staph suspected eg in influenza or measles
Use erythromycin if atypical pathogens suspected or penicillin allergic

Severe community acquired pneumonia of unknown aetiology

- *Neonate*: benzylpenicillin and gentamicin.
- *1 month to 18 years*: cefuroxime or co-amoxiclav (or benzylpenicillin if lobar pneumonia or S. pneumoniae suspected).

Use erythromycin if atypical pathogens such as mycoplasma (more common in children over 5 years) or *Chlamydia* suspected or penicillin allergic. Add flucloxacillin if *Staphylococcus* suspected.

Fits, febrile convulsions, and funny turns

A careful history is crucial. Epileptic fits may take many forms:

Grand mal (tonic/clonic) Loss of consciousness and shaking of all limbs.

Petit mal ('absences') Child pauses in speech or other activity and is unaware of episode.

Focal fit Involves 1 part of body (progression to grand mal = Jacksonian march).

Myoclonic fit May be violent and includes drop attacks.

Infantile spasm (Salaam attack) May involve truncal flexion and cause a fall.

Temporal lobe epilepsy Numerous bizarre presentations.

The fitting patient

The child who is still fitting on arrival to hospital is likely to have had a prolonged seizure and needs urgent attention.

- Give O_2.
- Secure the airway. If teeth are clenched, do not try to prise them open to insert an airway. Instead, if the airway is obstructed, try a nasopharyngeal airway (📖 p.325).
- Give IV lorazepam (0.1mg/kg) or if venous access is unsuccessful, per rectum (PR) diazepam (0.5mg/kg) or buccal midazolam (0.5mg/kg).
- Check bedside strip measurement of venous/capillary blood glucose (BMG) and treat hypoglycaemia with IV 0.5g/kg dextrose (5mL/kg of 10%).
- Treat fever >38°C with rectal paracetamol.
- If fits continue, follow the algorithm for status epilepticus (📖 p.690).

After the fit has finished

Reassess Airway, Breathing, Circulation. Continue O_2 and place in the recovery position. Check for injuries and perform regular observations.

First fit Refer for investigation of possible causes. U&E, blood glucose, Ca^{2+}, Mg^{2+}, FBC, and urinalysis will be required.

Subsequent fit If appropriate, check serum anticonvulsant level and arrange for GP/outpatient clinic to receive the results and adjust dose appropriately. Allow home patients with known epilepsy who have fully recovered and have no obvious cause for the fit (eg meningitis, hypoglycaemia).

Febrile convulsions

These are grand mal seizures lasting <5min and secondary to pyrexia of febrile illness. Commonest cause of fits between 6 months and 5 years, affecting 3% of children. Although 30% recur, only 1% go on to develop epilepsy in adult life. By definition, children already diagnosed as epileptic, do not have febrile convulsions, but 'further fits'. Treat patients who arrive fitting with O_2, airway care and IV lorazepam, PR diazepam or buccal midazolam as described opposite. Check BMG and T°. Give PR (or if conscious, oral) paracetamol (15mg/kg). Examine thoroughly for a source of infection (particularly meningitis) and perform an infection screen: U&E, FBC, blood cultures, MSU, CXR and LP. Consider discharging children aged >2 years with second or subsequent febrile convulsion, and obvious benign and treatable cause for pyrexia, with appropriate treatment. Liaise with GP to consider arranging for parents to administer rectal diazepam or buccal midazolam to terminate future febrile fits. Admit children aged <2 years, those with first febrile fits, and those with serious infections or an unknown cause of pyrexia.

Approach to the febrile child aged <3 years

Usually symptoms and signs of illness are non-specific. General aspects of behaviour and appearance provide the best guide as to whether a serious illness is likely. The degree of fever and response to antipyretics is not helpful. Up to 5% of those who present with fever will have bacteraemia. Admit any febrile child <3 years who appears unwell/ miserable.

Febrile infants (>38°C) aged <3 months are especially difficult to assess and require admission for a 'septic screen' (FBC, serology, blood cultures, urine culture ±CXR, lumbar puncture (LP). Discuss with a neonatologist the need for IV antibiotics in babies aged <28 days.

Young children aged 3 months–3 years who have a clear focus of infection and appear well should be treated as indicated. If there is no clear focus of infection, consider short-term admission in a paediatric facility.

Funny turns

Only a minority of reported 'funny turns' are epileptic fits. Most require referral and investigation. The history is crucial.

Infants Irregular and varying depth of respiration during sleep is normal, but can cause parental alarm. Self-limiting apnoeic or cyanotic episodes may be due to: fits, inhaled FBs, near-miss cot death, gastro-oesophageal reflux and laryngeal spasm, or arrhythmias (eg SVT).

Toddlers Breath-holding attacks commonly accompany frustration. They may cause the toddler to turn blue, lose consciousness, and even have a brief fit. Reflex anoxic episodes ('pallid syncope') are due to excess vagal stimulation in illness or after injury. Bradycardia, pallor and loss of consciousness is occasionally accompanied by a short fit.

Older children Syncope on exertion should prompt consideration of aortic stenosis, SVT, coarctation or hypertrophic cardiomyopathy. Vasovagal episodes and hyperventilation also cause 'collapse'. Atypical or unheralded collapse or seizures may be a feature of inherited long QT syndrome, and is associated with torsades de pointes. Obtain an ECG in any child who presents with collapse or 'first fit'.

Status epilepticus

Definition a fit (or consecutive fits without complete recovery between) lasting >30min. The duration of the seizures is often underestimated because the intensity of the jerking diminishes with time and small amplitude twitching may be easily missed.

Status epilepticus usually involves tonic-clonic fits and as in adults, is associated with significant mortality (≈4%) and morbidity (up to 30% have long-term neurological damage). Prompt treatment with termination of the fit is crucial to ↓ these risks.

Causes meningitis, head injury, altered drug therapy, or non-compliance in known epileptic child, metabolic disturbances, encephalopathy (including Reye's syndrome), 'febrile status', poisoning.

Treatment algorithm for the fitting child[1]

- Open and maintain airway and give O_2.
- Do not prise open clenched teeth—consider nasopharyngeal airway.
- Rapidly obtain venous access and check BMG.
- Give lorazepam 0.1mg/kg IV over 30–60sec* (if no venous access: give 0.5mg/kg diazepam PR or buccal midazolam 0.5mg/kg).
- Treat hypoglycaemia with 0.5g/kg dextrose (5mL/kg of 10%) IV.
- Apply pulse oximeter and send blood for investigations (see below).
- Check T°: if >38°C give paracetamol 15mg/kg PR.

If seizure continuing at 10min
- Repeat lorazepam 0.1mg/kg IV over 30–60sec* (or if vascular access still not obtained, give paraldehyde 0.4mL/kg PR in the same volume of olive oil or 0.9% saline).
- Get senior help and call for senior ED/anaesthetic/PICU help.

If seizure continuing after a further 10min
- If not known to be taking phenytoin: start phenytoin infusion 18mg/kg IV* over 20min (monitor BP and ECG) or if already on phenytoin, give phenobarbital 20mg/kg IV* over 10min.

If seizure continuing after a further 20min
- Paralyse, intubate and ventilate using IV thiopental (induction dose 4mg/kg) and consider a thiopental infusion.
- Transfer to ICU/PICU for ventilation and EEG monitoring.

Investigations: BMG and blood glucose, U&E, Ca^{2+}, Mg^{2+}, PO_4^{3-}, LFTs, FBC, ABG/capillary gas, blood cultures, coagulation screen, CXR. If taking anticonvulsant(s): check serum level(s). Obtain CT scan of head if intracranial disease is suspected (unless clinically meningitis), in which case treat immediately—📖 Meningococcal disease, p.666).

---

1 See *APLS Manual* 4th edn, 2005.
* Intraosseous route is an alternative.

Diabetic ketoacidosis

Diabetic ketoacidosis will usually present to the ED in a child who is known to be diabetic, but occasionally it can be the first presentation of DKA. The child will present with features including altered conscious level, polyuria, polydipsia, nausea, vomiting, and abdominal pain. Children with DKA can die from cerebral oedema (unpredictable and has 25% mortality), aspiration pneumonia, or hypokalaemia. All of these are avoidable with appropriate treatment.

Be very careful not to misdiagnose the abdominal pain of DKA as a 'surgical abdomen' or to dismiss the child as 'hyperventilating' (the ↑ respiratory rate is due to profound metabolic acidosis). Call senior ED and paediatric staff when DKA is suspected.

Causes First episode of DKA in a previously well child. In a child with known diabetes, lack of insulin, change of therapy, and intercurrent viral illness can cause DKA. Fever suggests sepsis (fever is not part of DKA).

Treatment algorithm for the child with DKA[1]

- Open and maintain airway if not fully conscious and give high flow O_2.
- Attach cardiac monitor (look for tall T-waves) and record CRT/BP.
- Rapidly obtain venous access and check BMG (remember BMG often underestimates blood glucose in DKA) and estimate weight.
- Take blood for glucose, U&E, FBC, VBG (and ketones if available).
- If evidence of shock (tachycardia, prolonged CRT, hypotension), give 10mL/kg 0.9% saline as a bolus; repeat as required up to 30mL/kg.

Confirm the diagnosis of DKA

- Check history with child and parents: polyuria, polydipsia; vomiting, abdominal pain, drowsiness, and ↑ respiratory rate.
- *Biochemical*: high glucose (>11mmol/L); acidosis (pH<7.3, bicarbonate <15mmol/L); glycosuria and ketonuria.

Involve senior paediatric ± PICU staff

- Assess level of dehydration (mild <3%; moderate 5% (dry mucous membranes/↓ skin turgor); severe 8% (sunken eyes, ↑ CRT, shocked and needed fluid bolus) and record in ED notes.
- Involve PICU if very young (<2 years), severe acidosis (pH<7.1), severe dehydration or ↓ conscious level (cerebral oedema, ↑ risk of aspiration).

Further care

- Do not start insulin until IV fluids have been running for *at least 1hr*—earlier insulin therapy is associated with ↑ cerebral oedema.
- Do not administer bicarbonate except on specialist PICU advice.
- Follow local protocols for continuing fluid replacement, but remember that over-infusion of fluid is associated with cerebral oedema.
- Aim for replacement of fluids and potassium over 48hr or longer.

---

1 See http://www.bsped.org.uk/professional/guidelines/docs/DKAGuideline.pdf for full details.

Urinary tract infection (UTI)

UTI in children requires prompt investigation, since progressive renal failure and hypertension may occur insidiously. 35% have proven vesico-ureteric reflux: early treatment may help to prevent renal failure. UTI may present in a variable and non-specific fashion. Consider and exclude UTI as part of the initial approach to any ill child presenting to the ED.

Presentations

Older children typically present with lower abdominal pain, dysuria, frequency, offensive urine, haematuria or fever. However, dysuria and frequency do not always reflect UTI. Children <3 years old often present unwell with fever and irritability, but no specific signs. Infants may present with poor feeding, vomiting, and failure to thrive.

Examination

Always check the BP and feel for loin tenderness (pyelonephritis) and abdominal masses (polycystic kidneys).

Investigation

Obtain a clean catch specimen of urine for urinalysis, microscopy, culture and sensitivity. This can prove to be quite difficult, depending upon the age of the child. Try one of the following approaches:

Neonates and infants
- Clean the perineum with sterile water, then tap with 2 fingers just above the symphysis pubis (ideally 1hr post-feed) and catch the urine which is forthcoming, trying to avoid the first few millilitres.
- Clean the perineum as above and use a urine collection pad according to the manufacturer's instructions.
- Suprapubic aspiration is useful if the baby is seriously ill. Clean the skin with antiseptic solution, then using sterile gloves and an aseptic technique, insert a 21G needle in the midline 2.5cm above the pubic crest and aspirate urine.

Toddlers and older children
- Co-operation will enable an MSU to be obtained (in the male, gently retract the foreskin (if possible) and clean the glans first; in the female, separate the labia and clean the perineum front to back, first).
- If the child is uncooperative, try a urine collection pad or bag.

Dipstick urinalysis at the bedside will reveal the presence of blood, protein, sugar, bilirubin, ketones or nitrite. A positive nitrite test is accepted as good evidence of UTI. Urine pH is not usually helpful, for although pH <4.6 or >8.0 may reflect infection, it may also be due to various acid-base disorders. Urinalysis may be normal, despite bacteriuria. Urine microscopy allows a search for pyuria and bacteriuria (highly suggestive of UTI) and an accurate assessment of other constituents (see Table 15.7). Perform FBC, U&E, blood glucose, and blood cultures if septicaemic, loin pain or ↑ T°.

Treatment

- *Children with suspected pyelonephritis or who appear toxic*: resuscitate as necessary with IV fluids (📖 p.663) and refer for admission and IV antibiotics (eg cefotaxime). Infection with beta lactamase producing *E. coli* is said to be increasing, and some recommend at least one dose of gentamicin, pending sensitivities. Give antibiotics for 10 days.
- *Symptomatic children with abnormal urinalysis (proteinuria or haematuria)*: start a 3-day course of antibiotics PO (trimethoprim or cefalexin—dose according to age, refer to *BNFC*). Encourage plenty of oral fluids and complete voiding of urine. Offer advice to the child and parents (eg avoid tight underwear, use toilet paper wiping from front to back).
- *Organize paediatric follow-up to receive results of MSU and to arrange subsequent investigations*: this may include U&E, blood glucose, ultrasound scan (USS) and a variety of other tests (eg isotope renography and micturating cysto-urethrography), according to local policy.
- Recurrent UTIs with anogenital signs may be due to sexual abuse.

Table 15.7 Urine microscopy findings and their significance

Red cells	Normally <3/mm^3
White cells	Normally <3/mm^3
Epithelial cells	Present normally: shed from urinary epithelium
Bacteria or fungi	Always abnormal, reflecting infection or specimen contamination
Casts	Hyaline casts—comprise Tamm–Horsfall protein: may be normal, but ↑ in fever, exercise, heart failure, after diuretics
	Fine granular casts—may be present normally, eg after exercise
	Coarse granular casts—abnormal, seen in various renal disorders
	Red cell casts—imply glomerular disease and glomerular bleeding
	White cell casts—occur in glomerulonephritis and pyelonephritis
	Epithelial casts—usually reflect tubular damage
Crystals	Phosphate, urate, and oxalate crystals may not be pathological, but are also seen in Proteus UTI and hyperuricaemia.

See the 'NICE Guidance on UTI in Children'. Available at: http://www.nice.org.uk/nicemedia/pdf/CG54quickrefguide.pdf

Renal failure

Causes of acute renal failure

Pre-renal Hypovolaemia (bleeding, dehydration, sepsis), heart failure, nephrotic syndrome.
Renal Haemolytic uraemic syndrome, glomerulonephritis, acute tubular necrosis, drugs.
Post-renal Obstruction following trauma or calculi.

Presentation and investigation

Presentation varies according to the cause. Emergency investigations include MSU for microscopy, culture and sensitivity, urine and plasma osmolality, U&E, blood glucose, FBC, albumin, LFTs, clotting screen, and ECG monitoring.

Treatment

Get expert help early. Pre-renal failure from hypovolaemia (urine: plasma osmolality ratio usually >5) should respond to treatment of the underlying condition and an IV fluid challenge (20mL/kg of 0.9% saline, ±colloid/blood products, depending on cause). Urinary catheter and CVP monitoring may help to assess fluid status. Urgent ultrasound can assess for obstruction of the urinary tract, the presence of stones and vascular filling status. ED treatment of renal failure focuses on hyperkalaemia and hypertension.
Hyperkalaemia Children presenting with hyperkalaemia (K+>7) in advanced renal failure may require emergency measures prior to dialysis. Obtain expert help. Give 0.5mL/kg of 10% calcium gluconate over 5min to stabilize the myocardium if there are ECG changes (widened QRS complexes or tall T waves). Give sodium bicarbonate 1mmol/kg IV and commence an IVI of glucose (0.5g/kg/hr) with insulin (0.05U/kg/hr). Consider nebulized salbutamol (2.5mg if <3 years; 5mg if 3–7 years; 10mg if >7years) or Calcium Resonium® 1g/kg PO or PR. Nebulized salbutamol, IV sodium bicarbonate, glucose/insulin all temporarily ↓ serum K+ by shifting it into cells: definitive treatment (dialysis) will still be required.
Hypertension Hypertension related to volume overload in renal failure may require IV nitrate therapy in the ED (as for pulmonary oedema), but otherwise seek expert help for further intervention.

Nephrotic syndrome

Most cases of oedema, heavy proteinuria and hypoalbuminaemia (±hypercholesterolaemia) are idiopathic ('minimal change nephropathy'). Presentation is diverse and includes: anorexia, lethargy, frothy urine, mild diarrhoea, abdominal pain, ascites, oliguria, peri-orbital, or genital oedema. The prognosis is generally good, but peritonitis, renal or cerebral venous thrombosis may occur. Check U&E, albumin, LFTs, FBC, complement, cholesterol and lipids. Refer for further investigation/treatment.

Haemolytic uraemic syndrome

Micro-angiopathic haemolytic anaemia, thrombocytopenia and renal failure of haemolytic uraemic syndrome typically affect infants/toddlers following a diarrhoeal illness (*E. coli 0157*, verocytotoxin, or shigella). The disease is also associated with SLE, HIV and various tumours. The child may present oliguric or anuric with ↓ conscious level due to encephalopathy. Mortality is >5%. FBC reveals anaemia with visible RBC fragments, thrombocytopenia, and leucocytosis. Coombs test is −ve. Urea and creatinine are usually ↑ and there may be electrolyte disturbances. Treat life-threatening hyperkalaemia as above and refer for possible dialysis and transfusion.

Haematuria

Dark or discoloured urine is frightening for both the child and parents. Although it may reflect haematuria, it may reflect other causes: very concentrated urine, beetroot, porphyria, conjugated hyperbilirubinaemia, free Hb or myoglobin (usually black, as seen in rhabdomyolysis and malaria), or drugs (Table 15.8).

Table 15.8 Possible alternative causes of discoloured urine

Drug/food	Colour
Rifampicin	Orange/pink
Desferrioxamine, senna, rhubarb	Brown
Methylene blue	Green

If haematuria is confirmed by urinalysis, obtain a full history, remembering to ask about preceding illnesses and trauma, foreign travel, drug history, and family history of renal or bleeding disorders. Full examination includes BP and a careful check for abdominal masses and oedema.

Causes of macroscopic haematuria

- UTI (including schistosomiasis).
- Glomerulonephritis.
- Trauma.
- Wilm's tumour.
- Bleeding disorder.
- Urinary tract stones.
- Drugs (warfarin, cyclophosphamide).
- Factitious.

Microscopic haematuria may be associated with: exercise, hypercalciuria or be familial.

Glomerulonephritis is often an immune reaction following an URTI due to β-haemolytic Strep infection 2–3 weeks previously. It may present with haematuria, oliguria ±hypertension and uraemia. A similar presentation can occur with Henloch–Schönlein purpura (📖 Purpuric rashes, p.664), SLE or Berger's disease (mesangial IgA nephropathy).

Investigation

Send MSU and obtain plain X-rays of the urinary tract if there is abdominal pain suggesting stones (relatively rare). Check U&E, blood glucose, FBC, clotting screen, and if significant bleeding (or if haematuria follows trauma) X-match. Further tests may be required (throat swab, urine, and serum osmolalities, viral titres, antistreptolysin-O, antinuclear antibodies, complement levels), but do not assist emergency treatment.

Management

Severe haematuria with clots requires resuscitation with IV fluids (±blood), but is uncommon in children, except after trauma. Treat associated severe hypertension or hyperkalaemia associated with renal failure as described opposite. Refer children with haematuria of non-traumatic origin to the paediatrician.

Poisoning in children

Paediatric poisoning may take many forms:
- Neonatal poisoning from drugs taken by mother prior to birth (eg opioids, benzodiazepines).
- 'Accidental' (unintentional) poisoning is the most common form of poisoning. It largely involves toddlers and pre-school children (boys > girls), who are at particular risk because of their innate curiosity and considerable indiscretion in putting things in their mouths. Children may be poisoned by any drugs that they can get their hands on, but also mushrooms, berries, plants, household items (eg disinfectant) and other objects misinterpreted as drink, food or sweets (eg button batteries).
- Inadvertent self-poisoning with recreational drugs (including alcohol and volatile agents).
- Iatrogenic poisoning by administration of the wrong dose ± wrong drug can happen with frightening ease. Paediatric dosage charts, calculators, obsessional checking, attention to detail and restriction of junior doctors' hours should help to prevent this in the ED.
- Deliberate self-poisoning in an apparent suicide attempt occurs in older children.
- Intentional poisoning by a parent, guardian, or carer is a sinister aspect of child abuse, which includes fabricated or induced illness (📖 p.772). The child may present in a bizarre fashion, with a non-specific illness, for which the diagnosis is not immediately apparent.

Approach

Follow the general guidelines described in 📖 pp.180–7 to treat poisoned patients, with initial attention to oxygenation (airway), ventilation (breathing) and circulation. Links to the National Poisons Information Service (www.toxbase.org Telephone 0844 892 0111) will provide advice for specific poisonings (📖 p.180). With notable exceptions (eg paracetamol, opioids, iron, and digoxin) there are few 'antidotes' available: treatment is often largely supportive.

Try to elicit the substance(s) ingested, the amount involved and the time since ingestion. The majority of ingestions are unintentional and the time to presentation is often short. Gastric emptying procedures are rarely performed, and should be considered only if a life-threatening amount of a drug has been ingested in the previous hour and the airway can be protected (📖 p.184). Avoid ipecac (ipecacuanha), which is ineffective in ↓ drug absorption and can be dangerous. *Never* try to empty the stomach following ingestion of petrol or corrosives (📖 p.205).

Charcoal

The role of charcoal (dose 1g/kg PO in infants; 15–30g in older children) in paediatric poisoning is limited by its lack of palatability. Attempts are currently being made to make charcoal more palatable, yet remain effective.

Prevention of paediatric poisoning

Background

Poisoning in children is very common. More than 40,000 children present to hospital in the UK each year, many of whom are admitted for observation. Thankfully, relatively few (10–15 per year) die. More than 75% of paediatric unintentional ingestions involve drugs and poisons in the home that are plainly visible to the child. Poisoning is particularly likely to occur at times of 'stress' (eg arrival of new baby, disturbed parental relationships, moving house) when there may be ↓ supervision and disruption of the usual routine. Perhaps partly for this reason, children who present with a first episode of poisoning are at ↑ risk of further episodes. It is therefore important to advise the parents of ways of preventing poisoning in children (see list below).

Official measures: packaging of drugs

Legislation has been introduced to try to tackle the problem of poisoning in children. Perhaps the most successful has been the widespread adoption of child-resistant drug containers. Unfortunately, it is not yet mandatory for these containers to be used for liquid drugs or potentially dangerous household items, such as bleach. Some drugs are presented in 'strip packaging', in the hope that an impulsive child would lose interest before gaining access to a significant quantity.

Advice for parents (consider providing a leaflet)

- Provide adequate supervision for toddlers and young children, particularly when visiting friends and relatives.
- Keep all medicines locked out of reach in a cupboard.
- Only purchase those drugs presented in child-resistant containers.
- Dispose of out-of-date drugs and those no longer required.
- Never refer to drugs as 'sweets' in an attempt to encourage the child to take them.
- Take medicines out of sight of the child to help prevent imitation.
- Keep all alcohol, perfumes, cosmetics, detergents, and bleaches out of reach.
- Ensure that all turpentine, paints, and weed killers are securely locked and inaccessible.
- Give away all toxic plants.
- Keep ashtrays and waste baskets empty.

Abdominal pain in children

The approach to the initial assessment and management of children presenting with abdominal pain is similar in many ways to that in adults (📖 p.504). Beware underlying 'medical' causes (eg DKA, pneumonia). Remember that disease processes may progress with great rapidity in children, therefore adopt a low threshold for referring children with abdominal pain to the surgical team. Whilst many of the common causes of abdominal pain are the same in children as in adults (eg 📖 Acute appendicitis, p.507), be aware of causes that are typically paediatric (eg intussusception). Likewise, certain causes of intestinal obstruction are seen almost exclusively in children.

Paediatric causes of intestinal obstruction

- Congenital (eg oesophageal/duodenal atresia, Hirschsprung's disease).
- Meconium ileus.
- Hypertrophic pyloric stenosis.
- Intussusception.
- Hernia (inguinal, umbilical).

Hypertrophic pyloric stenosis

Features

This condition is relatively common, typically presenting with effortless vomiting at between 2–10 weeks. It occurs more frequently in boys than girls and in first-born children. Vomiting becomes projectile in nature, with progressive dehydration and constipation. The vomit is not bile-stained. After vomiting, the baby appears hungry and keen to feed again. In advanced cases, there may be a profound hypochloraemic alkalosis, with associated hypokalaemia.

Diagnosis

Look for visible peristalsis. Abdominal palpation confirms the diagnosis if an olive-sized lump is felt in the epigastrium (most prominent during a test feed). If the diagnosis is suspected, but not proven clinically, resuscitate (as below) and arrange USS.

Management

Once diagnosed, keep the infant nil by mouth. Insert an IV cannula and send blood for U&E, glucose, and FBC. Commence fluid resuscitation under senior guidance and refer to the surgeon—operative treatment needs to be delayed until dehydration and electrolyte abnormalities have been corrected (this may take >24hr). Defer insertion of a NG tube for appropriately experienced staff.

Volvulus

This is associated with congenital malrotations, but may occur in other circumstances also (eg Meckel's diverticulum, adhesions from previous surgery). It can present with abdominal pain and other features of intestinal obstruction (vomiting, distension), sometimes with a palpable mass. Obtain an abdominal X-ray and refer promptly to the surgical team in order to maximize the chance of intervening to preserve bowel.

Intussusception

Telescoping of one segment of bowel into another may affect the small or large bowel, but most cases are ileocolic. Typically affects children aged between 6 months and 4 years. The child may suddenly become distressed, roll up into a ball, and appear unwell. Vomiting may develop and the child may pass a 'redcurrant jelly' stool. These features, however, together with pyrexia and a palpable mass, are not invariably present: sometimes the presentation is shock without obvious cause. X-rays may be normal or reveal an absent caecal shadow.

If intussusception is suspected, refer urgently to the surgical team. The diagnosis may be confirmed by air or barium enema, which may also be curative, by reducing the intussusception. A barium enema characteristically reveals a 'coiled spring' sign or sudden termination of the barium, but is contra-indicated if there is evidence of perforation.

Acute appendicitis (see 📖 p.507)

Consider this diagnosis in any child presenting with abdominal pain. Acute appendicitis can occur in children of all ages. It can be a difficult diagnosis to make, especially in the very young. 'Atypical' clinical presentation (eg diarrhoeal illness) is often associated with delayed diagnosis and an ↑ rate of perforation. Do not perform a rectal examination—in the unlikely event of this being considered essential, leave it to the surgical team.

Abdominal mass

There are many causes of abdominal masses in children, many of which may be relatively benign and asymptomatic:
- Full bladder.
- Full colon.
- Enlarged liver and/or spleen.
- Pregnancy in older children.
- Hydronephrosis.
- Hypertrophic pyloric stenosis (see opposite).
- Appendix mass.
- Intussusception.
- Volvulus.
- Neuroblastoma.
- Nephroblastoma (Wilm's tumour).

Intra-abdominal malignancy

Neuroblastoma and nephroblastoma may reach a large size before causing symptoms (eg haemorrhage into the tumour).

Neuroblastomas arise most commonly from the adrenal glands, but may occur at any point along the sympathetic chain.

Nephroblastomas (Wilm's tumours) arise from the kidneys and may present with haematuria.

All children with suspected malignant abdominal masses require CT scan and/or USS investigation—refer urgently to the surgical team.

Inguinal and scrotal swellings

Painless groin and scrotal lumps

The parents or child who discovers a lump may become very concerned. The absence of pain is to some extent reassuring, in that an acute surgical problem is unlikely. Ascertain when the swelling appeared, whether it changes in size or disappears, or whether there are any other symptoms.

Reducible inguinal hernia

Inguinal herniae in childhood result from a persistent patent processus vaginalis and are therefore indirect in nature. They are commoner in boys than girls and often bilateral. The history is typically of an intermittent swelling, which appears with coughing or straining. If the swelling can be demonstrated, it will be impossible to get above it. If it cannot be demonstrated, a thickened spermatic cord may be palpated (sometimes known as the 'silk sign'). Refer neonatal herniae for admission and surgery, refer infants and older children to a surgical clinic for elective surgery.

Painless irreducible inguinal hernia

Refer all irreducible inguinal hernias for admission and surgery (preceded by gallows traction in the infant).

Hydrocoele

This transilluminable painless scrotal swelling has similar aetiology to inguinal hernia. It appears gradually, rather than suddenly, and does not empty or reduce on palpation. Refer to a surgical clinic. An encysted hydrocoele of the cord may be impossible to distinguish from an irreducible inguinal hernia and therefore requires surgical exploration.

Undescended, retractile, or ectopic testis

Complete descent of the testis has yet to occur in 3% of term infants and 30% of premature infants. Arrange surgical follow-up if the testis cannot be brought down to the fundus of the scrotal sac: orchidopexy will be required if the testis fails to descend by 4 years.

Inguinal lymphadenopathy

This is on the list of differential diagnoses of painless inguinal swellings. Look for a potential source of infection in the leg and for involvement of any other lymph node groups.

Idiopathic scrotal oedema

An obscure allergic condition of the scrotal skin is possibly a variant of angioneurotic oedema. Redness, mild tenderness and oedema are not limited to one hemiscrotum. The testis is normal. The condition settles spontaneously, a process helped by antihistamines (eg chlorphenamine PO, doses: child 1–2 years require 1mg bd; 2–5 years require 1mg qds; 6–12 years require 2mg qds). If in doubt—refer.

Painful groin and scrotal lumps

Painful irreducible inguinal hernia

Likely to contain obstructed or strangulated small bowel. Confirm clinical suspicion of intestinal obstruction (pain, vomiting and abdominal distension) by X-ray. Resuscitate as necessary with IV fluids, give analgesia and refer for surgery.

Testicular torsion

Commonest in the neonatal period and around puberty. In the neonatal period the torsion is extravaginal in nature and often diagnosed late. Later in childhood, torsion of a completely descended testis is intravaginal due to a high insertion of tunica vaginalis. Undescended testes are also at particular risk of torsion. Classical presentation is with sudden onset severe pain and vomiting. Occasionally, the pain is entirely abdominal. Examination reveals a red, tender swollen testis. The opposite testis may be seen to lie horizontally, rather than vertically (Angell's sign). Fast and refer all suspected torsions for urgent surgery: exploration, untwisting and bilateral orchidopexy.

Torsion of the hydatid of Morgagni

This remnant of the paramesonephric duct on the superior aspect of the testis is prone to undergo torsion, causing pain and vomiting. A discrete tender nodule may be palpable. Refer, as surgical exploration and excision of the hydatid provides more rapid relief than the alternative conservative treatment (analgesia and rest).

Epididymo-orchitis

Unusual in paediatric age group, but may be associated with UTI. A painful swollen red testis and epididymis usually develops over a longer period of time, but may be difficult to distinguish from testicular torsion. Refer for an urgent surgical opinion.

Mumps orchitis

The diagnosis is usually apparent because of parotitis (📖 Childhood infectious diseases, p.222). Refer if there is doubt or symptoms are severe.

Henoch-Schönlein purpura

Occasionally, testicular pain may be one of the initial presenting complaints of Henoch-Schönlein purpura (see 📖 p.664).

Foreskin problems and zip entrapment

Phimosis

The foreskin may normally remain non-retractile up to age 5 years. Foreskin that remains non-retractile after this, which 'balloons' on micturition, or is associated with recurrent balanitis may benefit from surgery (preputial stretch or circumcision). Advise the parents to see their GP to discuss referral to a paediatric surgeon.

Balanitis

Balanitis produces redness, swelling, and even pus. Take a swab, check for glucose in urine and send an MSU. Treat with amoxicillin (10mg/kg PO qds) or erythromycin (10mg/kg PO qds). If redness and swelling involve the whole penis: refer for IV antibiotics.

Paraphimosis

Irreducible, retracted foreskin results in pain and swelling of the glans. As in the adult, cold compresses and lubricating jelly may allow reduction. If not, refer for reduction under GA.

Penile zip entrapment

Unfortunately, underpants do not completely protect boys (and sometimes men) from catching their foreskins in trouser zips. On many occasions the entrapment will be released quickly by the child or parent. On others, the child will present to the ED.

The optimal method to achieve release depends upon the entrapment

- 15% zip foreskin through the moveable part of the zip, so that it is simply caught between the teeth of the zip alone. In this case, achieve easy release by cutting transversely through the zip below the entrapment.
- 85% of entrapments involve the foreskin being caught between the teeth and the moveable part of the zip. Local anaesthetic (either injection using plain lidocaine or topical gel) may allow manipulation and release. If this fails, the least traumatic option is to divide the moveable part of the zip into 2 parts by dividing the central section ('median bar' or 'bridge') using bone cutters or wire cutters (use gauze to protect against parts of the zip flying off; Fig. 15.16). Older children and adults may tolerate this in the ED, but in younger boys referral for release under GA is sensible. Circumcision is rarely required.

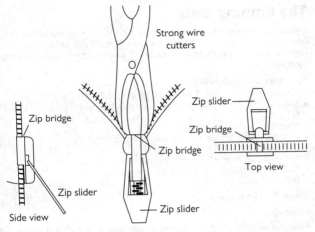

Fig. 15.16 Method to achieve release from zip entrapment.

The limping child

This common problem can cause diagnostic difficulty, particularly in the young child who cannot provide a history and is difficult to examine. It is important to try to exclude some causes of a limp that will require urgent treatment.

Consider the following

- Trauma (fractures, soft tissue injury, FB in foot, NAI).
- Specific hip problems (Perthes', slipped epiphysis, irritable hip— p.706).
- Infection (osteomyelitis, septic arthritis).
- Arthritis (Still's disease, juvenile ankylosing spondylitis).
- Osteochondritis (p.708).
- Referred pain from inflammatory process elsewhere.
- Malignant disease (Ewing's sarcoma, leukaemia).
- Sickle cell crisis (p.176).

Adopt the following approach:

History

Ascertain whether the problem developed suddenly (eg after trauma) or gradually. Enquire about recent illness and other symptoms, including joint pains elsewhere.

Examination

Check T°. If the child is walking, assess the gait. Carefully inspect all of the painful leg for erythema, swelling, deformity, and note the position adopted. Exclude a relatively simple problem, such as a FB embedded in the foot. Note any skin rashes. Palpate the limb for tenderness, joint effusions, and range of movement (compare with the other side). If the child will not walk, but can crawl without any apparent discomfort, this localizes the problem to below the knee (thereby avoiding the need to request 'routine' X-rays of the hips).

Investigation

If the child can walk, looks well, and there is no abnormality apparent on examination, consider providing analgesia and arranging to review after a few days, rather than undertaking all of the following investigations immediately. Ensure the parents are told that they should return earlier if the limp gets worse.

X-ray the tender or swollen part, particularly if there is a history of injury. If there is no obvious tenderness, X-ray the pelvis to include both hips. If the X-rays do not reveal a fracture, check *WCC* and *CRP* (or plasma viscosity/ESR). If the hip is implicated, but X-rays are normal, request *USS* of the hip (some experts prefer to use USS as the initial investigation). *MRI* is emerging as having a potentially useful role. Follow local ED protocols where available.

Management

Treat according to the cause (see opposite and pp.706–9).

Trauma

Treat according to cause, which may include a FB in the soft tissues. There may not always be a clear history of injury—this particularly applies to toddler's fracture (see 📖 Paediatric lower limb injuries, p.726).

Osteomyelitis

Acute osteomyelitis usually results from blood-borne spread of a distant pathogen (eg from the respiratory tract). *Staph. aureus* is usually responsible, with almost invariable involvement of the metaphysis of a long bone (most commonly proximal or distal femur, or distal tibia).

Features ↑ T°, lethargy, localized tenderness (which may be misdiagnosed as trauma). Septic shock may occur (especially in infants).

Investigations ↑ WCC, ↑ CRP, ↑ ESR >50mm/hr (but all may be normal initially). X-ray changes occur after ≈10days.

Treatment If suspected, refer for admission, IV antibiotics ± surgical drilling/drainage.

Septic arthritis

Most commonly, *Staph. aureus* infection in the hip or knee. Occasionally secondary to penetrating injury but usually haematogenous spread from a distant site. Constitutional symptoms, fever and joint pain occur. A joint effusion may be clinically evident. Joint movement is likely to be severely impaired. Investigations may reveal ↑ WCC, ↑ CRP and ↑ ESR. Refer for urgent confirmatory joint aspiration and treatment.

Non-septic arthritis

Multiple painful joints are more likely to be due to a juvenile arthritic process (eg RA or ankylosing spondylitis) than septic arthritis. Pain felt in several joints frequently accompanies a variety of infections and other diseases, eg rubella, rheumatic fever, Henoch–Schönlein purpura. Refer to the paediatrician for further investigation.

The painful hip

The limping child may be able to localize pain to the hip, but hip pain may be referred to the knee. Hip problems causing a limp include trauma, infection and other disorders as in 📖 The limping child, p.704. Specific hip problems include:

Perthes' disease (Legg–Calvé–Perthes' disease)

Aseptic necrosis of the upper femoral (capital) epiphysis presents with a painful limp in children aged 3–10 years. Boys are affected more than girls (M:F = 4:1). 15% are bilateral. Aetiology is unclear, but Perthes' disease is often grouped with the osteochondritides (📖 p.708). Often ↓ range of hip movement due to pain. FBC, CRP, ESR, and blood cultures are normal.

X-ray changes reflect stage of disease and are progressive (as opposite):
1 ↑ joint space on medial aspect of capital epiphysis (compare sides)
2 ↑ bone density in affected epiphysis (appears sclerotic)
3 Fragmentation, distortion (flattening) and lateral subluxation of upper femoral epiphysis (leaving part of the femoral head 'uncovered')
4 Rarefaction of the adjacent metaphysis in which cysts may appear

Treatment Refer for specialist assessment and treatment. Most cases respond satisfactorily to conservative therapy.

Slipped upper femoral (capital) epiphysis (Fig. 15.18)

This sometimes occurs during puberty and has been attributed to hormonal imbalance. It occurs in children (particularly boys: M:F = 3:1) who have one of 2 body types: obese with underdeveloped genitalia or tall, thin rapidly growing adolescent with normal sexual development.

Presentation A child aged 10–16 years may develop a painful limp suddenly or gradually. Often there is a history of trauma. The leg may be slightly adducted, externally rotated, and shortened. Movement of affected hip is ↓ compared with the other side (esp. abduction and internal rotation).

X-ray Obtain AP pelvis and lateral hip views ± 'frog-leg' views. Subtle slips may only be seen on lateral view. Larger slips will be obvious on all views. Look for Trethowan's sign: a line drawn along the superior border of the femoral neck normally cuts through the epiphysis (see Fig. 15.18).

Treatment Refer to orthopaedics for internal fixation ± manipulation.

Complications Avascular necrosis, chondrolysis, and osteoarthritis.

Irritable hip ('transient synovitis')

Common cause of sudden painful hip and limp in children of all ages. Aetiology is unclear, but many cases appear to follow a viral illness. Presentation varies from a slight limp to great difficulty WB. X-rays are normal. USS may show a hip effusion and allow aspiration for microscopy and culture. (Apply tetracaine cream over the hip before USS).

Pyrexia, ↑ WCC, ↑ CRP (and/or ↑ ESR/plasma viscosity) suggest infection.

Treatment If significant physical signs (significant pain, ↓ movement, difficulty weight-bearing) or there is evidence suggesting infection, refer to the orthopaedic team for admission for rest, traction and further investigation. If physical signs are not dramatic and X-rays and blood tests normal, discharge with NSAID, advise rest and review within a few days.

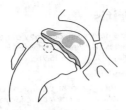

Fig. 15.17 Changes in the hip in Perthes' disease.

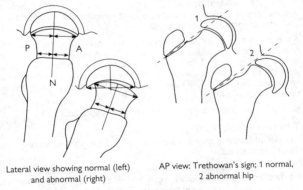

Lateral view showing normal (left)
and abnormal (right)

AP view: Trethowan's sign; 1 normal,
2 abnormal hip

Fig. 15.18 Slipped upper femoral epiphysis.

Osteochondritis

This term is applied to a heterogeneous array of non-infectious disorders affecting various epiphyses. They may be divided into 3 groups, according to the proposed aetiology (see Table 15.9).

Crushing osteochondritis

Apparently spontaneous necrosis of an ossification centre occurs at a time of rapid growth. This is followed by new bone formation.

Perthes' disease—see 📖 The painful hip, p.706.

Scheuermann's disease Fragmentation of low thoracic/upper lumbar vertebral epiphyseal plates of adolescents results in chronic back pain and a 'round-shouldered' kyphotic appearance. X-rays show anterior wedging of vertebral bodies, with sclerotic notches (Schmorl's nodes) on inferior or superior vertebral borders. Diagnostic criteria are >50° of kyphosis and wedging in 3 adjacent vertebrae. Treat symptomatically with NSAID and refer for orthopaedic follow-up.

Kohler's disease Avascular necrosis of the navicular affects children (particularly boys) aged 3–5 years. A painful limp develops, with tenderness on the dorsum of the foot over the navicular. The sclerotic fragmented navicular seen on X-ray is also seen in many asymptomatic children. Treat symptoms with rest, NSAID and orthopaedic follow-up. If symptoms are severe, consider BKPOP.

Kienbock's and Freiberg's disease—usually affect young adults

Traction apophysitis

The pull of a strong tendon causes damage to the unfused apophysis to which it is attached.

Osgood-Schlatter's disease Traction apophysitis of the tibial attachment of the patellar tendon is especially seen in boys aged 10–15 years. Anterior knee pain after exercise is characteristic. The tibial tuberosity is prominent and tender. The pain may be reproduced by attempted extension against resistance.

X-rays are not always needed, but show an enlarged and sometimes fragmented tibial tuberosity. Treat symptomatically with NSAID and orthopaedic follow-up. Most settle with conservative measures.

Johansson–Larsen's disease (Sinding Larsen's disease) Traction apophysitis of the lower pole of the patella in young adolescents results in local tenderness. Treat with rest, NSAID and orthopaedic follow-up.

Sever's disease Traction apophysitis of the calcaneal attachment of the Achilles tendon occurs in 8–14-year-olds. The resulting limp is associated with local calcaneal tenderness. X-rays may reveal a fragmented sclerotic calcaneal apophysis. Treat with rest, NSAID, a heel raise and orthopaedic follow-up.

Osteochondritis dissecans

A piece of articular cartilage and adjacent bone become partially or completely separated as an avascular fragment. The cause is believed to be an osteochondral fracture from repeated minor trauma. The lateral aspect of the medial condyle of distal femur is the most commonly affected site. Intermittent pain, swelling and joint effusion result. If the fragment becomes detached as a loose body, locking or giving way may occur.

X-ray Demonstrates the fragment or defect.

Treatment Refer the locked knee immediately. Treat the remainder with rest, consider crutches, and arrange orthopaedic follow-up.

Table 15.9 Classification of osteochondritis

Type of osteochondritis	Bone affected	Eponym
Crushing osteochondritis	Femoral head	Perthes' disease (📖 p.706)
	Vertebrae	Scheuermann's disease
	2nd metatarsal head	Freiberg's disease
	Navicular	Kohler's disease
	Lunate	Kienbock's disease
	Capitulum	Panner's disease
Osteochondritis dissecans	Medial femoral condyle	
	Talus	
	Elbow	
	Metatarsal	
Traction apophysitis	Tibial tuberosity	Osgood–Schlatter's disease
	Lower pole of patella	Johansson–Larsen's disease
	Calcaneum	Sever's disease

Major paediatric trauma

The background

Trauma is the largest single cause of death in children: ≈500 deaths/ year in the UK (Table 15.10). As in adults, blunt injury in children is far more common than penetrating injury. The number of deaths in children after trauma is dwarfed by the number who sustain serious injuries. Most serious injuries result from road traffic collisions and falls.

Table 15.10 Causes of trauma deaths in children

Road traffic collisions	48%
Fires	15%
Drowning	12%
Hanging	8%
Falls	8%
Non-accidental injury	5%
Other	4%

>70% of paediatric trauma deaths occur in the pre-hospital setting. Most of these children are either dead when found or have sustained overwhelming injuries. The greatest potential for reducing trauma deaths clearly lies with injury prevention. However, there is enormous potential to reduce the number of permanently disabled children by early identification of injuries and expert treatment. The best outcome results from involvement of senior and experienced staff at an early stage. Prompt recognition of the seriously injured child is crucial to this.

Pattern of injuries

Anatomical and physiological differences mean that the pattern of injuries in children differ considerably from those in adults. Compared with adults, children have: smaller physical size, a relatively larger head, more compliant bones, a higher ratio of surface area to body weight, epiphyses. Experience and an awareness of the patterns of paediatric injury will assist resuscitation efforts. The smaller size and physical proximity of internal organs frequently results in the dissipated forces causing injuries to multiple structures (multiple injuries). The compliance of the bony thoracic cage in children allows significant underlying organ injury without rib fractures. Similarly, certain injuries not uncommon in adults (eg rupture of thoracic aorta), rarely occur in children.

Injury prevention

Terminology

The term 'accident' implies an unforeseen unintentional event, one which occurs by chance. The implication is that 'accidents' cannot be prevented. However, there is considerable evidence to suggest that 'accidents' are far from random events, but are relatively predictable and amenable to prevention. For this reason, medical experts now prefer to avoid use of the terms 'accidents' and 'accident prevention' and refer to 'injury prevention' instead.

Background

Injuries to children tend to occur more frequently in certain groups and at certain times:
- Boys sustain more injuries than girls.
- Injuries are associated with social deprivation.
- Injuries often occur at times of family stress and change (including marital disharmony, moving house and holidays).

Prevention theory

Prevention of injury does not simply refer to physical injuries, but poisonings also. Injuries and/or the effects of injuries may be prevented in a number of different ways:

Primary prevention measures stop injuries occurring. For example, the installation of fences around domestic swimming pools may reduce drowning, locked medicine cabinets might prevent inadvertent poisoning.

Secondary prevention measures reduce the extent of harm caused by an injurious event. The most obvious examples are helmets, seat belts, and air bags in the context of road traffic collisions.

Tertiary 'prevention' includes most forms of first aid and hospital treatment, and aims to limit the effect of an injury after it has already happened (eg surgery to stop intra-abdominal haemorrhage, antidotes for certain poisons).

Prevention strategies and the role of ED staff

The focus of hospital staff treating injured patients has understandably always been the injuries themselves ('tertiary prevention'). In addition to any possible issues of NAI, ED staff need to consider how future injuries to children might be prevented (eg by discussing with parents the benefits of bicycle helmets). In the context of an individual child, it may sometimes be appropriate to contact the GP/health visitor with a view to seeing if interventions might prevent future injuries to a particular child and siblings.

More general interventions include:
- Leaflets and posters in the waiting room to target a captive audience
- Media involvement on certain issues, such as minimizing the risks of fireworks and sparklers

Further details of children's injuries and injury prevention are available from the Royal Society for the Prevention of Accidents (www.rospa.org.uk) and the Child Accident Prevention Trust (www.capt.org.uk).

Resuscitation of the injured child

The priorities in managing major paediatric trauma (Airway, Breathing, Circulation) are the same as in adults (📖 p.320). Staff accustomed to treating adults may have difficulty with equipment sizes and drug doses. Estimate the child's weight (📖 p.633). Call for help as soon as a seriously injured child arrives (or is expected) in the ED—senior ED doctor, ICU/PICU doctor and surgeon (preferably paediatric). It is often very helpful to seek the help of a paediatrician to assist with vascular access and, calculation of drug doses, particularly for pre-school children.

Airway with cervical spine control

Clear and secure the airway (suction and adjuncts) and provide O_2. If the airway is obstructed, use jaw thrust (not head tilt/chin lift) and call for expert help (senior ED/PICU/ICU) as intubation may be required. Ensure that manual immobilization of the cervical spine is maintained, whilst a patient airway is being obtained. When the airway is secure, an appropriately-sized hard collar with tape and sandbags should be used until injury to the cervical spine has been excluded.

Breathing

Quickly exclude and treat life-threatening chest injuries. Children are prone to swallow air, placing them at risk of massive gastric dilatation (can cause ↓ BP and subsequent aspiration): consider an orogastric tube.

Circulation with haemorrhage control

As in adults, hypotension is a late sign of hypovolaemia. Look carefully for other evidence: tachycardia, tachypnoea, agitation, lethargy, pale cold skin with ↓ capillary refill time (best elicited on the sternum). Obtain venous access (consider the intra-osseous route) as described on 📖 p.640. Treat hypovolaemia by stopping haemorrhage (splinting fractures, applying pressure to wounds, prompt surgery for internal haemorrhage) and giving IV fluid/blood resuscitation. Give a 10mL/kg IV 0.9% saline bolus rapidly and reassess. If there is no clinical improvement, give a further 10mL/kg crystalloid IV fluid bolus and repeat if necessary up to 40mL/kg. Remember that over-aggressive fluid replacement may worsen the situation if the patient is suffering from internal haemorrhage. If further fluid is required, give blood products (whole blood 20mL/kg or 10mL/kg packed cells) and request fresh frozen plasma (FFP) and platelets from the laboratory for massive transfusion.

Disability

Make a rapid assessment of the child's neurological status (📖 p.356).

Exposure

Early complete inspection is mandatory, but subsequently cover the child as much as possible in order to ↓ anxiety and prevent excessive heat loss.

Analgesia (📖 Analgesia in specific situations, p.280)

Analgesia is often forgotten or not considered early enough, even with major injuries. Prompt and adequate analgesia given to injured children will gain their confidence, enhancing assessment and treatment. Give IV analgesia titrated according to response. Do not use IM or SC analgesia.

In *severe pain* give morphine IV
- Up to 100 mcg/kg over 5min if 6–12 months.
- Up to 200 mcg/kg over 5min if >12 months.

Certain fractures are amenable to LA nerve block techniques (eg femoral nerve block for femoral shaft fractures—📖 p.304). Nasal diamorphine (📖 Analgesia in specific situations, p.280) and Entonox® (📖 Analgesics: Entonox® and ketamine, p.278) may also be useful for analgesia before IV access is available.

Parents

Remember the parents' needs: allocate a member of staff to this task (📖 p.278). Children who have suffered a traumatic event are at risk of developing post-traumatic stress disorder—inform the parents or guardians about this. Briefly describe possible symptoms (sleep disturbance, nightmares, difficulty concentrating, and irritability). Suggest to the parents/guardians that they contact the child's GP if symptoms persist beyond one month (NICE Clinical Practice Guideline 2005 (see http://www.nice.org.uk/nicemedia/pdf/CG026fullguideline.pdf)).

Considerations in paediatric trauma

Spinal injury

Cervical spine injury is relatively uncommon in children, but keep the whole spine immobilized until history, examination ± X-rays exclude injury. Injuries in children tend to involve upper (C1–3 level), rather than lower cervical spine. Remember that rotatory subluxation may cause significant cervical spine injury without fracture: the clue is combination of injury, neck pain and torticollis. Interpretation of cervical spine X-rays in younger children is frequently complicated by pseudo-subluxation of C2 on C3 and of C3 on C4. If in doubt, continue immobilization and obtain an expert opinion.

The paediatric spine is inherently more elastic so momentary inter-segmental displacement may endanger the cord without disrupting bones or ligaments. This can result in spinal cord injury without radiological abnormality (SCIWORA). Usually there are objective signs of injury, but these can be delayed. Therefore, if children present with transient neurological symptoms after neck injury, make sure you assess them carefully. Exclusion of significant injury requires an alert child with normal spinal and neurological examination with no painful distracting injuries and normal radiology (rarely the case for the seriously injured child).

Head injury

Of those children who die from trauma, most succumb to head injuries. Anatomical differences should be borne in mind. In infants, unfused sutures allow the intracranial volume to ↑ with intracranial haemorrhage, causing relatively large bleeds and even shock. Similarly, scalp wounds in infants and young children may bleed profusely and result in significant hypovolaemia. Assessment of children may prove difficult. An isolated episode of vomiting after minor head injury is a frequent occurrence. To assess level of consciousness, use the standard GCS (📖 p.361) for children aged ≥ 4 years; children aged <4 years require an adapted scale (📖 p.717, which contains further details about head injuries in children).

Chest injury

Significant thoracic visceral injuries may occur without rib fractures. There is a relatively high incidence of pulmonary contusion. Children have little respiratory reserve and can desaturate quickly. If a chest drain is required to treat a pneumothorax or haemothorax, use a size appropriate for the size of the child (as indicated by Broselow tape).

Abdominal and pelvic injury

Look for hypovolaemia. Abdominal palpation cannot yield useful information until child's cooperation and confidence are gained. Restrict any PR and PV examinations to the senior surgeon. USS and/or CT scan has replaced DPL. Gastric tubes are useful to treat the air swallowing and gastric dilatation prevalent in injured children. Insert an appropriately-sized urinary catheter if urine cannot be passed spontaneously or if accurate output measurement is required (eg after severe burns).

Burns

Burns and smoke inhalation from house fires still cause death in many children each year. Even more frequently, children present with scalds from hot or boiling liquids. The majority of these results from simple incidents in the home: ensure that treatment includes injury prevention advice for parents (p.711). Remember that some (occasionally characteristic) burns may reflect NAI. Assessment and treatment of the burned child follows similar lines to those in adults; urgent priorities include securing the airway (with an uncut ET tube) and adequate analgesia (p.320). IV fluid requirements in major burns depend upon the extent of the burn (use Lund–Browder charts, p.391) and clinical response (see p.390).

Drowning and submersion incidents

Children continue to die from drowning each year despite improved swimming education. Their high surface area to body weight ratio makes them prone to hypothermia. Cardiac arrest after immersion warrants prolonged resuscitation (p.259). Presume cervical spine injury and immobilize the neck. Prolonged submersion (>8min), no respiratory effort after 40min of CPR, persistent coma, persistent pH<7.0, persistent PaO_2 <8kPa imply a poor prognosis. Hypothermia favours a better prognosis. Of those who survive after hospital CPR, 70% make a complete recovery.

Wounds in children

Older children may allow wounds to be explored, cleaned, and sutured under LA, providing they are given appropriate explanation (sometimes it is worth demonstrating on teddy first) and a parent is allowed to stay with them. Injection of LA is least painful if a fine needle is employed and the LA is warmed, buffered and injected slowly. Some children, however, do not tolerate LA. Whilst some superficial wounds may be cleaned and closed (steristrips or tissue glue) without anaesthesia, often sedation or GA is needed. Anaesthesia is needed to allow adequate exploration and cleaning of the wound and to ↓ risks of infection and tattooing from embedded dirt. Never allow the lack of co-operation to compromise treatment, particularly with facial wounds, where wound closure under GA may produce the best cosmetic result.

Ketamine

Ketamine can be used in the ED as an alternative to GA and provides excellent analgesia for undertaking minor procedures in children (p.278; see http://www.collemergencymed.ac.uk/CEM/Clinical%20Effectiveness %20Committee/Guidelines/Clinical%20Guidelines/default.asp). Ketamine should only be used by clinicians experienced in its use and capable of managing any airway complications. Ketamine is *contraindicated* if:

- The child has had a full meal within 3hr.
- There is a high risk of laryngospasm (active respiratory infection, active asthma, age <12 months).
- There are severe psychological problems (cognitive or motor delay or severe behavioural problems).
- Cardiovascular disease (congenital heart disease, cardiomyopathy, ↑ BP).
- Significant head injury or neurological disease, porphyria, hyperthyroidism.

Head injuries in children

The principles of head injury management in children are the same as in adults (📖 pp.362–7), but there are some important differences (including the assessment of conscious level in small children).

Causes of head injury

Most head injuries in children are due to falls, but few of these cause serious injury. Severe head injury is often the result of a child running out in front of a vehicle. Some deaths are caused by NAI (📖 p.731), especially in babies who have been shaken violently, dropped, or thrown.

Assessment of a head-injured child

History

Record details of the injurious event, the time it occurred and the condition of the child before and after injury. Ascertain if the child was previously well. In particular, elicit any history of fits or bleeding disorder. An infection can render a child prone to falls and also cause subsequent symptoms: a small child who vomits after a fall may be suffering from otitis media rather than the effects of a head injury.

Determine the condition of the child immediately after injury: if he cried at once, he did not lose consciousness. Record if he was unconscious, confused or drowsy (and for how long) and whether he vomited or was unsteady or dizzy. Ask about headache. Remember to take into account the fact that a child might normally be asleep at the time he is examined.

Examination

Do not use the standard adult GCS (📖 p.361) in children aged <4 years—instead use the adapted scale opposite. Exclude hypoglycaemia. Note whether the child looks well and is behaving normally. Measure pupil size and check reactivity. Examine the head for signs of injury, but also look for injuries elsewhere. Check T° and consider co-existing illness, such as ear, throat, or urinary infections, or occasionally meningitis.

Management of head injury in children

When faced with a child with severe injuries summon senior help and follow standard resuscitation guidelines (📖 p.364). If there is any suspicion of NAI, involve the paediatrician at an early stage (📖 p.734).

Indications for immediate CT scan (see www.nice.org.uk)

Any 1 of: witnessed loss of consciousness for >5mins, any amnesia lasting >5mins, abnormal drowsiness, >2 discrete episodes of vomiting, clinically suspected NAI, post-traumatic epilepsy, GCS <14/15 or for an infant <15/15 on ED assessment, suspected open or depressed skull injury or tense fontanelle, any sign of basal skull fracture, focal neurological deficit, infants with bruising, swelling or laceration >5cm, dangerous mechanism of injury.

Admission or discharge

Admit and observe children with continuing symptoms or signs, skull fracture or if mechanism of injury suggests serious trauma (eg fall from upstairs window). When contemplating discharge, ensure that adequate supervision from a responsible adult is available. Provide the parent/guardian with a verbal explanation and a written advice sheet (📖 p.367, or see www.sign.ac.uk or http://guidance.nice.org.uk/index.jsp?action=download&o=36265).

Glasgow Coma Scale (children)

The 'Eye' and 'Motor' components of the GCS are similar as for adults (📖 p.361), but a modified 'Verbal score' is used in small children. The paediatric version of the GCS is shown in Table 15.11 (see www.nice.org.uk). Assessment of the best verbal response is likely to require assistance from parent/guardian/carer.

Table 15.11 Paediatric version of the Glasgow Coma Scale.

	Score
Best eye response	
Eyes open spontaneously	4
Eye opening to verbal command	3
Eye opening to pain	2
No eye opening	1
Best verbal response	
Alert, babbles, coos, words, or sentences to usual ability	5
Less than usual ability and/or spontaneous irritable cry	4
Cries inappropriately	3
Occasionally whimpers and/or moans	2
No vocal response	1
Best motor response	
Obeys commands or has normal spontaneous movements	6
Localizes to painful stimuli or withdraws to touch	5
Withdrawal to painful stimuli	4
Abnormal flexion to pain (decorticate)	3
Abnormal extension to pain (decerebrate)	2
No motor response to pain	1
Total	3–15

In pre-verbal or intubated patients, the 'best grimace response' may be used in place of the 'best verbal response', as shown in Table 15.12.

Table 15.12 'Best grimace response'

	Score
Spontaneous normal facial/oro-motor activity	5
Less than usual spontaneous ability and/or only responds to touch	4
Vigorous grimace to pain	3
Mild grimace to pain	2
No response to pain	1

Transient cortical blindness after head injury

Occasionally, children present with blindness immediately or soon after an apparently minor head injury. The mechanism is unclear, but in most cases blindness resolves spontaneously within a few hrs. In the meantime, arrange a CT scan to exclude intracranial haematoma.

Paediatric fractures and dislocations

Many paediatric fractures are similar to those in adults and prone to similar complications. Bones in children differ from those in adults in two important respects: they have epiphyses and are softer (hence fractures are more common than significant ligament injuries). Certain types of paediatric fractures reflect these differences:

Greenstick fracture An incomplete fracture in which one cortical surface of a bone breaks, whilst the other side bends.

Torus ('buckle') fracture Another form of incomplete fracture characterized by a buckling of the cortex.

Plastic deformation ('bowing deformation') Traumatic bending of long bone shaft without visible fracture occasionally occurs in young children.

Epiphyseal injuries

Injuries to the traction epiphyses are avulsion injuries (eg peroneus brevis insertion into the base of the 5th MT).

Injuries to the pressure epiphyses at the end of long bones adjacent to the articular surface have been classified into 5 types—the Salter-Harris classification (see Fig. 15.19):

- *Type I*: the epiphysis separates or slips on the metaphysis.
- *Type II*: a small piece of metaphysis separates with the epiphysis (commonest type).
- *Type III*: a vertical fracture through the epiphysis joins that through the epiphyseal plate.
- *Type IV*: a fracture passes from articular surface through the epiphyseal plate into metaphysis.
- *Type V*: a crush injury to the epiphyseal plate (X-rays may be normal).

Note that Salter–Harris types I and V may not be apparent on the initial X-ray. Undisplaced type I fractures often affect distal tibia and fibula and may present with circumferential tenderness around the growth plate. Treat with POP and immobilization according to clinical findings.

Epiphyseal growth plate injury

A concern specific to any epiphyseal injury is that premature fusion of a growth plate may result, with resultant limb shortening and deformity. The risk correlates to some extent with the mechanism of injury and amount of force involved. The different Salter–Harris fractures carry a different level of risk of long-term growth plate problems. The risk is low for types I and II (particularly if undisplaced), moderate for type III and highest for types IV and V. Problems are usually averted if Salter–Harris type III and IV injuries are accurately reduced and held (eg by internal fixation). Type V fractures are notoriously difficult to diagnose and often complicated by premature fusion: fortunately they are relatively rare.

Dislocations

Dislocated joints are relatively unusual in children. Most commonly involved are the patella (📖 p.726) or the radial head ('pulled elbow'— 📖 p.724). Similarly, due to relative strengths of bone and ligament, injuries to ligaments are much less common in children than in adults.

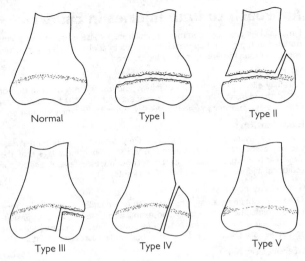

Fig. 15.19 Salter–Harris classification of epiphyseal injuries.

Approach to limb injuries in children

Limb injuries are very common in children. Whilst most of the points outlined in the general approach to trauma in adults may be successfully applied, certain modifications may be required.

History

Carefully elicit the mechanism of injury. The history may be confused or not forthcoming: try to establish a rapport with the child (and parents) nevertheless, in order to gain the child's confidence for the examination.

Examination

Search for evidence of a fracture (swelling, deformity, bony tenderness) and any associated neurovascular injury. Remember the adage that the most easily missed fracture is the second fracture: examine also for additional injuries to adjacent bones and joints.

Is an X-ray required?

If in doubt, obtain an X-ray. The ease with which children's bones fracture and the difficulties with history and examination mean that it is sensible to adopt a low threshold for requesting X-rays. Ensure that two views at right angles are taken (eg AP and lateral), including associated joints.

Interpreting X-rays

Many fractures are subtle and easily missed. To minimize the chance of this occurring, visually trace around the cortex of each bone, looking for any irregularities. Interpretation of paediatric X-rays is complicated by the presence of various ossification centres and accessory ossicles. Both are commonly mistaken for fractures (eg the olecranon epiphysis, the os trigonum and bipartite patella). Ossification centres appear and fuse in a relatively predictable fashion, although the rate at which this occurs varies slightly from child to child (see Table 15.13). Knowledge of this process, combined with experience of seeing many paediatric X-rays, greatly assists interpretation. If in doubt about an X-ray, obtain a second opinion (there is no justification for X-raying the uninjured side to see what 'normal' is). As an additional safeguard, most EDs now operate a policy of all X-rays being reported by a radiologist within 24hr.

Treatment

Give prompt, appropriate analgesia (📖 p.713). Follow the treatment suggested for specific fractures (📖 pp.722–7). Many undisplaced fractures will unite satisfactorily with a period of immobilization in POP (eg fractured distal radius), collar and cuff (eg fractured radial head) or broad arm sling (eg fractured clavicle). Minor angulation at the fracture site can be accepted, particularly in young children. Often, however, angulated fractures require MUA.

Compound fractures and dislocations

Give analgesia and give IV antibiotics (eg cefuroxime 25mg/kg slow IV bolus) and ensure tetanus cover. Take a digital photograph of the wound and keep it covered to minimize the risk of infection. Apply a dressing, splint the injured limb and refer the patient to the orthopaedic surgeon.

Table 15.13 Ossification centres

Centre	First appears	Fuses
Humeral head	0–6 months	18–21 years
Capitulum	3–6 months	14–16 years
Medial epicondyle	4–7 years	18–21 years
Lateral epicondyle	9–13 years	14–16 years
Trochlea	9–10 years	14–16 years
Radial head	4–5 years	14–17 years
Distal radius	6–12 months	17–19 years
Olecranon	9–11 years	13–16 years
Distal ulna	4–5 years	16–18 years
Capitate	birth–3 months	—
Hamate	birth–4 months	—
Triquetral	1–3 years	—
Lunate	2–4 years	—
Trapezium	2–4 years	—
Trapezoid	3–5 years	—
Scaphoid	3–5 years	—
Pisiform	9–12 years	—
1st MC base	1–3 years	14–17 years
Femoral head	birth–6 months	15–19 years
Greater trochanter	3–4 years	17–19 years
Lesser trochanter	11–14 years	15–18 years
Distal femur	birth	17–20 years
Patella	2–6 years	4–8 years
Proximal tibia	birth	15–18 years
Distal tibia	birth–6 months	14–17 years
Proximal fibula	2–4 years	16–19 years
Distal fibula	birth–1 year	14–17 years
Posterior calcaneum	5–8 years	13–16 years
Central calcaneum	birth	13–16 years
Talus	birth	—
Navicular	2–3 years	—
Cuneiform bones	1–3 years	—

These dates are subject to individual variation. In general, epiphyses in girls fuse before those in boys.

Paediatric upper limb injuries: 1

Some fractures and dislocations are common in both adults and children and are treated similarly. Certain injuries are either specific to children or are treated differently in children: these are described in the next six pages. Paediatric fractures are painful and need appropriate immobilization and analgesia (📖 p.713).

Clavicle fracture

Common in children and adults alike. Treatment is similar: oral analgesia, broad arm sling and fracture clinic follow-up. Even if X-rays do not appear to show a fracture, treat as for a fracture. Warn parents about a developing lump (callus).

Shoulder injuries

Shoulder dislocations are relatively rare in children. Salter-Harris types I and II epiphyseal fractures may occur in the proximal humerus: refer to the orthopaedic team if significant displacement or >20° angulation. Otherwise, give analgesia, collar and cuff, and fracture clinic follow-up.

Humeral shaft fracture

Check particularly for radial nerve injury. Remember to consider NAI especially if <3 years old or fracture is spiral. Treat as for adults (📖 p.459).

Supracondylar humeral fracture

Follows a fall on an outstretched hand. Swelling may be considerable. Check for associated neurovascular deficit (particularly brachial artery, median and radial nerves). 25% of supracondylar fractures are undisplaced and may not be obvious on X-ray, although a joint effusion will be seen. Most fractures are displaced, angulated or rotated. The extent of angulation (both in sagittal and coronal planes) is easy to underestimate. Viewed from laterally, the capitulum normally makes an angle of 45° with the humeral shaft (see Fig. 15.20). The anterior humeral line (drawn along the front of humeral shaft on the lateral view) normally passes through the middle of the ossification centre of the capitulum in the distal humerus. Also, the normal carrying angle (seen in AP view) is 10°. Record radial pulse frequently and consider compartment syndrome.

Treatment provide analgesia and refer for manipulation under GA if:
- Neurovascular deficit: operation is urgent if circulation is compromised.
- >50% displacement.
- >20° angulation of the distal part posteriorly (see Fig. 15.21).
- >10° medial or lateral angulation.

Refer others for observation and admission if there is much swelling. If no significant angulation, displacement or swelling, discharge with analgesia, a collar and cuff under a body bandage (elbow at 90° with confirmed radial pulse present) and fracture clinic follow-up. Consider using a padded back slab POP if significant pain is present.

Complications malunion with persistent deformity, stiffness (including myositis ossificans), neurovascular deficit (eg Volkmann's contracture).

Supracondylar humeral fractures

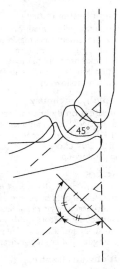

Fig. 15.20 Normal lateral view—the capitulum makes an angle of 45° with the humeral shaft.

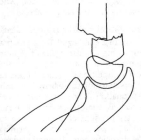

Fig. 15.21 Supracondylar fracture with >20° angulation and ~50% displacement.

Paediatric upper limb injuries: 2

Lateral epicondylar epiphyseal injury

Salter–Harris type II injury may follow a fall on outstretched hand. The elbow is swollen, with ↓ movement and maximum tenderness on the lateral aspect. X-rays demonstrate the fracture, which may be displaced by the pull of the forearm extensors, requiring surgical reduction. Treat undisplaced fractures with a long arm back slab POP, collar and cuff at 90°, analgesia and fracture clinic follow-up.

Medial epicondylar epiphyseal injury

Maximal tenderness is apparent on the medial side of the elbow. Check carefully for ulnar nerve damage. Refer immediately if the ulnar nerve is involved, or if the fracture is displaced. Treat undisplaced fractures with analgesia, collar and cuff at 90° under clothes (confirm radial pulse is present) and fracture clinic follow-up.

Radial head/neck fracture

The radiocapitellar line is drawn down the axis of the proximal radius on the lateral view of the elbow and should bisect the capitellum. Failure to do so suggests occult radial neck fracture or radial head dislocation. Most of these fractures can be managed satisfactorily with analgesia, collar and cuff (some prefer a broad arm sling) and fracture clinic follow-up (📖 p.450). Refer to the orthopaedic surgeon if there is significant angulation.

Elbow injury without obvious fracture

Treat elbow injuries where there is clinical suspicion of fracture, but none seen on X-ray, along the same lines as for an undisplaced fracture (analgesia, collar and cuff, and fracture clinic follow-up). This includes children who have ↓ range of movement and whose X-rays show an elbow effusion ('fat pad sign')—see 📖 p. 450.

Subluxation of the radial head ('pulled elbow')

A direct pull on the arm of a child aged 1–5 years may result in the radial head being pulled out of the annular ligament ('nursemaid's elbow'). The child then refuses to use the arm. If there is a characteristic history, there is no need to X-ray. The traditional reduction technique involves flexing the elbow to 90°, then supinating the elbow fully. However, manipulating the elbow into full pronation may give a better reduction rate (www.bestbets.org.uk). A click is sometimes felt or heard during reduction. If full pronation fails, try full supination and leave for 10min. Allow the child to play and watch: he will usually use the arm again soon. If he does not, obtain X-rays and senior help. Repeat manipulation can be done once, but if that does not lead to a rapid improvement in function then place the arm in a sling, give analgesia and plan to review in 1–2 days. The elbow may reduce spontaneously or may need further manipulation. Rarely, repeated manipulation is unsuccessful until sedation is given. After successful manipulation advise the parents to avoid pulling the arm forcefully. A pulled elbow may recur up to about age 5 if the arm is pulled, but after that the child should have no long term problems with the elbow.

Radius/ulna shaft fractures

Radius and ulna shaft fractures often cause significant displacement or angulation: provide IV analgesia, immobilize in a broad arm sling, obtain X-rays and refer for manipulation under GA. Never accept an isolated forearm shaft fracture without X-rays demonstrating the entire radius and ulna, otherwise a Monteggia or Galeazzi fracture-dislocation may be missed (☐ Forearm fractures and related injury, p.448).

Distal radial fracture (including Salter–Harris type II injuries)

A common fracture in all ages of children (and adults) after a fall on an outstretched hand. The fracture results in localized tenderness and variable swelling. Check carefully for a second injury (eg involving the thumb or scaphoid). X-rays will demonstrate the fracture and allow assessment of the need for MUA.

Moderate displacement or slight angulation may be accepted (particularly in younger children): if in doubt, obtain a senior opinion.

Minimally displaced or undisplaced greenstick, buckle or torus fractures commonly occur just proximal to the distal radial epiphysis. Treat with analgesia, elevation, a backslab forearm POP (extend this above the elbow in children <2 years or it will fall off) and arrange review and plaster completion at 24hr. Children who present with discrete tenderness over the distal radial growth plate, but without a fracture apparent on X-ray should be treated identically to those with a radiological proven fracture— presume a growth plate injury (sometimes a subperiosteal haematoma can be seen on ultrasound). Beware osteomyelitis (☐ The limping child, p.704), which can cause tenderness over the distal radius and be mistaken for trauma.

Removable splints For co-operative children (usually >4 years old) with torus/buckle fractures of the distal radius, an alternative option is to use removable splints. Parents and children report better functioning and fewer days off school. Splints should be retained until pain wears off (usually <3 weeks) and follow-up is not required if pain settles as expected.

Scaphoid fracture

Despite being uncommon, particularly in younger children, seek clinical evidence of scaphoid fracture in any child with wrist/forearm injury and obtain scaphoid views if appropriate (☐ p.442). Treat radiologically evident and suspected fractures as for adults as described in ☐ Carpal bone fractures and dislocations, p.442.

Metacarpal and phalangeal injuries

Treat these injuries along similar lines to those described for adults (☐ Hand fractures and dislocations, p.436). Remember, however, that children may not tolerate manipulation under LA: anaesthetic help may be required.

Paediatric lower limb injuries

Hip fracture

Children rarely sustain neck of femur fractures similar to those seen in adults. In the pre-adolescent child, trauma may precipitate a slipped upper femoral epiphysis (📖 The painful hip, p.706). Younger children who have been subjected to considerable violence may suffer a Salter–Harris type I injury to the proximal femoral epiphysis—carefully exclude other injuries and refer to the orthopaedic surgeon.

Femoral shaft fracture

May be spiral (the majority) or transverse, depending upon the mechanism of injury. Considerable energy is required to produce a femoral fracture: check for other injuries. Resuscitate as necessary with IV fluids and provide nasal diamorphine (📖 p.281) or IV opioid analgesia (📖 p.280). Perform a femoral nerve block (as described on 📖 p.304) to provide additional analgesia, using 0.2mL/kg of 0.5% plain bupivicaine (1mg/kg). Allow 20min for this to work, then apply skin traction. Gallows traction may be used on infants and children <2 years, but is best erected on the ward. A spiral fracture in a non-ambulatory child suggests child abuse—swelling is often not dramatic.

Knee injuries

Knee ligament injuries are rare in children compared with adults: suspect a fracture or epiphyseal injury instead. This is a reflection of the relative strengths of ligament and bone in the child. So, for example, an injury which might cause anterior cruciate ligament rupture in the adult will often produce avulsion of its tibial attachment in the child. This tibial plateau fracture will produce a haemarthrosis and will be apparent on the lateral X-ray. Provide analgesia and refer to the orthopaedic surgeon.

Patella fractures

Do not confuse a congenitally bipartite patella for a fracture. The small bony fragment in a bipartite patella lies superolaterally and has rounded edges.

Patellar sleeve fractures are not uncommon in children and adolescents. These osteochondral fractures typically result from high impact jumping activities or sports. Suspect clinically if there is local pain and tenderness and an inability to actively extend the knee. Radiographs can be misleading as only a small bony fragment is avulsed, usually from the inferior pole, but a large part of the articular surface is removed with it, but is impossible to see on plain X-ray. Provide analgesia and splintage and refer to the orthopaedic team for MRI to confirm the diagnosis ± ORIF.

Patella dislocation

This is seen relatively frequently in children and is treated in a similar way to that in adults (see 📖 p.476). Examine the X-rays carefully as associated osteochondral 'chip' fractures of the undersurface of the patella occur relatively frequently in children.

Tibial shaft fracture

Treat most fractures as for adults: splintage, IV analgesia, and referral for elevation and admission. Compound fractures require IV antibiotics and wound surgery. Displaced or angulated fractures require MUA and POP; undisplaced fractures respond to treatment with above knee non-WB POP and subsequent mobilization using crutches.

Toddler's fracture

Minor trauma in 1–4-year-olds may result in characteristic spiral undisplaced distal tibial fractures. These may not be apparent on the initial X-rays: localized warmth and tenderness with a history of trauma may suggest the diagnosis in the otherwise wide differential of the limping child (📖 p.704). If a fracture is visible on initial X-rays treat by rest in a POP and arrange fracture clinic follow-up. If the diagnosis is made without a visible fracture, treat in POP and review clinically and radiologically at 10 days: further X-rays may then demonstrate a long strip of periosteal tibial new bone formation. Continue to treat according to symptoms.

Ankle injuries

Ankle ligament injuries are less common than in adults, but are treated similarly (as are ankle fractures—📖 p.486). If there is no fracture apparent on X-ray, but there is much tenderness over the distal tibial or fibular epiphysis, treat as a growth plate injury (undisplaced Salter–Harris type I fracture) with BKPOP, crutches, elevation, analgesia and fracture clinic follow-up.

Calcaneal and other foot injuries

See 📖 Foot fractures and dislocations, p.488.

Child abuse

The boundaries of what defines acceptable behaviour and what constitutes child abuse are open to some debate and are certainly affected by historical and cultural factors. For example, corporal punishment, once considered normal and usual, is now unacceptable. The extremes of child abuse, however, are easily defined.

Types of child abuse

- Physical abuse (NAI)—including bruises, fractures, wounds, and burns.
- Sexual abuse.
- Poisoning.
- Suffocation.
- Neglect or emotional abuse.
- Fabricated and induced illness (previously known as 'Munchausen syndrome by proxy').

Prevalence

It is impossible to be sure how common child abuse is. It is generally agreed that it is much more prevalent than was previously believed. 4% of children are brought to the attention of professional agencies for suspected abuse. It is believed that ≈0.1% of UK children suffer severe physical abuse each year and it has been estimated that 100–150 child deaths occur each year as a result of abuse by parents or carers.

Aetiology

Child abuse affects both boys and girls. The first-born child is most frequently affected. Infants and young children are at most risk of serious injury or death, partly reflecting their physical vulnerability. The abuser is often a parent or cohabitant of a parent, more commonly male and may have suffered abuse themselves as a child. Sometimes the child may be targeted because they are unwanted (eg 'she should have been a boy'). Whilst the abuser may be a young parent with unrealistic expectations and living in difficult social circumstances (unemployment, drug abuse), often they do not conform to this standard description. Child abuse affects all levels of society. Clear links between domestic violence and physical abuse of children have been identified. Children whose parents have mental health problems may be more vulnerable to abuse and neglect.

Role of the junior emergency department doctor

Managing the child and family where there is suspected child abuse is an extremely delicate skill, requiring considerable tact and experience. The role of the junior doctor is to consider the possibility of child abuse and to involve a senior doctor at an early stage. Recent NICE guidance is available at http://www.nice.org.uk/nicemedia/live/12183/44872/44872.pdf

The suspicious history

Certain features should alert the doctor to the possibility of child abuse:
- Injuries inconsistent with the history given.
- Injuries inappropriate for developmental age (eg a baby aged <3 months 'rolled off a bed').
- Changing history of injury, or vague history, lacking vivid details.
- Delay in seeking medical attention.
- Abnormal parental attitudes (eg apparent lack of concern for child).
- Frequent ED attendances.
- Occasionally, children provide an account of abuse.

Presentation of child abuse: 1

Physical child abuse is commonly referred to as NAI. Children may present with a variety of injuries, which may occur singly or in combination.

Bruising

Children naturally sustain bruises during minor incidents as part of 'growing up'. Bruising over the knees and shins is a normal finding in children, particularly toddlers, who are also prone to sustaining injuries to their foreheads and chins as a result of falls. Older children frequently sustain bruises over the lateral aspect of their elbows and hips, during normal play and sport activities. As well as considering the possibility of NAI, remember that bruising may occur as part of an unusual pathological disease process (eg Henoch–Schönlein purpura, haemophilia, ITP, leukaemia, and other causes of thrombocytopenia). A Mongolian blue spot is an innocuous congenital finding on the lower back of some young children (especially non-Caucasians), which may be confused with bruising.

The following features should prompt consideration of NAI:
- Bruising in unusual sites (eg medial aspect of upper arms or thighs).
- Multiple bruising of different ages (very difficult for the non-expert to judge) at less common sites.
- Uncommon injuries bilaterally.
- Finger 'imprinting' (eg grip complexes around upper limbs or slap marks).
- Imprints or marks from other objects (eg belt, stick).
- Human bite marks (probably adult if canines >3cm apart: ensure photographs next to a ruler are planned after admission).
- Petechiae on the face may reflect smothering and asphyxiation (it has been previously suggested that 2–10% of SIDS may have been smothered), but remember that petechiae also occur with forceful coughing or vomiting.

Wounds and burns

Children commonly sustain wounds and burns unintentionally. However, deliberately inflicted burns are found in a significant proportion of physically abused children.

The following suggest the possibility of NAI:
- Torn frenulum of upper lip (can also reflect a 'normal' toddler injury).
- Perineal wounds and burns (see sexual abuse 🛄 p.732).
- Small, deep circular burns with raised edges suggest cigarette burns.
- Hand, lower limb, and buttock burns may follow forced immersion in bath water that is too hot. These burns tend to be of the 'stocking and glove' type, without higher splash burns. Parts of the buttocks may be spared, where skin has been in contact with the bath, not the water.

Head injuries

Most head injuries result from unintentional incidents ('accidents'). In infants, they often result from the parent or carer dropping the child. The fractures caused by this tend to be single, linear, and involve the parietal bone.

Consider NAI if the following occur:
- Retinal haemorrhages (characteristic, but not diagnostic of shaking—they may also rarely be seen in CO poisoning, for example). In the context of NAI, retinal haemorrhages are often associated with subdural haematomas.
- Occipital skull fracture.
- Multiple, wide or comminuted fractures.
- Subdural haematoma in an infant or toddler.

Natural progression of bruises

Swelling and tenderness of bruising suggests relatively recent origin, but this is not very reliable. Accurate assessment of the age of bruising according to its colour is not possible, except that a yellow bruise is almost certainly >18hr old. Oft-quoted natural temporal progression of colour changes of bruising allows only a guess at the age of a bruise—avoid being drawn on this issue, which may have considerable legal implications. Instead, record the findings as accurately as possible: describe the colour, size, and distribution of the bruising. Usually a child suspected of having suffered physical abuse will also be examined by a relevant expert, such as a paediatrician and/or police surgeon (clinical forensic physician).

Presentation of child abuse: 2

Fractures

Certain fractures are very common in children. Pay attention to the history of injury and whether or not it appears to be consistent with the fracture(s) sustained. Multiple fractures of different ages (especially if previously undiagnosed and/or not brought to medical attention) should arouse suspicion of NAI. To help assess the approximate age of a bony injury, see Table 15.14.

Table 15.14 Natural progression of fractures

Presence of soft tissue swelling	0–10 days
Periosteal new bone formation	10–14 days
Loss of definition of the fracture line	14–21 days
Callus formaton	14–42 days
Remodelling	≈1 year

Remember that times vary according to the age of the child.

Consider NAI in the following fractures
- Multiple fractures of different ages.
- Rib and spinal fractures.
- Fractures in infants who are not independently mobile.
- Long bone fractures in children <3 years old.
- Epiphyseal separation and metaphyseal 'chip' fractures of the knee, wrist, elbow, and ankle. These Salter–Harris I and II injuries are associated with traction, rotation, and shaking.

A few rare bone diseases may mimic NAI
- Osteogenesis imperfecta (blue sclerae, dental abnormalities and brittle bones—autosomal dominant).
- Pathological fractures (through multiple cystic bone lesions).
- Rickets (enlarged, cupped epiphyses, craniotabes, 'bow legs').
- Copper deficiency (eg Menkes' kinky hair syndrome).

Neglect and emotional abuse

There will be an element of emotional abuse as part of other forms of abuse, which may be manifest in the child in a variety of ways: behavioural problems, sleep disturbance, soiling, nocturnal enuresis. The neglected child may be dirty and unkempt, fail to thrive, and/or fall below the 3rd centile for height and weight. Occasionally, nutritional deficiencies may be extreme (eg rickets). Developmental milestones are often delayed (and may even regress).

Note the apparent attitudes of the parents/carers towards their child (eg critical and hostile or remote and unconcerned) and the child's attitude to the parents/carers (if in doubt as to whether this seems appropriate, ask an experienced nurse).

Sexual abuse

This may affect boys or girls and takes many forms, ranging from exposure to indecent acts through to rape. The abuser is often a male relative or carer who is well known to the child. The child may present in a variety of ways:

• Injury to the genitalia or anus.
• Perineal pain, discharge, or bleeding.
• Behavioural disturbance, enuresis, encopresis.
• Inappropriate sexual behaviour.
• The child may allege sexual abuse.
• Sexually transmitted disease (including anogenital warts).
• Pregnancy.

Accurately record statements made by the child 'word for word' using quotation marks. Do not pursue a genital examination, but involve a senior doctor at an early stage, who may wish to examine the genitalia using a colposcope, in collaboration with a police surgeon (clinical forensic physician). In the context of an allegation of recent sexual assault, the collection of forensic samples for DNA analysis is likely to be required.

Fabricated or induced illness (previously known as Munchausen syndrome by proxy)

A parent/carer may invent a history of illness in a child and fabricate physical signs to substantiate it. The history often involves one or more of the following: apnoeic episodes, fits, bowel disturbances, rashes, allergies, or fevers. Classically, the deceiver is the mother. The child may be made ill by administering drugs or poisons. If suspected, do not confront the deceiver, but take blood and urine samples for a toxicology screen and refer to the paediatric team.

Bear in mind that some parents may be naturally very anxious and may exaggerate symptoms, rather than deliberately fabricate them.

Management of child abuse

Role of the junior emergency department doctor

The junior ED doctor needs to be vigilant in considering abuse when initially assessing and treating children. Any suspicion of child abuse should prompt involvement of an expert senior doctor (paediatrician or ED consultant). In every hospital system there will be a designated doctor for child protection who should be available for advice. He or she will examine the child and arrange hospital admission for further investigations (eg skeletal survey) as necessary. Social Services and the police may need to be involved. The child may require examination by a police surgeon (clinical forensic physician) and samples/photographs obtained. Follow local procedures.

The chief consideration is the treatment and protection of the child, so do not delay treatment of painful or apparently life-threatening problems, whilst awaiting an 'expert'. Ensure that all documentation is legible and meticulous. Remember that if child abuse is considered likely, siblings may also be at risk.

UK law: The Children Act 1989

This act replaced previous statutes. Central to the Act is the concept that the welfare of the child is paramount. In the short term, the 1989 Children Act may be used to obtain orders to protect children. A variety of orders may be obtained:

Police Protection Order

A police officer has legal powers to take any child into 'police protection' for up to 72hr if deemed necessary for his/her own protection. This order may be used to prevent a child being taken away from the ED by a parent or guardian against medical advice.

Emergency Protection Order

This has replaced the 'Place of Safety Order'. A court order valid for up to 8 days may be obtained if the child is believed to be at significant risk of harm. Such an order would normally be requested by a social worker.

Child Assessment Order

This court order may be obtained in order to allow an assessment to be performed of a child who appears to be at risk of injury.

Care Order

This transfers the care of a child from the parent(s) to the local authority Social Services department. If a care order is in force, matters requiring parental consent should be referred to the social worker (not the foster carer).

Residence Order

This court order defines where a child should live and who has parental responsibility.

Child Protection Plan (replaces the 'Child Protection Register')

This register is kept by the social services. It contains a list of names of those children considered to be at current risk of harm. ED staff should be aware of how to access Child Protection Register information. Previous hospital case notes are also very useful in this respect. When searching for previous records, remember that many children may be known by several surnames.

Child protection conferences

A conference may be called by Social Services if it is suspected that a child has been abused. Child protection conferences should be held promptly and aim to define a protection plan for the future protection of the child and family. Unlike the criminal courts, where the onus is on the prosecution to prove abuse 'beyond reasonable doubt', child protection conferences will determine whether a child is deemed to be at risk of significant harm and whether a protection plan is required. Case conferences consist of a number of individuals, including: chairman (usually a senior member of the Social Services department), hospital consultant, GP, social worker, police, health visitor, teacher, education welfare officer, child abuse advisor, local authority solicitor. Parents are always invited and older children may also attend.

Child Protection and Substitute Child Protection and
Registers

Child protection registers

Index

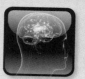